Core Concepts in Health

Fourth Edition

Core Concepts in Health

Paul M. Insel   Walton T. Roth

Mayfield Publishing Company
Palo Alto, California

Library of Congress Catalog Card Number: 84-062034
International Standard Book Number: 0-87484-675-7

Manufactured in the United States of America
10 9 8 7 6 5 4 3 2

Mayfield Publishing Company
285 Hamilton Avenue
Palo Alto, California 94301

Sponsoring editor: C. Lansing Hays
Manuscript editor: Marie Enders
Managing editor: Pat Herbst
Art director: Nancy Sears
Designer (interior and cover): Janet Bollow
Cover photograph: Mimi Fuller Foster
Technical illustrator: Judith McCarty
Production manager: Cathy Willkie
Compositor: Skillful Means Press
Printer and binder: Kingsport Press
Cover printer: Phoenix Color Corp.

Credits and Sources

Pages 7, 10-11 From the book *Become an Ex-Smoker* by Brian G. Danaher and Edward Lichtenstein. Copyright © 1978 by Prentice-Hall, Inc. Published by Prentice-Hall, Inc., Englewood Cliffs, NJ 07632.

Page 16 From Michael J. Mahoney, *Self-Change: Strategies for Solving Personal Problems* (New York: Norton, 1981).

Page 18 Donald M. Vickery, *Life Plan for Your Health* (pp. 17, 18). © 1978 by Addison-Wesley, Reading, Massachusetts. Reprinted with permission.

Page 27 Reprinted by permission; © 1981 by the New Yorker Magazine, Inc.

Page 29 Reprinted with permission from *Journal of Psychosomatic Research*, no. 227 (1967), T. H. Holmes and R. H. Rahe, "The Social Readjustment Rating Scale." Copyright © 1967 by Pergamon Press Ltd.

Page 45 Reprinted from *High Level Wellness* by Donald B. Ardell. Copyright © 1977 by Donald B. Ardell. Permission granted by Rodale Press, Inc., Emmaus, PA 18049.

Page 56 Reprinted with permission from *Science News* (November 5, 1983), the weekly newsmagazine of science; copyright © 1983 by Science Service, Inc.

Page 60 From *Essentials of Psychology*, 2nd ed, by Harriet N. Mischel and Walter Mischel. Copyright © 1977 by Random House, Inc. Reprinted by permission of the publisher.

Page 71 From *Self-Directed Behavior: Self-Modification for Personal Adjustment*, 2nd ed., by D. L. Watson and R. G. Tharp. Copyright © 1977 by Wadsworth Publishing Company, Inc. Reprinted by permission of the publisher, Brooks/Cole Publishing Company, Monterey, Calif.

Page 86 From *Getting Clear: Body Work for Women* by Anne Kent Rush. Copyright © 1973 by Anne Kent Rush. Reprinted by permission of Random House, Inc., and The Bookworks.

Pages 90-91 Condensed from *Giving Time a Chance: The Secret of a Lasting Marriage* by Ronna Romney and Beppie Harrison. Copyright © 1983 by Ronna Romney and Beppie Harrison. Reprinted by permission of the publisher, M. Evans and Co., Inc., New York, NY 10017.

Page 98 From *The Individual, Marriage, and the Family*, 2nd ed., by Lloyd Saxton. Copyright © 1972 by Wadsworth Publishing Company, Inc. Reprinted by permission of Wadsworth Publishing Company, Belmont, CA 94002.

Page 106 Reprinted from *Human Nature* (July 1978).

Page 113 From "Development of a Sex Anxiety Inventory" by L. H. Janda and E. E. O'Grady, *Journal of Consulting and Clinical Psychology*, 48 (1980), 169-75. Copyright © 1980 by the American Psychological Association. Adapted by permission of the authors.

Page 124 From *Our Bodies, Ourselves* by the Boston Women's Health Book Collective. Copyright © 1971, 1973, 1976 by the Boston Women's Health Book Collective, Inc. Reprinted by permission of Simon & Schuster, Inc.

Page 133 From *It's Your Choice* by Robert Hatcher et al. Copyright © 1981 by Irvington Publishers, Inc., New York..

Page 141 From "Study Refutes Claim That Vasectomy Is Health Hazard" by Allan Parachini. Copyright © 1984 by Los Angeles Times. Reprinted by permission.

Pages 147-48 From "Abortion and the Law," *Newsweek*, March 3, 1975. Copyright © 1975 by Newsweek, Inc. All rights reserved. Reprinted by permission.

Pages 175-76 From "Am I Parent Material?" by Carole Goldman, published by the National Organization for Non-Parents, 806 Reisterstown Road, Baltimore, MD 21208.

Page 178 From *Between Parent and Child* by Haim Ginott by permission of Macmillan, Inc. Copyright © 1975 by Maxmillan, Inc.

Page 191 Reprinted with permission from *Science News* (October 2, 1982), the weekly newsmagazine of science; copyright © 1982 by Science Service, Inc.

Page 193 From E. C. Hammond, "Life Expectancy of American Men in Relation to Their Smoking Habits," *J.N.C.I.* 43 (1969): 951-62.

Page 195 From "Now an Ex-Smoker" by Dr. Frank A. Oski, *New York Times*, January 12, 1984. Copyright © 1984 by The New York Times Company. Reprinted by permission.

Page 199 From "The Secondhand Smoke Issue" in *The Health Letter* (March 26, 1982). Reprinted by permission of Communications, Inc.

Page 200 From *The Social Animal*, 3rd ed., by Elliot Aronson. W. H. Freeman and Company. Copyright © 1980.

Pages 202-203 Copyright © 1984 by Consumers Union of United States, Inc., Mount Vernon, NY 10553. Reprinted by permission from *Consumer Reports* (August 1984), pp. 434-35.

(continued following the Index)

Contents

List of Boxes   ix
Preface   xiii
Introduction   xvii

Part One

Wellness Behavior

Chapter One

Health Behavior   3

Planning Life-Style Changes   5
Why Do I Behave as I Do?   5
How Can I Make a Change?   8
Avoiding Derailment   12
Maintaining Commitment   13
Troubleshooting   15
Health for Life   16
A Position of Tempered Enthusiasm   17
Behavior Features of the Following Chapters   19
  Health Behavior Outlook Scale   20
  Take Action   21

Chapter Two

Stress and the Social Environment   23

  Probing Your Emotions   23
Biological Versus Cultural Evolution   24
The Interaction Between You and Your
  Environment   27
The Stress Response   28
Psychosocial Stressors   32
The Role of Stress in Disease   38
Coping   41
  Stress and Coping Behavior Scale   47
  Take Action   48
  *Behavior Change Strategy: Type A Behavior
    Pattern*   48

Chapter Three

Mental Health   53

  Probing Your Emotions   53
What Mental Health Is Not   54

What Mental Health Is   54
Models of Human Nature   59
Human Problems   66
Promoting Mental Health   70
Getting Help   71
Approaches to Therapy   71
  Mental Wellness Scale   73
  Take Action   74
  *Behavior Change Strategy: Shy and Lonesome:
    Social Anxiety*   74

Part Two

Sexuality

Chapter Four

Sex and Intimacy   79

  Probing Your Emotions   79
Biological Differences and Variations   80
Vulnerability to Disease and Disorder   83
Culturally Induced Sex Differences: Sex Roles   85
Sex Differences and Individual Differences   87
Building an Intimate Relationship   89
  Intimate Relationship Scale   100
  Take Action   101
  Behavior Change Strategy: Sexual Dysfunction   101

Chapter Five

Sexual Responses   103

  Probing Your Emotions   103
The Role of the Nervous System in Sex   104
Stages of Sexual Response   109
Varieties of Sexual Experience   114
Variant Sexual Behavior   116
  Sexual Responsiveness Scale   119
  Take Action   120

Chapter Six

Birth Control   121

  Probing Your Emotions   121
Contraception   122

Sterilization   140
New Methods of Contraception   143
Abortion Methods   146
Abortion Complications   148
   Birth Control Behavior Scale   150
   Take Action   151

Chapter Seven

Pregnancy, Childbirth, and Parenting   153

   Probing Your Emotions   153
The Reproductive Process   154
Fetal Development   155
Changes in the Mother's Body During Pregnancy   159
The Importance of Early Prenatal Care   164
Exercise and Work During Pregnancy   165
Labor and Delivery   165
The Puerperium   169
Prospective Parents as Consumers in the Medical
   Marketplace   170
Parenting   176
   Family Planning Potential Scale   179
   Take Action   180

Part Three

Substance Use and Abuse

Chapter Eight

Tobacco   183

   Probing Your Emotions   183
The History of Tobacco   184
Tobacco Smoke   184
Immediate Effects of Smoking   187
The Smoking Habit   187
Behavioral Aspects of Smoking   188
Health Hazards of Smoking   190
Smokers' Effects on Nonsmokers   196
Other Forms of Tobacco Use   198
Other Opinions About the Health Hazards
   of Tobacco   198
What Can Be Done?   199

Benefits from Quitting   204
   Smoking Attitude and Behavior Scale   205
   Take Action   206
   Behavior Change Strategy: Quitting Smoking   206

Chapter Nine

Alcohol   209

   Probing Your Emotions   209
Alcohol and Behavior   211
The Metabolism of Alcohol   212
Immediate Effects of Alcohol   214
Medical Uses of Alcohol   215
Alcohol Abuse and Alcoholism   216
The Responsible Use of Alcohol   220
   Alcohol Behavior Scale   224
   Take Action   225

Chapter Ten

Other Psychoactive Drugs   227

   Probing Your Emotions   227
Factors Influencing Drug Effects   228
Major Psychoactive Drugs   230
Drugs and Delirium   242
Psychiatric Use of Drugs   242
   Psychoactive Drug Behavior Scale   245
   Take Action   246

Part Four

Physical Fitness

Chapter Eleven

Nutrition   249

   Probing Your Emotions   249
Nutrition and Nutrients   250
Adequate, Balanced Diets   253
Choosing a Daily Diet   257
Vitamin and Nutrient Supplementation   264
Hunger and Disease   267
The Future of Nutrition Research   271

Nutrition Behavior Scale 272
Take Action 273
Behavior Change Strategy: Nutrition 273

Chapter Twelve
Overweight 275

Probing Your Emotions 275
What Should You Weigh? 276
What Is Obesity? 276
What Causes Obesity? 278
How Can Weight Be Controlled? 285
Weight Control Behavior Scale 295
Take Action 296
Behavior Change Strategy: Weight Control 296

Chapter Thirteen
Exercise 299

Probing Your Emotions 299
What Is Physical Fitness? 300
Why Get into Shape? 300
How to Get into Shape: The Planning Stage 305
Implementing Your Program 306
What Is Enough? How to Maintain Fitness 313
Injuries 316
Fitness Behavior Scale 317
Take Action 318
Behavior Change Strategy: Exercise 318

Part Five

Consumer Health Issues

Chapter Fourteen
The Consumer and Medicine, Fads, and Quackery 323

Probing Your Emotions 323
The Scientific Tradition 324
The Past as Prologue 326
Orthodox Medicine 327

Alternative Approaches to Medicine 329
Quackery Today 332
Decision Making 334
Consumer Protection 336
Government Attempts to Reduce Health
Care Costs 338
Consumer Behavior Scale 341
Take Action 342

Chapter Fifteen
Prescription and Over-the-Counter Drugs 343

Probing Your Emotions 343
Primitive Drugs and Modern Drugs 344
Patent Medicines in America 344
Government Regulation of the Drug Industry 347
How New Prescription Drugs Are Tested 347
The Marketing of Over-the-Counter Drugs 348
Dangers of Self-Medication 348
How to Self-Medicate Safely 352
Emergency Treatment for Poisoning or Drug
Overdose 357
Possible Future Safeguards 357
Prescription and OTC Drug Behavior Scale 360
Take Action 361
*Behavior Change Strategy: Monitoring and
Managing Medication* 361

Chapter Sixteen
Medical Diagnosis 363

Probing Your Emotions 363
When to Go to the Doctor 364
Methods of Diagnosis 366
Principles of Diagnosis 375
Population Screening 376
Sabotaging the Diagnostic Process 378
Trends in Medical Diagnosis 378
Patient Responsibilities and Rights 379
Medical Diagnosis Behavior Scale 382
Take Action 383
*Behavior Change Strategy: Following Through with
Suggestions: Compliance and Adherence* 383

Part Six

Current Health Concerns

Chapter Seventeen
Cardiovascular Health   387

Probing Your Emotions   387
The Cardiovascular System   388
Major Forms of Adult Cardiovascular Disease   388
Cardiovascular Disease, Personality, and Life-Style   401
Heart Diseases in Children   402
   Cardiovascular Health Behavior Scale   403
   Take Action   404
   *Behavior Change Strategy: Behavioral Management of
      High Blood Pressure*   404

Chapter Eighteen
Cancer   407

Probing Your Emotions   407
How Many People Develop Cancer?   409
What Causes Cancer?   409
Detection and Diagnosis   416
Prevention   418
   Cancer Risk Behavior Scale   422
   Take Action   423

Chapter Nineteen
Infection and Immunity   425

Probing Your Emotions   425
Pathogens   426
Diagnosis of Pathogenic Diseases   430
Infection: The Breaching of Defenses   430
Immunity   438
Immune Mechanisms   438
Recognition of Foreign Cells   446
Immunology of Cancer   447
Allergies   448
Autoimmune Disease   451
Do the Emotions Affect the Immune Response?   451
   Immunity Behavior Scale   452
   Take Action   453

Chapter Twenty
Sexually Transmitted Diseases   455

Probing Your Emotions   455
Causes of the Prevalence of Sexually Transmitted
   Diseases   456
What the Individual Can Do   456
Major Sexually Transmitted Diseases   460
Other Sexually Transmitted Diseases   471
   STD Behavior Scale   472
   Take Action   473

Chapter Twenty-One
Aging   475

Probing Your Emotions   475
The Goal of Gerontology   476
Theories of Aging   481
The Ethics of Tampering with the Aging Process   484
Life-Extending Measures   486
Aging: A Positive Experience   492
   Aging Attitude Scale   493
   Take Action   494

Chapter Twenty-Two
Death and Dying   495

Probing Your Emotions   495
What Is Death?   496
Why Is There Death?   496
Denying Death in America   496
The Process of Dying   498
The Hospice   500
Dead Bodies as Resources   500
Grief   501
Coming to Terms with Death   502
   Death and Dying Attitude Scale   508
   Take Action   509

Index   511

Boxes

Chapter One
Health Behavior

The Health Diary 7
Personal Contracts for Change 10
The SCIENCE Mnemonic Formula for Personal
   Problem Solving 16
Ages of Health Advancement 18

Chapter Two
Stress and the Social Environment

Notes and Comment from *The New Yorker* 27
Student Stress Scale 29
Life Events: An Update 30
Test Anxiety and Stress 38
Social Support Scale 42
Relaxation 45

Chapter Three
Mental Health

Sampling America's Emotional Health 56
Maslow on Self-Actualization 60
Erik Erikson's Stages of Psychosocial Development 65
Suicide Among College Students 66
A Self-Change Program: How to Go About It 71

Chapter Four
Sex and Intimacy

Woman—Which Includes Man, Of Course: An Experi-
   ence in Awareness 86
Love That Lasts a Lifetime 90
Compatibility Quiz 92
Four Components of Love 98

Chapter Five
Sexual Responses

A Brief History of the Kiss 106
Myths About Sex 107

The Sexual Anxiety Inventory 113
Kinds of Sexual Contact 117
Homosexuality 118

Chapter Six
Birth Control

Attitudes Toward Birth Control 124
Planned Parenthood 128
Assessing Risks 133
What Are the Costs of Having Children? 135
Study Refutes Claim That Vasectomy Is Health
   Hazard 141
Abortion—The Hard Question 147

Chapter Seven
Pregnancy, Childbirth, and Parenting

Rh Negative Blood 165
Routine Delivery Procedures Some Parents Would Like
   to Change 171
Sudden (Unexplained) Infant Death Syndrome 174
Am I Parent Material? 175
How to Win Without Losing 178

Chapter Eight
Tobacco

Trends in U.S. Cigarette Use, 1965-1980 190
"Light" Cigarettes: Deadly as Ever 191
Smoking and Life Expectancy 193
Smoking Used to Be Good for Me 195
The Secondhand Smoke Issue 199
The Strength of Commitment 200
Gum to Help You Stop Smoking 202

Chapter Nine
Alcohol

The Discovery of Alcohol 212
Early Indications of Alcohol Abuse 218
Alcohol-Related Social Problems in the United
   States 219

College Students' Ten Most Common Reasons for
    Drinking Alcohol   220
The Autobiography of an Alcoholic   221

Chapter Ten
Other Psychoactive Drugs

Why People Use Drugs   230
Nonmedical Drug Use   234
Caffeine   236
Cocaine Survey Points to Widespread Anguish   239
The Marijuana Problem   241

Chapter Eleven
Nutrition

How to Tell the Truth About Nutrition   255
How to Keep the Natural Goodness in Food   256
Additives: Friend or Foe?   259
How to Cut Down on Sugar   260
Where's the Nutrition?   261
Junk-Food Fans in the Health-Food Ranks   264
A Sheepish Trend: U.S. Eating Patterns Become
    Animalistic   266
The Vitamin C Controversy   268

Chapter Twelve
Overweight

Anorexia Nervosa and Bulimia   284
25 Tips from the Diet Center   288
Evaluating a Fad Diet   289
Play Plans for Exercise and Weight Loss   292
Eating for Health   294

Chapter Thirteen
Exercise

Running to Olympus   302
Commercial Health Clubs   308
Physiological Benefits of Warm-Up   309

The Five Principles of a Safe and Effective Exercise
    Program   311
Steroids   312
That "Extra Effort" Can Hold You Back   315

Chapter Fourteen
**The Consumer and Medicine, Fads,
and Quackery**

Recognized Specialties and Subspecialties of Allopathy
    and Osteopathy   328
How to Cut Health Care Costs   330
Taking Responsibility   336

Chapter Fifteen
Prescription and Over-the-Counter Drugs

The Placebo—An Ethical Problem   345
Using Over-the-Counter Drugs   349
Drugs and Alcohol   354
Aspirin Use   356

Chapter Sixteen
Medical Diagnosis

How to Choose a Doctor   367
Guidelines for the Wise Use of Medical X Rays   372
Getting a Second Opinion   380
Patient's Bill of Rights   381

Chapter Seventeen
Cardiovascular Health

Heart Surgery May Not Be Necessary   391
Lowered Cholesterol Lowers Heart Disease   392
A System for Estimating Your Risk from High Blood
    Pressure   394
Climbing Stairs Is Best   398
What You Should Know About Heart Attack   400
The Warning Signs of Stroke   401

Chapter Eighteen
Cancer

Cancer and Personality   413
Interferon Research: New Hope for Cancer Control   415
If You Won't Read These 7 Signals of Cancer . . . You
   Probably Have the 8th   418
Breast Self-Examination   419
Breast Cancer Surgery: From Radical to
   Conservative   420
Testicle Self-Examination   421

Chapter Nineteen
Infection and Immunity

The Common Cold   431
Sickle-Cell Disease   432
Strange Alliance: Legions of Bacteria Created to Serve
   Man   437
The Mind as Healer   441
A Pictorial History of Events in Infection Immunity   444
Keeping Up with the Genetic Revolution   450

Chapter Twenty
Sexually Transmitted Diseases

Doctoring VD Stereotypes   458
The VD National Hotline   460

Dealing with Sexually Transmitted Diseases   462
Twenty Prominent Victims of Syphilis   464
Acquired Immune Deficiency Syndrome (AIDS)   469

Chapter Twenty-One
Aging

Aging and Health: An Anthropological Point of
   View   479
Parent Abuse   483
Senility   487
Gray Power   488

Chapter Twenty-Two
Death and Dying

Definitions of Death   498
Elements of a Hospice Program   502
About Memorial Societies   503
Life After Death: The Growing Evidence   506

Preface

More than ten years have passed since we sat in our offices at Stanford University and contemplated writing a textbook that would shift the emphasis from the lay person's reliance on traditional medicine to the individual's active role in maintaining his or her own health. In those ten years a revolution has evolved within our culture that makes our professional association with health promotion exhilarating as well as tempestuous.

The revolution is a massive shift in societal and personal values away from reliance on doctors and institutions for well-being toward a self-reliance based on our own values and life-styles. Health has become a matter of personal decision. Self-responsibility suddenly is paramount.

With the first edition of this book in 1976, we probed experimentally in several new and promising directions. We shifted the emphasis from merely listing factual information regarding health issues to guiding the reader toward a process of self-inquiry. Knowing what is best for our health does not always lead to behavior that promotes wellness. Why we behave the way we do regarding our health became the focus of our book. Reflecting our emphasis on the individual's role in maintaining health, we provided a series of personal health inventories and questionnaires to help each reader assess his or her own health behavior and to bridge the gap between factual information and students' values. At the same time, we did not ignore the contributions of the traditional health and medical sciences. Scientific foundations remain integral to informed personal decision making. Innovative chapters on our social environment, the problems of aging, cultural and psychological values of death and dying, and rapidly changing sex roles were presented to describe processes underlying specific health behaviors. In succeeding years these topics became integral components of the health curriculum.

We find personal health a fascinating subject, as full of contrary opinions and complex events as the rest of human experience: Our book has reflected this. We have used an open, magazine format to avoid typical textbook torpor. The earlier editions were fun to read without in any way lowering academic expectations. Boxes, short quotations, fine photographs, and a running glossary all contributed to a solid yet provocative presentation.

The success of the first three editions of *Core Concepts in Health* has been gratifying. Thousands of instructors and tens of thousands of students have used our book in their classes, and instructors have remained unusually loyal in using the book over and over again. New books with formats and coverage that parallel ours have appeared, and we believe the quality of personal health texts in general has risen dramatically in recent years. We are very pleased that our text contributed so significantly to the direction that new books have taken. We are all winners here; we all benefit from increased attention to the quality of educational materials in our field.

Features of the Fourth Edition

The fourth edition of *Core Concepts in Health* builds on the features that so strongly attracted readers' interest in the past three editions. We continue to experiment with innovative teaching materials that have been tested and confirmed by gifted teachers in our profession.

We have also experimented with a different graphic approach by using color illustrations. We regard color illustrations as a valuable, functional support to our text. Health and well-being are positive concepts needing expression in illustrations as vibrant and as realistic as possible. Life *is* colorful! We want our text's pages to invigorate us as does our living. Color helps us overcome the usual monotony of the textbook medium. We hope the color makes you smile, and cry, and feel as you think about what the text is saying, for effective health education touches all these sensibilities and thoughts at once.

Beyond the motivating use of color in the illustrations lies something else. Our color illustrations have been created by the very best illustrators in the country. Every piece in this book has been recognized by the graphics arts profession and applauded for its originality and graphic effect. The images are not always pleasant. Neither is life always sweet. We have included images that may be making an ironic statement because we find much of human behavior ironic, complex, often contradictory, sometimes injurious. Rather than impose our captions on these dramatic images, we hope the viewer will stretch to puzzle out his or her own interpretations.

The structure of each chapter has been modified slightly in the fourth edition. Our organization emphasizes individual responsibility. We work toward a goal of self-understanding and self-inquiry by bringing together an exploration of values with practical health information. Affective and cognitive elements for us are the yin and yang of health education.

1. *Probing Your Emotions:* The chapter-opening questions explore emotional issues to highlight awareness of feelings that can affect the cognitive information within each chapter.
2. *Self-Assessment:* At the end of each chapter, the reader is asked to complete a brief questionnaire that assesses attitudes and behaviors linked to the chapter content. The reader can locate his or her score on a wellness scale, which gives a chapter-by-chapter summary of each reader's health *and* potential for wellness.
3. *Take Action:* Sometimes the worst thing we can do is discover a truth about our own life or our values, realize we should do something about our self-discovery, but *do* nothing. At the end of each chapter, we specify actions the reader might take to improve wellness. We also encourage the keeping of an extended journal to reinforce the self-understanding that should be accumulating as this book is studied.
4. *Behavior Change Strategy:* Models for altering some behaviors that prevent individuals from achieving maximum health are presented at the end of appropriate chapters to simplify important or complex issues.

The text has been updated, an absolute necessity because health issues constantly change. Major beliefs, like the role of salt in blood pressure problems or the predisposition of certain personalities to cardiovascular disease, change frequently. Sometimes the change is 180 degrees from earlier belief. Sometimes the change is driven by our health technology: Diabetics now live on insulin identical to human insulin, but it is produced by bacteria called *E. Coli*, which have been genetically manipulated! Every page of this text represents the state of the art in living with good health.

We have streamlined the book by eliminating some longer boxes and asides. New boxes on topics of current interest or controversy have been added. We have retained the popular running glossary, in which words are defined on the text page when they are first encountered. Cross-references to the glossary appear in the index, where the location of defined words is indicated in boldface type.

In recent years, there has been an explosion of personal inventories or questionnaires, many of them having dubious origins or questionable utility. We have limited our use of these to major points where their utility is highly valuable. We have also tried to use instruments whose long-term use is educationally valid. You should not, after filling out answers to several purposeful questions, find yourself saying, "So what!"

The *Instructor's Resource Guide,* prepared for the fourth edition by Gerald F. Braza of the University of Utah and Kathleen Braza, is again available. This instructor's manual enjoys a reputation as the best manual of its kind for innovative and caring instructors. It is much more than a collection of test items. It includes student learning objectives keyed to the relevant pages in the textbook. Numerous learning activities use various teaching techniques—from research projects to group-facilitated discussion topics. A full range of test questions is included for each chapter. A major feature of the *Instructor's Resource Guide* is its collection of behavioral action handouts, which supplement the health appraisals in the textbook. This edition contains an extensive annotated listing of films, books, and other resources of potential interest to instructors and students.

Finally, we have innovations made possible by computer. All the test items in the *Instructor's Resource Guide* are contained in software compatible with major microprocessors. The software allows each instructor to select specific questions; generate several versions of the same test, with answer keys; and enlarge the test item data bank by adding new questions.

A Note of Thanks

More than most books, this text represents a truly collaborative effort by many thoughtful and hard-working people. To them all—contributors, advisors, and reviewers—we are most gratefully indebted.

Academic Contributors

Alfred Amkraut, *Infection and Immunity*

John H. Brennecke, *Mental Health*

Brian Danaher, Ph.D., *Health Behavior*

Thomas Fahey, Ph.D., *Exercise*

Christopher Gillin, M.D., *Mental Health*

Ralph Grawunder, Ed.D., *Aging; Death and Dying*

Lieselotte Hofmann, *Introduction; Stress and the Social Environment*

Marcia Seyler Insel, *Sex and Intimacy; Pregnancy, Childbirth, and Parenting*

Paul M. Insel, Ph.D., *Cardiovascular Health; Cancer; Stress and the Social Environment; Overweight; Health Behavior; Tobacco*

Robert E. Kime, Ph.D., *The Consumer and Medicine, Fads, and Quackery*

Norman Kretchmer, M.D., PhD., *Nutrition*

Marshall Kreuter, Ph.D., *Health Behavior*

Bea Mandel, R.N., M.P.H., *Sexually Transmitted Diseases*

William Van B. Robertson, M.E., Ph.D., *Nutrition*

Donald G. Ross, Boxed Material

Walton T. Roth, M.D., *Medical Diagnosis*

Carl Thoresen, Ph.D., *Overweight*

Jared Tinklenberg, M.D., F.A.P.A., *Tobacco; Alcohol; Other Psychoactive Drugs*

Mae Tinklenberg, R.N., R.P.N.P., *Birth Control*

Joseph B. Trainer, M.D., *Sexual Responses*

Jack Turner, R.Ph., *Prescription and Over-the-Counter Drugs*

Academic Advisors and Reviewers

W. Henry Baughman, Western Kentucky University

Don Brobst, San Jose City College

Judith E. Brown, University of Minnesota

Geral Dene Burdman, University of Oregon

Roy Burwen, San Francisco State University

Elaine Bush, Palo Alto Medical Foundation

David Chenoweth, Medical Datamation

Barbara Combs, City College of San Francisco

Thomas M. Davis, University of Northern Iowa

Darwin Dennison, State University of New York at Buffalo

Kathy Doyle, Eastern Illinois University

David F. Duncan, Southern Illinois University at Carbondale

Muzza Eaton, Brooklyn College

William Faraclas, Southern Connecticut State College

Kevin Foley, Suffolk County Community College

Keith Fraker, Valley Medical Center, Stanford University

Sharon Garcia, Diablo Valley College

Bruce Goodrow, Mankato State University

Michael Hamrick, Memphis State University

Sandy Kammerman, Eastern Illinois University

Richard Kaye, Kingsborough Community College

Robert E. Kime, University of Oregon

Mark J. Kittleson, Youngstown State University

Lloyd Kolbe, University of Texas Health Science Center

Alfred Kouneski, Montgomery College

John Leary, State University of New York at Cortland

Lorna and Aubrey McTaggart, San Diego State University

Monroe Pastermack, Diablo Valley College

Adolf Pfefferbaum, Stanford University

Valerie Pinhaus, Nassau Community College

Darlene Pleszewicz, Ohio State University

Marion B. Pollock, Long Beach State University

James H. Price, University of Toledo

Jane E. Richards, University of Northern Iowa

Stephen Roberts, University of Toledo

Laurna Rubinson, University of Illinois at Urbana-Champaign

R. Allen Rude, Foothill College

Robert Russell, Southern Illinois University

Richard W. St. Pierre, Pennsylvania State University
Albert J. Stunkard, University of Pennsylvania
Kenneth Swearingen, Saddleback College
Frances Thomas, Lane Community College
Robert F. Valois, Eastern Illinois University at Charleston

Barbara Wells, University of Virginia
Carol Weston, University of Wisconsin
Barbara Wilks, University of Georgia

Paul Insel
Walton T. Roth

Introduction

Measure your health by your sympathy with morning and Spring.

Thoreau

The next time you ask someone "How are you?" and get the automatic response "Fine," be grateful. If that person told you how he or she actually felt—physically, emotionally, mentally—you might wish you had never asked. Your friend might be one of the too many people who live most of their lives feeling no better than just all right, or so-so, or downright miserable. Some do not even know what exuberant health is. How many people do you know who feel great most of the time? Do you?

Health is considerably more than the absence of a minor or major illness. It is partly biological status, a matter of how well all the body's component parts are working. It is partly a consequence of behavior, a reflection of our ability to coexist with other people. And it is partly a product of personal and philosophical values, intimately tied to our concept of self—what we think we ought to be and what we think we really are.

Over the last 50 years, a growing understanding of the biological aspects of health has led to some exciting and startling technological advances in the battle against disease. Advances in immunology, for example, have resulted in the control in a few decades of many of the ills that plagued our ancestors for centuries. It is clear, however, that we cannot reasonably expect future technological advances to be of such magnitude. The great breakthroughs of tomorrow will almost certainly come in the behavioral sphere—that is, in a greatly expanded understanding of why we behave as we do and, more particularly, how we can go about changing behavior that is harmful to our health.

Staggeringly large numbers of the health problems that pervade this country are self-inflicted. They are rarely self-inflicted with the aim of self-destruction; they are more commonly the result of ignorance and confusion and apathy. The purpose of this book, then, is to inform, to clarify, and to dispel indifference.

The Meaning of Health and Disease

To James Thomson, the Scottish poet, health was "the vital principle of bliss." To the World Health Organization, it is ideally "a state of complete physical,

mental, and social well-being and not merely the absence of disease or infirmity." To psychiatrist Alexander Lowen, writing in *Pleasure: A Creative Approach to Life* (1970), health is "the truth of the body."

A bit more matter-of-factly, scientist and author René Dubos, in *Man, Medicine, and Environment* (1968), views health as a way of life that enables imperfect human beings "to achieve a rewarding and not too painful existence while they cope with an imperfect world." According to this definition, the fashion model, the Jesuit priest, the cattle rancher, the Mafia don, the oil tycoon, and the rock singer all will have different views of what health means because their physical and mental needs, their aspirations and hopes, their stresses, and their vulnerability to disease differ. They can measure their health generally by how well they are able to function within and adapt continually to their constantly changing environments.

Most people think of disease as an organic illness like cancer or a mental dysfunction like schizophrenia. But the word *disease* means only "not to feel at ease"; its meaning is not implicitly limited to abnormal or deadly conditions. The modern medical establishment itself is beginning to revise somewhat its view of disease. It is coming to understand that a "diseased" person can be suffering from an organic or a psychic disease, a real disease or an imaginary one, or one that may jeopardize life or simply put a damper on its enjoyment. In other words, you are healthy when you are in harmony with your outer and inner environments; you are sick when discord becomes the rule.

The stresses of life, if severe enough to defy adjustment, can be just as great a threat to health as physical and chemical forces, bacteria, and malnutrition. Body and mind are inseparably liked in a biochemical unity, and virtually every disease involves an interplay between them. Good medical care implies concern for more than the body or a certain part of the body; it implies concern for the whole person and for his or her total environment. As the famed Canadian physician Sir William Osler once said, "It is more important to know what sort of patient has a disease than what sort of disease a patient has."

To be healthy is to have the ability, despite an occasional bout of illness, to live with full use of your faculties and to be vigorous, alert, and happy to be alive even in old age. Perhaps the most poignant description of health you will ever find is one by British author Katherine Mansfield, who, when she was dying of tuberculosis, wrote in the final pages of her journal:

> By health, I mean the power to live a full, adult, living, breathing life in close contact with what I love—the earth and the wonders thereof—the sea—the sun. . . . *I want to be all that I am capable of becoming, so that I may be* . . . there's only one phrase that will do—*a child of the sun.*

Can Disease Be Completely Conquered?

The biochemical makeup of human beings has remained essentially static for some 100,000 years. So have the diseases that afflict human beings. These diseases are universal and unchangeable. Diseases that prevail in modern industrialized countries plagued prehistoric people too and have not completely by-passed today's primitive societies. What has changed is the prevalence of various diseases, both physical and mental, from one historical era to another, from one geographical area to another, and among different social groups. For instance, although all human beings presumably can get cancer, there are enormous differences in the incidence of various forms of cancer between one area and others and from one social group to another.

Affluence, no less than poverty, can bring on a host of diseases. *Diseases of civilization* and *pathology of inactivity* are not just empty phrases. Scientists have marshaled a vast amount of evidence in all the technologically advanced nations to show that a major factor of illness among people of all ages is the way of life they follow.

Some 2,500 years ago Hippocrates wrote, "It is changes that are chiefly responsible for diseases, especially the greatest changes, the violent alterations both in the seasons and in other things." Because human beings cannot adapt quickly enough, biologically and socially, to their changing environments, changing times, changing cultures, or even to the changes in everyday existence, the complete conquest of disease remains a dream. Yet the battle goes on.

Although the so-called advanced countries boast of having achieved the highest standards of health in history, they are nevertheless driven to spend more and more money to control disease. And, as René Dubos has pointed out in his disturbingly titled book *Mirage of Health* (1959), "For too many life in the modern world is a passive experience or a lonely struggle, the wounds of which are reflected not only in damage to the blood vessels of our brains and our hearts but also in the very loss of hopes."

The highest rates of suicide, death from violence, and drug addiction are found not in the less developed countries where life is harsh and filled with uncertainties, but in countries with the greatest material wealth, the greatest political stability, and the most advanced social legislation. Life in technologically advanced societies has additional perils. The same modern skills that have prevented and controlled certain diseases of Western civilization have also deprived Western populations of their natural immunities, making them exceedingly vulnerable when virulent germs do attack, as they frequently do. No medical magic is ever likely to rid the world of microbes: They are awesomely prolific, highly adaptable, and all over the place. Yet, contrary to the warnings of advertisers that countless germs are seeking us out with demonic fervor, the truth is that we are of comparatively minor interest to the vast microbial world. Relatively few species cause or are capable of causing disease. When those microorganisms that do seem to have a grudge against us invade and multiply, our bodies sometimes launch so many defenses that the result is overkill, which may be more harmful to us than the invaders themselves.

Four health problems—atherosclerosis, cancer, arthritis, and combined bronchitis, asthma, and emphysema—have become major killers and cripplers in the United States, Western Europe, and Japan. They owe much of their prominence to the fact that the infectious diseases that once killed so many people at a young age have largely been conquered. It is older people who primarily suffer from these four diseases, thanks, quite possibly, to their prolonged exposure to overrich diets, heightened stress, and filth in the atmosphere that vies with the microbial filth of the worst nineteenth-century slums.

The so-called new diseases (for instance AIDS—

Acquired Immune Deficiency Syndrome—Alzheimer's disease, herpes, and hemorrhagic fevers) are really not new. Apparently some of them existed in the past but were not spotted until diagnostic techniques became more refined and physicians began to be more inclined to report unusual ailments to their colleagues. Further, changes in ecology, technology, and life-styles may be giving organisms that perhaps have long existed undercover a chance to come to light. When these agents are brought together with the host and the environment in a new way, a new ailment is created. Some of these mysterious maladies seem to occur only in certain geographical areas, and some have thus far afflicted only a few people.

The notion that scientific medicine (the germ theory and the antibacterial drugs in particular) deserves *all* the credit for the dramatic decrease in death rates since 1900 is widespread but incorrect. Death rates from infections of various kinds had begun to decline in North America and in Western Europe long before specific methods of therapy were introduced and before the germ theory of disease had even been demonstrated. In our enthusiasm for the role science has played in controlling epidemic diseases, we overlook the various campaigns for purity —purity of food, water, and air—launched by humanitarian movements that were trying to wipe out the social evils of the industrial revolution.

Another popular idea is that the tremendous increase in life expectancy in the Western world during the past century has been the result of improved health of people during adulthood. Not so. What really has made all the difference is the spectacular drop in infant mortality. Until the mid-nineteenth century, only one-half of all children born in the United States reached their fifth year—precisely the figures that currently apply to some areas of the Third World. In earlier days, the figures were even more appalling. England's Queen Anne, who reigned in the early eighteenth century, was probably exceptionally unlucky: Sixteen of her seventeen children died as babies, and the sole survivor succumbed before he was 12 years old. Today, in economically developed countries, 97 percent of newborns survive to adulthood because they have been spared the killing infectious diseases. Life expectancy *at birth* has almost doubled, and more people survive the first half-century than in

the past, but the life expectancy of, say, a 45-year-old white American man in the 1980s is scarcely greater than it was in 1900. This man can expect to reach about 70 or 71 years of age—barely more than the biblical "threescore and ten" and a gain of only three years over 1900. An American woman does somewhat better: She can expect to live 77 years, a gain of seven years.

The Lure of Longevity

The possibility of finding a fountain of youth, a definite means of prolonging life, has teased the imagination for hundreds of years. Every living creature has a maximum life span, and the human being who occasionally lives beyond 100 lives longer than any other mammal (except perhaps the elephant and the whale). About a century ago there was a widespread belief that human beings could, with the aid of medical wizardry, extend their life span to 150 or 200 years. Today, although some health (particularly health-food) buffs cling to that belief, most sober-minded scientists see no immediate prospect of appreciably prolonging human life. Consider, however, this observation—from *The Stress of Life* (1956)—by Dr. Hans Selye, an outstanding pioneer of medicine:

> What makes me so certain that the natural human life span is far in excess of the actual one is this:
>
> Among all my autopsies (and I have performed well over one thousand), I have never seen a person who died of old age. In fact, *I do not think anyone has ever died of old age yet.* To permit this would be the ideal accomplishment of medical research. . . . To die of old age would mean that all the organs of the body had worn out proportionately, merely by having been used too long. This is never the case. We invariably die because one vital part has worn out too early in proportion to the rest of the body. Life, the biologic chain that holds our parts together, is only as strong as its weakest vital link. When this breaks—no matter which vital link it be—our parts can no longer be held together as a single living being.

It is, of course, doubtful that anyone would want to prolong his or her life if doing so meant extending misery and pain or if it meant living in an environment so noxious or a culture so dispiriting that one could not live fully and creatively. But does long life *have* to mean long suffering?

Among the healthiest and most long-lived people of the nearly four billion in the world are the very few—probably less than 0.1 percent—who live in such isolation that they are totally without medical care and health knowledge. Unmolested by outside influences, they are rarely ill, lead vigorous lives even in old age, and enjoy a longevity that would be considered unusual in a medically coddled society. Their superb health can be attributed largely to their adaptation to their various environments, environments that are physically harsh yet tranquil. Their diets, too, may have much to do with their enduring vitality, although (or because) they are a far cry from the fare of their affluent contemporaries in other lands. They thrive on whatever is available, and those who live on a monotonous diet consisting mainly of durra (a cereal grain) appear to do just as well as those who live on beans, unpolished rice, vegetables, and fruit or on such delicacies as lizards, emus, kangaroos, ants, nuts, and wild yams. The diets of the most long-lived of these people have three things in common: They are low in protein (by our increasingly questioned standards), high in roughage, and limited in amount.

When people who are very old but still spry are asked how they've managed to live so long, they come up with highly diverse and often zany answers, like never washing their hair, or eating only peanut butter and bananas, or working up a sweat every day, or washing their faces in cold water at the crack of dawn. Such whimsy aside, researchers have found that those who are extremely old and, importantly, relatively fit have certain characteristics in common: For instance, they remain active, are moderate in all things, eat lightly and simply, rarely worry, are serene and free from fear (especially the fear of death), and have a sense of humor.

It is possible that, in societies like ours, people are conditioned to *think* that rapid physical and mental decline is inevitable in the later years of life and that not many can overcome this conditioning. Brainwashed to accept the stereotype of the elderly as saggy, stooped, and not quite "all there," they adopt the sedentary, unchallenging life that contributes so much to premature aging—and rust out rather than wear out. Although it is true that some degenerative change occurs, the person who has followed sensible living habits throughout his or her earlier years and who feels love and a sense of purpose is not likely to go downhill fast. Encouraging, too, are recent studies suggesting that, except for mathematical material, older people can learn and retain what they learn just as well as or better than the young.

The American Medical Profession

The principles that guide the medical profession (and the other sciences) have been described as "intellectual integrity and objectivity, tolerance, doubt of certitude, recognition of error, unselfish engagement, sense of belonging, and recognition of priorities" (André Courand, "Preface," in Jean Hamburger, *The Power and the Frailty: The Future of Medicine and the Future of Man,* 1973). The lay public, as well as certain members of the medical profession, would claim that some doctors are not bound closely enough by these principles. Many Americans feel that the Hippocratic Oath has been changed into the Hypocritical Oath, that the doctor with the bedside manner has become the doctor with the six-bedroom manor. They complain of depersonalized care, high medical costs, and unnecessary treatments. Yet they flock to their physicians in ever greater numbers.

If money spent on health is any criterion, America ought to be the healthiest nation on earth. We spent more than $322 billion on health care in 1982, and the cost is rising about 10 percent each year—making the price tag in 1985 over $400 billion. If the indirect costs of disability and premature death are added to the direct costs of prevention, detection, and treatment, the total expenditure for illness skyrockets. The Social Security Administration reported that in 1980 that cost had already reached $378 billion, with illness causing working men and women to lose the equivalent of 2.3 million years of work.

Inflation is only partly responsible for the steepness of our current health care bill—a bill that has, since 1965, risen more than twice as fast as prices. We must also take into account that we are getting more health care than we did a decade or so ago. But the main reason for rising health costs is alleged to lie elsewhere.

According to Robert Claiborne (in "The Great Health Care Rip-off," *Saturday Review,* Jan. 7, 1978, p. 10),

> The individuals and groups that provide care—notably, the hospitals—and the organizations through which we pay for it—notably, Blue Cross—operate under incentives that reward inefficiency and outright waste. As a result, while a minority of Americans still get less health care than they need, collectively most of us get (and pay for) more, and more elaborate, care than we need—often, more than is good for us.

Unfortunately, we Americans have, by and large, come to believe that we should leave our health in the care of our doctors. We run to the doctor for dozens of minor ailments from which we could recover perfectly well on our own. Sir William Gull, a celebrated nineteenth-century physician, was not just being funny when he said, "Medicines do most good when there is a tendency to recover without them." Recent studies have shown that, after taking placebos (chemically inactive substances), roughly 30 percent of patients with physical ailments and 40 percent of those with psychiatric illnesses report that they feel better; even medically useless surgery—which reportedly accounts for about half of the surgery performed in the United States—can make patients feel better. What these findings suggest is that perhaps 70 percent of all patients who visit doctors would get well without medical help. Were the public to stop wasting doctors' time and talents on frivolous complaints, doctors' waiting rooms would be about as overcrowded as the Senate on the fifth night of a filibuster.

Take the common cold. There is a joke among doctors that "a cold lasts 4 days or 96 hours, depending on the treatment." Why bother to treat a cold then? Back in the 1700s, a French wag named Nicolas Chamfort suggested an answer: "The threat of a neglected cold is for doctors what the threat of purgatory is for priests—a gold mine." For a cold without complications, antibiotics and aspirin will do nothing more than time and chicken soup (or a more interesting therapeutic measure like a teaspoon of cayenne pepper with a double shot of whiskey) will do.

A number of physicians admit that many of the standard treatments they prescribe for minor ailments are contrary both to the principles of scientific medicine and to common sense. The therapeutic measures attack the *symptoms* that the disease causes, not the *cause* of the disease. These symptoms frequently reflect how the body's natural system of defense is battling the disease-causing agent, and thus the progress of the disease is obscured by the treatment. That can be dangerous if what first appears to be a minor ailment turns out to be a major one.

"Man has an inborn craving for medicines. . . . It is really one of the most serious difficulties with which we have to contend," Sir William Osler said. Today's doctors do not seem to be seriously trying to contend with that craving, and the pharmaceutical industry is far from eager to see them do so. Drug companies are not charitable institutions. They are in business to make a profit, and make a profit they do.

In 1980 Americans swallowed some 21,000 tons of aspirin, either plain or in combination formulations. That's about 55 billion tablets, or an average of 245 tablets per person. This tonnage has, if anything, increased.

There are now more than 5,000 prescription drugs and 100,000 over-the-counter drugs available. Every 24 to 36 hours, from 50 to 80 percent of American adults gulp down at least one prescribed drug. America's total bill for legal drugs is now more than $35 billion a year. Some of the drugs for which we pay all this money are harmful, and most of them do little or no good.

In ancient China personal physicians were paid only for keeping their clients healthy, not for curing them. We, too, have preventive medicine—in the form of insurance and taxes, public health agencies, and periodic examinations. And community health centers are slowly coming into their own, making health education and qualified medical advice accessible to thousands of people formerly excluded by poverty and geographic isolation. With adequate modes of preventive medicine, it is possible that half the hospitals we now fill could shut down. The prevention of disease is frequently far less expensive than the treatment of disease, but present health care is still focused on curative medicine. Dr. Robert S. Mendelson, who quite rightly calls himself "a medical heretic," goes so far as to say, "I believe that more than 90 percent of Modern Medicine could disappear from the face of the earth—doctors, hospitals, drugs, and equipment—and the health of the nation would immediately and dramatically improve" (*Male Practice,* 1981).

When he was president of the Rockefeller Foundation, the late Dr. John Knowles claimed that expensive life-saving techniques are preferred to simple prevention "for three obvious reasons: First, acute curative medicine is more interesting intellectually. Two, it's more gratifying emotionally. . . . Three, it's much more rewarding financially." Another physician, Dr. John R. Miles, points out that true progress lies in prevention and that "viewed in this light, organ transplantation might be described as the most brilliant surgical irrelevance of the century." Many physicians feel that the overall cost of one chancy heart transplant ($100,000 or more) might be better applied to preventive medicine.

When your body really needs help to heal itself, the doctor who applies his or her hard-won expertise intelligently can be a highly useful resource. In his *Aphorisms,* Hippocrates wrote of the doctor:

> Life is short, technique takes a long time to acquire, the right moment is fleeting, personal experience is deceptive, decision is difficult. The doctor should not be content to merely take appropriate action himself: he has to make sure that the patient, the surroundings, and even the outside influences all collaborate on the cure.

Remember that doctors have a crushing responsibility. They often deal with matters of life and death, knowing that 9 times out of 10 they are basing their decisions on probabilities, not certainties. And, actually, every doctor works at least part of the time in a fearful solitude. Do not expect your doctor to work miracles. Regard your doctor, advises Dr. Leonard Tushnet, not "as a wizard but as a mortal man who sees in the world a microcosm of ailments. And because of his specialized vision remember that he is shortsighted" (*The Medicine Men,* 1971). Many alternative healers, or "New Age" practitioners, tend to be just as shortsighted as orthodox physicians. It is all too easy to become a "holistic health junkie," going from treatment to treatment in search of some radical cure.

If you trust your doctor, if he or she does not treat you like a child or an idiot and answers all your questions candidly, then you are probably getting the best medical care for you. If you feel you are not getting that, change doctors. There are lots of good ones around.

The Healthy American?

Americans claim the highest standard of living in the world (not to be confused with the best quality of life), yet more than half of the adult population is chronically ill. Three major chronic diseases—arthritis, heart disease, and diabetes—partially incapacitate more than 22 million Americans. Arteriosclerosis, a disease almost unknown in some countries, kills some 2,000 Americans every day and hospitalizes thousands more. Our infant mortality rate ranks fifteenth in the world. Half of our hospital beds are occupied by psychiatric patients. The anxiety state, as a clinical syndrome, is the primary diagnostic problem in general medicine. Of the roughly 80 million Americans who are overweight, more than half are classified as obese; even a great many children are at least 10 percent overweight.

About three-fourths of all Americans are not living out their normal life spans, and those who do are likely to spend their waning years in pain and misery. Such a depressing state of affairs could largely be avoided if we were to adopt more sensible living habits. Yet few Americans make any effort to recognize, let alone accept, responsibility for their own health. Nutrition is one of the many examples. Why, in the face of a wealth of solid evidence that many of our illnesses are directly related to long-term dietary indiscretion, do we persist in eating as we do?

One of the reasons is our ceaseless pursuit of efficiency, which leads us to seek out more and better Instafast Taste-Tempters. Another, ironically, is our misguided notions of what kinds of food and how much we need to sustain good health. What we eat—along with a lot of the other weird things we do—might also have something to do with what is eating us. We can literally create our own diseases, diseases that are by-products of a mind that holds and will not let go of feelings of fear, worry, anger, hate, and the like.

However disturbing some of the statistics on the health of Americans may be, and however much our minor ailments are manufactured by the media into major afflictions, we are hardly a nation of invalids. As Dr. Lewis Thomas points out in *The Medusa and the Snail* (1979),

> We do not seem to be seeking more exuberance in living as much as staving off failure, putting off dying. We have lost all confidence in the human body. . . .
>
> Despite the persisting roster of still-unsolved major diseases . . . most of us have a clear, unimpeded run at a longer and healthier lifetime than could have been foreseen by any earlier generation. . . . We will still age away and die, but the aging, and even the dying, can become a healthy process.

The Option of Optimum Health

Optimum health: You cannot get it from your doctor, the hospital, your guru, your lover, a wonder drug, or a miracle food. You can get it only through what the Chinese call *tzu-li keng-sheng,* or regeneration through your own efforts. If expending such effort sounds like too much of a hassle, bear in mind that once you have optimum health, everything in your life becomes much less of a hassle.

Given the treatment it deserves, your body can fully use its remarkable capacity for healing itself and for protecting itself against most injuries, whether they are inflicted by nature or by your own civilization.

There is no one path to optimum health. Because you are a unique individual, you have unique transactions with both the world you've made for yourself and the world that you had no hand in making. True insight can be gained only by being honest with yourself, by tuning in to what your body is trying to tell you, and by having the wisdom and respect to listen.

Core Concepts in Health

Part One

Wellness Behavior

Chapter One

Health Behavior

To a very large extent our health is a direct result of how we live, love, work, and interact with others and with our environment. In short, health is a reflection or product of how we behave.

All of us behave in some ways that promote our own health and in other ways that put our health at risk. It is not enough only to be knowledgeable about risk of illness, however. We also need to understand ourselves and why we behave as we do. The purpose of this chapter is to lay a foundation for understanding how we can maintain *wellness behavior* and how we can change *risk behavior.*

Human beings are remarkably well equipped to adapt to environmental conditions. Each of us has an awesome potential for adapting to various social and physical circumstances. We also have an equally strong potential for avoiding adaptation.

The word *potential* is critical here because human behavior is by no means easy to control. Consider for a moment all the possible reasons a person might offer to "explain" why he or she overeats: enjoyment of the taste of food, family or cultural influences, a belief that overeating cannot be controlled, the abundance of available snack foods, stress at school or on the job, and so on. Not only is the list likely to be quite long and to differ from person to person, but it will also show how these presumed factors interact to encourage overeating. By acknowledging the complexity of human behavior, we are less likely to succumb to simplistic, "magic pill" answers. Statements attributing behavior to "willpower" and "self-control" (or the lack thereof) are both simplistic and vague. In fact, "willpower" rationalizations may actually undermine a person's attempt to change.

Chapter Contents

PLANNING LIFE-STYLE CHANGES

WHY DO I BEHAVE AS I DO?
Self-monitoring and data collection
Self-assessment and data analysis

HOW CAN I MAKE A CHANGE?
Set specific goals
Make a personal contract
Establish rewards

AVOIDING DERAILMENT
Using your health diary
Self-management

MAINTAINING COMMITMENT
Shape your expectations
Recruit support

TROUBLESHOOTING
Overcoming barriers
Outside sources of help

HEALTH FOR LIFE
Plan for a lifetime
Change the environment around you

A POSITION OF TEMPERED ENTHUSIASM

BEHAVIORAL FEATURES OF THE FOLLOWING CHAPTERS
Probing your emotions
Behavior scale
Take action
Behavior change strategy

Boxes

The health diary
Personal contracts for change
The SCIENCE mnemonic formula for personal problem solving
Ages of health advancement

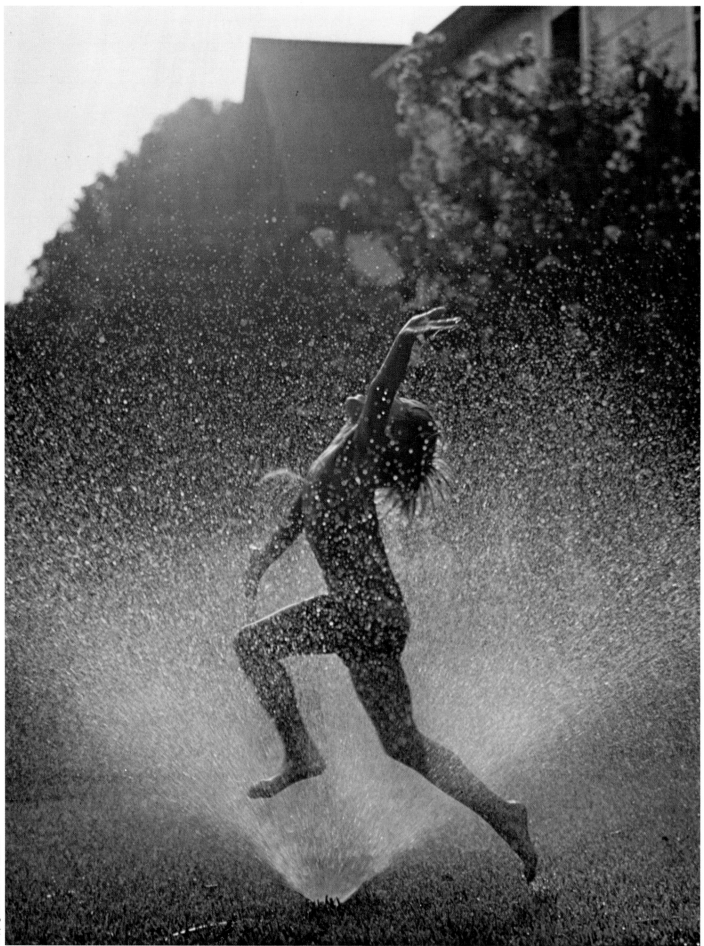

4

Wellness behavior
Behavior with a strong element of prevention that supports optimal health.

Risk behavior
Behavior that threatens health: for example, smoking or overeating.

Health diary
A record of behaviors and events thought to be associated with a particular health situation.

Planning Life-Style Changes

The Chinese are fond of saying that even the longest journey begins with a single step. Dr. Donald Ardell of Golden Gate University in San Francisco has developed 14 steps toward achieving a wellness life-style. Each step is equal to one day. His 14-day plan builds awareness, supports positive motivations, and presents strategies for long-term life-style changes.

Day 1 involves your learning the concept of wellness and wellness life-styles. On day 2 you test yourself to establish a benchmark from which you will start a wellness program. On day 3 you learn how the medical system works: its problems, its capabilities, and its role in promoting positive health. Day 4 involves your awareness of cultural norms and social expectations; you examine how these pressures affect your wellness life-style. On day 5 you concentrate on imaging. You begin to develop an awareness of the meaning of being truly healthy and the consequences of a lifelong pursuit of wellness. For day 6 Ardell provides a perspective on personal responsibility. He suggests you become familiar with the important elements of personal accountability in a wellness life-style. On day 7 physical fitness becomes a prerequisite to a wellness life-style. The measures of exercise adequacy include frequency, intensity, and duration. On day 8 you learn to eat for performance and appreciate the principles of wellness dining. You discover the personal approaches to food that help you think and function at your best. Understanding the six ways people eat—only one of which promotes wellness—is part of Ardell's plan. On day 9 you learn the simple basics of stress. You should understand the effective strategies for minimizing the hazards and maximizing the benefits of stress. Day 10 involves the management of stress. You can develop the capability and incentive to practice relaxation techniques on a regular basis (see Chapter 2). You should be able to reverse the physical and psychological symptoms of excessive stress and learn the responses that are optimal for personal effectiveness. On day 11 you learn to use your visualization skills to rehearse and picture in your mind's eye how to manage your stress successfully. Ardell provides tips and visualization approaches that support creativity to enhance health. On day 12 you

investigate what Ardell calls "wellness vital signs." These include both objective and subjective measures of health, such as heart recovery rate and energy level. On day 13 Ardell suggests you may want to plan and undertake a heroic act such as participating in a marathon. He defines a heroic act as any physical activity undertaken after strenuous preparation. He points out that this step is purely optional. Day 14, the last day of the plan, is the day everything should come together. You should be able to integrate your knowledge and interest in the wellness concept into a systematic personal program. Figure 1–1 on the next page summarizes Ardell's approach.

Let us examine some of the behavioral skills or enabling factors that permit us to influence our own life-style. Skill in managing our own behavior is an enabling factor that is far superior to the elusive concept of self-control or willpower. Try to think of self-control as a skill that you can learn rather than a description of your character.

In the following discussion of behavioral techniques, you will learn how to identify and change negative predisposing, enabling, and reinforcing factors that may be influencing your behavior. Your chances for lasting success are directly influenced by how well you use these self-management techniques.

Why Do I Behave as I Do?

Before you consider ways of changing a particular behavior or habit, first find out all you can about it. Compile information about your behavior. Then analyze the information. What provokes the behavior? When are you most vulnerable? How do outside factors influence your behavior?

Self-Monitoring and Data Collection   Most behavior change experts ask their clients to begin by keeping careful records of the circumstances that surround a particular target behavior. These records are usually kept in a *health diary.* (See "The Health Diary," page 7.) This diary is a prerequisite for making changes later. Most people are not keenly aware of the situational factors that trigger their target behaviors. In a diary for weight loss, for example, you might keep records of the amount of food you consume, time of day, situation, location, and even the level of your hunger. By means of such information, diaries are frequently used to focus attention on the *frequency, intensity,* and *duration* of target behaviors. Later in this chapter we will examine ways in which your health diary will lead you to specific self-management strategies.

Select any habit, such as smoking, overeating, poor study habits, test anxiety, or any behavior that is creating a problem for you. Keep a diary for one or two weeks. With the detailed data you collect about this target behavior, analyze the internal and external stimuli that lead to this particular habitual response.

Self-Assessment and Data Analysis After you have collected information on a particular habit, analyze the data to identify patterns in your responses. Perhaps you are especially hungry late in the afternoon. Discover the time of day that hunger strikes. Do you find that you drink more alcohol at a party than anywhere else? Do you drink more at a beer bust with loud rock music than you drink at a quiet gathering with a few friends? Discover how you react to the environment or the situation. Do you find that you want a cigarette more after dinner than at almost any other time? Once you have identified the interaction between your feelings and external stimuli such as location, time of day, and situation, you can design strategies to divert your behavior into new directions.

Figure 1-1

1	2	3	4	5	6	7
LEARN THE RULES	TEST YOURSELF	THE MEDICAL SYSTEM	CULTURAL NORMS	HEALTHY IMAGE	SELF-RESPONSIBILITY	PHYSICAL FITNESS
Wellness Wellness life-styles	Personal benchmark	Problems Capabilities Wellness role	Social expectations Unwritten rules	Health awareness Positive results	Wellness accountability	Frequency Intensity Duration

8	9	10	11	12	13	14
EAT FOR PERFORMANCE	DYNAMICS OF STRESS	STRESS MANAGEMENT	VISUALIZATION SKILLS	WELLNESS VITAL SIGNS	BECOMING A HERO (OPTIONAL)	PERSONAL WELLNESS PLAN
Varied food patterns Personal approaches Six ways of eating	Basics of stress Stress phenomenon	Stress symptoms Relaxation techniques Optimal responses	Rehearsal Using your mind's eye	Key measures Baseline status	Strenuous preparation Challenge Marathon event	Integrating and implementing a personal program

Source: Adapted from *14 Days to a Wellness Life-Style* by Dr. Donald Ardell.

The Health Diary

One version of a health diary for smokers asks the smoker to collect information on both cigarettes smoked and smoking urges. These data are recorded on specially designed diary pages that allow the smoker to indicate the hour during which the cigarette was actually smoked and/or the urge occurred. *Every* smoking urge is evaluated for its intensity on a 1- to 5-point scale of intensity. If a cigarette is actually smoked following the smoking urge, then the rating (a number from "1" to "5") is *circled* in the diary in the appropriate time box. The example that follows illustrates a typical case.

Example: Suppose you have an urge to smoke at 2:10 P.M. and you rate it as a #4. You immediately take out your smoking diary and write the number 4 in the 2 P.M. time box for the appropriate day (see day 1 in the illustration). Let us assume further that you go ahead and smoke a cigarette as a result of that urge: then you simply circle the number "4" (④). At 5 P.M. you experience a #3 urge, but you choose not to smoke because it occurs during dinner. At 6:30, however, you have a #2 urge, so you go ahead and smoke at that time. All these data are presented in the example page. Be sure that you fully understand how to keep track of your data in this manner. Note that day 2 on the sample page is more completely filled out. It is possible for you to record the data for many urges and cigarettes in the spaces provided. At the end of each day, circle the total number of cigarettes smoked in the space at the top of the A.M. and P.M. columns. Also cross out those times when you were asleep. Be sure to list the important situations on the back. *Note:* Make sure that you

rate all the urges that precede each of the cigarettes you smoke. This is true even though you may feel that some of your smoking is so automatic that it seems almost unconscious. Force yourself to pay attention to the smoking urges so that you become more aware of your smoking habit.

Keeping track of smoking urges in this manner can be extremely helpful because urges precede the target behavior (smoking). Gaining awareness of the urges helps to provide the smoker with the opportunity to decide not to smoke lesser-

valued cigarettes. Of course, once someone stops smoking, only urges remain to be monitored!

Once the behavior has been monitored for a period of at least one to two weeks, it is time to identify patterns. Using Mahoney's mnemonic formula [page 16], the examination of patterns leads to game plans or strategies that can be used to attack urges and achieve the behavioral objectives.

B. G. Danaher and E. Lichtenstein
Become an Ex-Smoker

Example of a Filled-in Page from a Smoking Diary

FRONT

KEY SITUATIONS

Day ___1___ : WITH WINE AFTER LUNCH
WITH COFFEE AFTER DINNER

Day ___2___ : WHILE GETTING UP IN THE MORNING - HURRY
DURING BREAKFAST
DRIVING TO WORK & BACK HOME AT NIGHT
BUSINESS MEETING @ MID AFTERNOON
(PRESSURE)
TIRED LATE AT NIGHT

Day ___3___ :

BACK

Personal contract
A written document that details decisions,
long-term goals, and milestones against
which progress can be measured.

How Can I Make a Change?

If you have been participating in the exercises discussed thus far, you may have felt a need to make some change in your health behavior. By using a diary and other self-assessment tools, you have had the opportunity to identify important variables contributing to the problem. The next steps include establishing your behavior change program by setting a goal, making a personal contract with yourself, planning alternative responses, and developing a system of incentives and rewards to aid you in your efforts.

Set Specific Goals   Assuming that you now have some fairly definite ideas about where you are heading, the next issue is how you get there and how you keep on track along the way. A crucial step is to analyze your long-term goal and break it into several small progressive stages or "chunks." As you make changes you will need mileposts to measure your progress just as you would count the miles or cities you pass on a long trip. For example, if you have decided to quit smoking, you may decide to chart your course by eliminating two cigarettes a day each week until you are down to 10 cigarettes a day. At that time you may be ready to quit "cold turkey," but you have been able to measure your progress by small progressive changes. Similarly, a weight loss of 25 pounds can be easier to tackle if you think of it in five-pound chunks. Another strategy is to begin with what is *easiest* and then progress to more difficult stages. Carefully set goals that will increase the probability of your eventual success.

Make a Personal Contract   Once you have made your decision and developed a plan of action, it is helpful to summarize your plan in writing by means of a *personal contract*. See "Personal Contracts for Change," page 10. As a written document, a personal contract solidifies a mobilization of priorities, time, energy, and resources to reach your goals. The personal contract should note your decision, your long-term goal, and mileposts against which you can measure your progress. If you plan to lose weight, include "before" and "after" weights, clothing sizes, measurements, even photos. To help you begin, the contract should identify exactly what your first

step will be and on exactly what day and time it will take place. Ideally, you should plan to begin with the easiest task, and the time to begin is now!

You can include other behavior change strategies in your personal contract. How you plan to reorganize your time, rewards for following your plan, support from family and friends, and alternative responses are examples of tactics we shall discuss in further detail. But the important thing for you to remember is that the personal contract will assist you in being as specific as possible. In essence you can make a blueprint or guide for constructing the kind of life you want to live.

You may need a series of small contracts or one big one with a number of points. In either case, begin by identifying your first goal and then list subgoals. Be sure that your first subgoal includes a starting and completion date and time and clear description of what you hope to accomplish.

Establish Rewards   Think about how you induce yourself to tackle any difficult task. What is the ultimate payoff? Aside from the satisfaction of reaching your goal, you can add to the jackpot. As you begin, decide upon a reward you can earn with six months of diligent effort. On a slip of paper write down this award, place the paper in your wallet, and tell no one. Your reward could be a new bathing suit to show off your slender figure. It could be a bicycle purchased with the money you save by not buying cigarettes. Your "grand prize" does not have to be expensive, but it should be personally meaningful. Monetary rewards can be a motivator, and "rebates" are often used as incentives for attending and successfully completing smoking or weight-control classes. Sometimes competition can also serve as an effective incentive, especially if you are competing with yourself. Marathon training gets many runners out of warm beds on cold mornings.

It is important for you to decide when a reward has been earned. In some cases you may want to reward goal attainment. For example, plan to treat yourself to a movie you have been wanting to see after you have been able to finish your first three-mile race. In other cases, such as the day you hit a weight-loss plateau, reward yourself for good behavior. During any habit
(text continues on p. 12)

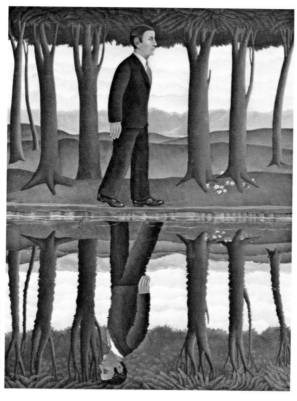

Personal Contracts for Change

All of us are familiar with the power of signed contracts. Documentation in black and white that commits our word, money, and/or property carries a strong impact and results in a higher chance of follow-through than casual, off-hand assurances or promises. Contracts can be used to try to change a health behavior if they include the time, date, and details of the change program. Some target behaviors, such as quitting smoking or losing extra pounds, lend themselves to contracts with very specific goals. Often a *witness* is also asked to sign the contract; this helps to set in motion the support and encouragement of a social network. A recent program in which all participants gave their formal commitment over citywide television resulted in much-higher-than-normal levels of change. Contracts reduce procrastination by specifying the dates and other details of the behavioral tasks and goals. They also act as reminders of a personal commitment to change. Here is an example of a behavioral contract for smoking.

Contract for Stopping by Yourself

Many people can stop smoking with little difficulty. In fact, they may have considerable experience with quitting in the past. If this corresponds to your smoking history, then you should follow the rules presented below.

Rule 1   Set a specific date and time for quitting, and write this in your personal contract. The time could be as early as three days from now or as far away as next week, whichever you prefer. This date and time (early in the morning or in the evening) should be listed in the target date box. Of course, you should follow through with the date, once chosen, and actually stop smoking at that time.

Rule 2   Three days before your target date, you should cut your daily smoking in half. For example, if you smoke 20 cigarettes per day, then you should reduce that total to only 10 cigarettes daily for the three-day period. Do NOT try to gradually reduce your smoking down to zero, however, because this will actually increase the value of each remaining cigarette and make your attempt to quit extremely frustrating. This rule is based on strong clinical evidence, so we urge you not to gradually go to zero cigarettes per day.

Rule 3   When you reach your target date, you may want to throw away all of your cigarettes. Some people like to make a ceremony out of this event. If you feel that you will panic unless you have cigarettes available somewhere (even if they are in the garage, the trunk of the car, or the attic), then you should follow your own inclinations. That is particularly true if these methods have been at least temporarily helpful to you in the past.

Rule 4   Try not to make too much out of quitting. Do not magnify it out of proportion because this may make you experience more stress and other withdrawal effects.

Rule 5   Once you have reached your target date and have successfully stopped smoking, remember to continue keeping track of smoking urges in your smoking dairy.

Contract for Stopping with Help from Others

The second method for stopping smoking involves arranging a contract with yourself and another person, preferably a trusted friend. The contract would involve a commitment on your part to stop smoking as of a particular date and hour following three days of reduced smoking—half the usual level— as was described in the previous section. In this case, however, you also build in an added incentive— the possible loss of money! The contract states that you [deposit a specified sum of money, which you will forfeit] if you fail to stop smoking. But you will receive portions of the deposit back as "payment" if you become an ex-smoker.

My Personal Contract for Quitting

I agree to stop all smoking on _____ at _____ . I understand that it
                          (target date)   (target time)
is important for me to make a strong personal effort at this particular time so that I can become a permanent ex-smoker. I sign this contract as an indication of my personal commitment to stop smoking on target.

_____   _____
(your signature)   *(date of signing)*

This contract arrangement can work without the help of others; you may act as your own banker for the agreement. But many people find that asking assistance of a friend helps them stick to their contract. Of course, it is important that this friend be trusted, because putting up your money and its repayment must be governed strictly by the written contract. This friend, the "banker" in your contract, should not be a smoker and should not attempt to tell you how to quit.

There are several rules for developing a contract with the help of others as a method for stopping smoking.

Rule 1   Risk an amount of money that would hurt you if it were forfeited. Five dollars would very likely be small and insignificant to you if it were lost; $50 or $100 is more significant!

Rule 2   Choose the banker with great care. He or she can be any nonsmoker you trust, who is willing to help by taking responsibility for keeping your deposit.

Rule 3   Once the contract is signed, stick to it. There should be no changes made in the target date and the monetary agreement, because changes undermine the effectiveness of this entire procedure.

Rule 4   Decide with great care what will be done with any forfeited money. The money must *not* go to your banker. Instead, it should be

---

(*Your copy*)   **Two-Party Contract for Quitting**

I agree to stop smoking on _____ at _____ . I have given the sum of
          (target date)   (target time)
$ _____ to _____ with the understanding that he/she will send the money
          (banker's name)
to _____ if I am unable to stop smoking according to this agreement. If I am
    (organization)
able to stop smoking completely for the first week after the target date specified above, I will at that time receive half of the deposit back. The remaining portion of the deposit will be returned after the second week of nonsmoking (two weeks from the target date).

_____ _____
          (your signature)   *(date)*

_____ _____
          (banker's signature)   *(date)*

(*Banker's copy*)   **Two-Party Contract for Quitting**

I agree to stop smoking on _____ at _____ . I have given the sum of
          (target date)   (target time)
$ _____ to _____ with the understanding that he/she will send the money
          (banker's name)
to _____ if I am unable to stop smoking according to the agreement. If I am
    (organization)
able to stop smoking completely for the first week after the target date specified above, I will at that time receive half of the deposit back. The remaining portion of the deposit will be returned after the second week of nonsmoking (two weeks from the target date).

_____ _____
          (your signature)   *(date)*

_____ _____
          (banker's signature)   *(date)*

---

payable to either a favorite charity or, even better, your least favorite organization—one you would hate to see get your good money! Write checks in advance with the name of the least favorite organization for the banker to hold, so that payment is almost automatic if you smoke. These strategies provide a powerful incentive for you to uphold the contract.

Rule 5   Use the contract presented here. One side should be signed by you and become your copy; it remains in this book. The other copy is kept by the trusted banker as his or her copy of the contract.

B. G. Danaher and E. Lichtenstein
Become an Ex-Smoker

change program there will be ups and downs. When progress is slow or uneven, be prepared to reward effort rather than accomplishments.

Develop a list of rewarding activities that are inexpensive and unrelated to food or alcohol—activities you can enjoy as much or more than snacking, smoking, or drinking. Treat yourself to a concert, buy a new softball, take a class in photography, go skating, or plan whatever appeals to you. Find out what works for you and be creative. You can identify and systematically influence reinforcing factors that affect your behavior.

Avoiding Derailment

As you go about making some long-term change in your health behavior, you will want to develop certain strategies for staying on track. Utilizing your health diary and various self-management techniques can help you avoid derailment.

Using Your Health Diary   We have already noted that keeping a health diary can help you examine specific incidents as well as related patterns of behavior. However, a diary's usefulness need not end here. It can also alert you to danger spots or weak points in your behavior change program that require different responses. Similarly, a diary can help to measure your progress in achieving goals.

Trace the Habit Chain   Using the data you gathered in the early stages of your habit change program, trace the chain of events—for example, from your purchase of snack foods or cigarettes to your consumption of them. There are numerous places along this chain at which you can choose an alternative response. What factors triggered your purchase of snack foods? Were you hungry when you went shopping? Did you see someone else smoking cigarettes? Did the smell of cigarette smoke trigger the urge? Did someone else offer you food or a cigarette? Did you respond to the bright packaging of cookies and candy in the supermarket?

Monitor Your Progress   Just as you might check off cities as you pass them on a long trip, you will want to keep track of your progress toward your goals by using the mileposts you have established. The best way to arrange for feedback is to keep a diary or log. Record your daily progress if you are working on a new exercise program. Each week chart your total progress on a graph. Because exercise is important to a sound weight-control program, you might chart your weekly weight on the same graph. It can be very motivating to watch your exercise level rise as your weight falls. Post your graph in a conspicuous place such as your dresser mirror or the refrigerator door. Objective feedback can be a reinforcing factor.

Self-Management   Despite our human frailties and the pressures of stress and other external influences, we all can exert a good deal of control over our lives. Think of self-management as a skill that you can develop if you allow yourself to be creative, perceptive, and flexible.

Control Environmental Stimuli   As you begin your habit change program, you may be especially vulnerable to environmental stimuli. If you have quit smoking, arrange to spend a good deal of your time in places where smoking is restricted and with nonsmoking friends. For example, go to libraries, movies, museums; eat lunch with a nonsmoking classmate and sit in the nonsmoking section of the cafeteria. Announce your intentions to friends and family. Ask them not to offer you food or cigarettes; and, if they must eat snacks, leave the room until they have finished. For a few weeks you may want to avoid social gatherings where you are especially tempted to overindulge in food, alcohol, or cigarettes. Carefully consider the roles that sight, smell, mood, situation, and accessibility play in triggering your response. You can control environmental stimuli or negative reinforcing factors by arranging to have food or cigarettes out of sight, out of the house, or in an inconvenient location.

Control Related Behavior   Avoid other habits that may be linked to the habit you are changing. For example, there are very definite links between alcohol and cigarettes, coffee and cigarettes, food and cigarettes, and food and alcohol. Some people are concerned about gaining weight once they have stopped smoking. Actually, only about one-third of former smokers gain weight. However, the way to manage this potential problem is to be aware that you can gain weight and to act accordingly. For a positive enabling factor, be careful to keep high-calorie snack foods out of the house and low-calorie foods accessible.

Plan and Rehearse Alternative Responses Try to anticipate temptation and plan alternative ways to deal with it. Inevitably, someone will offer you a cigarette. Mentally rehearse a polite refusal. At a party switch to a mixer to avoid encouragement to drink more alcohol than you feel you want. If you plan to eat out, decide ahead of time what you will eat and stick to your decision. You may also want to take low-calorie salad dressing and your own sweetener with you when you eat away from home. Don't be afraid to ask the chef to broil your meat rather than fry it. If boredom plays a significant part in your eating problem, develop new interests to get yourself out of the house or far away from food. Find a new hobby in which you use your hands. You want to identify activities that are incompatible with overeating. It's hard to eat popcorn and crochet at the same time!

If you absolutely must have some ice cream, go out and buy a single scoop and make it a real celebration. Do not buy a half gallon to keep in the freezer. Identify activities that are incompatible with your target behavior. With ingenuity you should be able to find some useful activities to help reduce your concentration on the target response.

Control Stress in Your Life Normal life events and the strain of ordinary living are common sources of derailment. However, stress is an inescapable part of modern life. You will want to analyze the present and potential sources of stress you encounter and the role stress may play in your problem habit. Chapter 2 of this book discusses stress and includes a stress scale (page 29) that will allow you to determine stress events and their probable intensity in your own life.

People sometimes use overeating, drinking, or smoking as stress management tactics. Plan to find less self-destructive ways to reduce tension. Many people,

for example, have found that regular exercise is an effective stress management strategy (see Chapter 13).

Maintaining Commitment

It is easier to maintain your commitment to a lasting behavior change if you establish positive but realistic expectations and ask others for assistance.

Shape Your Expectations Shakespeare wrote, "There is nothing either good or bad, but thinking makes it so." What we think or expect will happen often does, indeed, happen. If we are optimistic about ultimate success, the chances are good that our attitude will play a significant part in making us successful. However, it is also important to be realistic in our expectations. Lasting behavior change takes time. Because we are human, we will slip occasionally. But we can learn from our mistakes and from other people.

Expect Success Think thin. Think of yourself as a nonsmoker. Expect to succeed. Change your identity from a fat person to a thin person. How would a thin person react to a particular problem situation? Formerly overweight people often carry a "fat" self-image around with them for years after they have lost weight. This "fat person" is always eager to say, "I told you so!" Your expectations often shape what you actually do. Think of yourself as a thin person or a nonsmoker and begin to behave like one.

Expect Change to Take Time Fad diets may promise "instant" weight loss. However, weight loss is a long-term project that is accomplished one day at a time. Most people do not quit smoking on the first or even the second try. Expect change to take time, to have inevitable ups and downs, but plan to be persistent.

Forgive and Forget Suppose you actually do go on an eating binge. You can then conclude that you are, and always will be, "fat and ugly"; so why keep trying. Or you can look at the binge as something unfortunate, try to discover what set it off, and develop a plan to deal with similar situations should they occur again. Be forgiving of

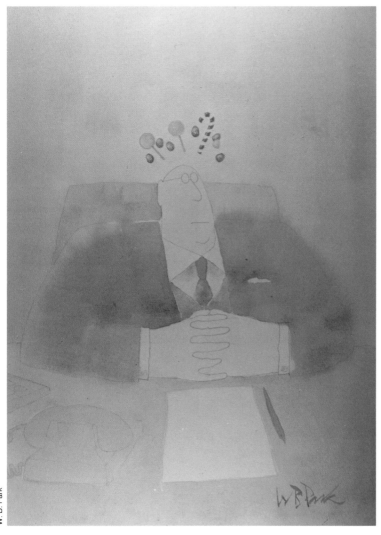

W. B. Park

any blunders. Observe what happened in a nonjudgmental way, and by all means try to avoid the self-destructive effects of guilt.

Use a Role Model   Find someone who possesses what you are striving for. This person might be a celebrity, sports figure, or someone you know. Why do you admire this person? How would this person respond to temptations? Talk to people you know who have successfully maintained aerobic fitness or weight loss or who have stopped smoking. What strategies have worked for them? How can you learn from their experience? People in public life occasionally share their struggles with alcohol and drugs, giving inspiration to many. Seek sources of inspiration to help you.

Recruit Support   Just as some people inspire us, so others can actively help us reach some of our goals. Asking a friend or relative for assistance helps you influence the enabling and reinforcing factors that affect your behavior.

Recruit a Buddy   There are many advantages of a "buddy system." If you examine the people with whom you spend your time, you are likely to find someone who is eager to make changes similar to those you have undertaken. You may have to look no further than your roommate, classmate, or family. Recruit one or more friends to participate in your plans for a life-style change. A buddy can serve as a sympathetic listener, someone who is interested in your progress. Beginning runners often find companionship and encouragement in the buddy system. It's easier to run on a cold morning when you know someone is expecting you, and a little friendly competition can be fun as long as it isn't taken too seriously. In a crisis situation ask your buddy to help you overcome the urge to smoke or gorge on snacks. Talking to a buddy can delay your response long enough for you to reconsider.

Recruit Support from Your Family and Friends   Life-style is a family affair, so encourage your whole family to get into the act. Others with whom you spend a lot of time are similar sources of support. Ask for specific

kinds of assistance. Encourage people to praise you when you have earned it, and encourage them to be active, interested listeners. And ask them to help you delay the decision to smoke or eat. Remind them not to advise or criticize you, not to offer you food or cigarettes, and not to feel rejected if you have to refuse something from them. Properly oriented, family, friends, classmates, and roommates can be a real source of reward, encouragement, and objective feedback. Ask for what you want and need. Nothing is more rewarding than to have people notice how hard you have worked. You can influence the reinforcing factors that affect your behavior.

Troubleshooting

If you encounter a serious problem in your behavior change program, try applying problem-solving skills and investigate outside resources that can help you with your problem.

Overcoming Barriers   When you have difficulty in implementing a life-style decision, it is helpful to consciously review and apply the stages of problem solving. Although most of us use these skills every day, when we stop to reassess our program in order to overcome a barrier, we often find that we have omitted one or more stages of the problem-solving sequence.

Recognize the Problem   First, you must recognize that a problem exists. For example, many beginning runners stop running after they have completed their initial training. What is the source of the problem? Some people train too rapidly and develop injuries. Others find that they cannot set aside enough time to maintain their activity. Still others lose motivation after their rate of improvement slows.

Acquire the Necessary Knowledge   Become better informed. For example, learn what aerobic fitness involves. Injuries can be prevented if you use the proper equipment, warm up adequately, do stretching exercises, and plan a graduated training program.

Mnemonic
A type of aid, such as a code, for remembering or memorizing.

The SCIENCE Mnemonic Formula for Personal Problem Solving·

S pecifying the general problem

C ollecting information

I dentifying patterns (possible causes)

E xamining possible solutions

N arrowing and trying

C omparing current and past progress

E valuating

Michael J. Mahoney
Self-Change

Generate Alternative Solutions and Evaluate the Consequences If the time your program requires seems to be the major barrier to successful maintenance, then examine your day. Time problems can be overcome if you set priorities and make choices. For example, list all of the possible times during the day when you could exercise. List all of the advantages and disadvantages related to each time. You might eliminate early morning because you hate getting out of bed any earlier than is absolutely necessary. You might dismiss exercising late at night because of a concern for safety. However, you could eliminate your concern over late-night safety by running with a buddy or using an indoor track. You might arrange to exercise during your lunch hour if showers are available. After you have completed your list of potential solutions, rank them in terms of their advantages and disadvantages. Select a likely alternative approach and use it. If adequate changes do not occur, then identify another alternative and use it. Of course, this is not a random trial-and-error approach because you should try to isolate effective approaches as you proceed. See "The SCIENCE Mnemonic Formula" above. If your best efforts still do not produce satisfactory results, seek outside help.

Outside Sources of Help   Habits such as sedentariness (a lack of moving around), smoking, or overeating are acquired over a lifetime and can be extremely difficult to change. Often these habits develop as the best response available at a particular time. Many people need outside help in overcoming such habits, and a variety of community and campus resources are available. On campus, courses in personal health, physical fitness, stress management, and weight control are often offered by the division of continuing education. The student health center or campus counseling center may also be a source of help.

Within the community, many low-cost services may be available through adult education classes, community school programs, local health departments, and private agencies such as heart, lung, and cancer organizations. Even hospitals are getting into the business of health promotion and life-style change. For further information about resources in your community, consult the Yellow Pages of your telephone directory, call your local health department, or contact the Information and Referral Service often sponsored by United Way.

Acquiring the necessary skills and using outside resources are two ways in which you can influence enabling factors that affect your behavior.

Health for Life

As you attain your goals, you will undoubtedly find that many positive changes take place. You may begin to enjoy new kinds of social activities and friends. Instead of the usual popcorn and candy at the movies every Friday night, you may occasionally find yourself at the ice skating rink. You may discover that you have things in common with new groups of people. Reach out to experience new people and new events. You may also find yourself accomplishing things you never thought possible. Enter and finish a race and wear your T-shirt proudly.

Plan for a Lifetime   Be proud of all that you have accomplished. Apply what you have learned about quitting smoking to your next self-improvement project.

Relapse
A return to previous behaviors or conditions after apparent progress.

Clinical program
Formal meetings with schedules and agendas.

Now may be a good time to tackle those 10 pounds you gained during your freshman year. Continue to watch for signs of *relapse*. Some ex-smokers still report a craving for cigarettes years after they have quit. Never be tempted to smoke "just one." Continue to weigh yourself weekly, and act immediately if you gain more than a pound or two. Cut back on what you eat for a week or so, and plan ahead for holiday seasons when food is overabundant and tempting. Remember your lifetime commitment to fitness. One day, one week, or one prolonged interruption in your program does not have to mean the end. Reorganize your life, recover from an illness or injury, and resume activity gradually and as soon as you can.

Change the Environment Around You   Use what you have learned about life-style change to help create an environment that supports healthful choices. Become an advocate of nonsmoking in public areas, more nutritious foods in vending machines, low-calorie lunches in the cafeteria, and showers for noontime exercisers. Talk your roommates out of keeping high-calorie snack foods around. Persuade your drinking buddies to play an occasional racquetball game instead of the usual Saturday night beer party. Become active in student government and lobby for better facilities, such as an indoor track or campus bicycle trails. Without being obnoxious, encourage someone else to quit smoking. Get involved in your community's health-enhancing activities, such as health fairs, no-smoking campaigns, or fun runs.

A Position of Tempered Enthusiasm

In this chapter on strategies for health behavior change, we must point out that much remains to be learned about how to help people alter their habits. All too often, early changes in a desired direction are rather quickly followed by a relapse. Researchers William A. Hunt, L. Walker Barnett, and Laurence G. Branch have examined the patterns of relapse following participation in programs for smoking cessation, alcohol abuse, and heroin abuse. The curves that follow the official termina-

tion of these programs are shown in Figure 1–2; they are remarkably similar and disappointing. While these curves reflect upon the performance of different participants undergoing programs of vastly different content and quality, they nonetheless underscore the point that the maintenance of behavior change remains the most difficult challenge of this field.

A second concern involves more widespread change. The vast majority of published research and descriptions in this field refer to *clinical programs* in which people from the general community are recruited to participate in a face-to-face gathering over the course of a program. Yet it is clear that clinical programs are too expensive and too few to accommodate the large number of people who want to make personal changes in their health habits.

Finally, it is impossible to provide a "cookbook" of health behavior change that includes specific "recipes" for changing all of your personal target behaviors. The field is too new and human behavior, fortunately, is too complex to permit such a simplified list of recommendations. Instead of searching for "the one

Figure 1-2   Relapse rate over time for heroin, smoking, and alcohol.

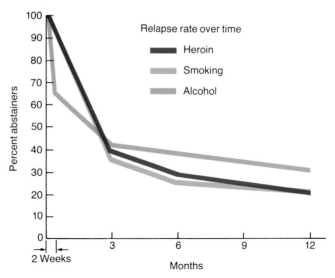

Ages of Health Advancement

In reality the nation's health has been improving for at least 200 years. These two centuries may be divided into three periods with reference to health. The first and by far the longest period was dominated by the effect of environment. The second, a brief period in the late 1930s and 1940s, witnessed the most important advances in medical care. Finally, we now find ourselves in an era in which life-style has come to the forefront. An understanding of the relative importance of environment, life-style, and medical care can be gained by an analysis of these three periods.

A study of death rates over the last century is a good place to begin. The accompanying figure illustrates the death rate for the United States and the times at which major medical advances became available.

Burn these facts into your mind:

■ Over 75 percent of the decline in death rate between 1875 and 1975 occurred *before* medicine's most significant discoveries became available. This decline actually began in the mid 1700s.

■ The discovery of antibiotics in the 1930s ushered in a period during which the decline in death rate was accelerated. This acceleration is usually credited to a number of significant medical advances which became available during this time.

■ The trend of several centuries came to an end in the early 1950s: the death rate stopped declining.

For the next 20 years there was no reduction in death rate and no increase in life expectancy for the population as a whole. For middle-aged males, life expectancy actually *decreased.*

■ This 20-year period of no progress coincided with the advent of high-technology medicine—coronary care units, heart surgery, and all the rest. It also coincided with a period of rapid rise in medical care costs.

■ Death rates began a modest decline in the early 1970s. This reflected a drop in the deaths due to heart attack and stroke. It coincided with reduced use of tobacco, less consumption of cholesterol and saturated fat, and increased exercise among Americans.

Thus the "miracles of modern medicine" taken as a group have had little to do with the decline in the death rate. They simply do not go together historically.

Donald M. Vickery
Life Plan for Your Health

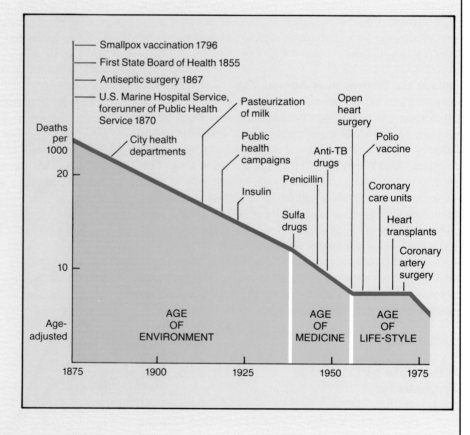

answer," then, it is better to look into selected topics and the lines of inquiry described below and to consider these ideas as initial steps in your process of personal problem solving.

Behavior Features
of the Following Chapters

As we have seen, all of us have a choice and a role in determining our own health by shaping our own behavior. The chapters that follow contain information on the complex psychological, social, and physiological elements that affect wellness and disease. A great many facts are presented in these chapters. However, even when we know the facts, we do not always act on our knowledge. For this reason special emphasis is given to these two questions: Why do we behave the way we sometimes do even at the risk of losing our wellness? How can we behave in order to promote our wellness?

This book, then, is a journey in personal self-discovery. You must become actively involved in your own health behavior. In order to clarify and highlight what you can do, *Core Concepts in Health* includes four features that help to personalize its factual material: Probing Your Emotions, Behavior Scale, Take Action, and Behavior Change Strategy.

Probing Your Emotions   Successful learning requires not only the understanding and retention of factual data; it also requires an emotional response. You must ask yourself how you *feel* about various health issues. Consider the person who wishes to avoid disease and understands that excessive use of alcohol can cause gastrointestinal damage. Understanding the need for moderation does little good if that person continues to

get drunk three times a week. Probing Your Emotions appears at the beginning of each chapter. It is a list of questions that focuses on your feelings concerning key issues to be discussed in the chapter. It is not a test—there are no right or wrong answers—and your responses will not be graded. Your emotions and attitudes are the topics here. After you have read the chapter, reconsider your initial emotions and attitudes.

Behavior Scale   The Behavior Scale that appears after the text portion of each chapter allows you to place yourself along a health behavior continuum. The scales do not provide perfect measurements; the items on them have not been tested for reliability or validity. However, they do have "face" validity. That is, on the face of it, they look to us to be appropriate in identifying certain behaviors and attitudes.

Take Action   Take Action is aimed at the student who would like to translate theory into practice. This section follows the Behavior Scale, and it invites you to do or experience something that will move you to the optimal position on the Behavior Scale and ultimately improve your health. You may, of course, have additional ideas of your own; if so, try them.

Behavior Change Strategy   Several chapters in this book conclude with a Behavior Change Strategy to help you begin to make changes. These strategies, as well as Chapter 1, provide detailed descriptions of general techniques that research has shown to be effective in eliminating unhealthful behaviors or improving healthy ones. The strategies can be the beginning of a path that you may wish to take. Remember, however, that this feature is only a general guide to your own self-examination. The rest is up to you!

Health Behavior Outlook Scale

Read the following statements carefully. Choose the one in each section that best describes you at this moment and record its score at the right. (For example, "energetic" has a score of 4.) When you have identified five statements, total your score and find your position on the scale.

5 high self-esteem
4 good self-esteem
3 adequate self-esteem
2 low self-esteem
1 little or no self-esteem

Score _____

5 exuberant
4 animated
3 passive
2 inhibited
1 withdrawn

Score _____

5 vigorously energetic
4 energetic
3 variable energy level
2 sedentary
1 lethargic

Score _____

5 very enthusiastic
4 enthusiastic
3 satisfied
2 dissatisfied
1 discontented

Score _____

5 consistently optimistic
4 basically optimistic
3 cautiously optimistic
2 generally pessimistic
1 depressed

Score _____

Total score _____

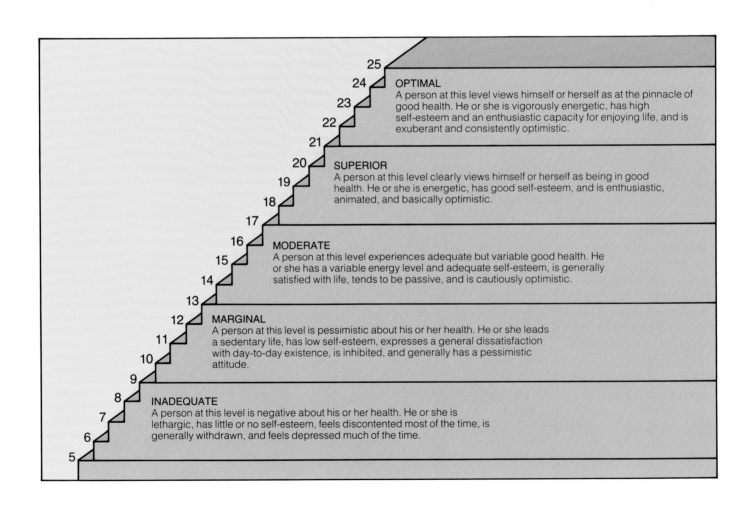

25
24   **OPTIMAL**
23   A person at this level views himself or herself as at the pinnacle of
22   good health. He or she is vigorously energetic, has high
21   self-esteem and an enthusiastic capacity for enjoying life, and is
     exuberant and consistently optimistic.

20   **SUPERIOR**
19   A person at this level clearly views himself or herself as being in good
18   health. He or she is energetic, has good self-esteem, and is enthusiastic,
17   animated, and basically optimistic.

16   **MODERATE**
15   A person at this level experiences adequate but variable good health. He
14   or she has a variable energy level and adequate self-esteem, is generally
     satisfied with life, tends to be passive, and is cautiously optimistic.

13   **MARGINAL**
12   A person at this level is pessimistic about his or her health. He or she leads
11   a sedentary life, has low self-esteem, expresses a general dissatisfaction
10   with day-to-day existence, is inhibited, and generally has a pessimistic
 9   attitude.

 8   **INADEQUATE**
 7   A person at this level is negative about his or her health. He or she is
 6   lethargic, has little or no self-esteem, feels discontented most of the time, is
 5   generally withdrawn, and feels depressed much of the time.

Take Action

Your placement level on the Health Behavior Outlook Scale will, we hope, encourage you to begin a process of self-exploration and self-discovery that you will continue. Reflect on the entire chapter's content and ask yourself how each point relates to your own life. Then take action:

1. Start a Take Action for Health notebook. List the positive behaviors that have helped to enhance your health. Consider what additions you can make to the list or how you can strengthen or reinforce the behaviors that have helped you. Don't forget to congratulate yourself for these positive aspects of your life. Next list the behaviors that block your achieving wellness. Consider each of these behaviors and decide which ones you can change. Begin with the easiest ones first.

2. Review the general techniques for accomplishing change that were presented in Chapter 1 and discuss them in class or with a close friend. What conclusions can you draw?

3. Find a person (or persons) who has the same problem you have (smoking, overweight, etc.). Invite that person to join you in a self-help strategy to deal effectively with the problem. Set specific goals, make a personal contract, and establish rewards.

4. Think about what troubled you most during the past week. In your notebook write down the names of three or four people who might be able to help you with whatever troubled you. If the problem persists, consider starting at the top of your list and talking to this person about it.

Chapter Two

Stress and the Social Environment

Probing Your Emotions

1. Take a moment to write down the circumstances involved when you last cried. What was the cause of your distress? What did you do to adjust to this stress? List as many coping techniques that you used as you can remember. Would you say that you successfully handled this stress? What constitutes successful adaptation to stress?

2. How assertively are you seeking solutions to stressful events? For example, think back to the last time you were really lonely. Did you go to bed and wait for the loneliness to go away? Is such a passive response good for you, or is it a rationalization for avoiding the problem? Did you do something more active? What? Was this act effective in relieving your loneliness?

3. You are one day away from a very important final examination. Although you have not prepared very thoroughly and you are very nervous, you decide to go to sleep early rather than cram all night. You have just made a coping decision. Is it a wise one? How about all those earlier coping decisions that you used to put off course preparation you should have been doing each week?

4. Late one night on the way home from the library you are startled by a man's figure in the shadows just off the sidewalk. You hurry on, wondering why your heart is racing. A few yards farther along you pass a young woman. For a minute you consider warning her about the man who startled you, but then you think you are unnecessarily alarmed and say nothing. The next day you learn that a woman was raped and beaten near the library last night. What would you have done in this situation? (After you have answered this question, consider Stanley Milgram's position on page 35 and reconsider your answer.)

Chapter Contents

BIOLOGICAL VERSUS CULTURAL EVOLUTION

THE INTERACTION BETWEEN YOU AND YOUR ENVIRONMENT

THE STRESS RESPONSE

PSYCHOSOCIAL STRESSORS
Social change
Crowding and urban life
The work environment and job choice

THE ROLE OF STRESS IN DISEASE
Social support systems and social stressors
The riddle of hypertension

COPING
Finding your stress point
Tuning down through diversion
Meditation and other techniques
Nutrition
Humor
A few other suggestions

Boxes

Notes and comment from *The New Yorker*
Student stress scale
Life events: an update
Test anxiety and stress
Social support scale
Relaxation

Stress
Something that disturbs a person's (or animal's) psychological or biological equilibrium.

Metabolic activity
Chemical and physical processes that involve the body's use of food to convert nutrients into energy and create molecules for tissue.

Homeostasis
Tendency of an organism to maintain conditions of stability and consistency in physiological functioning.

Adaptive reaction
A response by which a person attempts to improve his or her condition in relation to the environment.

2 To be alive is to be under *stress*. Biological stress and psychosocial, or cultural, stress are intertwined and integral to life itself. How we respond to the common and uncommon events and circumstances of our lives largely determines how healthful or destructive these situations will be. We would do well to remember these words of Marcus Aurelius: "If you are distressed by anything external, the pain is not due to the thing itself but to your estimate of it. This you have the power to revoke at any time."

Life is dependent, precariously so, on ceaseless *metabolic activity*. The body is constantly subject to the process of change, growth, degradation, and replacement. But, all the while, it tries to maintain a dynamic steady state, or *homeostasis*. Anything, whether internal or external, that disturbs this steady state threatens the organism. If that steady state is to be restored, adaptive reactions must take place. Life is, in a sense, one adaptation after another. Sometimes the *adaptive reaction,* or defense mechanism, is misdirected; the mind-body signals can misfire. The body's remarkable system of self-regulating checks and balances does not always work perfectly. If our responses to events and circumstances are too weak, it offers inadequate protection; if they are too strong, it overreacts, so that we harm ourselves.

Virtually all of us engage in a daily masquerade, constantly intermeshing with other people's needs, moods, assumptions, bodies, and demands. We get pushed around and pushed out of shape. To be natural, spontaneous, whole, and supportive in our socially conditioned world is hardly easy. Even those nonconformists who are far adrift from the cultural mainstream are usually not the free spirits they aim to be: They have merely traded one set of conventions for another, and they conform closely to this new set. And if free spirits are scarce, rarer still are those who can leaven their need for independence with commitment and compassion.

In our society, maintaining social relationships often takes priority over preserving physical health. We tend to behave as though our primary function is to fulfill the social roles that we have chosen or have been compelled to play. Yet the demands of these social roles, and of interpersonal relations, have given rise to some hefty biological challenges.

We have no grounds for saying point-blank that life is more stressful now than ever before, yet the fallacy of "the good old days" lives on. Granted, we live in a world of seemingly endless turmoil and inequity, a world in which, for instance, governments spend about the same amount of money every year on children as they dole out every two hours on deadly weapons. But history is filled with events and conditions so appalling as to defy our imagination. Many people in the past lived under such stressful circumstances as to make most of our own anxieties and discomforts pale by comparison. Today the mass media instantly and constantly inform us of ills all over the world, and this, added to our personal woes (real or imagined), may well give the impression that life has never before been so stressful.

Is life truly more stressful now than in the past? Why do some individuals become ill under mildly stressful conditions while others seem to thrive under considerable stress and some even seek more stressful situations? When is stress harmful and when is it harmless? What is your "stress point"? How can you gauge it and use it?

These questions do not have conclusive answers; the concept of stress itself is a source of controversy. Nevertheless, despite conflicting evidence and conflicting theories, it is clear that some of the stress in modern society is different in quality and quantity than it was in the past and that misdirected adaptations to the social environment can help trigger possibly unhealthful physiological reactions. It is also clear, however, that we can control to a surprising degree our responses to life situations, thereby not only preserving but also, perhaps, enhancing our physical and mental health.

Biological Versus Cultural Evolution

The human being, unlike any other organism, is the product of two evolutionary systems: the biological one, which is inborn, and the cultural one, which is learned. Culture consists not only of ideas, beliefs, and institutions but also of material objects and the know-how and technology to produce those objects.

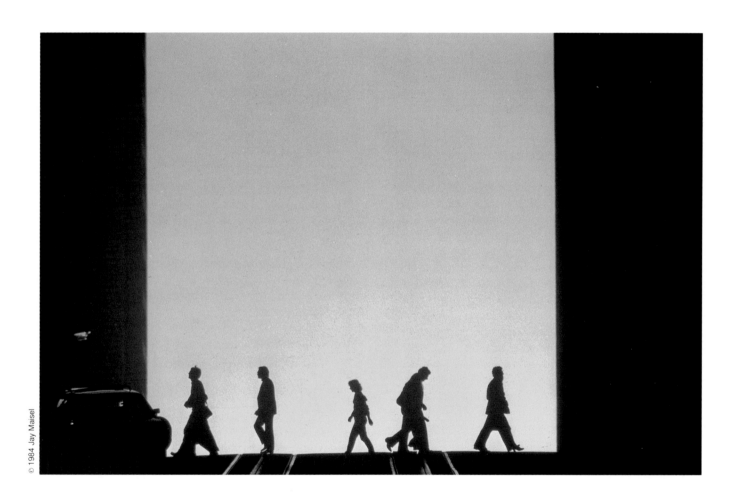

Cultural lag
A delay in the incorporation by social groups of social and behavioral patterns currently in use.

Gastrointestinal
Relating both to the stomach and to the intestines.

Central nervous system
The brain and spinal cord.

Neuroendocrine systems
Networks of interactions between the nervous system and the endocrine system.

Stimulus/stimuli (plural form)
Anything that causes an organism to respond.

Input overload
Excess of stimuli; stimulation to a point where a person can no longer respond to it.

In all the early stages of human development, technological progress moved incredibly slowly; human beings have lived with a hunting-gathering technology for over 90 percent of their existence. The machine technology, which has so dramatically changed life, appeared only in the last fraction of history. So while biological evolution has over the eons moved at an exceedingly slow but fairly steady rate, the rate of cultural change, suddenly picking up speed through technological innovations, has accelerated at an astonishing pace in a relatively brief time. The reason for this momentum is positive feedback—each innovation produces still other innovations. The time needed for translating a major scientific discovery into a usable product has been cut by about 60 percent since the turn of the century. For instance, it took 112 years for photography to be developed; the atomic bomb was produced in only six years. Except for TV, the major innovations that have changed our daily lives were all introduced between 1850 and 1940: the steamship, telegraph, railroad, electricity, telephone, automobile, radio, motion pictures, and airplane. The outstanding innovations that have appeared since 1940, such as nuclear power, missiles and satellites, and computers, have not greatly changed our *daily* lives, but they nevertheless affect us immeasurably.

With the appearance of each new technology comes a wave of cultural change. Our relationship with the natural environment is affected to various degrees by this change, but so too are our health, our belief systems, and our economic, political, and educational institutions. This change is typically uneven, with some parts of a culture altering drastically and others not at all. This unevenness, known as *cultural lag*, inevitably creates stress and disruption. It undermines the integration any culture needs if it is to function smoothly.

Minor and infrequent technological changes can be absorbed rather easily. But the rate of change characteristic of Western technology is so great that our hearts have trouble keeping up with our heads. We are experiencing what biologist John Platt, in his essay entitled "What We Must Do" (*Science* 166 [1969]: 1115), calls a "crisis of transformation":

The essence of the matter is that the human race is on a steeply rising "S-curve" of change. We are undergoing a great historical transition to new levels of technological power all over the world. We all know about these changes, but we do not often stop to realize how large they are in orders of magnitude, or how rapid and enormous compared to all previous changes in history. In the last century, we have increased our speeds of communication by a factor of 10^7; our speeds of travel by 10^2; our speeds of data handling by 10^6; our energy resources by 10^3; our power of weapons by 10^6; our ability to control diseases by something like 10^2; and our rate of population growth to 10^3 what it was a few thousand years ago.

Could anyone suppose that human relations around the world would not be affected to their very roots by such changes?

It has now become commonplace to talk about exponential curves—the acceleration of doubling rates of every kind. It is this change of scale that distinguishes our present from our past. And among the most startling changes of scale in our lives is that of numbers. Writing of the United States, sociologist Daniel Bell notes, in *The Coming of Post Industrial Society* (1973), that

the real change of scale between 1789 [when the Constitution was put into effect] and today . . . has to do with the number of persons each one of us *knows* and the number each of us *knows of*—in short, the way we *experience* the world. An individual today, on the job, in school, in the neighborhood, in a professional or social milieu, knows immediately hundreds of persons and, if one considers the extraordinary mobility of our lives—geographical, occupational, and social—during a lifetime one comes to know, as acquaintances or friends, several thousand. And through the windows of the mass media, and because of the enlargement of the political world and the multiplication of the dimensions of culture—the number of persons (and places) that one *knows of* accelerates at a steeply exponential rate.

With the rare exception of the happy hermit, the human being does not develop well physically or mentally or even remain quite sane unless he or she maintains close association with other people. But too many social contacts can be just as harmful as too few. What is safe depends not only on a person's genetic makeup and past experiences but also on the traditions, conventions, and values of the groups with which he or she is most familiar.

We have created a social environment that embodies vibrancy, diversity, and infinite possibilities on the one

Notes and Comment from *The New Yorker*

"I was going through the lobby of the Forty-second Street branch of C.U.N.Y. [City University of New York]—a shortcut—when I saw the sign announcing the lecture. . . . I was on my way to work. I'd waited for half an hour on a jam-packed subway platform for a downtown local at Eighty-first Street, then given up and taken a bus. There was an incident on the bus—accusations of pickpocketing, denials, tumult, delay—so I got off at Fifty-ninth Street and walked the remaining seventeen blocks. A man was running in and out of the traffic, laughing and gesticulating. He almost got hit. It was freezing cold; the temperature had dropped eight degrees during the night. I had been awakened in the morning by the wind flapping the window shades in my apartment, even though the windows were shut. The night before, I was supposed to go to a movie with a friend, but the friend had to work late and called me at seven-thirty to tell me so. I went alone. It was a Cinema 1, 2, 3, etc. My movie hadn't started. I stood waiting near the candy stand. An usher came up and demanded to know what movie I was waiting for. I told him. 'Wait in the upstairs lounge,' he ordered. Finally, the movie started. The place was almost empty. A man a few rows ahead kept turning around throughout the movie and staring at me. The film was about how miserable life can be. I went six blocks to a Burger King, sat at a small table. A disturbed-looking youth at the next table was smoking a cigarette. 'Do you have cigarettes?' he called to me, as if he hadn't. I went home. 'Beware—crime on this block is on the increase,' said a flyer taped to the vestibule wall. I opened my mailbox and found an appalling bill from Con Ed. When I was nearly asleep, I heard a car roar down the street, and a screech of brakes. Then there was a terrible crash: a solid hit. In the morning, I went to get a paper. The street was full of garbage, blown by the wind. Trash cans were rolling around. The woman running the newsstand screamed at me, accusing me of messing up her stack of papers. I read the paper on the crowded subway platform: toxic wastes were being discovered all over the country, and an increase in city transit fares was predicted. As I walked (after leaving the bus), I passed stores full of glittery awfulness. Finally, after an hour and a half of travel, I reached the C.U.N.Y. lobby, relieved to be approaching my office, and I saw the sign about the lecture. 'Stressors in the Workplace,' it said. 'Rm. 1629.'"

hand and frustration, fears, and infinite anxieties on the other. Through our culture, through our attitudes, economics, and technology, we have brought about unprecedented environmental changes. We are faced with trying to adapt to the accelerating stresses we ourselves have generated.

The Interaction Between You and Your Environment

A constant interaction between an organism and its environment is essential for maintaining life. Your own boundaries—that is, the limits at which your environment begins—are not only your skin and the membranous tissue lining your respiratory tract, your *gastrointestinal* tract, and your kidneys and urinary tract but also your organs of special sense.

Energy exchange is primarily associated with the skin, lungs, gastrointestinal tract, and kidneys. Information acquisition is mainly through the organs of special sense—the organs of vision, hearing, smell, and taste as well as special organs inside the body and within the skin that are receptive to touch, temperature, pressure, spatial orientation, and acceleration. These organs are closely allied with the *central nervous system* and, through it, with the *neuroendocrine systems*. This setup enables the human organism to draw conclusions about aspects of the environment that have no direct impact on it, that are removed in time and place. The whole human system finally becomes involved as the organism tries to organize adaptive responses to this "environment at a distance," an environment that, significantly, is largely composed of other people and the individual's social world.

Whenever these *stimuli*—sights, sounds, and smells as well as the actions and impositions of others—become too profuse or too varied, we are the victims of *input overload* (also called sensory, psychic, cognitive, or stimulus overload). The human being has a remarkable ability to adjust, biologically and socially, to a vast variety of living conditions, even apparently incompatible ones. This is good (it is how the human race has

Stressor
Any demand that gives rise to a coping response.

Fight-or-flight reaction
Physiological responses in which hormone secretion causes increases in heart rate, breathing rate, blood pressure, and perspiration.

Eustress
A stress state believed to be pleasant, even beneficial.

Distress
An unpleasant stress state believed to cause illness.

survived), but it is not all to the good. If we passively accept an overdose of stimuli, if we come to regard endless striving and competitive behavior, hostile personal relationships, overcrowding, and poisonous environments as acceptable and unchangeable, we are likely to suffer emotional stunting or warping, physical degradation, and personal and social degeneration.

Whether environmental stimuli intrude directly or indirectly, stress invariably will accompany them. Nearly all highly stressful situations throughout most of our history involved physical threats of some kind—hunger, excessive heat or cold, dangerous terrain, hazardous hunting. These called for exertion and endurance, and human beings emerged victorious through it all largely because of their superb biological equipment. Now many of the trappings of our future-oriented society, with its large numbers of people and its sedentary ways, present unfamiliar challenges to the human organism, although we perceive them as normal rather than novel.

Clearly, to live in a state of stress is unavoidable and indeed healthful; nonexcessive stress is just as natural as body temperature. Without stress we would be bored and listless and would lack adequate outlets for our creative and aggressive urges. The root cause of much mental illness is sheer boredom. Many whose lives are drab and uneventful are driven to risk-taking activities for the stimuli they offer. And while some people put themselves under extra stress out of vanity, or for kicks, or to prove something to themselves or to others, many stress-seekers find the exhilaration of a risky venture a means to self-fulfillment. (Mountain climbing, for instance, has been described as providing "elbow room for the soul.")

Human beings are dynamic creatures, designed to be on the move. Microbiologist René Dubos sums it up this way:

> Without exposure and response to stress, any organism—man in particular—stays where he is. All of biological history demonstrates without doubt that an organism too neatly adapted to too well-defined conditions has no chance in the long run. Unless he is capable of responding to change he will surely be displaced by another creature.

The stresses imposed by nature are probably less destructive than those we impose on ourselves and on others. Our modern world is obviously uniquely difficult in many ways. We have, for the most part, discarded the stoicism that enabled our forebears to endure hardships, lost the feeling of worth that comes from individual accomplishment, and no longer have a sense of permanent place in the social order. We tend to acquire a greater and greater number of things and at the same time feel our lives to be emptier.

Yet, in the final analysis, the *stressors* (physical and psychological stress-producing factors) that affect the greatest number of people have remained essentially the same throughout human history. The most common and often most potent stressors of all are disrupted interpersonal relations and any changes in an individual's personal circumstances.

Determine your own stress score from the "Student Stress Scale" on page 29. Then read "Life Events: An Update" on page 30.

The Stress Response

If you slip on a banana peel, watch a horror movie or a comedy, meet a celebrity or a long-absent friend, get a good grade or a mediocre one on an exam, attend a party, get caught in the rain, win or lose a game, run for a bus, or catch a cold, you are likely to experience only a mild, relatively harmless state of stress. If you get fired, discover you have diabetes, flunk four courses, get mugged, or win a million-dollar lottery, you will undergo much greater, potentially damaging stress. Whatever the situation—pleasurable or not, mild or severe—your body initially reacts in the same way the caveman's did when he faced a saber-toothed tiger: It interprets the situation as an emergency.

This immediate response, which alerts and prepares you for physical action, has been dubbed the *fight-or-flight reaction*. Though often absurdly inappropriate, it is part of our biological heritage. We may mask emotional turmoil in order to be socially acceptable, but our aroused physiological processes are indifferent to such niceties. Fortunately, the body has ways of cushioning this primary response, for if it should continue over a long period or become too generalized, the tissues of

Student Stress Scale

The Student Stress Scale* represents an adaptation of Holmes and Rahe's *Life Events Scale.* It has been modified to apply to college age adults and should be considered as a rough indication of stress levels and health consequences for teaching purposes.

In the Student Stress Scale each event, such as beginning or ending school, is given a score that represents the amount of readjustment a person has to make in life as a result of the change. In some studies people with serious illnesses have been found to have high scores on similar scales. People with scores of 300 and higher have a high health risk. Subjects scoring between 150 and 300 points have about a 50–50 chance of serious health change within two years. Subjects scoring below 150 have a 1 in 3 chance of serious health change.

To determine *your* stress score, add up the number of points corresponding to the events you have experienced in the past six months or are likely to experience in the next six months.

*Adapted from T. H. Holmes and R. H. Rahe, "The Social Readjustment Rating Scale," *Journal of Psychosomatic Research* 11 (1967): 213.

	Event	PAST		FUTURE
1.	Death of a close family member	☐	100	☐
2.	Death of a close friend	☐	73	☐
3.	Divorce between parents	☐	65	☐
4.	Jail term	☐	63	☐
5.	Major personal injury or illness	☐	63	☐
6.	Marriage	☐	58	☐
7.	Fired from job	☐	50	☐
8.	Failed important course	☐	47	☐
9.	Change in health of a family member	☐	45	☐
10.	Pregnancy	☐	45	☐
11.	Sex problems	☐	44	☐
12.	Serious argument with close friend	☐	40	☐
13.	Change in financial status	☐	39	☐
14.	Change of major	☐	39	☐
15.	Trouble with parents	☐	39	☐
16.	New girl or boy friend	☐	38	☐
17.	Increased workload at school	☐	37	☐
18.	Outstanding personal achievement	☐	36	☐
19.	First quarter/semester in college	☐	35	☐
20.	Change in living conditions	☐	31	☐
21.	Serious argument with instructor	☐	30	☐
22.	Lower grades than expected	☐	29	☐
23.	Change in sleeping habits	☐	29	☐
24.	Change in social activities	☐	29	☐
25.	Change in eating habits	☐	28	☐
26.	Chronic car trouble	☐	26	☐
27.	Change in number of family get-togethers	☐	26	☐
28.	Too many missed classes	☐	25	☐
29.	Change of college	☐	24	☐
30.	Dropped more than one class	☐	23	☐
31.	Minor traffic violations	☐	20	☐

Total _____

the body would be severely damaged, even to the point of death.

How do the body's adaptive defense mechanisms work and when do they stop working? No one has more thoroughly explored the biochemical and environmental facets of stress than Dr. Hans Selye, an endocrinologist and biologist. In *The Stress of Life* (1976), Selye defines *stress* as the common denominator of all the body's adaptive reactions; it is "the nonspecific response of the body to any demand made of it." The stress state, Selye believes, is "a state manifested by the specific syndrome, which consists of all the nonspecifically induced changes within a biological system."* It can be pleasant and curative (*eustress*) or unpleasant and disease producing (*distress*). The totality of changes in the body that help us adjust to constant internal and external changes is what

*Selye's concept of stress is not without critics. One of the major criticisms of Selye's theory is that the stress response, rather than being a nonspecific reaction, may in many cases be specific, with the specific stimulus being a psychological one. Selye's critics contend that psychological variables have been overlooked in his laboratory experiments. The progress of the refinement or extension of his theory can be followed in *The Journal of Human Stress.*

Life Events: An Update

In 1967 Drs. Thomas Holmes and Richard Rahe published the Social Readjustment Rating Scale (SRRS) in the *Journal of Psychosomatic Research*. The scale, composed of 43 life events, was thought to have great promise in predicting future illness events and became the basis for hundreds of publications in books, journals, magazines, and newspapers. The concept was intuitively a good one. If a person experiences an event or events that requires a substantial accommodation or readjustment in his or her life, the change may cause that person to be vulnerable to physical or mental disorders. Holmes and Rahe studied the case histories of numerous patients and extracted 43 events both desirable and undesirable that are likely to be disruptive. Examples of these life events are death of a spouse, divorce, marriage, pregnancy, troubles with the boss, an outstanding personal achievement, and Christmas. The researchers hypothesized that people experiencing one or more of

these events in a specified period of time would become ill. And, in fact, many investigators found that when they administered a life events scale to a patient population they indeed obtained higher life events scores than from a "normal" population. Unfortunately, it was difficult to tell from this type of study whether the patients' illness caused them to recall more life events or whether the greater number of life events caused their illness. Subsequent prospective studies either failed to predict future illnesses or obtained statistically significant associations that were so small that they could not be interpreted. Why has an obviously good intuitive idea failed to yield useful results? One answer is that an illness that has psychological antecedents is likely to be more complex than the assumptions leading investigators to expect a strong relationship between life events and illness. We don't know, for example, whether the person would have developed the illness even without experiencing a disrup-

tive life event. Another source of inquiry is the effects of the social environment on the development of physical and mental illness. No study of life events and illness has adequately taken account of the social environment despite the fact that the social environment has been shown to have powerful effects on behavior as well as on immunity to various illnesses. Social support, for example, has been shown to counteract the effects of negative variables. While the life events methodology has not produced expected results, that is, predictions of future illness events, mental illness itself successfully predicts future physical illness events. Results from many diverse studies are remarkably consistent in showing a strong positive association between emotional disturbance and physical illness. Thus the diagnosis of mental illness as a predictor of future physical illness events has succeeded where the life events methodology has failed.

Selye calls the *G.A.S.* (*general adaptation syndrome*), or stress syndrome.

The G.A.S. develops in three stages: the alarm reaction, resistance, and exhaustion. Normally active people often experience the first two stages in order to adapt to their various activities and to the demands made on them. During the resistance (or adaptive) stage the body begins to repair the damage sustained during the alarm reaction, and the stress symptoms diminish or disappear. But if the stress continues and the entire body is affected for a long time, the adaptation is lost. Exhaustion eventually culminates when the body runs out of energy. The effects of exhaustion can usually be reversed, because the body can activate its reserves of *adaptive energy*. These reserves are limited, however, and if they are spent, there is general exhaustion, and the individual dies from, for instance, aging hastened by an onslaught of stress. When the body's adaptation to stress through

biologic reactions is unsuccessful, it can develop what Selye calls diseases of adaptation (among them cardiovascular, kidney, blood vessel, and inflammatory diseases; mental disorders; ulcers; hyperthyroidism; and possibly cancer).

Whenever we are faced with a real or imagined threat, powerful hormones, which act as natural pep pills, are released into the bloodstream, and the sympathetic division of the *autonomic nervous system* gets the body ready for instant action. The autonomic nervous system (functioning in many respects independently of conscious thought) controls the organs and glands, regulating the heartbeat, the activities of the endocrine glands, and the temperature of the skin. It is made up of two parts, the *sympathetic* and the *parasympathetic* branches. When the body is stimulated by stress, the sympathetic branch mobilizes the body for action, and the parasympathetic branch calms it down, slowing the

G.A.S. (General Adaptation Syndrome)
A pattern of stress responses described by Hans Selye as having three stages: the alarm reaction, the stage of resistance, and the stage of exhaustion.

Adaptive energy
Limited body reserves that are activated when the body feels exhausted.

Autonomic nervous system
The nervous system that operates closely with the brain and spinal cord and regulates internal organs and glands.

Sympathic nervous system
A division of the autonomic nervous system that is active in emergency situations of extreme cold, violent effort, and emotional excitement.

Parasympathic nervous system
A division of the autonomic nervous system that is active in slowing metabolism and restoring energy supplies.

ACTH (adrenocorticotropic hormone)
A hormone formed in the pituitary gland, regulating the adrenal glands' outer region.

Endorphin
A chemical produced in the brain that has painkilling effects.

rapid heartbeat, drying the sweaty palms, and adjusting the temperature of the skin.

As soon as the brain signals that there's danger ahead, a complex series of chemical reactions takes place. The hypothalamus (a part located in the brain region at the base of the skull) stimulates the pituitary gland (located just below the brain), which in turn releases ACTH (*adrenocorticotropic hormone*) into the bloodstream, which conveys it to the adrenal glands, just above the kidneys. These glands then rush adrenalin, cortisone, and other "stress hormones" into the bloodstream, causing various useful changes: The pupils of the eyes enlarge to let in more light; hearing becomes more acute;

the heartbeat quickens; blood pressure rises; the digestive processes switch off; the liver transforms sugar from storage form (glycogen) into burnable form (glucose), and the glucose takes a swift trip to the muscles and the brain; muscle tone improves; the air passages in the lungs open up to admit more air; the arteries are flooded with red cells to help take in oxygen and cast off carbon dioxide; and brain peptides, called *endorphins,* which act like morphine but are far more potent, are released to provide relief from pain in case of injury. (See Figure 2–1.)

The effect of these reactions is to ready us for physical action. The trouble is that in civilized society the tense

Figure 2-1   The body's response to stress.

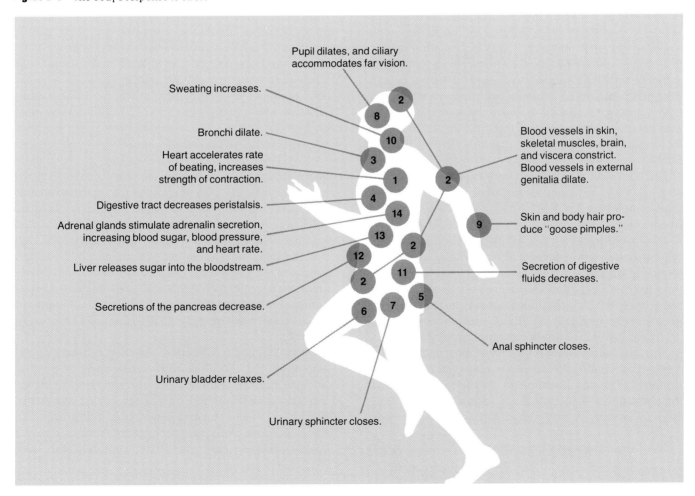

Pupil dilates, and ciliary accommodates far vision.

Sweating increases.

Bronchi dilate.

Heart accelerates rate of beating, increases strength of contraction.

Digestive tract decreases peristalsis.

Adrenal glands stimulate adrenalin secretion, increasing blood sugar, blood pressure, and heart rate.

Liver releases sugar into the bloodstream.

Secretions of the pancreas decrease.

Urinary bladder relaxes.

Urinary sphincter closes.

Blood vessels in skin, skeletal muscles, brain, and viscera constrict. Blood vessels in external genitalia dilate.

Skin and body hair produce "goose pimples."

Secretion of digestive fluids decreases.

Anal sphincter closes.

or competitive situations that continually arise usually cannot be handled by physical means. The result is frustration and, possibly, disability. (One of the reasons exercise is beneficial is that it accommodates rather than ignores the body's frequently revved-up state.) If the body's rapid mobilization for combat takes place too often or is too prolonged (sometimes continuing long after the stressor has vanished), heavy or irreparable damage can occur.

How do you know when you are "over-mobilizing"? You can spot the danger signals of stress. According to Selye, these signs are irritability, hyperexcitation, or depression; a pounding heart; dryness of mouth and throat; impulsive behavior or emotional instability; an urge to cry, run, or hide; inability to concentrate; feelings of unreality; dizziness or weakness; loss of energy and of joy in living; nonspecific ("free-floating") anxiety; "keyed-up" feelings; trembling or nervous tics; high-pitched, nervous laughter; stuttering; teeth grinding; insomnia; increased muscular movement and physical activity; sweating; frequent urination; diarrhea, queasy stomach, indigestion, or vomiting; migraine headaches; overeating or undereating; heavier smoking; increased use of tranquilizers, amphetamines, or other drugs; increased intake of alcohol; nightmares; and accident proneness.

The cumulative effects of stress begin in late adolescence, usually surfacing as full-blown disorders by the time people are in their forties and fifties. There are enormous differences in how little or much stress each of us can tolerate. A situation that might be very stressful to you could leave someone else utterly calm. Your tolerance depends largely on your genetic inheritance, your previous experiences, your ability to separate real from imagined or remembered psychosocial assaults, your unique response to stimuli and to the symbols associated with the stimuli, your philosophy of life, and how much social support you have. You might be able to ward off or at least lessen the effects of distress and disease by paying attention to the body's signals and then, whenever necessary, doing something about them. Says Dr. Howard A. Rusk, an authority on rehabilitation:

Every individual has his own stress point. If he goes a little

over, he is irritable, unhappy, and in the end inefficient. If he goes far over, he breaks. If he is below his stress point, he does not realize his true potential and have the great therapeutic satisfaction of accomplishment. If he goes far under, he vegetates. The individual who, through intuitive understanding and guidance, if necessary, finds his own specific stress point, finds his life is a happy and productive one.

Psychosocial Stressors

Whatever its virtues, our advanced technological society is not very congenial to our health and psychological well-being. It brings with it high stress levels, and change in these levels is not likely to occur soon. Neither is the adaptation that would be needed to tolerate such levels without ill effects. So people are largely on their own in undertaking to reduce undue stress. This calls for tough self-examination, because each person's circumstances and physical and emotional makeup are obviously different from anyone else's. How do you rate your tolerance of change, disruption, and uncertainty? What are some of the situations that you face now or are likely to face in the future that might require excessive adaptation and be potentially damaging to you?

Social Change   Such events as going to college, getting married, changing jobs, and moving to another area are common, but they can provoke considerable stress, especially if several occur at the same time or closely together. The cumulative impact of the pressures, decision making, and insecurities that are part of the normal events of life can have a great effect on health. Changes are often perceived as threatening, not because they are necessarily bad but because people have not learned to adapt to them adequately—that is, they don't know how to cope.

Even seemingly moderate social readjustments may take their toll. For instance, some years ago, when Navajo Indians were moved from their homes and located on reservations only a few miles away, their death rate from tuberculosis rose alarmingly. The Navajos' food, clothing, and hygiene were unchanged; their new physical setting was virtually the same

Disorientation
Confusion with respect to time, place or person.

Chronic
Describes a condition or disease that lasts a long time or recurs frequently.

Social anonymity
The state of being unrecognized as an individual by members of society.

---

as their old one. But the social disorganization was enough to overtax the adaptive capacities of many.

Migrants and immigrants of all races and countries are especially vulnerable to psychosocial stress. The rates of psychiatric hospitalization and illness events among these groups are ordinarily higher than those of other population groups. The risk of mental *disorientation* increases as newcomers face unfamiliar conditions, cultural differences, less social support, and pressures for assimilation, especially when there are no familiar groups to join. Migrants also appear to be more vulnerable to *chronic* diseases and infections than their contemporaries who stay put; and occupationally and geographically mobile people tend to have a higher incidence of coronary heart disease than more stable populations.

Anything that challenges one's values and beliefs is a source of stress. The social tumult of 1960s, which forced so many individuals to reevaluate their ideas and goals, generated stress in new forms. The women's movement, for example, has compelled both sexes to reinterpret feminine and masculine roles and interpersonal relations. But the new freedoms and competitiveness of women can be both heady and disturbing to them and potentially threatening to men. As more women enter the work force and more of them occupy executive positions, they are becoming as susceptible to peptic ulcers and cardiovascular disease as men are.

The youth cult so pervasive in the 1960s has lost some of its power (the young who warned their peers not to trust anyone over 30 are now themselves over 30 and doing some rethinking), but we remain essentially a youth-oriented culture. The young, if they think about old age at all, are afraid of getting old; and the old, who tend to think about their age too much, are often afraid of being abandoned and of dying. It is possible, though not easy, to overcome the stresses generated by these situations. One can develop a personal philosophy (and life-style) that reflects the pointlessness of a fixation on youth at the same time that it embraces the sense of wonder and spontaneity characteristic of youth.

Along with the devaluation of the elderly there has been a general loss of a sense of direction, of personal values and ideals, of spiritual comfort. Many people, finding themselves in limbo, are trying desperately to fill a spiritual vacuum. The result is an array of religious movements, pop psychologies, and occult practices, some of them so far out as to be dangerously disorienting. But out of this sweep of spiritual ventures and recharging techniques some helpful guidelines have emerged.

Crowding and Urban Life   About 75 percent of the people in this country are now bunched together on a mere 1.5 percent of the land. Over the years United States public-opinion polls have consistently shown that most of the residents of big cities would rather live in smaller ones. In the late 1960s and in the 1970s, some Americans indeed began moving out, from the center city and from the entire metropolitan area as well. But today, many of these rural residents are drifting back to the cities. Perhaps some found they had simply traded one set of stresses for another.

In 1890 the philosopher and psychologist William James wrote, "No more fiendish punishment could be devised, were such a thing physically possible, than that one should be turned loose in society and remain absolutely unnoticed by all the members thereof." With over 26,000 people residing within one square mile of New York City and over 15,000 in Chicago, in San Francisco, and in Philadelphia, perhaps living in a big city is just such a punishment for some people.

Some individuals feel lost, alienated, and helpless in this world of strangers, while others welcome the *social anonymity*. They savor a distinct sense of privacy. Others, paradoxically, feel so hemmed in by people that privacy is regarded as a rarely attained, though blessed, state. As a lonely character in a Jules Feiffer skit grumbles, "If only not being alone didn't depend on other people."

Cities act as magnets both for those who seek opportunity and for those who seek oblivion. To some the seemingly endless stimulation the city offers is intellectually arousing and full of untold excitements; to others it is numbing and dehumanizing.

Because they cannot scan, let alone process, the flow of urban stimuli, people attempt to protect themselves from overload by developing adaptive responses that

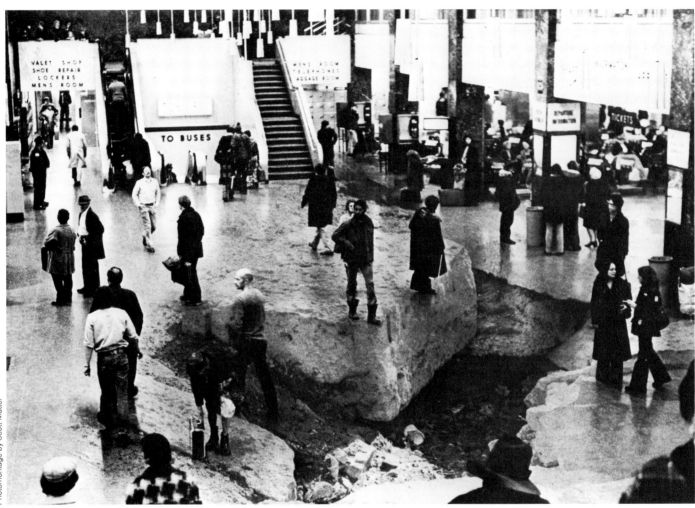

Photomontage by Scott Mutter

34

Serum cholesterol level
The amount of the chemical cholesterol in a given amount of serum in the blood. Cholesterol is related to hardening of the arteries.

Psychosomatic symptoms
Physical symptoms due to stress; may cause tissue damage.

---

streamline it. In doing so, however, they may also reject life-enhancing stimuli and become withdrawn, seemingly callous, and geared to a routine existence with little turmoil and many superficial relationships. It is not the stresses themselves that appear to account for the ills of urban living; it is the means people use to try to escape them.

In the view of social psychologist Stanley Milgram: "The ultimate adaptation to an overloaded social environment is to totally disregard the needs, interests, and demands of those whom one does not define as relevant to the satisfaction of personal needs, and to develop highly efficient perceptual means of determining whether an individual falls into the category of friend or stranger." In "The Experience of Living in Cities," Milgram cites a number of adaptive responses that enable city dwellers to shut out certain aspects of their environment. For instance, they give less time to each input; they screen out inputs that are of little personal importance (the drunk—or presumed drunk—on the sidewalk is ignored; people bumping into each other don't bother to apologize); they shift responsibility to another party ("It's none of my business"); and they discourage personal contact (phone numbers are unlisted; telephone receivers are left off the hook).

City life does not destroy the humanitarian impulse; it merely restrains it. In order to lead a reasonably well-ordered life, even the Good Samaritan would have to recognize the practical limitations of humanitarianism in the urban environment.

Cities have always stirred up conflicting reactions. Any argument favoring city life can be countered by an argument downgrading it. Similarly, although it is popularly believed that crowding is stressful and harmful to health, not every study supports this view.

The most crowded living conditions in the world are not found in the tenements of New York City, the sampan-houseboats in Hong Kong, or one-room houses in a Rio de Janeiro slum. They are found in the camps of the !Kung people in Africa's Kalahari Desert. (The exclamation point indicates a click, or suction stop, in the spoken language.) The !Kung, hunters and gatherers, deliberately arrange their camps so that the occupants are crammed into one tiny central area. Although the population density of their entire roaming area is one person per 10 square miles, they voluntarily form camps in which they occupy only some 180 square feet per person—or about 30 people to the room. The campers' arms and legs are usually touching, and the huts are so close together that people sitting at different hearths can hand food back and forth without getting up.

The health of the !Kung is apparently unaffected by this extraordinary group intimacy. They have low blood pressure throughout their lives, and their *serum cholesterol levels* rank among the lowest in the world (perhaps owing to their diet). Unlike crowded city dwellers, they not only have a great deal of supportive interpersonal contact but also are surrounded by an immense desert to which they can escape whenever they wish. In addition, they are free of discrimination, economic imbalances, constant competitive strife, noise and air pollution, and the multitude of other stressors of "advanced" societies.

Even in a modern culture like that of New Zealand, a survey of households has indicated that household crowding actually results in less stress. It was found that the greater the number of people living in a single dwelling, the less evidence there was of alcoholism, psychological disorders, and the use of mood-modifying drugs. The household residents—either relatives or long-term associates—apparently formed cohesive, supportive units that served as a buffer to environmental stress.

By contrast, other studies have indicated that crowding elevates the degree of physical arousal or stress, causing the entire human organism to suffer. Stress-related *psychosomatic symptoms* such as asthma and backpains show up, mental health deteriorates, blood pressure rises, and the heart rate increases. Moreover, interpersonal relations are damaged. and self-insight is severely hampered.

Many of the theories about the effects of crowding on human beings have been based on animal studies. Long-term crowding among deer, rats, lemmings, and other four-footed creatures has been shown to lead to lowered birthrates.

When long-term crowding is inevitable, many of the stresses can be modified. For instance, college dormitories arranged in suites—connected rooms occupied by three or four students—rather than corridor-style rooms

Alienation
The condition of being uninvolved in or
estranged from society.

can shield students from too much interaction. Even a small touch like pictures or mirrors on dormitory walls can make students feel less crowded, because pictures and mirrors give a feeling of added space.

The Work Environment and Job Choice   Just 2 percent of America's industrial establishments employ over 50 percent of the country's total civilian labor force. Some members of large, powerful, impersonal organizations join by choice, others out of necessity or because it is expected of them or because they want financial security and social status. But once they have become cogs in the machinery they may find they are deprived of personal satisfaction and are apt to plead, by way of lapel buttons, "I am a human being. Do not fold, spindle, or mutilate." When Studs Terkel was compiling material for his book *Working*, he asked 135 people from corporation presidents to elevator operators, "How do you like your job?" "I don't," most of them answered. According to the United States Department of Labor, 80 percent of the employees in this country are misemployed, working at the wrong jobs. Some promotions indeed reflect the Peter Principle: Employees are promoted from jobs they perform competently to higher positions until they reach a level of incompetence.

In offices, factories, and even executive suites, people complain more and more about their jobs, while their employers, who bitterly point out that the "work ethic" is dead, are forced to deal with rising rates of absenteeism—some of which may simply be a matter of goofing off, some the result of acute or chronic illness, with resentment and frustration perhaps at the core in either case. (Job complaints are almost universal; apparently only in China and Japan is the organization life reported as the ideal one.)

In all types of jobs, many employees claim to be *alienated* from their work: They feel trapped, overwhelmed by meaninglessness, self-estrangement, isolation, and powerlessness. Alienation is usually regarded as an affliction of the blue-collar worker, but in recent years thousands of executives have abandoned their jobs for work that may pay less but promises to be more rewarding. For instance, they have become artists, craftworkers, or singers, or have established agricultural communes.

One of the effects of alienation is sheer escapism. Thousands of assembly line workers and an equal number of executives daydream through their work. More than half admit they are working at only half their potential. Others escape through drugs and alcohol: Workers in some factories stay high on drugs during their entire shift, and many executives rely on the three-martini lunch to get through the day. In an effort to deal with work alienation, some organizations are embarking on "job enrichment" programs, giving each worker more varied tasks and allowing him or her a greater sense of responsibility for the finished product.

Clearly, excessive stress is the lot of almost every worker at some time. Job dissatisfaction, too little or too much responsibility, conflict with co-workers or with supervisors, lack of support, vague job expectations, and time pressure—all are stressors. When extremely aroused, a person is usually unable to do certain kinds of tasks as well as when he or she is less aroused. It is hard to do a complicated job, to think creatively, or to learn something new when under excess stress. For example, if you're nervous about an exam, you cannot absorb information as well as you could if you were less anxious. On the other hand, if you're taking an exam that is not too hard and that you are fairly well prepared for, being slightly "keyed up" will probably be helpful.

Monotony can be just as stressful as excessive activity. In a recent study of 2,000 male workers in 23 occupations, such traditional stressors as heavy work loads, long hours, and critical responsibilities were found to result in less physical illness, anxiety, and depression than less demanding jobs. Some corporation executives admit to deliberately stressing their employees because this seems, to them, the best way to get a job done. Emotional strain associated with job responsibility does contribute to ill health, however. For example, heart disease or ulcers frequently afflict police officers, fire fighters, taxi drivers, air-traffic controllers, and musicians on one-night stands. (A study of 100 police in Cincinnati unexpectedly showed that their most significant stressors were neither life-threatening situations nor the hostility they often encountered; instead, the stressors were those circumstances that undermined their sense of professionalism, such as a reprimand from a superior.)

Incidence
The rate at which something occurs.

Prevalence
The number of instances of a condition in a specified population at a given time.

Primitive
A word sometimes used to describe earlier, less "civilized" times; refers to cultures that are not technologically advanced.

Trauma
A wound or injury.

Genetic predisposition
Tendency to inherit.

Type A behavior
Type A behavior is exhibited in a complex of life-style characteristics including punctuality, impatience, inability to relinquish control, and aggressiveness.

Type B behavior
Type B behavior is relatively relaxed and easy-going.

---

cope and that resistance becomes even lower when he or she uses faulty coping techniques, techniques not relevant to the problem being confronted. We all have a finite amount of energy. If too much is expended in coping with the environment, there is less reserve for preventing disease. If life becomes too hectic, and our coping attempts fail, we get sick. Although major life events have often been cited as the most important factor in the onset of stress-linked disease, it is possible that the individual's effectiveness or ineffectiveness in adapting to daily, chronic irritants is the overriding factor.

Some doctors estimate that anywhere from 30 to 80 percent of their patients' illnesses are significantly linked to social and economic stresses on the one hand and to personal worries and circumstances on the other. Although the medical profession appears to regard the finding that disease can be socially generated as yet another breakthrough in modern medicine, medicine men in *primitive* cultures have long recognized that physical ailments can be expressions of emotional or spiritual distress or of snags in the web of social contacts. The medicine man was, in a sense, the world's first sociologist and its first psychiatrist; he did not erect an artificial wall between the social environment and the individual.

The traditional model of disease is that of infection or *trauma*—that is, a single cause for a specific ailment. But more and more scientists are beginning to accept the idea that even susceptibility to infectious diseases can be not merely a matter of exposure to an external source of infection; it has to be a reflection of environmental conditions that culminate in physiological stress. It is not, in other words, simply the germ that causes the disease but our relationship to the germ.

In the current model of disease, illness is regarded as having many causes. Among them are stressful environmental conditions, the person's perception that the conditions are stressful, the relative ability to adapt to them, *genetic predisposition* to a disorder, the degree of physical fitness, and the presence of a disease agent. In addition, according to one school of thought, unique personality profiles may be connected with such disorders as heart disease, asthma, arthritis, colitis, migraine and tension headaches, and even cancer.

For example, some apparently healthy individuals are at risk for developing heart disease but neither consider

themselves sick nor are so regarded by their families and friends. On the contrary, these people are so energetic and active that they give the impression of being unusually healthy. They are mentally alert, aggressive, always on the move, and highly productive. Their ability to fulfill valued social roles is also noteworthy. They frequently hold responsible managerial jobs, and most add to their job demands a host of family obligations and community activities. Despite these multiple pressures they rarely complain about anxiety or depression. Some go so far as to suggest that they thrive on challenges and deadlines. But do they really? These people, who have been studied extensively, tend to have heart attacks at a higher frequency and at younger ages than the general population. They are said to demonstrate *type A behavior*. Individuals who exhibit *type B*

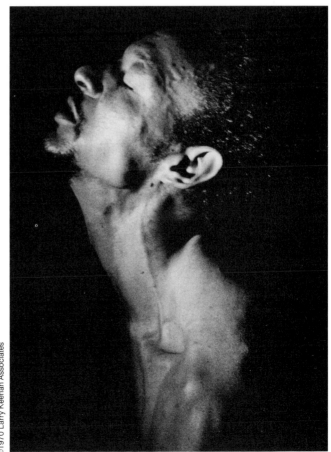

©1970 Larry Keenan Associates

behavior are more relaxed, relatively passive, and possibly better able to cope with stress and stressful environments. Recent research suggests that the most important difference in terms of cardiovascular health between type A and type B people is that the type A person is unable to relinquish control over almost any situation or environment. (See pages 48–51 and Chapter 17.) Dr. Carl Thoresen of Stanford University, in working with men identified as type A, recently demonstrated a reduction in heart attack rates using behavior therapeutic techniques that included teaching type A individuals how to relax.

A growing number of stress researchers maintain that, contrary to popular belief, certain types of relationships or situations are not inherently stressful and detrimental to health. For example, they point out that disease epidemics that were expected when Londoners were subjected to the horrors of being bombed during World War II did not materialize. Hardships cannot be unquestionably equated with a state of health. If you stop to think about it, you will realize that most people do not become disabled even when awful things happen to them. So exposure to stressors alone is not usually an adequate explanation for the onset of illness. Their impact seems to depend on three factors: the characteristics of stressful events (their magnitude, intensity, unpredictability, duration, and novelty); the individual's biological and psychological make-up; and the social supports available to serve as buffers.

Social Support Systems and Social Stressors   A term widely used these days is *social support systems*. These systems consist of the enduring interpersonal ties you have with groups of people—at home, at school, at work, and so on. These are people you can count on to give you emotional support, feedback, and assistance and resources when needed and with whom you share values and standards. We think of blood ties as the only ones that deserve to be called familial, but journalist Jane Howard, in researching family life ("All Happy Clans Are Alike: In Search of the Good Family," *Atlantic* [May 1978]: 37), concluded:

> Call it a clan, call it a network, call it a tribe, call it a family. Whatever you call it, whoever you are, you need one. You need one because you are human. You didn't come from

nowhere. Before you, around you, and presumably after you, too, there are others. Some of these others must matter a lot—to you, and if you are lucky, to one another. Their welfare must be nearly as important to you as your own. Even if you live alone, even if your solitude is elected and ebullient, you still cannot do without a clan or a tribe. . . .

> If our relatives are not, do not wish to be or [for] whatever reasons cannot be our friends, then by some complex alchemy we must try to transform our friends into our relatives. If blood roots don't do the job, then we must look to water and branches, and sort ourselves into new constellations, new families.

Determine your social support from community activities, friends, and relatives by completing the "Social Support Scale" on page 42.

The social position individuals or groups occupy can measurably affect their experience of stress and, it is assumed, their vulnerability to all sorts of disorders. The effects of exposure to stressful situations may be scaled down for anyone who is well bolstered by support systems, but the effects are ordinarily made worse when these systems are impaired. Three basic impairments in the social network can be singled out: social isolation, social marginality, and status inconsistency.

Social isolation is now believed to be a major factor in increasing the risk of disease. Some examples: disproportionately high rates of physical and psychiatric disorders occur in deteriorating socially shunned areas of the central city; people who live alone, uninvolved with other people or organizations, are especially vulnerable to chronic disease; institutionalized children, who commonly lack warm relationships with other people, often suffer from "failure to thrive"; and grief may contribute to ill health when social isolation is brought on by loss of a mate.

"Marginal" individuals are deprived of nourishing social contacts for various reasons, such as continuous residential and occupational mobility, isolated living conditions, broken homes, membership in a minority group that is spurned by the dominant majority. They have an increased vulnerability to ill health and other problems that may take many forms—schizophrenia, tuberculosis, multiple accidents, alcoholism, suicide.

If someone plays two or more distinct social roles

involving social expectations that are not compatible, he or she is burdened with status inconsistency and perhaps, as a result, ill health. Such an inconsistency may be, for instance, a discrepancy between education and occupation, between education and income level, or between age or sex and employment. Several studies indicate that extremely healthy workers have social backgrounds, interests, and goals that match their circumstances; and their educational, occupational, and family statuses are also consistent. Workers who are often ill, on the other hand, may have an educational or family status that does not match the sort of work they are doing.

The strength or weakness of social supports may figure prominently in rates of disease and of death. Single men (between the ages of 25 and 64) have a significantly higher death rate from heart disease than married men. Married people have lower death rates than single, widowed, or divorced people for a wide range of conditions. The states in this country that have high death rates for one cause appear to have high death rates for almost all causes. Death rates from all causes are low for certain religious groups, such as Mormons and Seventh Day Adventists. Social and cultural mobility tends to result in higher rates of coronary heart disease, lung cancer, depression, and pregnancy difficulties.

The Riddle of Hypertension   One of the most strongly debated issues among stress researchers is whether stress can cause hypertension (high blood pressure). Although hypertension can usually be controlled with drugs or diet or both (see Chapter 17), scientists still are not sure what causes some 90 percent of the cases. Many of the studies done so far are contradictory, and none has established a clear connection between stress and the development of hypertension. What is not in question is the harmful effect of stress on the course of the disease once it starts. The most consistently demonstrated relationship is one between excess weight and hypertension. It has been suggested that stress may induce hypertension indirectly by causing nervous appetite and thus an excessive intake of food, including salt.

The most recent studies lean strongly toward a stress-hypertension link. They point to connections between hypertension and job loss; type of job (air-traffic controllers have "incredible ranges" of blood pressure both on and off the job, besides being highly susceptible to ulcers); economic deprivation (this is cited as a primary factor in the high rate of hypertension among blacks); and crowding (according to one study, men in prison had higher blood pressures when forced to live in crowded dormitories—called "preferential housing"—than when confined to single cells).

Coping

As you can now see, the most potent stressors in your life are not the natural physical demands made on the tissues of your body, including such activities as healing wounds, fighting infections, and restoring lost blood, though these are obviously essential. It is the emotional stimuli you face day in and day out, particularly those that cause distress, that are the chief stressors—relentless, often insidious, potentially harmful. When you experience anger, fear, frustration, resentment, or envy, these nervous responses to the events and circumstances of your life evoke physical reactions that can affect you both immediately and, because of their cumulative power, far into the future. But the stressor itself is neutral. The effect of a stressor depends a lot less on what happens to you or on what you do than on how you take it.

Finding Your Stress Point   If you're at a party and drinking quite a bit, you tend to check—unless things really get out of hand—on how much liquor you have been consuming. You can pretty well tell when you are getting intoxicated, and if you are still rational, you will quit drinking or at least slow down. But at any time during your daily activities you can get intoxicated from your own stress hormones. Unless you are a rare person, though, you never think of checking these internal intoxicants. Hans Selye goes so far as to suggest that the drunkenness produced by stress hormones has caused society more harm than the alcoholic kind. Stress can become so constant that we become immune to its presence; physical symptoms and mental anxiety no longer produce noticeable discomfort.

Social Support Scale

Social support has been recognized for a long time in the behavioral sciences as an important adjunct to therapy. However, only recently has social support emerged among health care professionals as a moderator of stress, with high social support facilitating the ability to cope with stress and adapt to change and thus placing the vulnerable individual at lower risk for serious illness.

The social support scale (SSS) measures the extent to which a person receives or obtains social and psychological support from community activities, friends, and relatives. The score for the amount of social support obtained is found by adding all the numbers next to the boxes checked plus all the numbers circled. The following totals indicate high, moderate, and low support:

70 or more = HIGH SUPPORT, which suggests that you have a well-developed social support structure to counter the negative effects of stress.

40 to 69 = MODERATE SUP-PORT, which suggests that you have sufficient areas of social support to counter the negative effects of stress.

less than 40 = LOW SUPPORT, which suggests that you lack the minimum support structure to counter the negative effects of stress.

1. Do you belong to any of these kinds of groups? If YES, please indicate how much you take part in group activities. For example, VERY ACTIVE means you attend most meetings; SOMEWHAT ACTIVE means you attend meetings once in awhile; INACTIVE means that you belong, but hardly ever go to meetings.

HOW MUCH DO YOU TAKE PART?

	DO YOU BELONG?	INACTIVE	SOMEWHAT ACTIVE	VERY ACTIVE
a. A social or recreational group?	1☐NO 2☐YES→1☐		2☐	3☐
b. A labor union, commercial group, or professional association?	1☐NO 2☐YES→1☐		2☐	3☐
c. A political-party group or club?	1☐NO 2☐YES→1☐		2☐	3☐
d. A group concerned with children (such as P.T.A. or Boy Scouts)?	1☐NO 2☐YES→1☐		2☐	3☐
e. A group concerned with community betterment, charity, or service?	1☐NO 2☐YES→1☐		2☐	3☐

ASIDE FROM THE ABOVE GROUPS, DO YOU BELONG TO:

f. A church-connected group?	1☐NO 2☐YES→1☐		2☐	3☐
g. A group concerned with a public issue such as civil liberties, property rights, etc.?	1☐NO 2☐YES→1☐		2☐	3☐
h. A group concerned with the environment, pollution, etc.?	1☐NO 2☐YES→1☐		2☐	3☐
i. A group concerned with self-improvement that meets regularly?	1☐NO 2☐YES→1☐		2☐	3☐
j. Any other groups?	1☐NO 2☐YES→1☐		2☐	3☐

Describe them: _____

2. How many close friends (people you feel at ease with, can talk to about private matters, and can call on for help) do you have?

CIRCLE ONE: None 1 2 3 4 5 6 7 8 9 10 or more

3. How many relatives do you have that you feel close to?

CIRCLE ONE: None 1 2 3 4 5 6 7 8 9 10 or more

4. How many of these friends or relatives do you see at least once a month?

CIRCLE ONE: None 1 2 3 4 5 6 7 8 9 10 or more

5. About how often do you see any close relatives or friends?

5☐ MORE THAN ONCE A WEEK   4☐ ONCE A WEEK   3☐ A FEW TIMES A MONTH   2☐ ONCE A MONTH   1☐ LESS THAN ONCE A MONTH

6. How often are you on the telephone with any close relatives or friends?

5☐ MORE THAN ONCE A WEEK   4☐ ONCE A WEEK   3☐ A FEW TIMES A MONTH   2☐ ONCE A MONTH   1☐ LESS THAN ONCE A MONTH

7. How often do you exchange letters with any close relatives or friends?

5☐ ONCE A WEEK OR MORE   4☐ A FEW TIMES A MONTH   3☐ ONCE A MONTH   2☐ A FEW TIMES A YEAR   1☐ ONCE A YEAR OR LESS

It is, of course, harder to recognize and combat an internal foe than an external one, but it can be done. Most of us keep our minds so cluttered that we have a hard time even noticing the body's alarm signals, let alone assessing them accurately. If you ignore the stress signals, you habituate yourself to taking on a heavier load of stress rather than to searching for ways to lessen it. But you can learn to become alert to the signals that inform you that you are too keyed up and you can learn to tune down in time to avoid harm.

When you analyze your stress status, you should consider not only the total amount of stress but also whether there is proportionately too much stress in any particular part of you. If there is too much total stress, you need a rest; if there is too much lopsided stress, you need a diversion.

Tuning Down Through Diversion   Mental or emotional stress is best remedied by either physical or mental diversion. If you involve your whole body in some task, activate it through general stress (not distress), whatever is worrying or blocking you automatically loses some of its force because the proportions of stress have been altered. Jogging, swimming, cleaning the car, or just plain walking can help. Such voluntary activities often work better than merely resting. Or you can use a mental diversion to equalize the stress. If you consciously concentrate on something else, something pleasant, again whatever is troubling you will be erased or at least fade as you rechannel your thoughts. Solving a puzzle, reading, painting, going to a movie, or simply thinking about something pleasant can put a different perspective on your problems.

Meditation and Other Techniques   Highly perfected meditation practices, both sacred and secular, appear in almost every culture on earth. Yet until the last couple of decades, most Westerners dismissed them, particularly the centuries-old Eastern meditation techniques, as nonsense. But ever since so many Americans decided they needed to alter their consciousness and realized that they could indeed voluntarily regulate the autonomous nervous system, the United States has become host to a swarm of swamis and a glut of gurus. There are some frauds among them, but on the whole their mystical or semimystical techniques have been shown to have practical consequences. The benefits of self-induced, rather than drug-induced, altered states of consciousness are improved mental and physical health, enhanced ability to deal with stress, and heightened creativity. The various ways of letting go—for instance, transcendental meditation, yoga, Zen, autogenic training, biofeedback—have beneficial, measurable effects on such stress-related conditions as irregular heartbeats, hypertension, and migraine and tension headaches. Whether these methods, by reducing stress, can prevent such ailments is not known.

An integrated central nervous system reaction, sometimes called the relaxation response, appears to underlie the altered states of consciousness, which can restore energy at least as effectively as deep sleep. Intense immersion in these different states seems to lead to a completely new awareness, a recognition of a vast realm of new and infinite possibilities. This shift of consciousness, this emptying of the mind, is known as "losing your mind in order to come to your senses."

The essence of all systems of meditation is concentration—on a word, an object, or nothing—plus slow, rhythmic breathing. Once the meditator's mind has been quieted, once it quits flitting from one subject to another, the meditator experiences what is known as cosmic consciousness, transcendental awareness, or (in Zen) satori. Both attention and attitude are what count, whatever the method used.

Thanks to the evangelistic fervor of Maharishi Mahesh Yogi, transcendental meditation (TM) has become, as Adam Smith puts it, the McDonald's of meditation. Although it grew out of a mystical school of yoga and uses a Hindu devotional in its initiation ritual, its practitioners tend to ignore its religious trappings and thus usually feel comfortable with it. Because it is a simple technique that can be learned in about four hours of training, it has had an enormous appeal for Americans, who are accustomed to "instant everything."

Zen is another form of meditation about which an enormous literature is accumulating. Sometimes known as "the short path" to liberation, Zen is in fact a steep, strenuous course. Paradoxically, it is difficult because it is so simple (Zen is full of paradoxes). As a doorway to the superconscious, Zen can lead eventually (usually after years of practice) to a "state of no mind," a self without image. Its *koans,* or riddles, often used in conjunction with meditation, paralyze the usual logical thought processes. Zen is not for dabblers. Unless undertaken with rigorous discipline, it is useless and may even be risky.

Although the martial arts, such as karate, kung fu, and aikido, which are generally perceived as being combative and competitive, would seem to be an unlikely means of relieving stress, they can in fact be one of the best means. All those kicks and shouts and throws and breaking of bricks with the naked hand disguise the true meaning of these arts. A clue to that meaning can be found in the imperturbability of those who have mastered or nearly mastered them. Stress appears to be

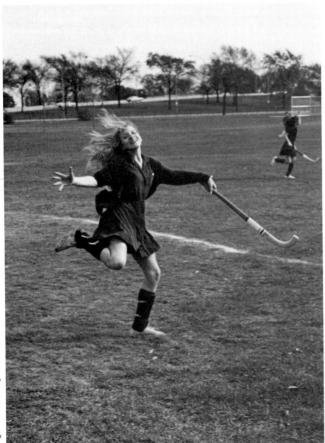

Roger Malloch, Magnum Photos

foreign to such people. They have learned how to relax, how to breathe, how to concentrate, and how to center themselves.

Nutrition   Anyone who is serious about handling stress is going to choose vitamins over Valium. Because a sensible diet has such a great bearing on general well-being, on making you feel your best, it can go a long way in protecting you from stress. A food can be a stressor if it harms the body in any way or makes it have to work harder. Many nutritionists now agree that certain substances are stressors for everyone, and at the top of the list are large amounts of caffeine and refined sugar. Both substances have the potential to trigger the stress response.

"Empty calorie" food, junk food, and highly processed and overrefined foods affect the body adversely not only by making metabolism and detoxification more difficult but also by lessening or destroying the appetite for more nutritious fare. And stored nutrients must thus be put to extra work to deal with such dubious fare in addition to going about their normal, intricate business of sustaining the body. Such foods rob the body of the very vitamins and minerals it most needs to combat stress: the water-soluble vitamins B complex and C and the minerals zinc, magnesium, calcium, and potassium.

If you are overindulging in coffee and sugar, junk food, and highly processed foods (as most Americans are), try cutting down on them, or, even better, not using them at all, and see if you notice a difference in your vulnerability to stress. By eating simple, whole foods, you will probably be getting all the antistress vitamins and minerals you need, without taking supplements.

Humor   Laughter is a built-in tranquilizer and healer. Laughter, the type we associate with good humor, can indicate a state of mental and physical well-being. It reduces stress and has a relaxing effect on the body. The enormous power of laughter was demonstrated by Norman Cousins, editor of the *Saturday Review,* when he was struck by a crippling disease. Told that he had one chance in 500 of surviving, he decided to be more than a passive observer. With the help of an open-minded doctor, he put himself on a program that

Relaxation

To evoke the relaxation response you need:

1. *A quiet environment*   One should choose a quiet, calm environment with as few distractions as possible. Sound, even background noise, may prevent the elicitation of the response. Choose a convenient, suitable place—for example, at an office desk in a quiet room.

2. *A mental device*   The meditator employs the constant stimulus of a single-syllable sound or word. The syllable is repeated silently or in a low, gentle tone. The purpose of the repetition is to free oneself from logical, externally oriented thought by focusing solely on the stimulus. Many different words and sounds have been used in traditional practices. Because of its implicity and neutrality, the use of the syllable "one" is suggested.

3. *A passive attitude*   The purpose of the response is to help one rest and relax, and this requires a completely passive attitude. One should not scrutinize his performance or try to force the response, because this may well prevent the response from occurring. When distracting thoughts enter the mind, they should simply be disregarded.

4. *A comfortable position*   The meditator should sit in a comfortable chair in as restful a position as possible. The purpose is to reduce muscular effort to a minimum. The head may be supported; the arms should be balanced or supported as well. The shoes may be removed and the feet propped up several inches, if desired. Loosen all tight-fitting clothing.

Eliciting the Relaxation Response   Using these four basic elements, one can evoke the response by following the simple, mental, noncultic procedure that subjects have used in my laboratory:

In a quiet environment, sit in a comfortable position.

Close your eyes.

Deeply relax all your muscles, beginning at your feet and progressing up to your face—feet, calves, thighs, lower torso, chest, shoulder, neck, head. Allow them to remain deeply relaxed.

Breathe through your nose. Become aware of your breathing. As you breathe out, say the "one" silently to yourself. Thus: breathe in . . . breathe out, with "one." In . . . out, with "one" . . .

Continue this practice for 20 minutes. You may open your eyes to check the time, but do not use an alarm. When you finish, sit quietly for several minutes, at first with your eyes closed and later with your eyes open.

Remember not to worry about whether you are successful in achieving a deep level of relaxation—maintain a passive attitude and permit relaxation to occur at its own pace. When distracting thoughts occur, ignore them and continue to repeat "one" as you breathe. The technique should be practiced once or twice daily, and not within two hours after any meal, since the digestive processes seem to interfere with the elicitation of the expected changes.

I have a technique which seems to work for me, and I do it every morning on rising, most evenings before retiring, and at any time during the day when I feel tense or uncomfortably "hyped." I have no idea whether it would work for anyone else, but I will mention it in case you might be interested. I simply sit comfortably in a chair, close my eyes, and (slowly) inhale and exhale as deeply and fully as I can. I try to feel myself relaxing, starting with my toes and feet and proceeding to my ears and head. (If you have never experienced fully relaxed ears, well, you're missing something. Like limp ears.) All this takes but two or three minutes, which I am willing to surrender for the calming effect it provides. On the other hand, the TM I learned years ago required 20 minutes every morning and night (before meals), and I found too many distractions disrupted that routine. While I do not expect to take up TM again (I also have difficulty relating to a mantra, levitations, and other trappings), I do respect the results which others report from employing this and other relaxation methods. In the future, I expect to devote more time to quieting than I do today, and to put greater effort into constructing an environment suited for and conducive to my own approach to stress management.

Donald B. Ardell
High Level Wellness

included huge dosages of both vitamin C and laughter and restored himself to health.

Novelist Erich Maria Remarque has observed, "Not to laugh at the twentieth century is to shoot yourself." Yet we Americans now seem to have a peculiarly low mirth rate in comparison with times past. Sometimes we cannot even recognize humor unless it is accompanied by canned laughter. But perhaps we should look at this situation the way essayist Frank Trippett does: "Plainly, no nation that has survived 95 Congresses and exalted the portrait of a soup can as a work of art and adopted John Wayne as an elder statesman can be written off as hopelessly serious" ("How to Raise the U.S. Mirth Rate," *Time* [April 3, 1978]: 94).

The comic perception offers a respite, however brief, from the tyranny of any situation you may find yourself in. It detaches you from both your situation and yourself. Don't allow yourself to be ultraserious, a slave to all the little dramas of your life. It's been aptly said that the cosmic consciousness is also a comic consciousness. (Zen is unique in bringing this out, for it is the only esoteric method that finds room for playfulness and laughter.)

A Few Other Suggestions You can burden your memory with too much information. There is a limit to how much it will hold without balking. One of the major sources of mental stress is trying to remember too many things. Forget the unimportant ones (they will usually be self-evident) and keep your memory free for those that are essential. Nor should you clog your mind with the debris of past events by reliving them. Clinging to experiences and emotions, particularly unpleasant ones, can be a deadly business. Let them go and keep your mind free and clear for what's happening now.

There is absolutely no point in trying to live in the abstract world of desire, turning down the reality of the present in favor of the unreality of the past, the future, or the ideal. The past cannot be recovered. We all know that, but we usually act as if we do not know it at all. We worry at it as though it were a hangnail ever reappearing to allow us to indulge in a sort of exquisite torture. As for the future, it can never exist as the future. And the ideal, if it were to become real, could never turn out to be the ideal as such.

Pleasure, or joy, is vital for optimum health. But it should not be regarded as simply a reward for something you do, or as a feeling that you can have only occasionally, or as something you must pursue. Rather than take an I'll-be-happy-when attitude (I'll be happy when I graduate, when I fall in love . . .), try to realize that pleasure is integral to being alive and that you yourself can create it every day of your life.

Anticipating an event can be a greater source of stress than the event itself. "I am an old man," said Mark Twain, "and I have known troubles in my life, most of which never happened." You know exactly what anticipatory stress is if you have ever spent a lot of time thinking about an exam. You may even have suffered from a stomach ache, skin rash, asthma, or hay fever or other allergies because of it. Immediately before the exam, you may have had cramps, diarrhea, or nausea. If you have prepared adequately for any exam, such symptoms are unlikely to be as severe if they even exist. If you simply do what is to be done, and don't think and think and think about it, you can save yourself a lot of distress. Procrastination is almost guaranteed to bring you distress, never eustress.

In spite of the flood of self-help books on the market, all of which in one way or another advise you about how to combat stress, there is no procedure manual, no ready-made success formula, that suits everyone. The simplest formula probably ever devised is "roll with the punches." Perhaps Hans Selye, in *The Stress of Life*, best sums up the philosophical implications of all the stress research that has been done:

> Stress is usually the outcome of a struggle for the self-preservation (the homeostasis) of parts within a whole. This is true of cells within an individual, of individuals within society, and of species within the whole animate world. After surveying the emotions which govern interpersonal relations (the thirst for approval, the terror of censure, the feeling of love, hate, gratitude, and revenge), we come to the conclusion that the incitement, by our actions, of love, goodwill and gratitude in others is most likely to assure our safety within society. Why not seek this consciously as a long-range aim in life? No other philosophy has the exquisite property of necessarily transforming all our natural but reckless egoistic impulses into altruism without curtailing any of their self-protecting value.

Stress and Coping Behavior Scale

Read the following statements carefully. Choose the one in each section
that best describes you at this
moment and record its score at the
right. (For example, "some stress but
coping well" has a score of 4.)
When you have identified five statements, total your score and find your
position on the scale.

5 highly productive
4 productive
3 efficient
2 inefficient
1 unproductive

Score _____

5 very decisive
4 decisive
3 somewhat hesitant
2 indecisive
1 easily confused

Score _____

5 free from symptoms of stress
4 some stress but coping well
3 slightly uncomfortable stress
2 heavy stress
1 severe stress

Score _____

5 quickly responsive to change
4 adaptable to change
3 tolerant of change
2 resistant to change
1 distressed by change

Score _____

5 regularly enjoys recreation
4 plans recreation time
3 has trouble getting away to relax
2 rarely makes vacation time
1 seldom enjoys vacations

Score _____

Total score _____

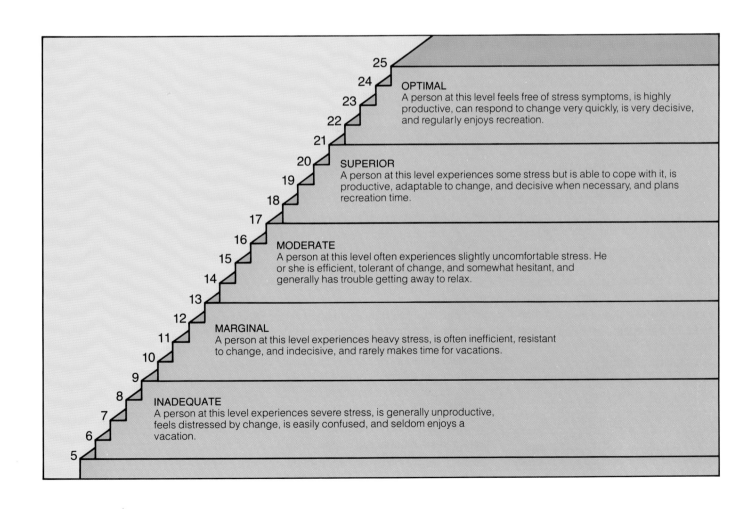

25
24 23 22 **OPTIMAL**
A person at this level feels free of stress symptoms, is highly productive, can respond to change very quickly, is very decisive, and regularly enjoys recreation.

21 20 19 18 **SUPERIOR**
A person at this level experiences some stress but is able to cope with it, is productive, adaptable to change, and decisive when necessary, and plans recreation time.

17 16 15 14 **MODERATE**
A person at this level often experiences slightly uncomfortable stress. He or she is efficient, tolerant of change, and somewhat hesitant, and generally has trouble getting away to relax.

13 12 11 10 **MARGINAL**
A person at this level experiences heavy stress, is often inefficient, resistant to change, and indecisive, and rarely makes time for vacations.

9 8 7 6 5 **INADEQUATE**
A person at this level experiences severe stress, is generally unproductive, feels distressed by change, is easily confused, and seldom enjoys a vacation.

Take Action

Your answers to Probing Your Emotions at the beginning of this chapter and your placement level on the Stress and Coping Behavior Scale will, we hope, encourage you to begin a process of self-exploration and self-discovery that you will continue. Reflect on the entire chapter's content and ask yourself how each point relates to your own life. Then take action:

1. Dr. Edmund Jacobson of the University of Chicago noted that people tense their muscles when they are stressed but don't realize they are doing it. He reasoned that if they can learn to relax, they can lower the stress they experience.

Think about a specific time when you felt anxious or stressed. Now take your pulse rate and record it in your Take Action notebook. Turn to page 45. Learn and practice the relaxation response. Immediately after relaxing the last muscle group, take your pulse rate and record it in your notebook, indicating the time, date, and conditions after which you took it. Was

there any difference in your pulse rate? If so and your pulse rate slowed, you may want to incorporate relaxation as a regular technique in your behavioral approach to stress.

2. Think about the next important test you will be taking. It might be a mid-term, final, or qualifying exam. Do you feel a bit anxious or fearful at the thought of it? If so, plan a systematic attack on the problem. Begin by reviewing "Test Anxiety and Stress" on page 38. Next design for yourself a personal program to reduce your anxiety about the upcoming exam. *Hint:* Are there any exams you don't feel anxious about? Also try combining the relaxation technique with your plan.

3. Think about all the different environments in which you function, including your classrooms, the student union, the dorm, your house. Are some more stressful than others? Make a list of the environments in order of the most stressful to the least stressful. Indicate next to each environment the reasons you think it is stressful or nonstressful. Now start

at the top of your list and record three or more ways to reduce the stressful impact these environments have on you.

4. Turn to the Student Stress Scale on page 29 and determine your score. Distinguish the events you can change from those you cannot change. List the former in your notebook and note how you are going to try to change them.

5. According to some health care professionals, social support can help people cope with stress and thereby lower their risk of serious illness. Find your level of social support on the Social Support Scale that begins on page 42. If your score is 40 or higher, congratulate yourself. If it is below 40, think of at least four specific ways in which you can seek increased social support. Then act on those specifics.

6. Read the following Behavior Change Strategy, and take the appropriate action.

Behavior Change Strategy

Type A Behavior Pattern

The term *type A* is used quite often in everyday discussion to refer to someone who is always working, hurrying, and pressing. A more technical definition is provided by Dr. David Jenkins of Boston University, the designer of the major pencil-and-paper inventory of type A:

The type A behavior pattern is considered to be an overt behavioral syndrome or style of living characterized by *extremes* of competitiveness, striving for achievement, aggressiveness (sometimes stringently repressed), haste, impatience, restlessness, hyperalertness,

explosiveness of speech, tenseness of facial muscles, and feelings of being under the pressure of time and under the challenge of responsibility. Persons having this pattern are often so clearly committed to their vocation or profession that other aspects of their lives are relatively neglected. Not all aspects of the syndrome or pattern need to be present for a person to be classified as possessing it.

There is also a type B pattern that describes the other end of the continuum. Type B individuals can also be quite successful and productive, but their behavior appears to be more flexible and less rushed, and they are

better able to achieve a daily mixture of work and nonwork activity.

Measurement   Type A was initially identified in clinical interactions of cardiologists with their patients (see "Are You a Type A?" page 49), and then it was systematized through carefully structured interviews. Additional tests have been developed, including an activity scale developed by David Jenkins. Dr. David Glass of the University of New York has adapted the Jenkins scale so that the type A characteristic of college students can be measured.

Health Implications Despite the fact that type A individuals have a significantly higher number of heart attacks than type B's, only a handful of studies have attempted to try to help type A's to moderate their tendencies—to move in the type B direction. Some investigators have recommended a training program that utilizes progressive relaxation procedures. Dr. Ethel Roskies of the University of Montreal has published two major reports that have provided at least preliminary grounds for some optimism that type A patterns can be moderated. With half of her test group of 27 middle-aged men, Roskies and her colleagues used a "behavior therapy" program that included extensive training in progressive relaxation and the monitoring of personal stress. The other half of the test group received psychotherapy complete with interpretations of current behaviors as signs and symptoms of unresolved childhood problems! Fortunately for the participants (but unfortunately for our understanding of the phenomena), the participants in *both* groups changed in the positive, or type B, direction.

Roskies and her colleagues concluded that some positive changes could be encouraged, but they also included the following caveat:

. . . the results of a few pioneer studies attempted to date . . . are provocative rather than definitive. The various researchers involved have all reported beneficial change following their respective interventions. Before we can begin to debate the ultimate clinical utility of these treatment effects, we must first establish their reliability.

It is not easy to recruit type A individuals into remedial treatment programs in order to help them to reduce various behavioral characteristics. This is largely because such characteristics have contributed to their work output. Roskies and others have managed to recruit participants by describing their programs as learning experiences that will enable business managers to be even more effective than before because they will learn how to make the level of their energy output commensurate with the demands of the tasks encountered. In other words, the inducement to change comes from maintaining or even improving performance while reducing the personal cost exacted by the performance.

To determine whether you are type A or type B, complete the following questionnaire.

Are You a Type A?

Dr. Ray Rosenman and Dr. Meyer Friedman at Mt. Zion Hospital in San Francisco have studied over 3,000 men who were classified according to whether they were one of two different types—type A and type B. After a follow-up period of 5½ years, type A's were seen to have a significantly greater number of heart attacks than type B's. Which type are you?

Following are 30 items defining type A and type B behavior. After you complete the questionnaire, you can score yourself to see what category you fall into. If you are a type A person and wish to become more of a type B person, what can you do to alter your behavior?

Instructions Read each of the following statements. Then circle one of the numbers *on each line* to indicate whether the statement is true or false *for you*. There are no right or wrong answers.

If a statement is definitely true for you, circle 1.

If it is mostly true for you, circle 2.

If you don't know whether it is true or false, circle 3.

If it is mostly false for you, circle 4.

If it is definitely false for you, circle 5.

	DEFINITELY TRUE	MOSTLY TRUE	DON'T KNOW	MOSTLY FALSE	DEFINITELY FALSE
1. I am more restless and fidgety than most people.	1	2	3	4	5
2. In comparison with most people I know, I'm not very involved in my work.	1	2	3	4	5
3. I ordinarily work quickly and energetically.	1	2	3	4	5
4. I rarely have trouble finishing my work.	1	2	3	4	5
5. I hate giving up before I'm absolutely sure I'm licked.	1	2	3	4	5

	DEFINITELY TRUE	MOSTLY TRUE	DON'T KNOW	MOSTLY FALSE	DEFINITELY FALSE
6. I am rather deliberate in telephone conversations.	1	2	3	4	5
7. I am often in a hurry.	1	2	3	4	5
8. I am somewhat relaxed and at ease about my work.	1	2	3	4	5
9. My achievements are considered to be significantly higher than those of most people I know.	1	2	3	4	5
10. Tailgating bothers me more than a car in front slowing me up.	1	2	3	4	5

	DEFINITELY TRUE	MOSTLY TRUE	DON'T KNOW	MOSTLY FALSE	DEFINITELY FALSE
11. In conversation I often gesture with hands and head.	1	2	3	4	5
12. I rarely drive a car too fast.	1	2	3	4	5
13. As a young person I preferred work in which I could move around.	1	2	3	4	5
14. People consider me to be rather quiet.	1	2	3	4	5
15. Sometimes I think I shouldn't work so hard, but something drives me on.	1	2	3	4	5
16. I usually speak more softly than most people.	1	2	3	4	5
17. My handwriting is rather fast.	1	2	3	4	5
18. I often work slowly and leisurely.	1	2	3	4	5
19. I thrive on challenging situations. The more challenges I have the better.	1	2	3	4	5
20. I prefer to linger over a meal and enjoy it.	1	2	3	4	5

	DEFINITELY TRUE	MOSTLY TRUE	DON'T KNOW	MOSTLY FALSE	DEFINITELY FALSE
21. I like to drive a car rather fast when there is no speed limit.	1	2	3	4	5
22. I like work that is slow and deliberate.	1	2	3	4	5
23. In general I approach my work more seriously than most people I know.	1	2	3	4	5
24. I talk more slowly than most people.	1	2	3	4	5
25. I've often been asked to be an officer of some group or groups.	1	2	3	4	5
26. I often let a problem work itself out by waiting.	1	2	3	4	5
27. I often try to persuade others to my point of view.	1	2	3	4	5
28. I generally walk more slowly than most people.	1	2	3	4	5
29. I eat rapidly even when there is plenty of time.	1	2	3	4	5
30. I usually work fast.	1	2	3	4	5

Scoring Instructions.   To find out whether you are type A or type B, compare your answers with those on the scoring sheet. Note which of your answers are A's and which are B's. Give yourself plus 1 point for every A item you have circled. Add these pluses for a total A score. Give yourself *minus* 1 point for every B item you have circled. Add these minuses for a total B score. Give yourself *minus* 1 point for every Don't Know item you have circled. Divide the Don't Know number by 2. The difference between all your plus scores and all your minus scores is your total. Type A's are described as aggressive, ambitious, competitive, restless, and often working against deadlines. Type B's appear to be much more relaxed. They are less aggressive and competitive. Type A's are more vulnerable to heart attacks than type B's. The following table indicates whether you are an A or a B.

```
+15 to +30 = Definite A
+ 1 to +15 = Moderate A
  0 to −15 = Moderate B
−16 to −30 = Definite B
```

Here is an example of scoring: If you circled nine A items, you would have a subtotal A score of + 9. If you circled 15 B items, you would have a subtotal B score of −15. If you circled 6 Don't Know items, you would divide −6 by 2, which would give you a subtotal Don't Know score of −3. The difference between −18 and + 9 is your total, −9. Your score indicates you are a moderate B.

ANSWERS–SCORING SHEET

	DEFINITELY TRUE	MOSTLY TRUE	DON'T KNOW	MOSTLY FALSE	DEFINITELY FALSE
1. I am more restless and fidgety than most people.	1 = A	2 = A	3	4 = B	5 = B
2. In comparison with most people I know I'm not very involved in my work.	1 = B	2 = B	3	4 = A	5 = A
3. I ordinarily work quickly and energetically.	1 = A	2 = A	3	4 = B	5 = B
4. I rarely have trouble finishing my work.	1 = B	2 = B	3	4 = A	5 = A
5. I hate giving up before I'm absolutely sure I'm licked.	1 = A	2 = A	3	4 = B	5 = B
6. I am rather deliberate in telephone conversations.	1 = B	2 = B	3	4 = A	5 = A
7. I am often in a hurry.	1 = A	2 = A	3	4 = B	5 = B
8. I am somewhat relaxed and at ease about my work.	1 = B	2 = B	3	4 = A	5 = A
9. My achievements are considered to be significantly higher than those of most people I know.	1 = A	2 = A	3	4 = B	5 = B
10. Tailgating bothers me more than a car in front slowing me up.	1 = B	2 = B	3	4 = A	5 = A
11. In conversation I often gesture with hands and head.	1 = A	2 = A	3	4 = B	5 = B
12. I rarely drive a car too fast.	1 = B	2 = B	3	4 = A	5 = A
13. As a young person I preferred work in which I could move around.	1 = A	2 = A	3	4 = B	5 = B

	DEFINITELY TRUE	MOSTLY TRUE	DON'T KNOW	MOSTLY FALSE	DEFINITELY FALSE
14. People consider me to be rather quiet.	1 = B	2 = B	3	4 = A	5 = A
15. Sometimes I think I shouldn't work so hard but something drives me on.	1 = A	2 = A	3	4 = B	5 = B
16. I usually speak more softly than most people	1 = B	2 = B	3	4 = A	5 = A
17. My handwriting is rather fast.	1 = A	2 = A	3	4 = B	5 = B
18. I often work slowly and leisurely.	1 = B	2 = B	3	4 = A	5 = A
19. I thrive on challenging situations. The more challenges I have the better.	1 = A	2 = A	3	4 = B	5 = B
20. I prefer to linger over a meal and enjoy it.	1 = B	2 = B	3	4 = A	5 = A
21. I like to drive a car rather fast when there is no speed limit.	1 = A	2 = A	3	4 = B	5 = B
22. I like work that is slow and deliberate.	1 = B	2 = B	3	4 = A	5 = A
23. In general I approach my work more seriously than most people I know.	1 = A	2 = A	3	4 = B	5 = B
24. I talk more slowly than most people.	1 = B	2 = B	3	4 = A	5 = A
25. I've often been asked to be an officer of some group or groups.	1 = A	2 = A	3	4 = B	5 = B
26. I often let a problem work itself out by waiting.	1 = B	2 = B	3	4 = A	5 = A
27. I often try to persuade others to my point of view.	1 = A	2 = A	3	4 = B	5 = B

		DEFINITELY TRUE	MOSTLY TRUE	DON'T KNOW	MOSTLY FALSE	DEFINITELY FALSE
28.	I generally walk more slowly than most people.	1 = B	2 = B	3	4 = A	5 = B
29.	I eat rapidly even when there is plenty of time.	1 = A	2 = A	3	4 = B	5 = B
30.	I usually work fast.	1 = A	2 = A	3	4 = B	5 = B

Chapter Three

Mental Health

Probing Your Emotions

1. Recall your most depressing day in the last month. List some of the steps you took to get over the blues. They might have been active—like going for a walk or seeing a movie—or passive—like going to bed. Why are these activities effective for you?

2. What is the difference in how you would feel if you
   a. broke your arm and sought treatment from an orthopedist
   b. suffered from depression and sought treatment from a psychiatrist
Seeking outside help for a broken arm is obvious, but many people feel mental problems should be "handled" by the individual. What is the source of this curious difference in attitudes?

3. Matt and Marsh are brothers majoring in pre-med. Both fail their chemistry midterm examination. Marsh is depressed for two weeks; Matt is disappointed but doesn't see it as a big deal and tells Marsh to take it in stride. Why do you think they handle the situation so differently? What are some of the sources of their adjustment differences?

4. Probably all of us have been rejected by someone else (friend, parent, lover) at least once. What was your reaction to such a rejection? What did you feel? What did you do?

Chapter Contents

WHAT MENTAL HEALTH IS NOT
WHAT MENTAL HEALTH IS
MODELS OF HUMAN NATURE
The biological model
The behaviorist model
The Freudian model
The humanist model
Implications of the four models
HUMAN PROBLEMS
Rejection and alienation
Anxiety and depression
Stress and conflict
Manipulation
PROMOTING MENTAL HEALTH
GETTING HELP
APPROACHES TO THERAPY
Biological therapy
Behavior therapy
Psychotherapy
Psychoanalysis
The humanist-existential therapies
Transactional analysis
Group therapy and the encounter group
   movement

Boxes

Sampling America's emotional health
Maslow on self-actualization
Erik Erikson's stages of
   psychosocial development
Suicide among college students
A self-change program: how to go about it

Normality
The mental state attributed to the majority
of people in a population at a given time.

Statistical concept
A concept that is derived from a branch of
mathematics that has to do with probability.

Self-actualized
An adjective describing a person who has
achieved the highest level of growth
according to a hierarchy developed by the
psychologist Maslow. When people are
self-actualized, they are motivated by what
the self chooses freely.

3 Mental health is a function of continuous interplay between human beings and their environment. The environment serves as the source of everything material that we require for life. It also places adaptive requirements on us and constrains what we can do. But the interaction is not one-sided. In using environmental resources, we also alter our own world. We not only are shaped by our encounters with the environment, but we also shape that environment. Our mental health seems to be influenced by our biology, psychology, and life experiences. Our heredity and environment set us on our course.

Any definition of mental health is fraught with controversy, but some definitions seem to be better than others. What follows is our own perspective on mental health.

What Mental Health Is Not

Mental health is not the same as *normality*. Normality is a *statistical concept*. Normal is whatever state most of the people in a population are in a given time. What is normal for a Manhattan store clerk might not be normal for a Nigerian sorcerer. If we take normality as a standard of health we are quickly led to the ridiculous. By this standard, an official in a Nazi concentration camp who felt guilty for mass murders would be less healthy than one who did not. We would also have to call Galileo mad (some people did) for seeing the solar system as we now know it to be.

Never having had professional help does not necessarily mean that a person is mentally healthy. Similarly, nothing is necessarily "wrong" with someone who has had psychotherapy, although many still think there is. (When the press announced that Senator Thomas Eagleton had at one time been under the care of a psychiatrist, he was forced to withdraw as a 1972 candidate for the vice-presidency.)

Nor can we say that adjustment to society or to "reality" is a sure sign of mental health. What if the society is sick? Whose "reality" is the one that is healthy? Many of the greatest leaders of this and other societies have been people who refused to adjust to what they considered wrong. One could say that they "adjusted" by trying to change what they did not like, but they did not accept things as they were.

We cannot say a person is mentally ill or mentally healthy on the basis of symptoms alone. Healthy people may still have problems, and unhealthy people may not show any symptoms. Some pathological killers have seemed mild-mannered and harmless right up to the minute they started killing.

Not even everlasting happiness is a positive indication of mental health. In the first place, no one is happy all the time. Healthy people have ups and downs, too. But they are exceptional largely in their ability to experience their feelings, no matter what these are—joy, sadness, excitement, grief, frustration, anger, satisfaction.

Finally, although healthy people are able to function in all the areas of their lives—love, play, work—not all people who are able to function are healthy. This ability to function totally has sometimes been taken mistakenly as *the* standard for mental health.

What Mental Health Is

In recent years, people have come to think of wellness as much more than just not being sick. Wellness is a positive quality. Abraham Maslow studied healthy, *self-actualized* people who seemed to be realizing their full potential. In *Toward a Psychology of Being* (1962), he listed the qualities that they share:

They are able to deal with the world as it is, not as it should be.

They are able to accept themselves, others, and nature.

They experience more profound interpersonal relations.

They have a continuing freshness of appreciation for what goes on around them.

They are able to direct themselves independently of the culture and environment.

They trust their own senses and feelings.

They are creative.

They are democratic in their attitudes.

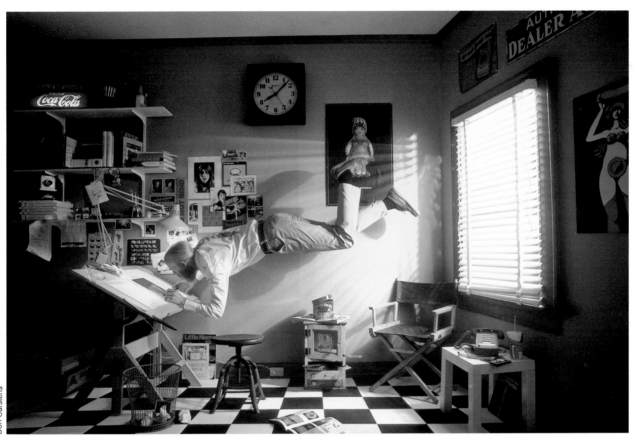

Don Carstens

Sampling America's Emotional Health

The mental health of the American citizenry is a subject of enduring scientific interest, and at least four major surveys have been conducted during the past 30 years to estimate the rate of psychological dysfunction in the general population. Estimates from those surveys have ranged from a low of 10 percent to a high of over 80 percent. In 1979, the National Institute of Mental Health (NIMH) in Rockville, Md., began the largest and most systematic survey of psychiatric disorders ever—covering 20,000 households in five U.S. cities—and the preliminary findings from three of the sites offer some challenges to psychiatric dogma.

The most surprising report is that the highest rates for most psychiatric disorders were found among young adults—primarily among those between 25 and 44 years old and secondly among 18- to 24-year-olds. The researchers anticipated that the oldest group (those over 65) would report more illness, having lived more years at risk; but the elderly showed the highest rates only for general intellectual impairment. Most serious psychiatric illnesses—including schizophrenia, panic disorder, obsessive-compulsive disorder, depression, anti-social personality and alcohol dependency—were much more common among younger adults. According to NIMH epidemiologist Darrel A. Regier, a director of the

study, these data are difficult to interpret with confidence; they may reflect a sampling bias or the fact that older people fail to report problems more often (perhaps because they forget). However, Regier adds, the data also raise the possibility that a true historical increase in mental illness has taken place over the past few generations.

The scientists also found that the most common problem in American society today is alcohol dependency, which affected one of every seven adults surveyed. This runs contrary to the widely held view that depression is the most prevalent psychological disorder. Phobias, too, were found to be somewhat more common than depression, which ranked third and was diagnosed in about 5 percent of the population. Drug abuse was the fourth most prevalent disorder, and not surprisingly, it was found largely among the 18- to 24-year-olds.

The survey data were gathered from interviews with more than 11,000 adults living in Baltimore, St. Louis, and New Haven, Conn., by researchers at Johns Hopkins University, Washington University and Yale University, respectively. According to the preliminary report . . . the data were remarkably consistent across all three sites. Other findings include:

■ Men had slightly higher rates of mental illness than did women, con-

tradicting another common view—that women are more susceptible to emotional illness. The survey only included 15 selected disorders, however, so that the prevalence rates may not accurately reflect the total psychiatric disability in the community, the researchers note. As other studies have suggested, women and men suffer from different disorders. Men were five times as likely to have alcohol problems and antisocial personality, where women were twice as likely to be depressed and reported many more cases of phobia—including agoraphobia . . .

■ Blacks and whites had equal overall rates of illness. Blacks had slightly higher rates for drug dependence and phobia; whites had slightly higher rates for anorexia nervosa and depression.

■ There was no association between bereavement and depression.

■ City dwellers had modestly higher rates of mental illness than did those from rural areas. Those with a college education had modestly lower rates than those without.

Data from an additional 7,000 interviews in Los Angeles and North Carolina, now being compiled, are expected to provide information on distress in Hispanic and rural communities.

Science News

Authenticity
Genuineness.

Neurotic needs
Needs that are unrealistic because they are out of proportion, inappropriate, or too rigid.

Outer-directed
An adjective describing a person who looks to others for guidance in how to behave.

Inner-directed
An adjective describing a person who has an inner set of rules about how to behave.

Self-image
The mental pictures that people have of themselves.

Sidney Jourard, in "The Invitation to Die," suggests some of the causes of wellness:

> In the average person, the one who is not sick, higher-level (beyond normality) wellness appears to ensue from such events as having one's individuality respected and acknowledged . . . i.e., being listened to with understanding and of being touched. Being heard and touched by another who "cares" seems to reinforce identity, mobilize spirit, and promote self-healing.

What are the qualities mentally healthy people seem to have? We shall try to define mental health by describing several of these qualities.

Very small children have the quality of being "real." They respond in a genuine, spontaneous way to whatever happens. When people are genuine, they have no pretenses. They are not phony, and they do not need to censor their words or actions. They do not plan what they say or how they act to get approval or to make an impression. They are, instead, un-self-consciously themselves here and now. This quality is sometimes called *authenticity*.

Mentally healthy people are also realistic. They know the difference between what is and what should be. They also know what they can change and what they cannot. Many times unrealistic people get stuck with their idea of what should be. This habit makes them unable to accept what is and forces them to spend great amounts of energy trying to push the world and the people in it into a shape that comes close to their ideal picture of it. Realistic people accept evidence that contradicts what they believe or want to believe, and, if it is important, modify their beliefs accordingly.

Healthy people know what their needs are and do what they must to satisfy them. They do not pretend to be helpless. They also do not waste energy trying to satisfy *neurotic needs*. Neurotic needs are needs that do not promote personal growth. They also can never be satisfied because they are masquerading for some other (perhaps unknown) needs. The unknown needs remain unsatisfied, no matter how many times the known (neurotic) needs are met.

Healthy people take responsibility for their own feelings and actions. They do not mistake their own feelings for someone else's actions. They do not blame others for their own actions. For example, it is both more responsible and more honest to say, "I'm feeling rattled," than to say, "You're trying to confuse me." A person who no longer says, "He made me do it," or, "It was all her fault," is also moving toward personal responsibility.

Being free and autonomous is another characteristic of mentally healthy people. Freedom is more than simply not being controlled by something or someone outside. Many people, for example, shrink from being themselves and expressing their feelings because they fear disapproval and rejection. They are unable to act freely and respond only to what they feel as outside pressure. This behavior is called *outer-directed*. *Inner-directed* people are sensitive to their natural impulses and responses, and they trust them. They are not afraid to be themselves. Free people act because they choose to act, not because they are driven or pressured. When a free person says yes, it is not because he or she is afraid of displeasing someone. When free people say no, it is not because they are afraid to say yes. Free people also respect the rights of others to be free.

Mentally healthy people have a good *self-image*. This means that they have positive mental pictures and positive good feelings about themselves, about what they are capable of, and about the roles they play. People with good self-images like themselves, and they are better able to like others genuinely. They are also likely to live up to their positive feelings about themselves, which, in turn, reinforces these feelings. Having a good self-image is based on a realistic assessment of one's own worth and value and capabilities. It does not mean being "stuck on yourself."

Healthy people can be comfortable with silence and with being alone. Some people feel they must have a radio or stereo going constantly to drown out the silence. Others cannot stand to be alone and feel they must always be surrounded by people. Still others require definite signs of civilization, lights, hamburger joints, gas stations, anything, just as long as they do not feel alone. These people are likely to be running away from something within themselves, feelings that they cannot face. Healthy people often seek solitude and silence to refresh and renew themselves. A time away, whether it is in the next room or on a remote beach, also seems to make it possible for many of these people to continue

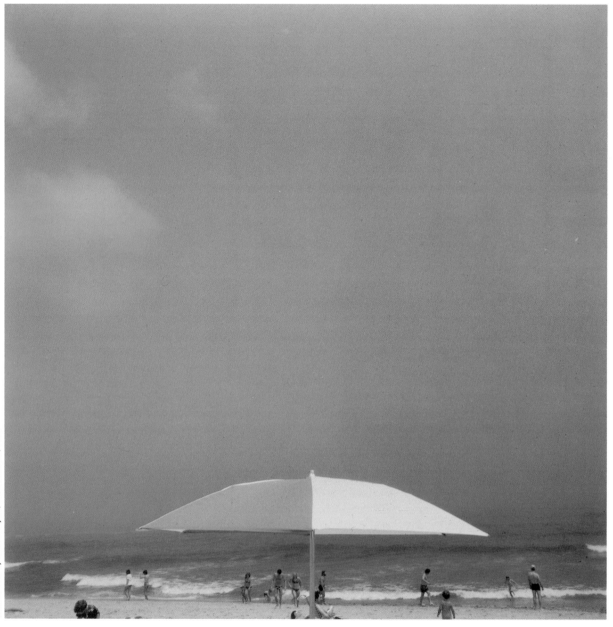

Untitled work by Michael Myers, Massachusetts, 1980

Emotional intimacy
A closeness between people that includes a mutual awareness and influence of feelings.

Perceptiveness
The ability to notice things.

to be more open and responsive to the stimulation of people and activity when they return.

Healthy people are capable of physical and emotional intimacy. Their senses, feelings, and body processes are not blocked. They are open to the pleasure of touching intimately and to the risks and the satisfactions of being close to another person in a caring, sensitive way. Intimate touching means "good sex," but it also means something much more. It means intense awareness of both your partner and yourself in which contact becomes communion and communication and a shared joy. *Emotional intimacy* can exist only when two people openly and honestly share their feelings.

Being aware of feelings and being able to express them are also characteristics of mentally healthy people. Part of the reason small children seem so real is that they know instantly how they feel, and so does anyone who is around them. Many adults and older children have been taught to hide their feelings from themselves and from others. Indeed, in this culture, learning to disguise feelings is often considered to be part of growing up. It would be healthier for children (and adults) if they were encouraged to recognize and handle their emotions rather than to hide or deny them. A child who is crying, for example, is crying for a real reason. If he or she is forced to stop crying, at least two things may happen (and possibly more). The child may doubt the truth of the feelings because of being told to stop them. And he or she will have to physically react against them to shut them off. To stop crying, the child must tighten the chest and diaphragm muscles. The result for the child is likely to be confusion (between what is felt and what "should" be felt) and long-lasting physical tensions. Being aware of true feelings and being able to express them in appropriate ways is perhaps one of the most hard won of the qualities associated with mental health.

Being self-actualized is another indicator of mental health. As Maslow studied healthy people, he decided he would have to stop thinking of creativeness in conventional terms. He found that many healthy people are not great poets, scientists, musicians, or leaders. Instead, they are people who live their everyday lives in creative ways: "A first-rate soup is more creative than

a second-rate painting." He saw in these people a special kind of *perceptiveness*, something psychologist Carl Rogers called "openness to experience." In *Toward a Psychology of Being*, Maslow suggested that self-actualized creativeness was

in many respects like the creativeness of *all* happy and secure children. It was spontaneous, effortless, innocent, easy, a kind of freedom from stereotypes and clichés. And again it seemed to be made up largely of "innocent" freedom of perception, and "innocent" uninhibited spontaneity and expressiveness. Almost any child can perceive more freely (than any adult) without a priori expectations about what ought to be there, what must be there, or what has been there.

Self-actualized people are not frightened by the unknown. They do not feel it necessary to reduce uncertainty or avoid it. They are in fact attracted to the unknown. They do not share conventional ways of seeing certain things as opposites. For example, they do not see selfishness and altruism as opposed to each other. They also have "lack of fear of their own insides, of their own impulses, emotions, thoughts." They seem to be what Rogers called "fully functioning persons." None of these qualities is the result of a superhuman effort. These people do not become "higher" beings. They are simply not inhibited in being themselves.

Models of Human Nature

How and what people see is determined largely by the model, the picture of reality, that they carry in their minds. Students of human behavior have proposed at least four different models of behavior: the biological, behaviorist, intrapsychic, and humanist models. It is important to note that these models are not mutually exclusive. Concepts from each may form the individual's view of reality.

The Biological Model   The biological model recognizes that human beings are animals with an evolutionary history that has shaped not only their anatomy and physiology but their behavior and their emotions. The

Maslow on Self-Actualization

Abraham Maslow, a psychologist representative of the humanistic movement, assumes that man is basically good, and that growth motivation helps the individual to progress toward *self-actualization*—the full realization of one's human potential. In Maslow's view, behavior is goal-directed and purposeful and is motivated by higher needs for self-actualization and growth as well as by more primitive biological needs. Maslow arranges motives in a hierarchy ascending from such basic needs as hunger and thirst through safety and love needs to needs for esteem, understanding, aesthetic order, and ultimately, self-actualization.

One of his greatest interests was the study of self-actualization. He selected such people as Lincoln, Jefferson, and Einstein, whom he judged to be highly self-actualizing, and suggested (1968) that the following attributes are most characteristic of them:

1. Perceive reality accurately
2. Accepting of self, of other people, and of the world
3. Spontaneous and natural
4. Concerned with problems outside themselves and capable of retaining a broad perspective
5. Need and want privacy and solitude; able to depend on their own potentialities
6. Autonomous; fairly independent of extrinsic satisfactions (such as popularity and reputation)
7. Capable of a continued freshness of appreciation of even the most commonplace everyday experience
8. Experience mystic ("oceanic") feelings in which they feel out of time and place and at one with nature
9. Have a sense of identification with mankind as a whole
10. Form their deepest ties with relatively few others
11. Unprejudiced and respectful of all others; truly democratic

12. Ethical; can discriminate between means and ends
13. Thoughtful, unhostile sense of humor; can laugh at the human condition (but not at a particular person)
14. Creative and inventive, possess a naive and unspoiled freshness of approach
15. Able to have some detachment from their culture; can recognize necessary changes in society

Harriet N. Mischel and Walter Mischel
Essentials of Psychology

characteristics that make people "human"—such as their gregariousness, intelligence, and ability to communicate by language—are just as much a part of their biological heritage as the characteristics that they superficially share with other mammals, including a backbone, hair, and breast feeding. All of these characteristics, behavioral as well as physiological, have evolved over millions of years and have enabled the species to survive the threats to existence that face all living creatures—threats such as predators, disease, and extremes of heat and cold. Humans have not survived because they are the fastest or strongest or because they are blessed with the keenest senses. Rather, humans have survived because of their curiosity and intelligence, their social structures, and their ability to share old traditions and new information within and among generations.

In its more philosophical aspects, the biological perspective of human nature views human behavior and social life in the context of evolution and in the context of ecological adaptation and survival.

In its modern version, the biological viewpoint is that human behavior is the joint product of both its biological heritage and the individual's personal history in the broadest psychological and cultural context. It is not a question of nature or nurture but both.

In its more clinical aspect, the biological perspective views human behavior and psychopathology from the perspective of genetic inheritance, biological mechanisms, and individual historical psychodynamic and cultural influences. Genetic factors appear to influence individual personality, temperament, and certain specific abilities in such areas as mathematics, music, and athletics. Remarkable similarities, for example, have been found in identical twins who share the same genes but who were raised apart, often without knowledge of each other's existence. There is also considerable evidence that genetic inheritance may predispose some individuals to certain types of mental disorders, such as manic-depressive illness and *schizophrenia*. If a parent is a *manic-depressive*, for example, the risk of the

Schizophrenia
A mental disorder that involves a disturbance in thinking and in perceiving reality.

Manic-depressive
A person suffering from a mental disease that is characterized by cycles of depression and mania. During the manic phase of the disease, people may be hyperactive, elated, and irritable.

Stimulus-response bit
A conceptual unit consisting of sensory input to the organism and the response that input produces.

Stimulus/stimuli (plural form)
Anything that causes an organism to respond.

Conditioning
The simplest type of learning in which a new stimulus-response connection is made.

Reinforcer
A reward or punishment, depending on how it is perceived.

Behavior modification
A technique that rewards desired behavior and punishes undesired behavior

Desensitization
A technique that reduces fear by gradually increasing exposure to the thing that is feared.

---

disorder in a child is increased about four times. This does not mean that all or even most children of manic-depressives will develop the illness, and it does not mean that all mental illnesses have been proven to have a genetic basis. But it does clearly indicate that biological factors have to be considered in the etiology of mental disorders.

The Behaviorist Model The behaviorists focus on the scientific method. They differ from the biologists in emphasizing function instead of structure. They focus on how something reacts rather than on how it is put together. The "atoms" the behaviorists work with are *stimulus-response bits,* bits of behavior that can be measured. The groundwork for the behaviorist model was laid in the late nineteenth century when Ivan Pavlov found that he could train (condition) a dog to salivate in response to various signals. About 60 years ago, in *Psychological Care of Infant and Child* (1928), John Watson first set forth the theory: "The time has come when psychology must discard all reference to consciousness. . . . Its sole task is the prediction and control of behavior."

In other words, psychology was to be a science, just like any other science. Watson reasoned more or less as follows: Scientific study is objective observation of facts that can be measured. What a person feels, senses, perceives, thinks, dreams, or imagines cannot be measured; hence it cannot be included in any scientific study. Some behaviorists carry this thought a step further and assume that what they cannot measure does not exist.

In the behaviorist model, all behavior is constructed out of stimulus-response bits. Any action that can be seen is a direct response to a *stimulus,* either past or present. The process is purely reactive. Individual differences are only the result of different past stimuli. A human being is a sort of pinball machine with a memory circuit. If we can measure the strength of a rat's motivation to get food by the number of hours it has been deprived of food, we can, according to B. F. Skinner, a prominent behaviorist, measure a person's motivation the same way.

Behaviorists generally assume that there is no such thing as human nature. They consider a person at birth to be a *tabula rasa,* or blank slate, completely moldable

and without features. He or she can be molded, or shaped, in any way by learning, and learning means *conditioning.*

Conditioning is a simple process. If you want a certain behavior in a pigeon or a person, you reward that behavior whenever it occurs. This procedure is called positive reinforcement. If you do not want a certain behavior, you either punish it, called aversive conditioning or ignore it. A *reinforcer* is a reward or a punishment.

Mental health from the behaviorist viewpoint is a matter of learning, or conditioning. A person can be only what he or she has been programmed or conditioned to be. If the organism is not functioning efficiently, it must first be deconditioned, then reconditioned. So far, most nonlaboratory attempts to apply behaviorism have been directed to solving highly specific problems such as fear of heights or fear of snakes. *Behavior modification* and *desensitization* are the methods most often used. Behavior modification is the rewarding of desired behavior or the punishing of undesired behavior or both. Desensitization usually involves reducing fears by gradual exposure to the feared stimulus or by associating the stimulus with pleasurable stimuli. Skinner does not believe in using punishment. He feels that using re-

Untitled work by Michael Myers, 1980

Psychoanalysis
The psychological theory originated by Sigmund Freud or a therapy that is based on Freud's theory.

Motivation
The plan or force that pushes an organism to a goal.

Unconscious
That which is in the mind but is out of awareness.

Consciousness
The part of mental activity that one is aware of.

Archetype
A recurring theme or pattern with threads of common experience.

Persona
In Jungian theory, the mask or face we present to the outside world.

Shadow
In Jungian theory, the hidden, unconscious parts of the mind.

Defense mechanisms
Mental devices for controlling anxiety.

Armoring of the ego
Defense mechanisms that have become fixed personality characteristics. These mechanisms act like armor in protecting the self from anxiety.

---

wards works better and avoids the possibility that punishments may so disturb or anger the subject that learning is blocked altogether.

The Freudian Model Sigmund Freud and *psychoanalysis* are so closely associated that we can hardly think of one without the other. Freud was medically trained, first as a physiologist, then as a neurologist. Later he became a psychiatrist. His first model for human nature was biological. His theories eventually took him very far from that view, but he always hoped to find the link that would tie up psychoanalysis and the physical sciences.

Freud was primarily interested in *motivation*. Why do people act in such strange and unpredictable ways? Why, with all the power of reasoning humans have, do they continue to behave as if they have none?

Freud believed that the answers to those questions were in the *unconscious*. Most of us give reasons for our behavior or what we think are reasons. The real reasons, however, are hidden from *consciousness*. This idea is the center of the Freudian model: Human behavior is determined by unconscious motivations.

This psychic determinism, in Freud's view, is so complete and thorough that there is no such thing as an accident in human behavior. Everything we do or say has some meaning in terms of inner motives. It is a persuasive idea. Consider how often and widely the phrase *Freudian slip* is used to mean "slip of the tongue." The implication is that such a slip reveals inner intent and that the unconscious is expressing itself, whether the conscious would or not.

The unconscious does not, however, express itself directly; it speaks symbolically. Meaning is hidden and revealed at the same time. To find out what the unconscious is saying, one must interpret the symbols. In one of the most familiar and classic examples of Freudian symbolism—the phallic symbol—any cylindrical object, a pencil, a hose, a snake, is likely to represent a penis. Symbolism is also the basis of Freudian dream analysis. The analyst tries to decipher and interpret the symbols of the dream, explaining what each symbol actually stands for in the dreamer's life.

Some psychoanalysts who were followers of Freud later deserted Freud's camp. Alfred Adler believed that what motivates human behavior is not, as Freud suggested, sexuality but the will to power. Otto Rank believed that the significant event of a person's early life is the trauma of birth and that all later activities are attempts to return to the womb.

Two of the deserters—Carl Jung and Wilhelm Reich—seem particularly interesting to many people now because some of their theories fit the humanist model of human nature.

Carl Jung tried to understand human nature in the largest possible context. He looked for significant principles and relationships in cultures as well as in individuals. And he looked in such areas as philosophy, theology, music, dance, art, mythology, and anthropology. It became clear that there were widely differing images of human nature. He also found threads of common experiences: similar themes in the myths, legends, symbols, tendencies, and cultural patterns of different cultures. These recurring themes or patterns he called *archetypes*. He believed that the psyche has three parts: a personal consciousness, a personal unconscious, and a collective unconscious. The collective unconscious runs throughout the species and contains the archetypes. Jung also believed that the psyche has two sides. One side is the *persona* (which is the Latin word for "mask"). This side is the "face" the person presents to the world, the role he or she assumes to meet social demands. The other side is the *shadow*, the hidden side of the psyche.

Wilhelm Reich, almost alone among former followers of Freud, did not reject the idea that sexual repression is central to neurosis. What he did reject totally was Freud's belief that *defense mechanisms* are necessary to health and that the individual's instinctual demands must give way to the demands of society. He emphasized that repressions and other defense mechanisms are the neuroses and that only sexual freedom can eliminate neurosis from society.

Reich's ideas about neurosis seem to be significant to an increasing number of people. He stressed the formation of problems in the muscles of the body in response to conflicts in early childhood. In *Character Analysis* (1949), he called this process the *armoring of the ego:* "The armoring of the ego takes place as a result of the fear of punishment, at the expense of id energy, and contains the prohibitions and standards of parents and teachers."

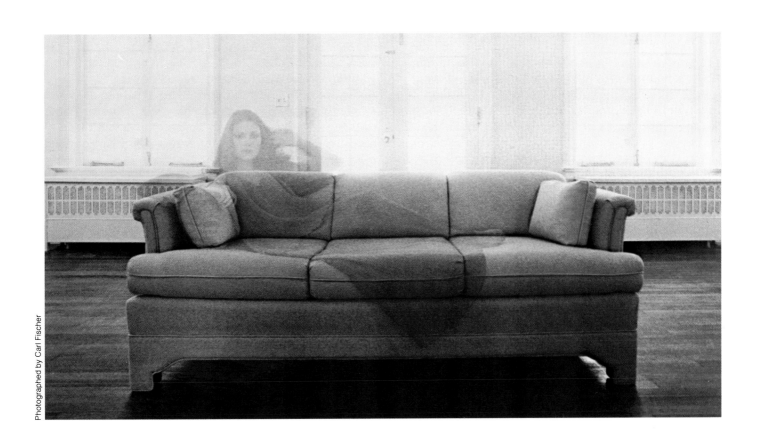

Photographed by Carl Fischer

63

Role playing
Acting the part of another person or the
part of another side of one's self as in a
play. This process is a psychotherapeutic
technique usually used in a group setting.

The immediate purpose of armoring is to block feeling, originally sexual feeling. Blocking sexual feeling, however, becomes the basis for blocking other feelings—love, hate, anger, anxiety. A person usually blocks feelings by tightening the stomach muscles and holding the breath. Reich called habitual ways of blocking repressed feelings character armor, or muscular armor.

The Humanist Model In *Toward a Psychology of Being*, Abraham Maslow, formerly a behaviorist, wrote:

> There is now emerging over the horizon a new conception of human sickness and of human health, a psychology that I find so thrilling and so full of wonderful possibilities that I yield to the temptation to present it publicly even before it is checked and confirmed, and before it can be called reliable scientific knowledge.

Maslow then listed the assumptions of this new model:

1. People have a biologically based inner nature that is "natural" and partly unchangeable.
2. Part of this nature is unique to each individual and part is shared by all humans.
3. We can study this inner nature scientifically and discover what it is like.
4. This inner nature seems not to be evil. It is either "neutral, or positively 'good.'" The possibilities of human nature "have customarily been sold short."
5. "Since this inner nature is good or neutral rather than bad, it is best to bring it out and to encourage it rather than to suppress it."
6. Denying or suppressing this inner nature causes sickness.
7. This inner nature is easily overcome by "habits, cultural pressures, and wrong attitudes toward it."
8. Even though denied, this inner nature "persists underground forever pressing for actualization."
9. Discipline, deprivation, frustration, pain, and tragedy are desirable to the extent that they "reveal and foster and fulfill our inner nature."

It is easier to see Maslow's central points if we contrast his model of human nature to two other views. The first is the traditional viewpoint of Western religion: Humans are born evil; and what is natural is probably corrupt. Since humans are naturally evil, the task of education is to constrain them, to correct by force their deviant ways and make them behave in good ways.

The second view is the one that sees people as only empty machines, nothing to begin with. A person can only become something by being molded or hammered into shape. Humanness is not necessarily a part of the mechanistic model; it must be programmed into the individual by parents and teachers.

Humanists feel that both of these approaches do violence to the individual and prevent him or her from becoming self-fulfilled. "Trust what is natural in yourself and others" is the humanist attitude simply stated.

One of the humanist assumptions is that what keeps a person from being happier or more effective or more successful is a block, something that makes it impossible for the person to use inborn qualities. It has nothing to do with personal shortcomings or defects. We are all functioning at a fraction of our potential. Freeing blocked energy is an important goal for many humanists. To be self-actualized in the humanist model is to be using all the faculties, all the talent, all the awareness, all the power that we all already have within ourselves.

Another humanist assumption is the unity of the self and of the self with nature. If we fragment ourselves or split ourselves in two (for example, into mind and body or flesh and spirit), we create unnecessary conflict and confusion. In line with this thinking, humanists see the human organism as something that grows from its own center according to a natural pattern, not as a house constructed with bricks and mortar from outside plans.

Humanists believed that people can overcome earlier conditioning and can take full responsibility for their own choices that they make freely. They believe that people are most alive when they are most aware. Further, they do not believe that people are the same as rats. Humans are unique and cannot be understood by way of animal experiments. Subject matter for psychology should be chosen because it is relevant to human life, not because it is easy to quantify.

Neurosis is a split. It is a split between the individual and his or her feelings. And it is a split, according to humanistic psychiatrist R. D. Laing, between the true, inner self and the false, outer self, the one that emerges when children lose their spontaneity. What happens is that children give up being themselves and begin trying to be the people their parents or others want them to

Erik Erikson's Stages of Psychosocial Development

From Erikson's point of view individuals develop through stages, and in each stage they meet a psychosocial crisis that is characteristic of it. In the first stage, children are confronted with the issue of trust versus mistrust, particularly in their relationships with their mothers. In resolving this issue, children develop enduring attitudes related to how safe the world is, how nurturant a place it is, and how freely they are able to offer affection to others. The solution to this crisis—as well as to the others—determines the extent to which people will develop. Erikson is a psychoanalyst who focuses on the psychosocial development of the individual in a framework of broad social and cultural forces. His ideas have had a tremendous impact on concepts of human nature. One of the most interesting of these is that there is an *identity crisis in adolescence.*

Adolescence is the time when individuals are struggling with various contradictions within themselves. A boy, for example, might like to appear tough and masculine in front of his peers. He might also

be drawn toward activities he views as feminine, such as art, music, and dancing. If he is unable to resolve the clashing elements within himself, he will suffer from what Erikson calls "identity diffusion." He will not have succeeded in "finding himself." The "search for identity" is part of adolescence in our culture. People can find themselves too early and close the door on rewarding experiences and experimentation that could lead to later personal fulfillment. For

example, the girl who marries the boy next door after high school graduation and raises a family right away does not give herself a chance to explore life's potentials. Erikson suggests that all people must generate for themselves individual central perspectives and directions that give them a meaningful sense of unity and purpose and that integrate the remnants of their childhoods with the expectations and aspirations of adulthood.

Age	Psychosexual stage	Important persons	Psychosocial crisis
0–1	Oral	Mother	Trust vs. mistrust
1–3	Anal	Parents	Autonomy vs. shame
3–5	Phallic	Family unit	Initiative vs. guilt
5–12	Latency	Neighborhood and school	Industry vs. inferiority
12–17	Adolescence	Peer groups	Identity vs confusion
17–22	Genital	Close friends; sex partners	Intimacy vs. isolation
Middle adult		Work associates; shared household	Generativity vs. self-absorption
Older adult		Mankind	Integrity vs. despair

Source: Based on Erik Erikson, *Childhood and Society*, W. W. Norton, New York, 1963.

be. Sometimes the strategy fails. Even the false self cannot always meet the demands and expectations of others, and madness results.

Learning—and education—in the humanist model is learning by doing, by direct experience. *Role playing* and taking part in both simulated experiences and real situations are preferred over such standard practices as listening to lectures and reading texts. Feeling an experience is more real and more whole than thinking about it. Humanists believe that thinking can interfere with feeling.

Implications of the Four Models Reality is never simply what we see; it is in large part what we have learned to see. Each person sees the events of his or her everyday life according to some model. The model

could be modern European or Chinese or Hopi or any one of hundreds of others. Even time and space are based more on models of perception—learned through language—than on some tangible reality "out there."

The four models of human nature we have described all come out of the same overall cultural tradition. Even though they seem to differ hugely, each of us can probably see glimmers of our own experience in each one. Perhaps the questions to ask are "Which of these models seems to fit my own experience of life? Which one matches most closely how I see myself and the people I know?"

We all experience problems. What are these problems? Being rejected, depressed, anxious, manipulated —these are a few of them. And how we see them is likely to depend on which model of reality we find

Suicide Among College Students

Approximately 1,000 college students take their own lives each year. Figures indicate that the incidence of suicide is twice as high among college students as it is among people of the same age who are not in college. Often scholastically superior, the suicidal student seldom attempts suicide because of academic difficulties or pressures. Rather, the motive is most often the failure to develop or maintain a close interpersonal relationship, usually with someone of the opposite sex. Warning signals associated with suicidal behavior include withdrawal, depression, loss of appetite, and a dramatic loss of interest in studies or other previously enjoyed activities. The student may stay alone in his or her room for long periods of time, neglecting both grooming and personal hygiene. Because the suicidal student seldom seeks professional help, it is important that these warning signals be recognized, so that help can be obtained.

Currently there are over 200 suicide prevention centers throughout the United States. Typically, the counselor—either a professional or a trained volunteer—will try to gain the caller's confidence by listening in a caring, nonjudgmental way. Once the caller has been helped through the immediate crisis, an effort is made to refer him or her to someone who is professionally qualified to provide more long-term guidance and support. With long-term help, the distressed individual may explore alternative ways of handling the stresses that initially triggered suicidal thoughts.

most believable. Models of reality influence approaches to therapy, too.

Human Problems

People do not have to be crazy or sick to have problems in living. We all have them. Even the more extreme symptoms of "mental illness" are not that different from common experience. For example, one standard of sanity is whether or not a person is in touch with reality. What is in touch, however, varies considerably from person or person, even among "normal" people. It even varies from time to time for the same person.

Some people, however, may be totally unable to test their perceptions and beliefs against reality. When this inability occurs, they will suffer illusions and delusions and be considered *psychotic*. Someone is also described as psychotic if he or she acts in a bizarre way. Standing on a street corner commanding troops that are not there is an example of bizarre behavior. *Neurotic* behavior, on the other hand, covers a wide range—from what is taken to be "normal" to such *obsessive* or *compulsive* acts as changing clothes eight times before going outside. Compulsive smoking or talking or eating are not as obvious perhaps because they are more common, but they are still compulsive—and neurotic. Some people withdraw by sleeping far more than they need to. Some people are especially likely to have accidents because of self-destructive wishes. Most of us shut off feelings, although the extent varies, and at times this can be an effective coping device (a healthy response to

stimuli overload). We may do it through tension or tics or smoking or drinking, or in any of a thousand other ways. All are generally responses to the same few basic difficulties, some of which seem to be part of the culture itself. Whether or not the behavior is labeled neurotic seems to depend largely on the degree of behavior and on who is doing the labeling and for what purpose. For one view of the spectrum, see Figure 3–1. Note also the incidence of various mental disorders according to age in Figure 3–2.

Rejection and Alienation   Almost all of us have been rejected at some time or another by someone—parent, friend, lover. It is a painful experience. Some have been rejected not because of what they are themselves but because they are members of certain religious, ethnic, or other minority groups. Women are thought by some to be inferior to men and are rejected on that basis. Many people reject children. At least as many do the same to older people, although for different reasons.

People react very intensely to being rejected. They go to great lengths to avoid even risking it. George Bach and Ronald Deutsch, authors of the book *Pairing* (1971), think that the fear of rejection is a major stumbling block to most people in trying to establish relations with members of the opposite sex. They describe role-playing exercises that help people to live through the fear and the experience of rejection. These exercises are conducted by a group leader who helps people be more aware of what they are feeling and doing, and also helps them to communicate their wants more openly and clearly. Unfortunately, most people do not have such precise

Psychosis
A severe mental disorder in which there is a distortion of reality. Symptoms might include delusions or hallucinations.

Neurosis
The presence of anxiety or other symptoms in a person who is able to perceive reality without major distortions.

Obsessive
Pertaining to thoughts that recur despite one's wish to think about something else.

Compulsive
Pertaining to actions that one feels compelled to perform in spite of mental opposition.

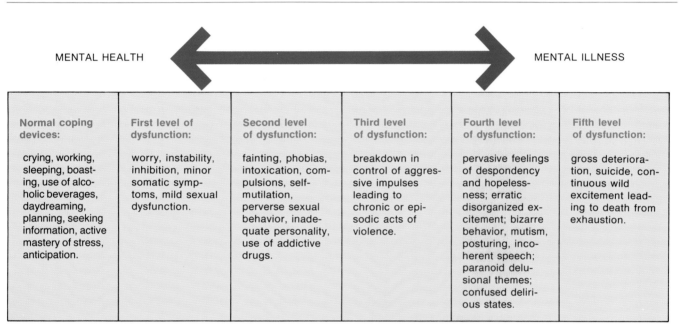

MENTAL HEALTH   MENTAL ILLNESS

Normal coping devices:	First level of dysfunction:	Second level of dysfunction:	Third level of dysfunction:	Fourth level of dysfunction:	Fifth level of dysfunction:
crying, working, sleeping, boasting, use of alcoholic beverages, daydreaming, planning, seeking information, active mastery of stress, anticipation.	worry, instability, inhibition, minor somatic symptoms, mild sexual dysfunction.	fainting, phobias, intoxication, compulsions, self-mutilation, perverse sexual behavior, inadequate personality, use of addictive drugs.	breakdown in control of aggressive impulses leading to chronic or episodic acts of violence.	pervasive feelings of despondency and hopelessness; erratic disorganized excitement; bizarre behavior, mutism, posturing, incoherent speech; paranoid delusional themes; confused delirious states.	gross deterioration, suicide, continuous wild excitement leading to death from exhaustion.

Figure 3-1   Menninger's unitary concepts of mental disorder: one view of the spectrum of mental stress.

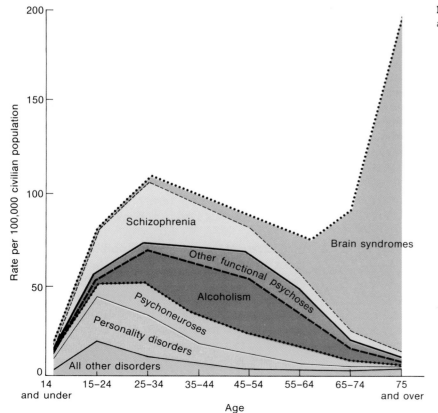

Figure 3-2   Incidence of mental disorders according to age.

Alienation
The condition of being uninvolved in or estranged from society.

Anxiety
A sense of real or imagined danger that causes physical and mental distress.

Repressed
Ideas or feelings that forces in the mind keep out of consciousness; unconscious ideas or feelings.

Depression
A prolonged feeling of dejection and low spirits often accompanied by an inability to act.

---

and specific help, and each rejection makes risking it the next time more difficult.

The sense of being "a stranger, alone and afraid, in a world I never made" runs throughout the lives of many people. Some are alienated from society. Others are alienated from nature or, perhaps most disquieting, from themselves.

Alienation may arise from a problem within the self. It may reflect a lack of internal harmony. It may also be that the person who feels alienated does so because he or she does not have a strong sense of self. If you had to change yourself into someone you did not feel like being in order to earn your parents' approval, you cannot possibly feel like yourself. In a sense, you are left without the only person you can completely identify with, and you are alienated.

Anxiety and Depression   Fear is a subjective response to something definite—a tangible present threat. If you hear strange noises coming from your basement at night, you feel fear. You might also have a feeling of fear without being able to identify what you are afraid of. Then the feeling is called *anxiety*. According to psychoanalytic theory, the source of the fear in an anxious person is unconscious. The impulses or feelings that lie behind the fear are *repressed*, but the feeling of anxiety is a sign that this defensive maneuver has not been completely successful. The possibility that these impulses or feelings might surface gives the person a sense of impending disaster. The behaviorists emphasize that fears are learned and that situations similar to the original painful ones can produce fear. The distinction between fear and anxiety is unimportant to behaviorists because their therapy is a kind of retraining that does not seek unconscious roots for feelings.

Depression may refer to prolonged sadness or to an absence of all feeling. Depression may be the result of a loss—for example, the loss of one's love or the loss of one's confidence in his or her ability to work—or, like anxiety, it may have no apparent source. For psychoanalysts the unknown source is an unconscious one, related to experiences of loss in childhood and infancy. Although explanations of this type may be valid in certain cases, some kinds of depression seem to be related to chemical disturbances in the brain.

Stress and Conflict   Pressure, tension, frustration, or conflict may place a person under stress. Stress is not just a condition of the mind. Its effects are felt throughout the body because it forces the body to draw heavily on its reserves of energy. It is not possible to avoid stress completely, but certain environments and life-styles are quite stressful. Some people are better able than others to tolerate the conditions that produce stress. These people are usually the ones who are most in touch with their own feelings. (See Chapter 2 for a fuller discussion of stress.)

Conflict can take place at a number of levels. Psychologist Kurt Lewin studied the most obvious form—that which takes place consciously. In *A Dynamic Theory of Personality* (1935), he identified three kinds of situations that create conflict:

1. *Approach-approach.* The approach-approach situation is one in which the person is forced to choose between two (or more) alternatives that are equally attractive. The person cannot have both (or all).
2. *Avoidance-avoidance.* Avoidance-avoidance is a situation in which the choice is between two (or more) equally unattractive alternatives. The person must choose one and cannot reject both (or all).
3. *Approach-avoidance.* Approach-avoidance is a situation in which each choice a person has carries with it both good and bad. No matter how the person chooses, something unpleasant will be one result of the choice.

Often we are not aware of our conflicts because they involve repressed feelings. Often we are not even aware of the tension that conflict, repression, and anxiety create. Whether we are aware of it or not tension exists in the nervous system and in the muscles.

Manipulation   Manipulation is a problem that comes up most often and obviously in relations between people. If one person tries to control another person by deception, that is manipulation. A person is also being a manipulator when he or she tries to control whether or not someone feels pleasure or pain. To ask for something or to demand it is not manipulation, but to get it by trickery or game playing or subtle coercion is. Manipulation usually involves deception. It always

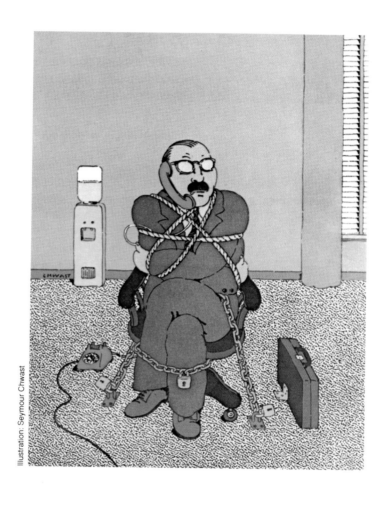

involves treating the other person as a thing, an object, rather than a person. In this sense, manipulation is one form of violence.

Everett Shostrom, in his book *Man the Manipulator* (1968), characterizes eight types of manipulators:

1. The Dictator, who pretends to be stronger than he really is, dominates, and gives orders.
2. The Weakling, who "forgets, doesn't hear, is passively silent."
3. The Calculator, who "deceives, lies, and constantly tries to outwit" others.
4. The Clinging Vine, who wants to be led and taken care of.
5. The Bully, who "controls by implied threats."
6. The Nice Guy, who "kills with kindness."
7. The Judge, who "distrusts everybody and is blameful, resentful, slow to forgive."
8. The Protector, who "spoils others, is oversympathetic, and refuses to allow those he protects to stand up and grow up for themselves."

(See Figure 3–3 for Shostrom's suggestion concerning manipulative potentials and actualizing people.)

Promoting Mental Health

There are many things that we as individuals can do to promote our own mental health. We can try, first to all, to be ourselves. By doing this, we can eliminate many of the anxieties that stem from being phony or putting on a false front. We can try to be realistic in terms of our needs, goals, and responsibilities. Just as very few people are totally self-sufficient, very few are totally helpless. We can try to be open to new ideas, to creative ways of viewing and responding to ourselves and outside stimuli. We can, most of all, be kind to ourselves. Each of us has certain capabilities and strengths, and all of us possess value and human worth. If we like ourselves, we become more comfortable with being alone sometimes, with enjoying silence, with taking time

Figure 3-3 The actualizing person as a combination of four complimentary potentials, all developed usually out of former manipulative potentials. You may not agree with the choice of examples, whose lives demonstrated these potentials in certain ways. Perhaps you can choose your own candidates.

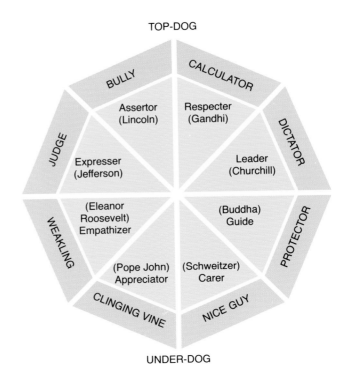

A Self-Change Program: How to Go About It

There is a definite sequence in deliberate self-direction. Most self-change programs comprise the following steps:

1. Selecting a goal.
2. Specifying the behaviors you need to change in order to reach the goal. These are often called the *target behaviors.*
3. Making observations about the target behaviors. You may keep a kind of diary describing those behaviors or count how often you engage in them. You discover the events that stimulate your acts and the things that reward them.
4. Working out a plan for change, which applies basic psychological knowledge. Your plan might call for gradually replacing an unwanted action with a desirable one. You might change the way you react to certain events. You might arrange to be rewarded for certain behaviors.

5. Readjusting your plans as you learn more about yourself. As you practice analyzing your behavior, you can make more and more sophisticated and effective plans for change.

D. L. Watson and R. G. Tharp
Self-Directed Behavior:
Self-Modification
for Personal Adjustment

---

out to renew our own strength. And as an added benefit, we ultimately strengthen our interactions with other people and our environment.

These, then, are just some of the things that we can do individually to help promote our own mental health. However, there are also actions that we can take collectively to improve the mental health of others. Consider social problems such as sexism, racial discrimination, poverty, and noise and how each can affect mental health. Collectively, we can become better informed and more vocal on the issues, take political action, join organizations, and participate in programs to alleviate specific problems that affect mental health.

Getting Help

People are gradually accepting the idea that sometimes a person needs outside help to handle personal and interpersonal problems. The process is very slow, however, and often the people who most need help are the most unwilling to get it. These people draw a distinction between having an emotional problem and a physical one. To seek help for one, whether it be warts or pneumonia, is smart. To seek help for the other is shameful, a sign of weakness.

More and more people are seeking help, however, and for a great variety of reasons. Couples having problems in their relationship are finding that they can learn new ways to communicate their feelings to each other. Families are discovering that the so-called generation gap disappears when all the family members can say what they feel and know they have been heard. In groups, people are learning more about how others see them. They are also learning to be more aware of themselves, and of what they say and do. People are learning in many ways to improve their relationships with others. Some people just want help in learning new ways to grow.

Getting help, for whatever reason, does not have to cost a fortune. Many clinics have what is called a sliding scale of fees. The individual pays only what he or she can afford. Some insurance plans pay for certain kinds of therapy. If you want or need help either in solving problems or in learning or growing, find out what the possibilities are. If you do not know where to start, first identify, if you can, the kind of help you want. Then ask your physician or clergyman or a county health office or a Family Service agency where you can go to get it.

Approaches to Therapy

Earlier in this chapter we discussed four models of human nature: (1) the biological, (2) the behaviorist, (3) the intrapsychic, and (4) the humanist. Each of these models suggests a different approach to dealing with problems of living. Biological therapy makes sense in the biological model. The behaviorist model reduces all behavior to stimulus-response bits and its matching therapy is called behavior therapy. Psychoanalysis, the technique first practiced by Freud, is the intrapsychic method. The humanist model produces the humanist-existential therapies as well as group therapy and encounter group methods. Transactional analysis does not fit any of these categories precisely. All the therapies

Phobia
An exaggerated and often inexplicable fear.

Psychotherapy
Healing by psychological means.

Therapist
A person trained to treat or rehabilitate others without using surgery.

except biological therapy are psychotherapies. None of them is "pure." They all borrow from each other, at least in part.

Biological Therapy Biological therapists most commonly use two techniques. They either give drugs to treat symptoms of mental disorders or give electroconvulsive shock treatments. Drugs are useful in treating schizophrenia and certain kinds of depression. For example, lithium has been found to control and prevent manic-depressive episodes. To a certain extent anxiety can be relieved by tranquilizers, but these drugs can easily be overused and can lead to neglecting other ways of alleviating anxiety. Shock therapy sometimes produces rapid improvement in depressions of later life that fail to respond to any other kind of treatment.

Behavior Therapy Behavior therapy is directed toward a specific problem, and the symptom is considered to be the problem. The symptom is removed, usually in one of three ways. The therapist may reward desired behavior or punish undesired behavior. The therapist may also cut down a patient's excessive sensitivity to a stimulus by applying the stimulus in small doses or in company with a stimulus that has an opposite effect. A person who has a *phobia* (excessive fear) of harmless snakes is taught to relax and then to imagine small snakes in a secure container. When this imagining can be done without fear, the person goes on to imagine more frightening snakes while remaining relaxed. In a stepwise manner therapy progresses to a point where live snakes can be handled calmly.

Psychotherapy Most forms of *psychotherapy* are "talking cures." The patient, or client as he or she is sometimes called, either talks while the *therapist* listens or talks with the therapist as the therapist guides the conversation. Several of the humanist therapies, however, rely on body manipulation techniques or on a combination of these with talking. Many of these therapies grew out of the work of Reich. They are not as common or as widely practiced as the following therapies are.

Psychoanalysis Psychoanalysis takes a long time, sometimes several years, and it can be quite expensive. Its aims are broad and ambitious, often including a change of personality structure. The patient is encouraged to say out loud whatever thoughts come into his or her head. The analyst listens and occasionally asks questions and interprets what the patient is saying. The analyst remains in the background, helping the patient to gain insight into his or her own problems.

The Humanist-Existential Therapies Many different approaches come under the heading of humanist-existential therapies. Client-centered therapy, also called Rogerian therapy after its founder, Carl Rogers, is one approach. The therapist, called a counselor or facilitator, does not interfere with the client and does not make judgments. His or her purpose is mainly to mirror what the client is saying and help him or her to sort, focus, and clarify feelings and thoughts. Gestalt therapy is another approach. In this therapy, the therapist may aggressively attack the person's defenses or encourage him or her to role play conflicting parts of his or her personality. Humanistic therapies work with individuals, couples, families, and groups.

Transactional Analysis Transactional analysis, commonly referred to as TA, is usually directed toward specific problems. The client sets a limited goal and works toward it by using specific plans the therapist suggests. People are helped to look at the self-defeating "scripts" they live by, and then to change them.

Group Therapy and the Encounter Group Movement Encounter groups and therapy groups focus on communication. The aim is for people to be real and honest with each other at the moment they are together. Group members are encouraged to stop being polite and to "level" with each other. They are expected to honestly and openly express their feelings, whether these be positive or negative.

Mental Wellness Scale

Read the following statements carefully. Choose the one in each section that best describes you at this moment and record its score at the right. (For example, "spontaneous" has a score of 5.) When you have identified five statements, total your score and find your position on the scale.

5 open to new experiences
4 accessible
3 informal
2 formal
1 hostile

Score _____

5 open to criticism
4 tolerates criticism
3 resists criticism
2 offended by criticism
1 dictatorial

Score _____

5 spontaneous
4 independent
3 self-sufficient
2 dependent
1 closed-minded

Score _____

5 up front/undisguised
4 honest
3 trustworthy
2 deceptive
1 dishonest

Score _____

5 self-confident
4 secure
3 stable
2 insecure
1 unstable

Score _____

Total score _____

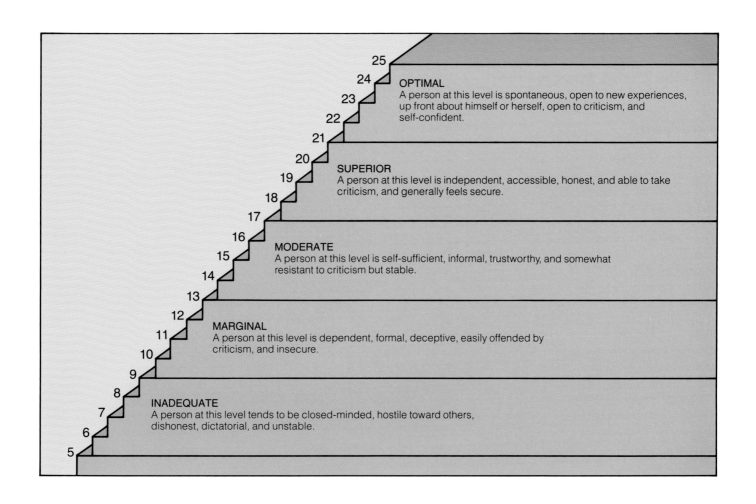

25
24
23
22
21
20
19
18
17
16
15
14
13
12
11
10
9
8
7
6
5

OPTIMAL
A person at this level is spontaneous, open to new experiences, up front about himself or herself, open to criticism, and self-confident.

SUPERIOR
A person at this level is independent, accessible, honest, and able to take criticism, and generally feels secure.

MODERATE
A person at this level is self-sufficient, informal, trustworthy, and somewhat resistant to criticism but stable.

MARGINAL
A person at this level is dependent, formal, deceptive, easily offended by criticism, and insecure.

INADEQUATE
A person at this level tends to be closed-minded, hostile toward others, dishonest, dictatorial, and unstable.

Take Action

Your answers to Probing Your Emotions at the beginning of this chapter and your placement level on the Mental Wellness Scale will, we hope, encourage you to begin a process of self-exploration and self-discovery that you will continue. Reflect on the entire chapter's content and ask yourself how each point relates to your own life. Then take action:

1. Most students have had the experience of writing lengthy papers on various topics. One topic they rarely write about is themselves. Yet this is an excellent way to explore feelings and attitudes and gain insight into aspects of yourself you rarely think about. Write your personal biography. Let your mind freely wander. Continue writing until the well runs dry.

Write anything you want to as long as it relates directly to you and your innermost feelings. When you finish consider showing it to a close friend or someone whose reactions might be valuable.

2. Answer each of the following questions in three sentences or fewer: Who am I? Who would I like to be? What are the similarities between the person you perceive yourself to be and the person you would like to be? What are the differences? What conclusions can you draw from this assignment?

3. "Peak experiences" as described by Maslow are happiest moments, most fulfilling moments, ecstatic moments, feelings of complete freedom, feelings of soaring, and so forth. People who are self-actualized

report having these feelings often. How frequently do you have such feelings? Keep track of them in your Take Action notebook for one month. Fully describe these moments of rapture so that you can review them later.

4. List the positive behaviors that help you adapt to change and remain open. Also list those behaviors that block your openness and adaptation to change. Consider how you can strengthen your existing positive behaviors and reduce the blocking behaviors. Don't forget to congratulate yourself for your positive behaviors.

5. Read the following Behavior Change Strategy, and take the appropriate action.

Behavior Change Strategy

Shy and Lonesome: Social Anxiety

Many people experience significant personal difficulty in getting along with others—particularly members of the opposite sex. This problem is usually referred to as shyness or loneliness, but researchers have coined several alternative labels such as social inhibition, heterosexual anxiety, social anxiety, and interpersonal anxiety.

College-student dating has been given the greatest amount of research attention probably because of the easy access to likely clients who are experiencing acute difficulties initiating new friendships. In collecting questionnaire data from 479 students enrolled in an introductory psychology course at Stanford University, Horowitz and French (1979) found that 5 percent of the sample, or about 25 students, could be classi-

fied as lonely. The researchers found that the most common problem for these lonely college students involved inhibited sociability. A more specific listing of the statements of lonely students is presented in the table on the next page.

Of course, it should come as no surprise that physical appearance plays a major role in terms of friendship development—but looks are often given too much credit or blame in this regard. A variety of subtle social skills is needed to initiate and then sustain human relationships. These skills include appropriate eye contact, sense of humor, reflection, facial expression, initiating topics in conversation, maintaining the flow of conversation by asking questions, and so on.

One general plan of treatment assumes a *skills-deficit perspective,* and it teaches college students how to use these interpersonal skills to

greater personal advantage by means of videotape feedback and modeling (practice exercises). Practice-dating programs in which both partners know that their interaction has been scheduled for practice and self-improvement help extend modeling well beyond the clinic into "real world" social settings.

A slightly different approach stems from the perspective that people know well enough what to do to make and keep friends—the problem of social inhibition comes from the anxiety that reduces a person's ability to perform key social skills. Reduced performance produces even greater self-doubt and anxiety, which only interferes further with later performance to produce a vicious circle of damaging experiences. With this approach people for whom anxiety plays a key role receive special training in relaxation skills and other stress management strategies—

perhaps in conjunction with the more complex and time-consuming anxiety-reduction procedure known as *systematic desensitization.* More details about these methods can be found in Chapter 2.

In most cases shyness and loneliness are not unidimensional, not easily diagnosed as being only a problem of skills or a problem of anxiety. Most programs assume that *both* skills and anxiety play a role, and these programs provide a comprehensive treatment that includes modeling, structural practice, and stress management components.

Programs usually begin with a self-monitoring phase in which all facets of a person's daily routine are noted in a diary format somewhat similar to the one found in Chapter 1. The Social Activity Diary shows how a coding scheme (noted in the key) can be used to help keep track of the pattern of social contacts, the amount of time spent in effective studying, and the amount of time wasted each day. These patterns are monitored for at least one week so that general trends can be identified.

Depending on the particular program, the shy person is then told

to make better use of "wasted time" and to begin to practice some of the skills he or she has learned in the class or clinic in the least troublesome (anxiety-producing) situations. This tactic might be translated into an assignment (and behavioral contract) to initiate brief, nonthreatening conversations with same-sex classmates on an academic topic (the upcoming midterm or the homework assignment, for example). Once these conversations are successfully accomplished, then the next phase of the program could encourage practice of discussions that involve more personal subjects (personal opinions about nonacademic topics). Later assignments might involve members of the opposite sex. The individual steps would form a type of hierarchy, incorporating topics, people, and places, from least to most difficult. The person would accomplish these steps by using a consistent theme of practice, modeling, and stress management skills while moving up the hierarchy.

One final point is in order regarding the role of a person's living situation. Research has shown that students—both male and female—

Statements Identifying Lonely College Students

It is a common problem for me to . . .

☐ Make friends in a simple, natural way.

☐ Introduce myself to others at parties.

☐ Make phone calls to others to initiate social activity.

☐ Participate in groups.

☐ Get pleasure out of a party.

☐ Get into the swing of a party.

☐ Relax on a date and enjoy myself.

☐ Be friendly and sociable with others.

☐ Participate in playing games with others.

☐ Get buddy-buddy with others.

Source: Adapted from L. M. Horowitz and R. de S. French, "Interpersonal Problems of People Who Describe Themselves as Lonely," *Journal of Consulting and Clinical Psychology* 47 (1979):762–64.

who live off campus may well have to take a more assertive role in initiating social contacts and developing friendships than students who live on campus. This is because living off campus is often more isolated than the highly concentrated social environment on campus.

SOCIAL ACTIVITY DIARY

	DATE: 11/16		DATE:		DATE:	
	AM	PM	AM	PM	AM	PM
12		I, I, W				
1		A, W				
2		S				
3		S				
4		S				
5		I, I				
6		W				
7		W				
8		S				
9		S P, P				
10	I, I, S	S				
11	S	W				

KEY

P = Social phone call
I = Social interaction (at least 5 minutes)
A = Social activity
S = Study time
W = Wasted time

Sexuality

Chapter Four

Sex and Intimacy

Probing Your Emotions

1. What boundaries exist for you because of your sex? List the behaviors that because of your gender (a) you are expected to perform, (b) you are allowed to perform, (c) you are forbidden to perform. Circle the expectations or limitations that bother you, and think of how they might be resolved.

2. Do you remember specific events from your childhood that clearly defined for you what it meant to be a member of your sex? When did you first start to accept different behaviors for each sex? If you raise your own children, how are you going to handle their acquisition of sex roles? What disadvantages would your children have if they were raised without any clearly described sex roles?

3. What advantages come with marriage and other intimate relationships? What proportion of these advantages come only from your own thinking and emotions? What proportion come from parental and societal expectations? Is there anything inappropriate about accepting traditional marriage roles?

4. Suppose a close friend tells you that he or she is homosexual. How would you react? Would you feel threatened? Would your friendship undergo any changes? Would you still talk about the same things with your friend? Could you talk freely about sexual behavior with your friend?

Chapter Contents

BIOLOGICAL DIFFERENCES
AND VARIATIONS
Genetic differences
Gonadal differences
Hormonal differences
Somatic differences

VULNERABILITY TO DISEASE
AND DISORDER

CULTURALLY INDUCED SEX
DIFFERENCES: SEX ROLES
Adult responses to childhood sexuality
Sex-role learning

SEX DIFFERENCES AND
INDIVIDUAL DIFFERENCES

BUILDING AN
INTIMATE RELATIONSHIP
How to select a compatible intimate
Conflict management: Learning to fight
Developing a sexual relationship
Marriage
Dissolution of marriage
Alternatives to marriage

Boxes

Woman—which includes man, of course:
   an experience in awareness
Love that lasts a lifetime
Compatibility quiz
Four components of love

Genitals
The reproductive organs, especially the external sex organs.

Chromosomes
Threadlike structures in the nuclei of cells. They split as cells divide and carry the genetic material that causes the new cells to be like the original cell.

Ovum (Egg)
The female reproductive cell. The egg is generated in the ovary, and after it is fertilized it develops into a new member of the same species as the parents.

Ovary
One of the two female sexual glands in which the ova (eggs) and hormones are formed. Each ovary contains a mass of vascular fibrous tissue that contains a number of follicles, each enclosing an ovum.

Sperm
The male reproductive cell that serves to impregnate the ovum.

Testicle
The male reproductive gland, the source of sperm and androgens (hormones that develop and maintain masculine characteristics).

Zygote
The cell resulting from the fusion of the ovum and the sperm; the fertilized egg.

Gene
The portion of a DNA molecule that contains the information necessary to synthesize an enzyme; carries the chromosomes in the zygote (the cell formed by the union of sperm and egg) and determines gender.

Gonads
Sexual organs; ovaries are the female gonads, and testicles are the male gonads.

---

4 When a baby girl is born, her femaleness is apparent in the most simple, direct, and natural way. Her vulva is plainly visible and plainly part of her. In the same way, a newborn baby boy wears his sex openly in the form of his penis and testicles. Within minutes the baby's tangible sex identity is covered by a diaper, and within hours the baby is wearing its sex in a symbolic form, an ID bracelet—pink beads for a girl, blue for a boy.

This encounter between culture and nature and between the symbolic and the organic continues throughout life. The baby does not know or care whether its beads are blue or pink. But once out of infancy, he or she will be expected to show signs—styles of dress, grooming, movement, gesture, language, and speech—that will allow others to read his or her sex instantly.

Adults will reinforce the child's sex identity by responding one way if they see the child as female, another way if they see it as male. The child will also find numerous sex-role taboos, the warning signs that "boys don't do that" or "girls don't do that." These patterns all become part of the child's consciousness. They are learned, then the child forgets that they were learned, and finally they are assumed to have been there always.

Studies of other cultures have shaken many of our assumptions about sex identity: Behavior considered masculine in one culture can be considered feminine in another. This fact means generally that the details of sex identity are cultural and arbitrary, not natural and organic. Some sex differences are part of our biological makeup—differences in cell structure, in hormone production, in body characteristics, and, of course, in *genital* structure. Beyond that, some studies have shown certain average differences. Females appear to have greater verbal ability, and males, greater mathematical and visual-spatial ability and more combativeness. But average differences between the two sexes are generally not as great as individual differences within each sex.

Our ability to see people as they are has also been cramped, at least until recently, by the either-or, all-or-nothing nature of the old models and the old assumptions. Biologically as well as psychologically, no one is all male or all female.

Biological Differences and Variations

In the nucleus of every cell of a woman's body is a pair of *chromosomes* of a type that we call X. Every cell in a man's body has a pair of unlike chromosomes, one X and one Y. The *ovum*, or egg, formed in a woman's *ovary* contains a single sex chromosome, and it is an X chromosome. Each *sperm* formed in a man's *testicles* also contains one chromosome, but about half the sperm cells have X chromosomes, and half, Y chromosomes.

This 50-50 distribution of X-chromosome and Y-chromosome sperm cells is the key to the 50–50 distribution of male and female babies (actually about 52-48). If the egg (X chromosome) is fertilized by an X-chromosome sperm, the new cell formed (called a *zygote*) will have an XX pair of chromosomes, and so will every cell formed from it by cell division, and the baby will be female. If the egg (X chromosome) is fertilized by a Y-chromosome sperm, the new cell formed will have an XY pair, and the baby will be male.

There are four major kinds of biological sex differences, which we call *genetic determinants,* and three of them stem from the difference between XX and XY chromosomes. The four determinants are *genes*—presence of XX and XY chromosomes; *gonads*—presence of ovaries or testicles; *hormones*—secretion of estrogen and progesterone or of testosterone; and *somatic features*—differences in size, musculature, bony structure, skin, and metabolism.

Usually the newborn baby can be identified easily as male or female on the basis of gonads alone, and its genetic sex is likely to confirm this identity. As the baby matures, its hormone secretions and body characteristics are likely to develop in accordance with its genes and gonads, but there are some possible variations.

Genetic Differences   Males normally have XY chromosomes, and females, XX chromosomes. Occasionally, however, there may be too few or too many of either X or Y. Several combinations that are considered abnormal occur.

Hormones
Chemical substances formed in one part of the body and carried to another part where they stimulate certain responses. Sex hormones stimulate and promote the development of sex characteristics. Male hormones as a group are called androgens, the most abundant of which is testosterone; female hormones belong to two major groups, estrogen and progesterone.

Somatic features
Physical characteristics.

Fertilization
The initiation of biological reproduction, as, for example, when the sperm and ovum unite to form a zygote (fertilized egg).

Secondary sex characteristics
Any of various genetically transmitted anatomical, physiological, or behavioral characteristics, such as voice quality, abundance of facial hair, or breast development. Secondary sex characteristics first appear in humans at puberty and differentiate the sexes without having a reproductive function.

Puberty
The stage of maturation in which a person becomes physiologically capable of sexual reproduction.

Menstruation
The process by which blood and dead cell debris is discharged from the uterus through the vagina at approximately monthly intervals after puberty and until menopause.

Ovulation
The release of the egg (ovum) from the ovaries.

XXY The individual is male, but at puberty the penis stays small, and female breast buds develop. Surgery and treatment with hormones can make it possible for the person to live a relatively normal life.

XYY Sensational news stories have surrounded claims that males with XYY chromosomes are inherently superviolent people. But in 1969 Fred Sergovich, a geneticist, reported that males with XYY chromosomes are quite common and that most of them lead normal lives.

XO The XO combination of chromosomes is called Turner's syndrome. The zero stands for no chromosome. The individual remains physically a little girl all her life. She does not mature, having a short stature, small breasts, ovaries that do not function, and an infantile uterus. She never menstruates. Her cells have what is called a mosaic pattern. They are not all alike but show various duplications and losses. Some sort of mental defect is common.

XXX Triplication of the female chromosome, the XXX pattern, is similar to Turner's syndrome, and here, too, the individual is sterile.

Continued research on the identification of chromosomes and on long-term effects of changes in the chromosomal makeup of individuals may help us to understand some of the more subtle differences between the sexes.

Gonadal Differences The presence in every human cell of at least one X chromosome strongly supports the idea that we are all basically female. All of us, male and female, did in fact have exactly the same genitals up to about the seventh week after *fertilization;* genitals were then more female than male in form. After the seventh week, if the embryo is male, the part of the embryo's genitals that corresponds to the vaginal opening begins to close up, except for a small portion that becomes the opening of the urethra. The part corresponding to the labia becomes the scrotum, the sac that encloses the testicles, and the part corresponding to the clitoris becomes the penis.

Nearly 10 percent of male infants are born with undescended testes; a much smaller percentage of females are born with a testis in each labium; and very rarely an individual is born with an ovotestis (a sex gland containing both male and female tissues), which can be determined by surgical exploration.

Hormonal Differences Growth and development is genetically controlled in two ways. The genetic code directs certain glands to produce the right hormones in the right amounts at the right times; the code also ensures that the appropriate tissues will be receptive to the action of those hormones. At birth a girl has complete female genitals, and a boy, complete male genitals, although they are infantile in size and form. The girl's glands make small amounts of estrogen and progesterone, which are the female sex hormones, and the boy's glands make small amounts of testosterone, the male sex hormone.

When children are about seven years old, the production of these hormones increases sharply.

At about age nine, on the average, girls begin to acquire what are called *secondary sex characteristics.* Breast buds begin to develop, and downy hair appears in the pubic area and the armpits. Baby fat in the waist and abdomen begins to disappear, and the hips begin to fill out. At about ten to twelve, boys develop their secondary sex characteristics: pubic hair, a deeper voice, disappearance of baby fat in the waist and abdomen, and growth of chest and shoulders. These changes are generally referred to as *puberty,* although people do not always agree on the exact meaning of that word.

Puberty continues for perhaps three or four years. During that time the genitals of both boys and girls grow to adult size. Pubic hair becomes coarser and denser, taking a vertical diamond shape in males, a fan shape in females. Coarse body hair appears on many boys and some girls. Girl's breasts develop. When a girl's ovaries begin to produce eggs and a boy's testicles begin to produce sperm, puberty gives way to adolescence.

In girls the signals of the beginning of reproductive capacity is the first *menstruation* (menarche), although the first *ovulation* (release of an egg from an ovary) is

Ejaculation
An abrupt discharge of fluid, especially of semen, from the penis.

Semen
A viscous, whitish secretion of the male reproductive organs; the transporting medium for sperm.

Wet dream
An erotic dream accompanied by sexual climax.

not believed to occur until about a year after the first menstruation. At the end of the nineteenth century, the average age of menarche in the United States was just under 17. Today it is 12.8 and it is still decreasing. Thus for each new generation, adolescence lasts a little longer.

The male equivalent of ovulation is the production of sperm. As with females, the external signal that reproductive capacity—the *ejaculation* of *semen*—is about to begin probably comes before the actual production of sperm. The first ejaculation may occur during an erotic dream, and thus is called a nocturnal emission, or *wet dream*. Puberty characteristics of both males and females are illustrated in Figure 4-1.

Figure 4-1 Physical characteristics of puberty.

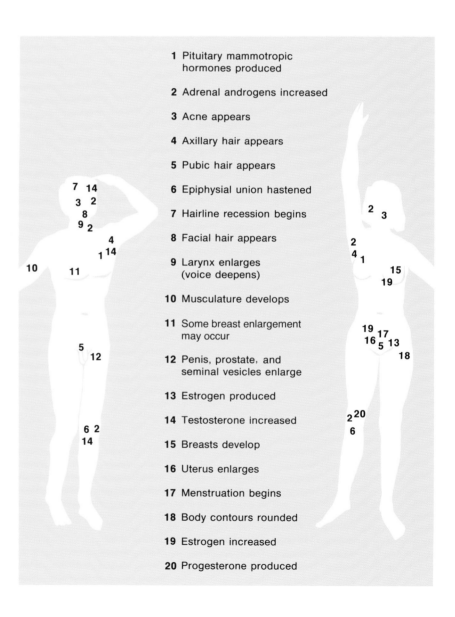

1 Pituitary mammotropic hormones produced
2 Adrenal androgens increased
3 Acne appears
4 Axillary hair appears
5 Pubic hair appears
6 Epiphysial union hastened
7 Hairline recession begins
8 Facial hair appears
9 Larynx enlarges (voice deepens)
10 Musculature develops
11 Some breast enlargement may occur
12 Penis, prostate, and seminal vesicles enlarge
13 Estrogen produced
14 Testosterone increased
15 Breasts develop
16 Uterus enlarges
17 Menstruation begins
18 Body contours rounded
19 Estrogen increased
20 Progesterone produced

Acne
An inflammatory disease of the oil glands, characterized by pimples usually on the face and often on the chest and upper back.

Metabolic rate
The speed at which the body carries out the chemical changes involved with nutrition. The term refers both to the use of food and energy to make larger molecules such as proteins and to the breakdown of molecules into simpler substances or waste matter releasing energy for other processes.

Average life expectancy
The length of life a person can expect to live (barring accidents), based on the average age of death. In the United States, average life expectancy is 70 years for males, 78 years for females.

Somatic Differences   Body characteristics—size, musculature, bony structure, skin, and metabolism—are the most immediately obvious and familiar biological sex differences in a society such as ours.

Size   Human males are generally bigger and heavier than human females. This statement concerns the *average,* however, and no one has any trouble recalling many exceptions.

Musculature   Human males are (on the average, again) stronger than human females. Muscle growth is increased by using the muscles, as when one works against a greater and greater load, and by male hormones. Professional weight lifters frequently make use of injections of testosterone in training for contests. Muscle size is what makes strength. A woman and a man with muscles of exactly the same size are exactly equal in strength.

Bony Structure   The male skeleton is usually larger than the female. Long bones grow at their ends, and during puberty and adolescence the female hormone estrogen arrests such growth faster than the male hormone testosterone does.

Male and female skeletons differ slightly in shape, a difference that is probably controlled in the chromosomes. The bones of the shoulder girdle are heavier in the male, and the pelvis is narrower. In the female the shoulder girdle is narrow, and the hips are full. The female elbow is sharper than the male because the bones are shaped differently. In the female the ring finger tends to be longer than the index finger; the reverse is true in the male.

Skin   Male and female skin look the same in infancy and throughout most of childhood. Puberty brings on several changes. *Acne* is the most noticeable of these changes, and acne is almost universal in pubescent and adolescent males. It is caused by the secretion of large amounts of male hormone. It also occurs in a young female when her body does not make enough estrogen to counterbalance its production of male hormone. Acne consists of an accumulation of a mixed fatty material

called sebum, which is produced by the sebaceous glands of the skin of the face, chest, and upper back.

As males mature, their skin grows thicker and coarser. They have relatively thick eyebrows and heavy facial hair; coarser and often darker hair on the chest, back, arms, and legs; and pubic hair extending from penis to navel.

Females grow luxuriant head hair and tend to have pale, fine body hair that is almost invisible except for a few wisps around the areolas (the dark areas around the nipples), a moderate amount in the armpits, and pubic hair in a fan shape.

The distribution of fat in males and females differs markedly. The layer of fat just under the skin is usually thicker in females, enough so that the insulating function of the skin is changed. Female skin becomes warmer in warm weather and colder in cold weather than male skin. Normal amounts of fat tend to be deposited in the breasts, the lower abdomen, and the buttocks in the female; and in the lower abdomen and (less so) the upper chest in the male. (Excesses of fat, of course, will fill up spaces all over the body of either sex.)

Metabolism   Males have a higher *metabolic rate* than females, meaning that they use more oxygen and produce and lose more heat. To transport the oxygen, males have about 5 million red cells per cubic milliliter of circulating blood, females about 4.5 million.

Vulnerability to Disease and Disorder

Many diseases occur mainly in one sex, and males are the most vulnerable. This imbalance is well illustrated by survival statistics. As many as 140 male embryos are formed for each 100 female embryos, and by birth the ratio in the United States and Great Britain is 105 males to 100 females. By age 20 the numbers are equalized and females begin to outnumber males. The *average life expectancy* in the United States is 71.8 years for males and 81 years for females. At age 85 there are twice as many females as males. In other words, for every 100 females at that age, there are only 50 males.

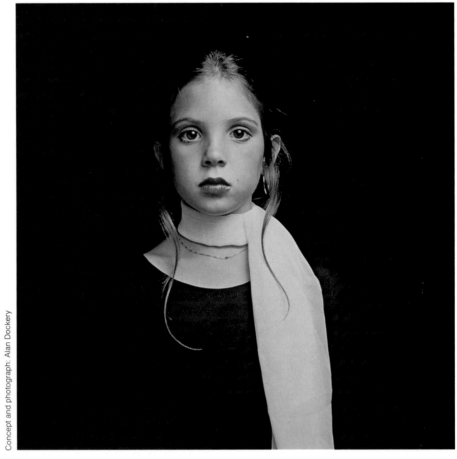

Congenital
Existing at birth, an effect of heredity or fetal environment.

Premenstrual tension
Stress occurring during the last 7 to 10 days of the menstrual cycle, possibly due to a change in the processing of sodium in the central nervous system, and often accompanied by head- and backaches, depression, and irritability.

Sex role
A pattern of behavior expected by society for members of one's sex.

Sex-role learning
Learning the socially accepted pattern of behavior for one's sex.

Males are more likely to have hemophilia, an inherited disease in which the blood does not clot normally within the body. Males are much more likely to have pyloric stenosis, a disease in which an overactive infant develops an oversized, continuously active muscle at the outlet of the stomach, with the result that eating leads repeatedly to vomiting. Surgical correction must be made. Eye defects and speech defects are also more common in males.

On the other hand, females are four times as likely to suffer from *congenital* dislocation of the hip and from patent ductus arteriosus, a defect in the development of heart and blood vessels in which blood is diverted away from the lung and back into major circulation. This condition prevents the blood from receiving a full supply of oxygen and causes what is called a "blue baby."

The foregoing are only a few examples of diseases that seem to be more common to one sex than another. Even the same disease may have different effects for the two sexes. In the male, rheumatic fever more often may lead to a disorder of the heart valves; in the female, to a disorder of motion control in the brain.

Culture sometimes influences biology. For example, certain diseases may be widespread in one culture and scarce or even absent in another. In much the same manner, culture can subject more males than females, or more females than males, to diseases that are not biologically sex-linked. Our culture places on males heavy expectations of achievement, aggressiveness, drive, and competitiveness. The impact of failure on a man's self-image is often catastrophic, with the result that drinking, smoking (until recently), and suicide have generally been more common among males. At one time the ulcer and the coronary could almost have been considered male diseases. As women demand and get more opportunities to compete equally, these "male" diseases may be found to increase among females.

Premenstrual tension affects, according to various estimates, from 30 to 90 percent of the adult female population. During the last 7 to 10 days of their menstrual cycle, these women experience discomforts that may include headache, backache, a sense of mid-abdominal fullness and pelvic heaviness, and, most frequently, retention of from 2 to 10 pounds of water. Anxiety, depression, fatigue, irritability, and greater likelihood of crying may accompany these discomforts. Many women also report an increased sex drive during this time, as well as a craving for sweets and for salty food.

Researchers currently believe that premenstrual stress is caused by an excess of estrogen relative to the amount of progesterone available. The hormone imbalance affects the distribution and excretion of sodium (from salt) and water in such a way that the breasts become more swollen and the abdomen fuller. Gravity acts on the excess fluid, causing the legs and feet to swell. The shift in fluid is what is responsible for the fullness and discomfort, while a change in the processing of sodium in the central nervous system may have a part in the emotional effects.

Culturally Induced Sex Differences: Sex Roles

A *sex role* can be defined as the ways in which a person of a certain sex is expected to behave in a certain society. The learning of sex roles is so powerful that a male raised as a female will consider himself female and will have the personality traits accepted as female in his culture. The same is true of the female raised as a male. These findings are the results of a study done in Baltimore by Money and Hampson (1955). In this study, the genetic sex of a number of pseudohermaphrodites (people who appear to be male but have ovaries or appear to be female but have testicles) was determined by chromosome identification. Researchers found that regardless of genetic sex, each subject had the sex identity assigned in his or her upbringing.

Sex-role learning begins early. Several studies show that mothers, perhaps because they believe girls are more fragile and thus need more care and concern, smile at, talk to, and touch their female infants more than their male infants, beginning when the infant is two days old.

Perhaps because they receive more overt affection in infancy, girls are evidently more affectionate than boys, both toward their peers and toward adults. They are freer to touch not only adults but also peers of both sexes. However, if a girl's behavior appears too warm, open, or uninhibited to her parents or to other adults, they may

Woman—Which Includes Man, of Course: An Experience in Awareness

There is much concern today about the future of man, which means of course, both men and women—generic Man. For a woman to take exception to this use of the term "man" is often seen as defensive hair-splitting by an "emotional female."

The following experience is an invitation to awareness in which you are asked to feel into, and stay with, your feelings through each step, letting them absorb you. If you start intellectualizing, try to turn it down and let your feelings again surface to your awareness.

■ Consider reversing the generic term Man. Think of the future of Woman which, of course, includes both women and men. Feel into that, sense its meaning to you—as a woman—as a man.

■ Think of it always being that way, every day of your life. Feel the ever-presence of woman and feel the nonpresence of man. Absorb what it tells you about the importance and value of being woman—of being man.

■ Recall that everything you have ever read all your life uses only female pronouns—she, her—meaning both girls and boys, both women and men. Recall that most of the voices on radio and most of the faces on TV are women's—when important events are covered—on commercials—and on the late talk shows. Recall that you have no male senator representing you in Washington.

■ Feel into the fact that women are the leaders, the power-centers, the prime-movers. Man, whose natural role is husband and father, fulfills himself through nurturing children and making the home a refuge for woman. This is only natural to balance the biological role of woman who devotes her entire body to the race during pregnancy.

■ Then feel further into the obvious biological explanation for woman as the ideal—her genital construction. By design, female genitals are compact and internal, protected by her body. Male genitals are so exposed that he must be protected from outside attack to assure the perpetuation of the race. His vulnerability clearly requires sheltering.

■ Thus, by nature, males are more passive than females, and have a desire in sexual relations to be symbolically engulfed by the protective body of the woman. Males psychologically yearn for this protection, fully realizing their masculinity at this time—feeling exposed and vulnerable at other times. The male is not fully adult until he has overcome his infantile tendency to penis orgasm and has achieved the mature surrender of the testicle orgasm. He then feels himself a "whole man" when engulfed by the woman.

■ If the male denies these feelings, he is unconsciously rejecting his masculinity. Therapy is thus indicated to help him adjust to his own nature. Of course, therapy is administered by a woman, who has the education and wisdom to facilitate openness leading to the male's growth and self-actualization.

■ To help him feel into his defensive emotionality, he is invited to get in touch with the "child" in him. He remembers his sister's jeering at his primitive genitals that "flop around foolishly." She can run, climb and ride horseback unencumbered. Obviously, since she is free to move, she is encouraged to develop her body and mind in preparation for her active responsibilities of adult womanhood. The male vulnerability needs female protection, so he is taught the less active, caring virtues of homemaking.

■ Because of his clitoris-envy, he learns to strap up his genitals, and learns to feel ashamed and unclean because of his nocturnal emissions. Instead, he is encouraged to keep his body lean and dream of getting married, waiting for the time of his fulfillment—when "his woman" gives him a girl-child to carry on the family name. He knows that if it is a boy-child he has failed somehow—but they can try again.

Theodora Wells

---

be more worried than pleased. Boys often have a strong peer-group taboo against touching anyone with affection, although in adolescence this taboo fades with respect to girls.

Adult Responses to Childhood Sexuality Many parents still believe in the myth of childhood innocence, the notion that a child does not naturally want sexual stimulation. No other culture has such a myth, and it has existed here only since the 1830s.

Not surprisingly, adults do not keep the unreal picture they have of children to themselves; they present it to children, in the school and in the home, as the only way children can be. One consequence is that children sometimes try to live up to the myth. Reality imitates fantasy, and the child learns to live a lie. Another consequence is that parents often do not know how to respond when children behave in ways contrary to the myth and reveal sexual feelings or experiment sexually, as children naturally do. An earlier generation of parents

Heterosexual
Sexual orientation toward the opposite sex.

would have taken the child's sexuality as evidence of innate evil, and their response would have been to punish the child. Parents today are less apt to be openly disapproving.

One thing has not changed: The severity of the parents' response depends heavily on the sex of the child. Sexual experimentation by boys is not totally out of line with what our culture expects of males. The boy's father may even feel a twinge of secret (sometimes not so secret) pride—as long as the experiment is *heterosexual*. But if the experimenting child is a girl, her parents are more likely to feel shame and disgrace. Sexuality is less accepted for the female than it is for the male.

Certainly, parents are influenced by the very basic and reasonable fear that their daughter might be sexually assaulted. Parents traditionally feel it part of their duty to protect a girl from unwelcome sexual contact. But the fear does not end there. For many parents, the prospect of a girl's *choosing* to be sexually active may be equally threatening. There is still a widespread belief that a girl's virginity must be kept for her—against her wishes if necessary—and the keepers are her parents. The immediate reactions of individual parents to their children's sexuality may run the gamut from advice to denial to distraction, but there is a single general outcome: Girls generally are not allowed the same freedom as boys.

Sex-Role Learning   The most important models for sex roles are the parents. A second source of learning is the peer group. Boys are raised in one subculture, girls in another, and differences develop accordingly. Boys spend much of their time away from Mother's watchful eye. Boys are venturesome and learn by experience. Boys explore. Boys experiment, finding out what they want to know by firsthand testing of the external world. Boys are better problem solvers than girls, and they have a better feeling for spatial relationships. Boys are encouraged in physical exploits and in innovation and improvisation. Boys are more obedient to peer group pressures and less obedient to adult direction. Boys are likely to learn to be contemptuous of anything they see as girl-like.

Girls tend to stay closer to their mothers. A girl is reminded to tug down the hem of her skirt and to keep her knees together. Girls are not encouraged to be either venturesome or self-reliant. A girl is more often urged to feel that she dare not rely on her own impulses to guide her in what is presented to her (rightly or wrongly) as a potentially dangerous, threatening, and invasive world.

Thus, by age five, girls have learned to become more dependent and more obedient than boys. They follow orders better and are more likely to complete a school or household chore.

Studies cited by Bem and Bem (1971) showed that even as early as nursery-school age, boys ask more questions about how and why things work. In one study children were asked to suggest ways to improve toys. In first and second grade, boys did better on the fire truck, while girls did better on the nurses's kit. In third grade, boys did better on all toys. Other studies showed that in elementary school "girls were more likely to try solving a problem by imitating an adult, whereas the boys were more likely to search for a novel solution not provided by the adult."

Girls outperform boys in most schoolwork in the early grades, but the Bems suggest that this, too, is a product of sex-role training. Young children consider school "feminine." "In elementary school, with its large number of female teachers and its emphasis on being 'good' or docile, girls have a momentary advantage; pleasing the teacher and doing good school work are more appropriate for girls than for boys."

In the upper grades, boys gain the academic advantage, especially in mathematics; males score 60 points higher, on the average, in College Board examinations.

Sex Differences and Individual Differences

Every society fosters sex roles. They vary greatly from society to society, and some are more constricting than others. The most serious consequence of sex roles is that they destroy individual differences. Those differences tend to be repressed, to go undeveloped, to be undervalued when they do appear, and often simply to go unseen. The result is that only one part of each of us is given the chance to grow, and society as well as the individual is deprived of much variety. Until very

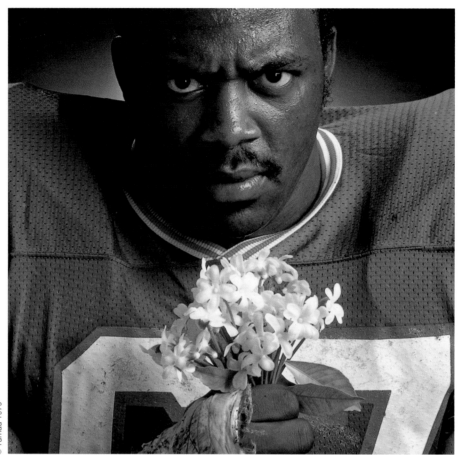

recently, it has hardly even been possible to study biological sex differences beyond the simplest—those that can be tested by such methods as chromosome identification—because the more complex biological patterns, if there are any, have been cloaked by cultural uniformity.

Building an Intimate Relationship

Ideally an intimate relationship evolves through a mutual sharing of inner feelings and private emotions. Its strength derives from a constancy of affection, trust, acceptance, dependability of emotional support, respect, willingness to make oneself available, and understanding. Intimates can reveal themselves without fear of being hurt. They may not always agree with each other, but they try to understand each other and work together toward mutual goals. An intimate relationship is a place to love, a world created by two people, and it exists only for them. It is unique because the people in it are unique.

Why then, if they are so wonderful, do so many relationships break up? Because the characteristics just listed are ideals; frequently those ideals are not achieved because of the participants' personalities and expectations. No relationship means the same thing to both people. Everyone has different needs, and everyone has different expectations of what an intimate relationship will supply. The relationships that have the best chance of surviving are those in which the partners become aware of their expectations and limitations and share them verbally with each other.

There are no rules governing what an intimate relationship is. To have one you must define and create it with someone else. It works better to know in advance what you want from a relationship. Certain characteristics of relationships do open up new worlds to the partners who create them. Worthwhile relationships recognize and protect the rights of both parties. They allow two people with equal rights to grow and share a view of the world that is greater than either sees alone.

Intimacy is not fusion, and each person in a meaningful relationship must allow the other the freedom to grow. Helping a partner to develop her or his full potential actually strengthens a relationship. Freedom to grow is also freedom to grow apart.

In addition to the right to grow, successful intimate relationships are characterized by certain other rights. Among the most important is the right to be oneself. Each of us is unique; we can only play our own part well. When one person demands that the other change to keep the relationship alive, it is already doomed. No one has the right to make another person change, unless he or she chooses to change. Furthermore, each partner has the right to be respected for being himself or herself, for being of value. Showing respect for an intimate entails listening to the other person, sharing his or her triumphs and problems.

Both people in a relationship also have the right to privacy. Everyone needs time and space to be alone, to sort out thoughts and feelings, to organize oneself, to tap one's own resources.

Still other rights are those of honesty and trust. Self-disclosure by partners is essential, but it must not put them in a position of jeopardy. Not being able to share attitudes and emotions closes off intimacy. The matter of trustworthiness is fragile and, if betrayed, often irreparable.

In intimate relationships, as in all other human interactions, rights go hand in hand with responsibilities. The healthiest relationships occur between people who take responsibility for themselves. Each takes responsibility for his or her own self-development, quality of existence, and personal identity. Passive members of relationships who do not take responsibility for themselves pose burdens to their partners. They let others make decisions for them; they protect themselves by never taking a position or never giving a response that is their own. There is always a price for yielding responsibility. If we surrender our responsibilities to the other person when we form a relationship, we violate ourselves, become less of a person, and undermine the relationship itself. We hold the other person liable for our losses, and our resentment eventually eats us up.

If one of the purposes of life is to celebrate it, the purpose of an intimate relationship is to celebrate life together. Nevertheless, from time to time remind yourself of this: No one can make you feel truly complete but yourself. No relationship, no matter how deep and sat-

Love That Lasts a Lifetime

Practically everybody remembers the first time of making love with a spouse. Practically nobody remembers the 373rd. Love stories are about falling in love, not staying that way.

One wonders what happens in a marriage that has lasted many years. Is there any excitement about staying in love? Can it remain romantic when you climb into bed with the same person night after night?

"It depends on what you mean by romantic," says one wife of 15 years. "If you mean that can't-keep-your-hands-off-each-other feeling, then no, you don't have that. It's actually better than that, because sex is no longer a performance. You can relax and enjoy what's happening. That's what makes it romantic to me. I know I'm loved by someone who really knows me. Nobody can beat that."

Of all the joys of familiarity, one of the most central is security. You learn to trust this person who handles your body and your emotions so intimately. You can let down the barricades and approach the experience with openness.

More than that, there is the security of having a shared history as lovers, a sense of safety about each other. Given the avalanche of sexual information available today, there is formidable pressure to "get it right." Husbands and wives have the comfortable knowledge of all the times their lovemaking has worked—as well as the knowledge that when it has not, nothing important changed in their relationship. "That's the advantage of being married," says Gina. "There are other things going on. If the sexual side isn't working, you've got everything else to hold you together until the problem is solved."

Whereas in the early stages of love the obsessive desire for each other closes out the rest of the world, intimacy between two people who have been married for many years has room to take in all facets of life. It can be exchanging a look over the head of your child or reaching out to take your husband's hand at the exact moment he reaches out for yours. Some of the most intimate moments in marriage are those spent just talking, at times when the disappointments of the world seem to have stripped away every defense and you are hurting. . . .

The core of intimacy is a profound knowledge of each other, and that knowledge takes years to develop. For husbands and wives who work at staying in touch—who listen to each other, who share what's going on whether it's fascinating or not—intimacy becomes a steadily increasing element of the marriage that enhances all other elements. Within the intimacy of marriage, sex becomes the physical expression of the unity of two people.

What frightens many people is the normal fluctuation of passion within the long time-frame of intimacy. When the fresh excitement of a new love begins to mellow into the gentler security of an established relationship, some people panic and try to find the newness again with somebody else. To make marriage work, you have to step forward into the territory of familiarity and discover, beyond novelty, the intimate warmth of making love with the person you know almost as well as yourself.

Faces do wrinkle, bodies do get pudgier, energy levels do recede, and most people do face an increasing number of niggling ailments. A

long-lasting love accepts all of these less than agreeable facts. It comes to terms with time. What binds the lovers together is not what they look like, but what they are.

If the physical need for each other feels less all-consuming as time goes by, it can still be intensely satisfying. If anything, it can be better, since like most other skills sex improves with practice.

There is a particular pleasure in making love for couples in the middle phase of their marriage when the world around them is the most demanding. The whole intricate machinery of jobs and household has to be kept functioning. The days are relentlessly busy, and in the middle of all this, making love can be an island of privacy. . . .

It isn't that sexual relationships in long-term marriages present no problems. A study of couples in successful marriages, published in 1978 by researchers at the University of Pittsburgh's Western Psychiatric Institute and Clinic, reported a frequency of sexual difficulties similar to that of couples studied by Masters and Johnson. Despite the problems, almost all of the individuals in the study reported that their sexual relationship was satisfactory. When it was good, the sexual sharing added to the overall sense of contentment and affection. When it wasn't, the rest of the relationship seems to have supplied enough warmth and understanding to make the difficulties less important.

Some therapists even feel that when a married couple does find sexual problems troubling enough to seek counseling, what may help the marriage more is not the improved techniques learned but the experience of sharing a mutual goal and working together, tenderly and lovingly, to achieve it.

When problems are not so acute, or when people feel they've hit a dull patch, many couples take time off by themselves. . . .

Going away together, alone, can provide a temporary return to that blissful first stage. "You have to go away," one wife says, "even if you just go downtown to a hotel. Otherwise you see the dust under the bed, the dishes in the sink and the briefcase in the hall. You have to leave all that behind."

When everything *is* left behind, all the energy that went into running a joint life can be turned into renewing the basis for it—the loving, continuing relationship of a man and a woman who have chosen to move through time together.

Those are the moments that sustain a marriage, and spouses committed to a long love build up their own private treasury. It can be lying together in a quiet room while dawn slowly lightens outside the window, holding hands under a restaurant table or coming together after a separation with fresh hunger for each other.

All are ways of making love.

Ronna Romney and Beppie Harrison
Giving Time a Chance

---

isfying, can assuage all hurts or ward off all bouts of loneliness. In a sense, we are all ultimately alone; sometimes the people we love can make it through to us, and sometimes they cannot, no matter how hard they try.

How to Select a Compatible Intimate   Employers use interview and psychological tests to see who is compatible with available jobs. Not a bad idea. How would you rate yourself—and the person you would like to be intimate with—on the following characteristics?

1. *Tolerance for differences.* A tolerance for differences in other people is more important than and overrides many of the variables listed below. Tolerance brings us a long way toward coping with differences of background, viewpoint, interest, and energy level. If you are able to grant your would-be partner a long leash that gives her or him plenty of freedom to enjoy your differences, and if that person can do the same for you, you have each made a rare find and should consider yourselves fortunate.

2. *Educational level.* College graduates have lower divorce rates than nongraduates, perhaps because they marry later and have had more time to compare choices. They also earn more money and are more likely to seek professional help for problems. Great differences in educational levels may mean great differences in know-how: in dealing with people, in power, in knowledge. (In the past men usually received more education than women did; fortunately that is changing.) However, if both partners are committed to grow, they may be able to solve problems of educational differences.

3. *Socioeconomic background.* Life-style depends partly on socioeconomic background. What are your and your potential intimate's attitudes toward money, social position, family background? Flexible people may be able to adapt to differences in types of neighborhoods, housing, clothes, transportation, recreation, and so on, but a big difference in socioeconomic background can make adjustment— either up or down—very difficult.

4. *Values and taste.* How do your values and tastes compare in terms of religion, politics, music, art, types of people? If either of you is not very tolerant, having similar values and tastes is a necessity.

5. *Self-esteem.* Do you respect and like yourself? What about your intended partner? The more one likes oneself, the more nourishment one can offer to another person and to an intimate relationship.

6. *Commitment to growth.* Commitment to growth is reflected in a willingness to expand one's world, to learn more about oneself, others, new ideas, and new activities. Without a commitment to growth, both the partners and the relationship can grow stale and stagnate. There is some risk in continuing growth because two people can grow apart. But growing apart is most likely when there is a big difference in interest and commitment to consider new ideas and experiences.

7. *Authority.* Do you and/or your would-be partner insist on making the final decision or having the last word? Collaboration is usually the best system. Although authority is almost never shared 50–50, it is probably best divided according to time and talent. Can the two of you do that?

8. *Energy level.* How do your energy levels compare? Do you like to laze around in the house all the time while the other person wants to be on the go constantly? A significant difference in energy levels can strain a relationship.   (*text continues on p. 95*)

Compatibility Quiz by Barbara Burtoff, M.S., Ed.

How compatible are you and your prospective mate? To find out, take this quiz and let your spouse-to-be do the same. Then compare your answers.

According to psychologist Karen Shanor of Washington, D.C., who helped put this quiz together, the more areas of agreement here, the less possible conflict in marriage.

However, she says, it is no fun to be married to a clone, so it is OK to have some disagreement—provided that you are able to compromise or, at least, agree to disagree.

This quiz is not meant to be a valid scientific measure of your compatibility. It was put together as an exercise to get you thinking about situations that can be difficult and cause stress in marriage.

The issues were chosen because they have specifically been mentioned by various couples who have sought counseling from Shanor.

This quiz can be taken by anyone, but it was primarily designed for those going into a first marriage, and for that reason, you'll find no questions referring to children and/or former marriages.

1. How many of the 10 items on this list do you have in common with your prospective mate: religion, career, same home town or neighborhood, friends, education level, income level, cultural pastimes, sports/recreation activities, travel, physical attraction?
   a. Almost everything on the list.
   b. Quite a few.
   c. A few.
   d. Almost none.

2. Would you prefer a relationship that is:
   a. Male-dominated.
   b. Female-dominated.
   c. A partnership.

3. What banking arrangement sounds best after marriage:
   a. Separate account.
   b. Joint account.
   c. Joint account, but some cash for each of you to spend as you please with no accounting.

4. If you share an account, whose responsibility should it be to balance the checkbook and pay bills?
   a. The man in the family.
   b. The woman in the family.
   c. Whoever is better at math and details.

5. If you inherited $10,000, would you prefer it to be:
   a. Saved toward a major purchase.
   b. Spent on something you could enjoy together such as a vacation.
   c. Spent on luxury items you could enjoy individually, such as a fur coat or golf clubs.

6. Where do you think you should spend major holidays?
   a. With his family.
   b. With her family.
   c. Alternating with his and her family.
   d. At your place and inviting the relatives.
   e. Just the two of you at home, or with friends, or off on vacation.

7. How frequently do you want to see your in-laws if they live in the same town?
   a. Only on special occasions and holidays.
   b. Twice a month.
   c. At least once a week.

8. How frequently do you enjoy talking with your own parents?
   a. Every day.
   b. Once a week.
   c. Once a month or less.

9. If you both have careers, what will be your priority?
   a. Marriage before career.
   b. Marriage equally important to career.
   c. Career before marriage; my spouse is going to have to be understanding.

10. If you are offered a career promotion with a hefty raise making your income much more than your spouse's but involving a move out-of-state, would you:
   a. Expect your mate to be agreeable to relocation.
   b. Try a commuter marriage; only seeing each other weekends or occasionally.
   c. Say "no" rather than move, money isn't everything.

11. If your new spouse sets aside one evening a week to go out with a friend or friends of his/her same sex would you feel:
   a. Jealous of the time away from you.
   b. Happy that he/she has friends.
   c. This should not go on; let your feelings be known.

12. If you've had a bad day at the office and come home feeling moody, would you prefer that your mate:
   a. Back off, get out of the way.
   b. Act sympathetic, be a good listener.
   c. Discuss the events that led to your mood, perhaps offering some alternative suggestions for dealing with the persons or problems that made you unhappy.

13. If your mate does something that makes you extremely angry, are you most likely to:
   a. Forgive and forget it.

b. Hurl insults.

c. Mention you are angry at an appropriate time, preferably when the anger is first felt and explain why without making derogatory accusations.

14. If you can't stand his/her friends and he/she can't stand yours, how will you deal with this after marriage? (You may choose more than one.)

a. Cultivate new friends that you both can enjoy.

b. See your friends by yourself and let him/her do the same.

c. Phase out the friends you knew before marriage; expect your partner to do the same.

15. If you and your spouse-to-be are different religions, would you expect to:

a. Convert before marriage.

b. Have him/her convert before marriage.

c. Take turns attending each other's place of worship.

d. Observe religious days separately.

e. Not worry about it; religion is not an issue in your relationship.

16. When do you want to start a family?

a. As soon as possible.

b. After you have spent a few years enjoying your relationship as a couple.

c. As soon as careers are firmly established.

d. Never.

17. What is your attitude about housework? (You may check more than one.)

a. It is unmasculine for a man to do it. A woman should do all of it even if she chooses to have a career.

b. It is fine for a man to help,

but only with certain tasks, such as mowing the lawn or taking out the trash.

c. If a woman works outside the home, cleaning should be shared.

d. Even if a woman does not work outside the home, cleaning should be shared.

e. A maid regardless, if it fits the family budget.

18. Before marriage, you go out as a couple several times a week. A few months after marriage, you realize that you are going out a lot less. Would you consider this:

a. OK. The pace was exhausting.

b. Dull. You worry that you are being taken for granted.

c. Not OK. You and your mate should make plans for some evenings out or evenings at home with friends.

19. You need to buy a new suit. Your spouse wants to come along. Would you see this as a sign of:

a. Interest in spending time with you.

b. Crowding your relationship.

c. Watch-dogging your taste or pocketbook.

20. How would you prefer to spend your annual vacation? (Check as many as apply.)

a. On a trip by yourself.

b. On a trip with your mate.

c. On a trip with your mate and another couple.

d. Visiting your relatives or in-laws at their homes.

e. At a beach relaxing.

f. Engaged in an active sport such as skiing, tennis camp, or hiking/camping.

g. Traveling to another city for sightseeing/shopping.

h. At home catching up on repairs, appointments, books, visits with friends.

i. I would rather take a vacation less frequently than once a year and spend this money on rent or mortgage, enabling us to live in a more convenient or prestigious neighborhood.

21. If you were hunting for a place to live, would you prefer being in:

a. The country.

b. The suburbs.

c. The city.

22. If your spouse-to-be had many loves before he/she met you, would you prefer that he/she:

a. Keep the details to himself/herself.

b. Tell you everything.

c. Answer truthfully, but only the questions you ask, such as what broke up each relationship.

23. If your new spouse is in a romantic mood and you are not, how would you be most likely to respond?

a. Communicate your mood; suggest another time.

b. Pretend you are feeling romantic.

c. Invent an excuse rather than communicate your mood.

Psychologist Karen Shanor Explains

1. The more you have in common, the more of your life you can share and enjoy together.

2. Research and experiences of many couples have shown that the equal relationship is most successful.

3 and 4. There is no one right answer. Decide what works best for you and creates the least tension in your relationship.

(continued on next page)

Compatibility Quiz (continued)

5. We've all learned early in life to spend our limited money in certain ways. For some, it's on clothes; for others, it's on home or travel. Unless we understand our priorities and communicate them to our partner, we can find ourselves in great financial conflict and tension.

6. Very often we expect others to celebrate holidays as we do and give them the same sense of importance as the family in which we grew up. This isn't always so. Be able to compromise on this one.

7 and 8. Some are happy going for years at a time without seeing relatives. Others intentionally buy the house next door and want to drop in every day. Most important here is to let your spouse know that he/she comes first before parents and in-laws.

9. Talk about career and marriage priorities. Can you be accepting of your spouse's choice if he/she considers time spent on work more important right now than time spent with you?

10. There is no one right answer. Decide what works best for you and creates the least tension in your relationship.

11. It's healthy to have friends. You can't realistically expect your mate to spend 24 hours around the clock with you. If you or your mate go off for a time with friends, it wouldn't be too mushy to kiss, hug, or otherwise reassure your mate by words or actions that he/she is still first in your life. A spouse needs to hear this.

12. There are times when answer A would be best; other occasions call for B or C. Be sensitive to your mate's mood. If you are the one in the bad mood, don't expect your mate to read your mind as to whether you need space, sympathy or discussion. Clue him/her in.

13. Answer C is best. Somewhere along the way, people have to learn how to express anger constructively.

14. Be careful here. If you make his/her old friends feel left out or unimportant, they could work on your prospective mate to break up your relationship.

15. If you have major differences on this one, you may want to consider terminating the relationship before committing to marriage.

16. It's impossible to have half a child. Compromise won't work on this one, so it is best to speak your mind before marriage.

17. The most successful marriages are the ones in which men and women do not limit themselves in the traditional masculine-feminine roles. The sharing of responsibility heightens a sense of trust, caring and cooperation.

18. Sometimes the pace during dating is frantic. It is nice to calm down, but not nice to settle down to the point that each of you is taking the other for granted. Marriage requires continual work if you are going to keep adventure and interest in the relationship.

19. Whether you see it as interest, crowding or distrust, communicate your feelings to your mate. If you'd

rather shop alone, let that be known too.

20. Agree upon your needs in advance of the annual vacation, or what should be a time of relaxation away from the daily grind will turn into a source of tension and arguments. There is nothing wrong with separate vacations if one of you wants to fish on the lake and the other enjoys sightseeing.

21. If you are set on a particular style of living and not willing to change it after marriage, speak up before you say, ''I do.''

22. In general, it is not a good idea to go into great detail about past relationships because they are not totally relevant to your current one. However, trust and honesty are very important. If your partner asks a question, answer honestly but think very carefully. If you are the one doing the questioning, ask yourself, ''Do I really want to hear this?''

23. There are times in your relationship when you may want to go along with your spouse's romantic feelings, but it is generally best to communicate in a nice way without making him/her feel rejected or unloved that you simply are not in the mood. Do suggest another time.

9. *Communication skills.* People are not mind readers. How are you at sharing when you are anxious and irritable? Can you say unpleasant things that need to be said? What about the other person? Can the two of you communicate positive feelings of praise, support, and empathy? Most important, can you really listen to each other? Communication skills are essential to a healthy relationship.

10. *Tolerance of intimacy.* Are you or the other person embarrassed or anxious about expressing your feelings and thoughts? Must you defend yourselves against closeness with jokes, teasing, planning escape routes through activities? What do the two of you really want and expect of a relationship with each other?

Conflict Management: Learning to Fight   In intimate relationships all kinds of conflicts appear to serve as springboards to arguments: differences in body clocks, tastes in music, furniture, style, politics, and neatness. Most of these conflicts, however, matter only when something deeper is wrong—something like one person's feeling used or exploited or jealous or taken for granted.

Anger is a reality in intimate relationships. It is not something to feel guilty about but rather an indication that there are strong feelings of dissatisfaction to work out. Expressing the dissatisfaction usually does not mean that the dissatisfied person does not love the other person. If that is the actual message she or he wants to impart, actions will show it and arguing won't help anyway.

People have denied their anger for centuries; women particularly have been taught to deny all aggressive feelings. But now therapists are recognizing the value of treating anger and conflict for what they are, and they are training clients in conflict management, a skill everyone needs. In discussions both people in a relationship should be able to express all genuine feelings. Not being able to handle criticism or anger is detrimental to the exploration of deep feelings and to the relationship itself. If you cannot express all your feelings, ask yourself whether this is the right relationship for you.

The point of a fruitful argument should be to clear the air and to discover more truth about the meaning of the

feelings two people have about each other. Combatants stake out the territory and seek some resolution of who's going to have control. Compromise may be the answer. Here are some suggestions for managing conflict.

1. Try not to start an argument unless you know what you are angry about. If you are jealous, don't pretend it's about not taking out the garbage. Don't argue just to get attention: That's too costly psychologically. It wears out both partners, and there are far more positive ways to endear yourself.

2. Try to determine whether your feelings and their intensity are appropriate to the issue. Don't dramatize just to make the debate more interesting.

3. Know what you want to accomplish. Are you just letting off steam? Just making a point? Will you insist on behavior change? Settle for a compromise? State your complaint and your desires simply and clearly. Then wait for a response.

4. Unless you intend to leave after discussing the problem, work toward a resolution and plan for a joint activity afterward.

5. Pick a time and place where you can both be open without embarrassing each other. Otherwise the issue is clouded; you can be attacked for being petty and unfair. Try making an appointment ahead of time for your fight. That will give you time to cool off and to build your case if it involves a persisting problem.

6. Allow enough time. Avoid jumping into an argument five minutes before you are scheduled to go out for a night on the town or you are expecting company.

7. Try not to lay on the guilt. Relating what you feel—anger, hurt—is more effective than blaming and accusing. And don't leave in the middle of an argument, a ploy the other person resents because you make her or him worry.

8. Do not let the situation overwhelm you. If you feel overpowered by the other person, say so and ask for the courtesy of speaking your mind without interruption. If you feel intimidated, say so. Remember, you are supposed to be equals.

9. Listen. See if your partner has acceptable reasons for her or his actions. Laziness, greediness, and

Institutional marriage
A marriage that emphasizes society's expectations.

Companionship marriage
A marriage that places mutual consent above society's rules.

selfishness are not good reasons. If you are the defendant, acknowledge what you hear by repeating the accusation to make sure it's clear.

10. Try corresponding by mail. Personal feelings can sometimes be more easily influenced by logic and rational thought with some emotional distance.

11. If you are the one confronted, do not immediately try to defend yourself or feel righteously indignant. Let the other person vent the wrath and get it out of her or his system. Stay open. Don't crumble in guilt or defensiveness. Don't close yourself off angrily. Don't deny the conflict.

Developing a Sexual Relationship The greatest amount of sexual activity takes place between married couples and, to an increasing extent, between couples who have some kind of commitment to each other but are not legally married. Sexual success will vary directly with the degree of intimacy that the partners achieve.

If personal intimacy can be attained first, there are usually fewer problems in developing enthusiastic, varied, and unself-conscious sexual relations. Circumstances sometimes dictate otherwise, however, and the two occur simultaneously, or even less fortunately, attempts at sexual relations precede those at intimacy.

Because early sexual experiences affect those that follow, it is critically important that they be as pleasurable and psychologically painless as possible. One disageeable experience, even with a person whom we love deeply, may provide a block to satisfactory sex that will persist over the years. Here we should try to realize that there is really no hurry, however urgent the feelings are. There is time and the stakes are high. There is no substitute for approaching the other person with consideration, awareness, and tenderness as well as with affection.

Marriage More than 94 percent of the population do, in fact, eventually marry. This figure is particularly interesting in view of the fact that a hundred years ago only 60 percent of the population married.

The real wonder is that a significant number of these people have the strength, courage, and adaptability to go on from an unrealistic start to a workable relationship, one characterized by mutual love, support, trust, and sharing.

More than half the couples who marry fare less well. The average length of marriages has now declined to less than six and a half years. Many factors work against marital success. Conflicts between job and home plague many couples. Employees are expected to give priority to demands of the job. The result is that a disproportionate share of marital responsibilities falls to the people staying at home (more often women), a situation that is inequitable and one that can generate a great deal of resentment. If both partners work, as has increasingly been the case in recent years, and the wife is still expected to carry the full burden of running the household, her resentment, coupled with her increased earning capacity, can give her both the motive and the means to relinquish the marriage.

Society as a whole drags far behind individual members in its concepts of marriage. We have not yet escaped the sex-role stereotypes of marriage. The traditional view of the "institution" of marriage seems to ignore the pattern of social change that actually exists, including women's striving for equality. According to the Bureau of the Census, no more than 7 percent of families meet the old stereotype of a husband out making a living and a wife living entirely in the home, housekeeping and raising children.

Slow though it may be, we can distinguish a steady and strong change from the old *institutional marriage* to *companionship marriage*. Institutional marriage has been a societally designated form of "success" (as it still is in much of the world), with little consideration for whether this is satisfactory to either participant. Companionship marriage, on the other hand, is predicated upon being the major source of personal and mutual satisfaction in most areas of life for both men and women.

Dissolution of Marriage A marriage may be dissolved by the desertion or death of one of the partners, but most often it is dissolved by divorce. Divorce is one of the most stressful events people can experience. Actually, it is more accurate to describe divorce as a series of stressful events: the deterioration of the relationship; the decision by one of the partners to dissolve the marriage and his or her announcement of that intent; the awkward period of living together after the announcement but before the separation; the separation; the legal procedures, and the granting of the decree. The impact divorce

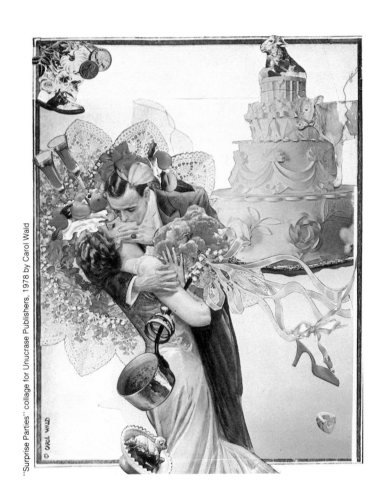

"Surprise Parties" collage for Unucrase Publishers, 1978 by Carol Wald

Four Components of Love

In marriage there is usually a fairly constant interplay of altruistic, companionate, sexual, and romantic love. The relative importance of these four components will, of course, vary for any given couple, with altruism or companionship or sex or romance being more prominent in some marriages than in others. The relative importance of these four components also varies for any couple with the duration of their marriage. In the very early stages of marriage, for example, the sexual and romantic components are generally predominant.

Obviously, the most significant influence on the relative prominence of one or another of the components of married love is the immediate love need of one or both of the persons in the relation. The love needs of a person will vary from time to time in a marriage, and these needs will not always coincide with the needs of the other person. But the societal expectation is that each will fulfill the particular need of his spouse, not because he

shares that particular need at that particular time but because he recognizes the need in the other. He provides the need as a love offering. On occasion such provision will be simultaneous and mutual; but more often it is alternate.

So long as, in the long run, there is a balance of at least the alternate form of love fulfillment in marriage—so long as a person feels that he is getting as much as he is giving and that the spouse is giving because he wants to rather than because he feels he must—the marriage should be happy and fulfilling.

Despite the mass-media emphasis on sex and romance, the companionate side of love—shared dependence, mutual respect, and "belonging"—probably has more to do with what the average couple experiences as conjugal love than does the passionate romantic attachment of a Romeo and Juliet. We must remember that part of the essence of the romantic attachment of Romeo and Juliet was its brevity. Romeo [and Juliet's] marital relation

may continue to include the passion and idealism of the romantic, sexual love of their youth—at least on occasion—but an increasingly important factor in their relation would be the satisfactions of shared responsibilities and experiences in meeting the practical demands of daily circumstance, in providing support and companionship to one another, and in loving and launching their children. These satisfactions would not only assume an added importance but might even come to constitute the chief basis of their relation. This fusion of romantic love (idealization of the love object), altruistic love (desiring the well-being of the love object), sexual love (in which the love object and the sex object are the same), and companionate love (or friendship) is the contemporary ideal of conjugal love in our society.

Lloyd Saxton
The Individual, Marriage, and the Family

has on human health is only hinted at in Table 4–1, which lists common symptoms of people experiencing a divorce.

More general reactions include anxiety, depression, grief, hostility, loneliness, and a sense of failure. The divorced person is likely to feel emotionally bruised and in need of *nurturance*. How these needs are met can

have a considerable effect on the success of the person's reentry into the "single" world, and a common reaction is to seek refuge in another marriage. All too often this solution merely recycles the original problem.

Alternatives to Marriage One of the most obvious alternatives to marriage is chosen by those who decide

Table 4-1 Common Symptoms of People Experiencing a Divorce

Symptom	Percent of people experiencing symptom at:		
	Decision	Separation	Decree
Sleep loss	16	27	11
Diminished health	15	26	12
Loneliness and melancholy	11	29	12
Decreased work efficiency	8	16	11
Decreased memory	6	11	6
Increased smoking	4	11	6
Increased drinking	1	5	4

Nurturance
Comfort and support in the interest of personal growth.

Homophile
Preference for the same sex; homosexual; gay.

---

to remain single. For others, however, a complicating factor in marriage and—especially—divorce is that the state is the third partner in the relationship. The obvious way to deal with this complication is to keep the state out of the relationship. Many people choose this route either because they do not want a legally sanctioned contract or because they have a kind of relationship not recognized by the state.

Single-Parent Household   Divorce, desertion, or death may leave a family with only one parent. Although some of the remaining parents remarry, a substantial number do not. Some single-parent households also result from pregnancies outside marriage or from single-parent adoptions, an increasingly accepted solution to the problem of finding parents for orphaned, abandoned, or otherwise parentless children.

Living Together   Especially among young people, there is a growing trend toward setting up housekeeping without any formal legal or religious sanction. Sometimes the mutual expectation is that this will be a temporary arrangement leading either to a friendly farewell or to a legal marriage. Some expect the same permanence conventionally expected of marriage. Children may or may not be part of the plan, but their arrival

usually increases the social pressures on the couple to legalize their union.

Homosexual Marriages   One aspect of the *homophile* (gay liberation) movement has been an increased effort to have same-sex unions accorded the same recognition as opposite-sex unions. The legal system has thus far refused to recognize such unions, and the antihomosexual backlash of the mid-1970s produced some state laws specifically denying gay marriages.

Group Marriages   Some people find a deeper emotional and sexual satisfaction in long-term relationships that involve more than two people. Group marriages often involve three partners and occasionally four. Sometimes an entire communal family is the marital unit.

The single-parent family and the couple living together show signs of becoming permanent parts of our social fabric. Homosexual and group marriages are rare, and the future of these forms of marriage seems uncertain. They are still largely experimental, but if they satisfy the needs of a significant number of the experimenters, they may become more popular. As bizarre as multiple-partner marriages may seem to many Americans, they are permitted in more than half the world's cultures.

Intimate Relationship Scale

Read the following statements carefully. Choose the one in each section that best describes you at this moment and record its score at the right. (For example, "prefers to talk rather than listen" has a score of 2.) When you have identified five statements, total your score and find your position on the scale.

5 listens without making snap judgments
4 listens without interrupting
3 listens but often interrupts
2 prefers to talk rather than listen
1 is unwilling to listen

Score _____

5 expresses inner feelings freely
4 expresses inner feelings cautiously
3 has difficulty expressing inner feelings
2 feels that expressing inner feelings is weakness
1 is incapable of expressing inner feelings

Score _____

5 responsive to the needs of others
4 sensitive to the needs of others
3 capable of meeting others' needs
2 uninterested in others' needs
1 incapable of responding to others' needs

Score _____

5 unbiased by traditional sex roles
4 not influenced by sex-role stereotypes
3 somewhat affected by sex-role stereotypes
2 strongly influenced by sex-role stereotypes
1 behaves according to sex-role stereotypes

Score _____

5 is tolerant of differences in others
4 can adjust to differences in others
3 prefers people of similar background
2 has problems with differences in others
1 is intolerant of differences in others

Score _____

Total score _____

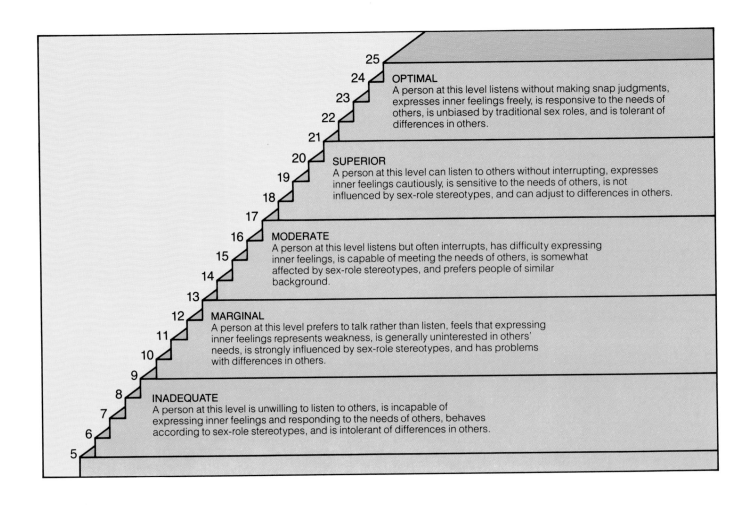

OPTIMAL
A person at this level listens without making snap judgments, expresses inner feelings freely, is responsive to the needs of others, is unbiased by traditional sex roles, and is tolerant of differences in others.

SUPERIOR
A person at this level can listen to others without interrupting, expresses inner feelings cautiously, is sensitive to the needs of others, is not influenced by sex-role stereotypes, and can adjust to differences in others.

MODERATE
A person at this level listens but often interrupts, has difficulty expressing inner feelings, is capable of meeting the needs of others, is somewhat affected by sex-role stereotypes, and prefers people of similar background.

MARGINAL
A person at this level prefers to talk rather than listen, feels that expressing inner feelings represents weakness, is generally uninterested in others' needs, is strongly influenced by sex-role stereotypes, and has problems with differences in others.

INADEQUATE
A person at this level is unwilling to listen to others, is incapable of expressing inner feelings and responding to the needs of others, behaves according to sex-role stereotypes, and is intolerant of differences in others.

Take Action

Your answers to Probing Your Emotions at the beginning of this chapter and your placement level on the Intimate Relationship Scale will, we hope, encourage you to begin a process of self-exploration and self-discovery that you will continue. Reflect on the entire chapter's content and ask yourself how each point relates to your own life. Then take action:

1. In 1967, 85 percent of the parents of college students in a CBS poll believed that all premarital sexual intercourse was morally wrong. But in a 1981 poll, 63 percent of such parents agreed with the statement, "If two people love each other, there's nothing morally wrong with having sexual relations." Interview three older students about their atti-

tudes toward students of the opposite sex living together. Contrast their attitudes with the attitudes of three much younger students. Are there any differences? If so, who or what do you feel is responsible for shaping attitudes?

2. Have you ever seen an ad in the newspaper advertising marriage and family counseling? Have you ever wondered what qualified someone to perform such services? Find out about the resources in your community for premarital and marital counseling. Does the state require counselors to be licensed? What requirements must the counselors have?

3. Think about your best friend. Analyze the elements that make this relationship so satisfactory. What elements are unsatisfactory? Make an

effort to talk to your friend about your recent thoughts.

4. List the positive behaviors or attitudes that help you feel good about your close relationships. Consider how you can strengthen those behaviors or attitudes. Then list the behaviors or attitudes that block your getting the most out of your relationships. Consider each of these behaviors and decide which ones you can change.

5. Take the Compatibility Quiz on page 92. Then read the psychologist's comments following it. In your notebook write down what you have learned that you were unaware of before.

6. Read the following Behavior Change Strategy, and take the appropriate action.

Behavior Change Strategy

Sexual Dysfunction

Most people will experience sexual dysfunction sometime in their lives. This often involves difficulty in becoming aroused or reaching orgasm. William Masters and Virginia Johnson, in *Human Sexual Response* (1970), estimate that approximately half of all married couples in the United States have experienced some form of sexual dysfunction. Single people have an even higher rate, a fact that is usually attributed to insecurity in their relationships and less familiarity with their partner's sexual preferences.

Male sexual dysfunctions include ejaculatory incompetence (difficulty in reaching orgasm); premature ejaculation (ejaculation earlier than desired); and erectile dysfunction, also known as impotence (the lack of a sustained erection for intercourse). Female dys-

functions include vaginismus (involuntary contraction of vaginal muscles that prevents entry by the penis); primary orgasmic dysfunction (a woman has never reached orgasm and is unable to do so); situational orgasmic dysfunction (a specific situation, partner, etc., prevents orgasm). Women with orgasmic dysfunction may be very sensitive, concerned, and frustrated; there should be no implication that they are "frigid" or uninterested in sex.

Sexual dysfunction may be caused by physical or psychological factors. Approximately 10 to 20 percent of all sexual dysfunctions stem from disease. Diabetes and heart disease, for example, may be an underlying cause of erectile dysfunction. Fatigue can cause problems that are temporary unless one becomes overly

anxious about future performance. Drugs, especially depressants such as alcohol, may also inhibit sexual responses. People experiencing sex difficulties should have a thorough physical examination.

Psychosocial causes of dysfunction include troubled relationships, lack of sexual skills, irrational attitudes and beliefs, anxiety, and psychosexual trauma. One outmoded traditional attitude holds that sex is an undesirable duty for women and pleasurable only for men. This kind of stereotypical thinking can create such anxiety for a woman that she cannot enjoy coitus and may, in turn, cause erection or ejaculation problems for the man.

Like other skills, sexual competence is learned. We learn what makes us and others feel good by talking with them about sex, reading about it, watching films, and experimenting. Many people, however, do not acquire sexual skills because they lack the opportunity to experiment or because even the thought of violating traditional mores creates overwhelming anxiety for them.

Sex Therapy   The behavioral treatment of sexual dysfunction concentrates on reducing performance anxiety, changing self-defeating expectations, and learning sexual skills or competencies. Masters and Johnson offer a two-week treatment program for couples, who live in residence at their clinic. Included in the program is "bibliotherapy" or treatment through the reading of self-help manuals. Examples of other techniques that have been effective follow.

A man who is unable to attain an erection learns to relax and receive sexual stimulation. The partners first massage each other without touching the genitals, using verbal instructions and guiding each other's hands in order to communicate. Genital manipulation follows after a few sessions. When erection is reliably attained, the couple does not immediately attempt intercourse because performance anxiety might develop. Instead, the partners follow a series of sexual activities that ultimately ends in intercourse. Masters and Johnson report that erectile dysfunction has been reversed in 72 percent of the couples treated.

Premature ejaculation is often treated by the "squeeze technique" in which the tip of the penis is squeezed when the man feels he is about to ejaculate. This technique is learned from a sex therapist. Gradually, the man learns to prolong intercourse without ejaculating. Masters and Johnson report that this technique is successful in 90 percent of the men treated.

Primary orgasmic dysfunction frequently occurs among women who feel that sex is dirty and may have been taught never to touch themselves. They are anxious about their sexuality and have not had the chance to learn through trial and error what types of sexual stimulation will excite them and bring them to climax. Most sex therapists prefer the use of masturbation to treat this problem. Masturbation provides women with a chance to learn about their own bodies and to give themselves pleasure without depending on a sex partner. Masturbation programs first teach women about their own anatomy by means of reading, discussion groups, and the use of a mirror. They experiment with self-caresses at their own pace, learning gradually to bring themselves to orgasm. The behavioral approach uses the reward or pleasure principle to counter negative or anxiety-provoking situations. Once a woman can masturbate to orgasm, she may need additional treatment to transfer this learning to sex with a partner.

Chapter Five

Sexual Responses

Probing Your Emotions

1. How confident are you of your own sexuality? Do you feel it is necessary to understand your own sexual needs and how your sexual response works? How does understanding your own sexual and intimate needs relate to your general health and wellness?

2. With respect to your sexual maturity, where do you feel you are at this stage in your life? Do you expect too much of yourself? Too little? What kinds of experiences would you like to have to make your life more sexually fulfilling?

3. What frustrations have you had regarding your own experience with your sexuality? What experiences make you angry, sad, or disappointed? Make a list of these; when you read the following chapter, keep this list to maintain a personal focus.

Chapter Contents

THE ROLE OF THE NERVOUS SYSTEM IN SEX
The pleasure center
The impact of feelings on the sex drive
The sexual response
The thalamus and sexual response
STAGES OF SEXUAL RESPONSE
Excitement stage
Plateau stage
Orgasmic stage
Resolution stage
VARIETIES OF SEXUAL EXPERIENCE
Intimacy needs
Sexual needs
VARIANT SEXUAL BEHAVIOR
Passive variance
Active variance

Boxes

A brief history of the kiss
Myths about sex
The sexual anxiety inventory
Kinds of sexual contact
Homosexuality

Old cortex
A small, hidden part of the human brain that governs the sense of smell. In lower vertebrates, the old cortex makes up most of the outside layer of the brain.

New cortex
The outside layer of the brain that appeared late in evolution (hence, new) and came to its highest development in human beings; controls complex behavior and mental activity.

Hypothalamus
An area at the base of the brain just below the thalamus.

Orgasm
The climax of sexual excitement; marked normally by ejaculation of semen by the male and by release of tumescence in the erectile organs of both sexes.

Septum
Dividing wall or membrane.

Hippocampal gyrus
Portion of the temporal lobe of the cerebrum, part of the new cortex.

---

5 The more we learn about the difference between what is naturally, biologically, inherently human and what is arbitrary or superstitious in our culture, the freer we are to create new codes that are more in harmony with human nature and less repressive of the individual spirit. To a great extent, this change is exactly what is happening in America today.

Nature gives us the impulse for sex, but culture organizes our perceptions, telling us with whom we can make love, as well as when, where, and under what conditions. Our training, besides telling us which people may be acceptable as sex partners, even tells us what traits in a person may be seen as sexually appealing. But something it does not always tell us is the "how." We are not born knowing how to make love. These activities must be learned, and not knowing does not make a person a sexual "failure."

The Role of the Nervous System in Sex

Erotic sensations are carried in a system of sensory nerves. You become aware of these sensations when the impulses from the sensory nerves are transmitted to the brain's pleasure center—which is in a part of the limbic cortex, or *old cortex*, so called because in the history of our species it evolved earlier than the cerebral cortex, or *new cortex*.

Reception of erotic sensory inputs stimulates increasing rhythmical motor activity in the body, and this activity feeds back additional inputs to the sensation, increasing it. Eventually there is an overwhelming electrical discharge from the *hypothalamus*, which is made more intense by the greatest possible motion. This final discharge—along with the other events it triggers—is the *orgasm*.

The Pleasure Center Neurophysiologists have identified the *septum* as both the center of pleasurable feelings in general and the center for the more specific pleasurable sensations of sex. The septum is located at the open end of a horseshoe-shaped structure called the *hippocampal gyrus*. The nerve cells follow a pattern around the gyrus corresponding to locations in the body from top to bottom. See Figure 5–1.

In the septum is the olfactory nerve, the nerve involved in the sense of smell. Next to the olfactory nerve are the nerves that receive impulses from the anogenital region. The nerves involved in sight and taste are also close to the ends of the gyrus. It is possible that this configuration helps to explain why the sense of smell plays such an important part in the sexuality of all mammals and why human sexual responses in particular are excited by sexual sights, tastes, and, to a limited degree, smells. It also explains why stimulation of the anogenital structures evokes arousal and fantasy.

The Impact of Feelings on the Sex Drive The hypothalamus, in its capacity as an apparatus that drives erotic sensory nerves, is extremely sensitive to emotional states. Izard and Tomkins (1966) have tried to classify these states. They described two ranges of positive emotions: interest to excitement; and enjoyment to joy. They also identified five negative ranges: fear to terror; anger to rage; shame to humiliation; distress to anguish; and contempt to disgust. The positive feelings, it was found, tend to increase the hunger and sex drives, and the negative feelings tend to interfere with hunger and with sexual arousal. Anger seems to block sexual feeling

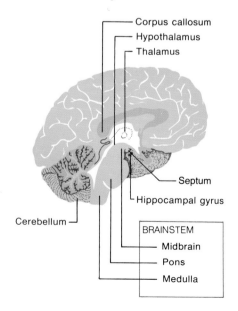

Corpus callosum
Hypothalamus
Thalamus

Septum
Hippocampal gyrus

Cerebellum

BRAINSTEM
Midbrain
Pons
Medulla

Figure 5-1 Parts of the brain responsible for sexual behavior.

Sensor
Something that responds to stimuli of some type.

Vulva
The external genital organs of the female.

Vagina
The canal in the female extending from the vulva to the cervix.

Clitoris
A small erectile organ at the upper end of the vulva; homologous with the penis.

Penis
The male organ of copulation and urination.

Receptor
A nerve ending specialized to receive or to sense stimuli.

Erection
The condition of erectile tissue such as the penis, clitoris, or nipples when filled with blood.

---

in a couple accustomed to sex, but apparently increases the sexual aggressiveness of the rapist.

The Sexual Response   Every person has a system of sexual *sensors* that consist of

1. Specialized nerve endings wherever skin and mucus membranes meet.
2. Specialized nerve endings adapted to sexual function in the nipples and areolas of the breasts.
3. General sensory nerve endings in the skin that respond sexually in the arousal state.
4. Muscle nerves that function sexually in the arousal state.
5. Sensory nerves in the hollow tubular structures of the genital system.

These sensors send erotic impulses to the brain if they are stimulated by a touch that is not too light (as tickling with a feather might be) or too harsh (as hitting might be) and if the drive function of the hypothalamus has not been shut off by negative emotions. We shall describe the items listed above in the approximate order in which they come into play.

The Mucocutaneous System   The mucocutaneous system has erotic sensory nerve endings in four areas:

1. At the margins of the eyelids.
2. Around the lips and just inside the mouth on the inner border of the lips and the front part of the cheeks. The presence of these nerve endings inside the mouth helps to explain why the sensuous kiss is often a deep kiss, with the tongue stimulating a greater and greater number of the interior nerve endings.
3. In the genitals. Erotic nerve endings are densely concentrated in the entire *vulva,* including the labia minora (the pink inner lips); in the urethra, especially at its opening; and around the opening of the *vagina,* although there are none inside the vagina. The *clitoris* has a tremendous concentration of these nerve endings, as many as there are in its male equivalent, the *penis.* In the male the concentrations of erotic nerve endings are greatest in the glans of the penis, especially at the tip, and most especially in the little tag of tissue just under the urethral opening called the frenulum. Friction at either the glans or the vulva

is likely to be painful rather than pleasurable if the person is not aroused. For some women direct pressure on the clitoris even during arousal is uncomfortable.

4. In the anus. The anus shares with the genitals all the sensations of arousal and stimulation, including the experience of orgasm. The presence of mucocutaneous nerve endings in the anus is probably the reason that some people prefer anal intercourse.

Pressure-Sensitive Receptors   In the walls of the expandable veins of the penile shaft and the clitoral shaft are nerve endings that are sensitive to pressure. *Erection*

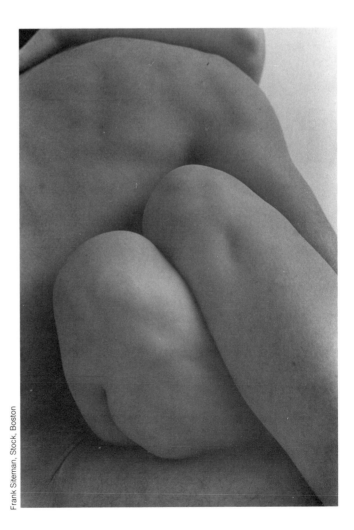

Frank Siteman, Stock, Boston

A Brief History of the Kiss

Classifications are entertaining but not especially illuminating. Types of kisses overlap and change through time, like dunes in the wind. A kiss that began with one intention may be transformed until its original meaning is lost.

For example, St. Paul may not have known what would come of his simple advice to "salute one another with an holy kiss," a brief admonition in Romans 16:16 that is repeated in Corinthians I and II. Over the centuries St. Paul's "holy kiss" was interpreted and reinterpreted, finding expression in a variety of religious rites—baptism, marriage, confession, ordination. The *osculum pacis,* or kiss of peace, was supposed to represent God's kiss of life and Christ's kiss of eternal blessing; thus believers could, with a kiss, transmit spiritual feelings and the chaste love of others.

In some Christian denominations the holy kiss was exchanged between the priest and the penitent; in others the clergy exchanged the kiss during special masses; members of the Greek Church exchanged the kiss on Easter Sunday. The holy kiss passed out of common practice after the Reformation, but it seems to be enjoying a renaissance in modern Catholic, Anglican, and Episcopalian congregations.

The kiss between bride and groom, which contemporary couples interpret as an expression of love and desire, had actually been part of pre-Christian pagan rites and meant that legal bonds were being assumed. The Catholics took the existing ceremonial kiss of legality and changed it into a transmission of the kiss of peace: from the priest to the groom, from the groom to the bride.

In a culture that reserved the kiss for ceremonial and religious occasions, the kiss of peace might have retained its austerity and chastity. But in Europe the kiss had erotic connotations, and the Church waged a continous battle against licentious kissing in the name of spiritual communication. A special instrument to convey the holy kiss was introduced in England in the thirteenth century: The osculatorium, a metal disc with a holy picture, was passed around the congregation. A clever suitor, however, would try to kiss the [disc] in the same spot his beloved had and thereby transmit a delayed, but profanely intended kiss.

By the Middle Ages the holy kiss had wended its way into secular activities—to confirm agreement or to reconcile enemies, for example. ("To kiss and make-up" may derive in part from such kisses of reconciliation.) To kiss was to convey one's intentions for the health and salvation of the other's soul, which could hardly be done if a grudge were unresolved.

Of course, where there are saints, there are sinners. Christ kissed mankind for salvation, but Judas betrayed with a kiss. The "Judas kiss" was a heinous sin, a reversal of all things good and loyal that the holy kiss signified. The Judas kiss, according to anthropologists Francis and Elizabeth Ianni, is still used among some Mafiosi. When a man has betrayed the group, his relative or a close friend ceremonially marks him for death with a kiss on the mouth. This kiss means "I still love you; this is not a personal matter but a business one." In the late 1600s, English fashions in kissing changed rather suddenly. Gestures of respect and reverence turned from kisses to bows, curtsies, hat lifting, and variants of arm waving; the kiss on the mouth or cheek was kept for members of one's social circle. Why the change? One reason may be the outbreak of plague in London in 1665, which panicked people about contagion. Another may be the decline of feudalism and the spread of commerce, trade, and travel, which created a larger network of business relationships and started to break up rigid social and economic hierarchies.

The middle- and upper-class social kiss of greeting held its ground through the seventeenth and part of the eighteenth century. Apparently it became a court fad of colossal proportions, because it became a target of satire by Molière, Congreve, and other writers. Lately, journalists and social scientists have observed that middle-class social kissing in America and England has become an epidemic. The no-contact "air kiss"—a lip smack in the vicinity of the cheek but never touching—is exchanged, it seems, at every opportunity.

Leonore Tieffer
The Kiss

Myths About Sex

Male genital size is related to sexual capability. Bigger is better.

Not so. Actually, size is irrelevant to sensitivity or satisfaction.

The male is erotic; the female interested only in reproduction.

Not necessarily so. Women may desire and have multiple orgasms, as many as 30. Men are somewhat limited.

The woman who does not reach orgasm as a result of vaginal stimulation has a sexual problem.

Not necessarily so. Erotic response cycles are completed in various ways. Some women do not respond to vaginal stimulation at all.

The best position for intercourse is the one with the man on top of the woman.

Not necessarily so. There is no one best position for everyone. The best positions are the ones the people involved decide on.

Physical performance suffers if the person has sex.

No evidence whatsoever to support this idea. It is just as likely that sexual activity relaxes an overly tense person.

The ability to have genital sex is lost in the aging process.

Depends. People can and do have sex in their 70s and 80s if and when both partners are interested enough.

Sexual intercourse is not recommended during the last three months of pregnancy.

Not true unless there is postcoital bleeding or evidence of membrane rupture or bleeding. Normal sexual intercourse can be continued throughout pregnancy.

Women experience two types of orgasm, "clitoral" and "vaginal."

All orgasms in the woman are physiologically identical.

Circumcision increases sexual sensitivity in the male.

There is no measurable difference in sexual sensitivity between males who have been circumcised and those who have not.

---

exerts pressure on these nerve endings of the pressure-sensitive system, and they send impulses that register as erotic and pleasurable.

Nipple-Areola System   Suckling is a sensation made pleasurable by nature to ensure its occurrence, as with the suckling infant. However, the pleasure becomes a sexual pleasure through learned behavior, as is true for other sexual sensors, with about a third of both males and females reporting sexually sensitive nipples. The nipples respond with erection and any touch, from light to heavy, may be pleasing.

All of these three primary systems—mucocutaneous, pressure-sensitive, and nipple-areola—show increased sensitivity during sexual arousal, and the stimulation of any may produce arousal.

Touch Receptors of the Skin   Sexual arousal changes the quality of the impulses sent by touch receptors from ordinary to erotic and pleasurable. When two people are in a highly charged state of mutual attraction, even the touch of a hand on an arm can evoke a profound sexual response. Any part of the body can become an erogenous zone if it is stroked. This fact is true not only of the obvious places like breasts, buttocks, thighs, and abdomen, but also of the head and neck, the cheeks, eyes, earlobes, shoulders, armpits, and almost any other

place; each individual has his or her own special places. The role of the hand in human sexual exploration and stimulation is greater than in any other species.

The Other Senses   The senses of smell, vision, hearing, and taste all have sexual significance. Pheromones are the specific sexual scents given off by animals; musk perfumes attempt to capitalize on this property. Vision seems to play a more important part in human sexual response than it does in other species and a more important part for human males than for human females, although this may be owing to the influence of culture. Even without smell or touch stimulation, human lovers seem to be greatly and sometimes instantly aroused by the sight of each other's bodies. This situation is true not only of the obvious case of total or partial nudity but also of almost any part of the body or expression of the body or movement of the body. A look in one's eyes can have a powerfully erotic impact. Similarly, the sound of a lover's voice can evoke a strong response. Sounds also help awareness of the partner's reactions and of one's own reactions—sounds of heavy breathing, moans, words, animal sounds, even screams. This awareness intensifies arousal. Taste is closely related to smell and is subject to some of the same cultural interference. When there is no interference, it can play an important part in arousal.

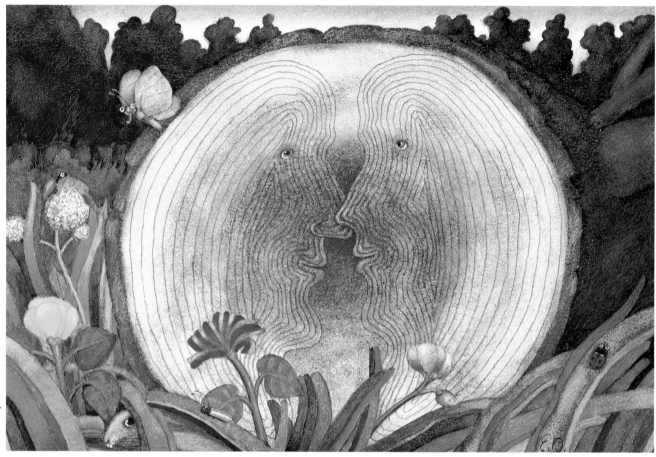

Postural muscles
Muscles that help to position the body.

Thalamus
The relay station for sensory impulses.

Excitement stage
The first stage of sexual response. During this stage the body first recognizes a sexual stimulus.

Plateau stage
The second stage of sexual response. During this stage there is heightened sexual arousal.

The touch receptors and the other senses are classified as secondary sensors. The secondary sensors either play a supporting role in sexual arousal, as vision does, for example, or change their function to a sexual one during arousal, as touch receptors do.

The Muscle Receptors   Muscle tension during sexual activity has been likened to an epileptic seizure. People clasp and grasp each other in a rhythmic pattern and strain together, all of which involves the *postural muscles.* Each set of postural muscles sends its sensory volley to add to the bombardment of the central nervous system. During the preorgasmic peak of activity there is coordinated rhythmic movement of the great mass of the pelvic and leg muscles, often augmented by contractions of the muscles of the pelvic floor. The latter tighten the vaginal inlet and the anus as well as the muscles at the base of the penis. During orgasm, there is slower sustained straining movement of the postural muscles, which contributes heavily to the sensation of that peak event.

The Visceral Receptors   The visceral receptors lie in the walls of all the hollow-tube pelvic structures—the vagina, uterus, and oviducts in the female; the prostate, vas deferens, seminal vesicles, and bulbous urethra in the male. Contraction of these structures is associated with the sensations of orgasm. See Figure 5–2.

Muscle receptors and visceral receptors can be classified as tertiary sensors. Their inputs, although important even in early stages of sexual activity, are greatest during orgasm.

The Thalamus and Sexual Response   The *thalamus is* the part of the brain stem that extends upward toward the new cortex. It is the part of the human being that registers either a deep sense of well-being or the opposite, a sense of profound uneasiness. It seems to function in both aggressive and sexual behaviors, being the receiving point for sexual sensory impulses.

Impulses from the sensory nerve endings travel through the spinal cord and enter the tract leading from the spine to the thalamus to find their first activation point. Some of the impulses are relayed down to the hypothalamus, some up to the old cortex, and some

back to the motor systems, where they induce salivation, genital activity, erection, and, in males, ejaculation.

Stages of Sexual Response

It is evident that sex can be anything from a simple genital event to a whole-person experience involving thought, idea, emotion, and basic neurobiological responses. Four stages of sexual response have been identified by William Masters and Virginia Johnson in *Human Sexual Response.*

Excitement Stage   Sexual excitement may begin with a thought or fantasy, with the perception in some way (sight, smell, touch, and so on) of a desirable sexual partner, or with the stimulation of an erotic sensory area. The excitement can be quite impersonal (as in casual sex or commercial sex); it can be personal (two people who find each other sexually attractive); it can be love-related or affectional. Notable among the many body responses at the *excitement stage* are widely opened eyes, rapid heartbeat and respiration, and flushed skin.

Plateau Stage   The nearness of an attractive partner or the development of a sexual fantasy can cause a progression from excitement to sexual arousal. During this *plateau stage* the surrounding world seems to recede and sexual tension increases. A set of initial signals is sent and received via posture, gesture, expression, and words. An embrace in the excitement phase becomes stronger and more passionate. Kissing moves from light and gentle to deep and often rough. The trunk and pelvis almost independently take on sexual motions. Sexual arousal quickly makes one single-minded. The heart races, breath is short, penis or clitoris erect, salivation increases. The hand begins to play its sexual part of exploration, and a mutual effort to struggle free of clothing proceeds.

While a voluntary or outside interruption could be accomplished earlier, during the plateau stage it is almost certainly too late. Verbal communication becomes segmented words or exclamations carrying an emotional tone rather than a discrete meaning. The only

Figure 5-2 The reproductive organs: (*a*) male; (*b*) female internal organs; (*c*) female external organs.

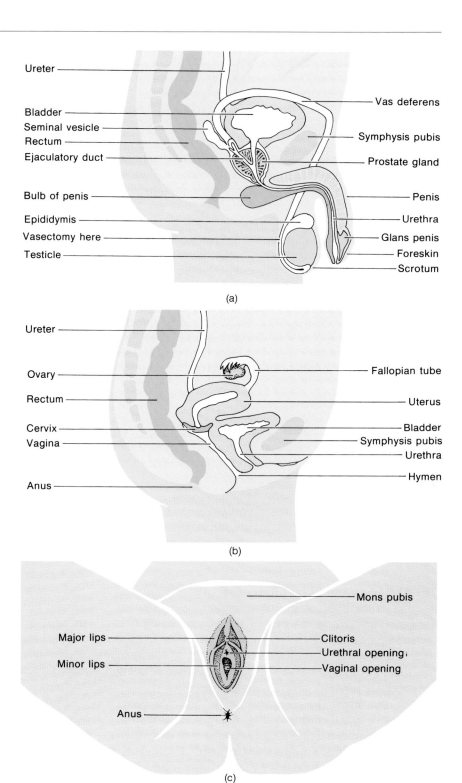

Ureter

Bladder
Seminal vesicle
Rectum
Ejaculatory duct

Bulb of penis

Epididymis
Vasectomy here
Testicle

Vas deferens

Symphysis pubis

Prostate gland

Penis

Urethra

Glans penis

Foreskin

Scrotum

(a)

Ureter

Ovary

Rectum

Cervix
Vagina

Anus

Fallopian tube

Uterus

Bladder
Symphysis pubis
Urethra

Hymen

(b)

Mons pubis

Major lips

Minor lips

Clitoris
Urethral opening
Vaginal opening

Anus

(c)

Copulation
Sexual intercourse.

Masturbation
Excitation of the genitals by means other than sexual intercourse.

Orgasmic stage
The third stage of sexual response. During this stage sexual excitement reaches a climax.

Resolution stage
The fourth stage of sexual response. During this stage extreme relaxation follows orgasm, and tension is absent

really purposive movements are carrying themselves forward to the next stage.

Orgasmic Stage   *Copulation* (see Figure 5–3) or *masturbation* moves at an accelerated pace during the *orgasmic stage*, and the sensitivity of the glans penis and of the clitoris increases. At some point a slightly spreading sensation reaches consciousness, and at this time an orgasm is usually inevitable. (One of the few things which preempts it is a foot cramp.)

Orgasm produces a generalized pleasure response that is initiated by a high voltage discharge in the brain stem. It lasts from about two to ten seconds and is accompanied by massive contractions of the trunk and limb muscles, by a maximum physiologic heart rate, and irregular breathing. This is reflected in the female by successive contractions of the tubes, the uterus, and the vagina; and in the male by contractions of the urethra, the vas deferens, the prostate, seminal vesicles, and the bulbocavernosus muscle. In the male these contractions marshall the components of semen, and ejaculation occurs.

The orgasm peaks with awareness only of the self and the monumental sensations pervading the whole body.

Resolution Stage   If the experience has been a good one (and what is good is different for each person) and if the orgasm has been complete, the extreme activity of copulation and orgasm is followed by extreme relaxation. In the *resolution stage*, tension is absent, and there is a feeling of satisfaction and well-being. Sleep comes easily. It is difficult for the male to become sexually aroused again until he has recovered, a process that may take a few minutes or a few hours. This time

Figure 5-3   A cross section of human intercourse.

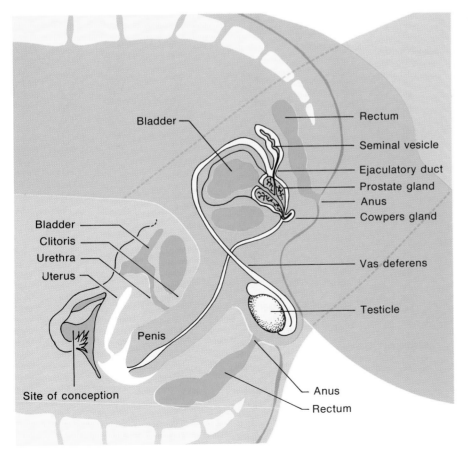

Bladder — Rectum
— Seminal vesicle
— Ejaculatory duct
— Prostate gland
— Anus
— Cowpers gland
Bladder —
Clitoris —
Urethra —
Uterus —
— Vas deferens
— Testicle
Penis —
— Anus
Site of conception
— Rectum

Refractory period
The period of time it takes for the male to
again become sexually aroused after
orgasm.

is known as the *refractory period.* The female may,
however, be ready for more sex and more orgasms.

In a study at the University of Pennsylvania almost
all women identified the sense of intimacy in this stage
as the most satisfying part of sex. Half the men agreed,
while the other half identified the orgasmic peak as the
most satisfying.

Figures 5–4 and 5–5 present simple diagrammatic
graphs of the male and female sexual response cycles.

This description of the stages of sexual response is

both idealized and oversimplified. It is not a plan to be
followed. In many real-life situations, the excitement and
enthusiasm, rather than being perfectly mutual, are
somewhat one-sided. Distractions, sexual problems, or
a large variety of other obstacles can and often do prevent
completion of copulation (or masturbation, in which the
most intense orgasms have been measured) or make it
less than satisfying. One partner may be insensitive to
the other's needs or may feel fearful or inadequate. One
or both of the partners may "perform" in a way unsat-

Figure 5-4   The male sexual response cycle.

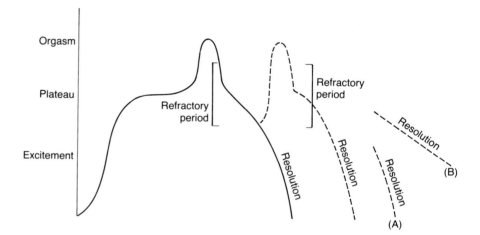

Figure 5-5   The female sexual response cycle.

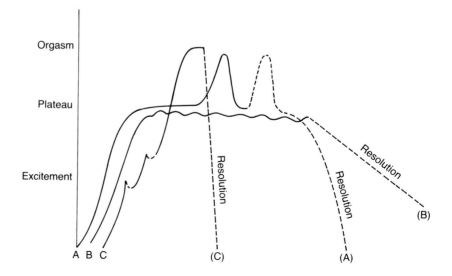

The Sexual Anxiety Inventory

While a little anxiety of the sort we experience on a first date can enhance sexual response, severe anxiety can block it. Factors like traditional sex-negative beliefs, psychosexual trauma, troubled relationships, irrational beliefs, and concerns about performance can all contribute to our sexual anxiety.

The following questionnaire, constructed by psychologists Louis Janda and Kevin O'Grady, will allow you to compare your level of sexual anxiety to that of other college students. Read each item and choose the answer, a or b, that best describes your feelings. Work rapidly and leave no item blank—even if the choice is difficult.

Then turn to the scoring key to interpret your answers.

Sexual Anxiety Inventory

1. Extramarital sex . . .
a. is O.K. if everyone agrees
b. can break up families

2. Sex . . .
a. can cause as much anxiety as pleasure
b. on the whole is good and enjoyable

3. Masturbation . . .
a. causes me to worry
b. can be a useful substitute

4. After having sexual thoughts . . .
a. I feel aroused
b. I feel jittery

5. When I engage in petting . . .
a. I feel scared at first
b. I thoroughly enjoy it

6. Initiating sexual relationships . . .
a. is a very stressful experience
b. causes me no problem at all

7. Oral sex . . .
a. would arouse me
b. would terrify me

8. I feel nervous . . .
a. about initiating sexual relations
b. about nothing, when it comes to members of the opposite sex

9. When I meet someone I'm attracted to . . .
a. I get to know him or her
b. I feel nervous

10. When I was younger . . .
a. I was looking forward to having sex
b. the thought of sex scared me

11. When others flirt with me . . .
a. I don't know what to do
b. I flirt back

12. Group sex . . .
a. would scare me to death
b. might be interesting

13. If in the future I committed adultery . . .
a. I would probably get caught
b. I wouldn't feel bad about it

14. I would . . .
a. feel too nervous to tell a dirty joke in mixed company
b. tell a dirty joke if it were funny

15. Dirty jokes . . .
a. make me feel uncomfortable
b. often make me laugh

16. When I awake from sex dreams . . .
a. I feel pleasant and relaxed
b. I feel tense

17. When I have sexual desires . . .
a. I worry about what I should do
b. I do something to satisfy them

18. If in the future I committed adultery . . .
a. it would be nobody's business but my own
b. I would worry about my spouse's finding out

19. Buying a pornographic book . . .
a. wouldn't bother me
b. would make me nervous

20. Casual sex . . .
a. is better than no sex at all
b. can hurt many people

21. Extramarital sex . . .
a. is sometimes necessary
b. can damage one's career

22. Sexual advances . . .
a. leave me feeling tense
b. are welcomed

23. When I have sexual relations . . .
a. I feel satisfied
b. I worry about being discovered

24. When talking about sex in mixed company . . .
a. I feel nervous
b. I sometimes get excited

25. If I were to flirt with someone . . .
a. I would worry about his or her reaction
b. I would enjoy it

L. H. Janda and E. E. O'Grady
Development of a Sex Anxiety Inventory

Coitus
Sexual intercourse.

Intimacy needs
Needs for companionship, mutual respect,
love.

The Sexual Anxiety Inventory (cont.)

Scoring Key

For each of the following answers, credit yourself with
a point of sexual anxiety:

1. b	6. a	11. a	16. b	21. b
2. a	7. b	12. a	17. a	22. a
3. a	8. a	13. a	18. b	23. b
4. b	9. b	14. a	19. b	24. a
5. a	10. b	15. a	20. b	25. a

In their studies with 95 males and 135 females, Janda
and O'Grady (1980) found the average score for
males to be 8.09 and the average score for females
to be 11.76. Approximately 2 of every 3 scores for
men fell within the range from 3 to 13. Approximately
2 of every 3 women's scores fell between 7 and 17.

Don't take your own score too seriously. You are
comparing it to only a small and rather unrepresen-
tative sample of individuals. But if you are concerned
about your score, you may wish to discuss it with
your professor.

---

orgasms; some have orgasms but not in *coitus;* some
do not have orgasms but still enjoy sex. One adaptive
technique is for the male to delay his orgasm. Another
is for the male to bring his partner to orgasm with his
tongue or his fingertip. Simultaneous orgasm is not very
common, and the use of "adaptive techniques" is more
the rule than the exception. Many partners find that if
they experience orgasm at the same time, they cannot
fully enjoy each other's orgasms. Their own experience
blots out awareness of the other's.

Because the whole nervous system is very much
involved, our sexual patterns quickly become a matter
of habit. The more things we can put into the automatic
range of function dictated by our series of self-images
and needs, the more comfortable we are. If we start off
a sex life badly, it has a great chance of falling into a
habit pattern of remaining bad. If we begin by cultivating
positive and satisfying habits, they, too, tend to sustain
themselves. Sex is thus both an automatic and a learned
behavior.

Varieties of Sexual Experience

Sexual activity in some species is highly stereotyped; that
is, there is only one pattern of courting behavior, one
mounting position, and little chance for variety. In
humans the possibilities for variety seem almost limit-
less. The human body is superbly suited for many kinds
of erotic contact, and the human imagination has an
amazing capacity to discover the possibilities.

Humans also create cultures, and those cultures may
declare certain forms of sexual expression taboo. Society
then has assumed the task of restraining many of the
organism's natural impulses.

Descriptions of all the possible forms of human sexual
experience would fill several books. We shall limit our
discussion to intimacy needs and sexual needs as they
affect various kinds of sexual experiences.

Intimacy Needs   Human sexual needs resemble, in
many respects, human *intimacy needs,* although it is not
unusual for a person to pursue one but not the other

---

isfying to the other. The lovers may be tired of each other
or unable to communicate sexually with each other.
Interpersonal conflicts also can diminish pleasure.

People sometimes feel that as they become more and
more sexually aroused they lose control. Sexual arousal
does, in fact, bring a shift from conscious, willed,
manipulative control to spontaneous, involuntary control. People who are unable to lose some voluntary
control often find sex a disappointing experience.

What factors determine timing of arousal and orgasm
are not fully known. There are cultural as well as
individual differences. For example, in some but not all
cultures women are slower in arousal than men.

Because the female orgasm is subject to such great
individual differences, the male must often adapt. Some
females have multiple orgasms; some have single

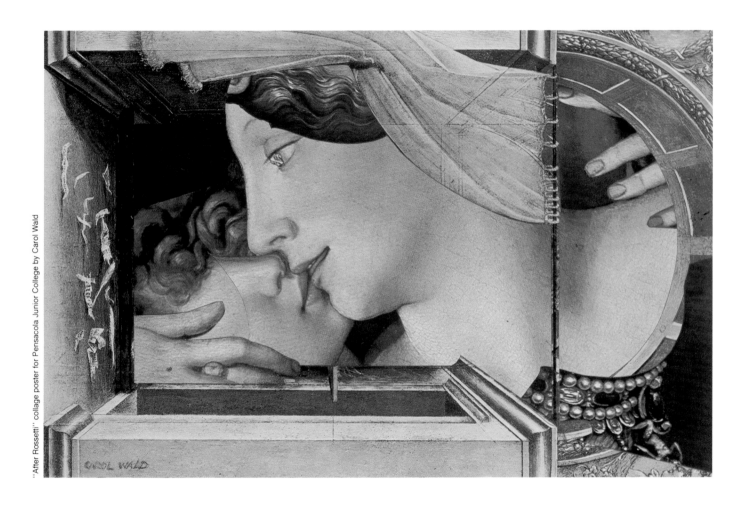

"After Rossetti" collage poster for Pensacola Junior College by Carol Wald

CAROL WALD

Sexual needs
Need for gratification of the sexual drive.

Autosexuals
People who confine their sexual activity to masturbation.

Homosexuals
People who confine their sexual activity to same-sex partners.

Heterosexuals
People who confine their sexual activity to opposite-sex partners.

Bisexuals
People who are able to enjoy either heterosexual or homosexual activity.

Catasexual
Adjective describing sexual activity with a nonhuman partner.

Variance
A deviation from cultural norms.

Voyeurism
Act of obtaining pleasure from watching sexual activity or nudity.

Exhibitionism
Act of deriving pleasure from exposing one's genitals.

Sexual taboo
A condemnation by society of certain sexual acts. Incest is a prime example of a sexual taboo.

Incest
Sexual union between people who are so closely related that their marriage is illegal or forbidden by custom.

---

or to pursue them in different directions. Intimacy needs have been classified as self-loving (autophilic), loving those like oneself—those of the same sex (homophilic)—and loving those unlike oneself—those of the opposite sex (heterophilic).

All three kinds of intimacy needs are part of growing up, and part of any whole person. Without the ability to love oneself, it is not possible to love others. Without the ability to love one's own kind, it is not possible to love one's opposite. Development in some people is arrested at the self-loving stage, and their attention remains turned inward on themselves. They give the appearance of loving only themselves, but, instead, they are really stuck because they cannot accomplish the task of self-love. Some people remain at the homophilic stage, the stage of loving those of their own sex, and

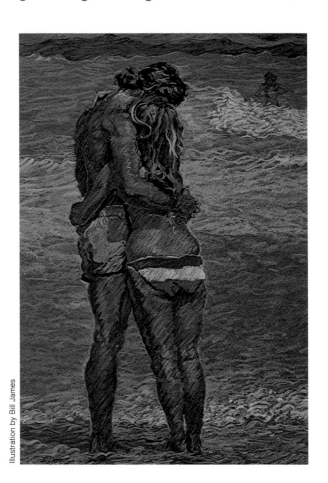

Illustration by Bill James

some people fail to move on to the heterophilic stage, which is love for the opposite sex. What happens in the development of these intimacy needs affects the development of sexual needs.

Sexual Needs   Paralleling the three kinds of intimacy needs are three kinds of *sexual needs* — *autosexual, homosexual,* and *heterosexual.* There are strong indications that humans naturally have all three kinds of needs. However, the power of culture to inhibit and to modify natural feelings is tremendous, and many individuals are exclusively autosexual, exclusively homosexual, or exclusively heterosexual. Autosexuals, because they cannot or do not want to relate sexually to other people, either confine their sexual activity to masturbation or have no sex life at all. Exclusively homosexual individuals, because they cannot or do not want to relate sexually to opposite-sex partners, either confine their sexual activity to same-sex partners or have no sex life. Exclusively heterosexual behavior is perceived as the norm in our society, but many behavioral scientists now believe it reflects the repression of other feelings, not their absence. An increasing number of people have begun to consider themselves *bisexual* —able to enjoy either heterosexual or homosexual activity—and some scientists believe that humans are a bisexual species.

Some sexual activity is labeled *catasexual.* In this kind of behavior the partner chosen is, instead of a person, usually a barnyard animal. Children raised on farms sometimes choose nonhuman partners, but this behavior is likely to be experimentation rather than a fixed pattern.

If all one's possible autosexual, homosexual, and heterosexual partners were listed, the list would include the name of every living person; it would be hard to imagine a greater range of possibilities. But as we shall see, cultural taboos can shorten the list drastically.

Variant Sexual Behavior

Sexual *variance* is a concept firmly embedded in the quickly shifting sands of cultural evolution. It changes from time to time and from place to place or within the

Kinds of Sexual Contact

Whether you believe there are two or 101 or 2,037 possible positions for human intercourse, you will find that all of them are variations of a few simple themes. In light of the earlier discussion of the erotic sensory system of the body, it will not be a surprise that in all but one of these themes organs other than genitals function as sex organs.

Orthogenital sex is coupling of the penis and the vagina. Countless variations are possible and may be enjoyable, even though many societies have at various times tried to enshrine one or another of these positions as *the* position.

Paragenital sex is sex in which one's genitals are in conjunction with a nongenital part of one's partner. A female can be masturbated by her partner; she can be the recipient of cunnilingus (licking of the clitoris and vulva); a male can be masturbated by his partner; he can be the recipient of fellatio (sucking of the penis); or he can be the active partner in anal coitus. All these acts are examples of paragenital sex.

Metagenital sex is sex in which a nongenital part of oneself is in conjunction with the partner's genital. A person who is masturbating his or her partner or who is in oral contact with the partner's genitals or who is the passive partner in anal coitus is engaging in metagenital sex.

Amphigenital sex is sex in which two partners are in simultaneous oral-genital contact with each other. This form of sex is often called "69" because the shapes of the numbers seem to suggest the partners' inverted positions with relation to each other. In a heterosexual pair amphigenital sex consists of simultaneous fellatio and cunnilingus. In a homosexual pair it consists of either mutual fellatio or mutual cunnilingus.

---

sample place. All of the kinds of sexuality we currently know of were seen and recorded in the Chinese pillow books and the *Kamasutra* of Vatsayana thousands of years ago. The sexual behaviors described below fall into the category of sexual variance; the variance is in cultural acceptability.

Passive Variance   The category labeled passive variance contains two rather mild forms of activity, *voyeurism* and *exhibitionism*. Technically, a voyeur is a person whose principal source of sexual pleasure is in looking at sex organs and sex acts. This behavior is difficult to identify and define, however, because it is hard to draw the line between what is accepted and what is not. It is not unusual for a healthy man to obtain pleasure and erotic stimulation from seeing a nude or partly nude woman. An entire industry is founded on that fact. And more than a few women enjoy looking at nude men. Voyeurs differ in that they often go to great lengths to satisfy a need that perhaps all of us have. Their activity is a problem when it involves an unwelcome intrusion into the privacy of another person. Much voyeurism seems also to be a *dis*connecting activity rather than a relating activity.

With exhibitionism, sometimes referred to as "indecent exposure," it is also hard to draw the line. Many people of both sexes and all ages sometimes find it erotically pleasurable not only to be nude but also to be aware that their bodies are being seen. But the classic exhibitionist—the man who whips open his raincoat to expose his genitals—is not interested in making personal contact with the people he exposes himself to. His act is distancing.

Active Variance   People who are actively variant usually have a strong sex drive and run afoul of a *sexual taboo* by choosing an excluded partner, by choosing a large number of partners, or by displaying more than the accepted amount of aggressiveness in their pursuit of pleasure.

Sexual Aggression   How much aggression is acceptable? Certainly rape is a crime, not necessarily because it is sexual but because it is violent. It is a direct and usually totally unprovoked attack on another person's right to choose whether or not to have sex and with whom.

Just how sex and aggression are related, if they are, is still not known. They may be connected in the temporal lobe of the brain. We do know that the sexual receptors sometimes respond erotically to sensations that are supposedly painful. Some people have woven an entire sexual life-style out of the aggressive aspect of sex, calling it by such names as "sadism and masochism" or "bondage and discipline."

Incest   According to anthropologists, every known present-day society has *incest* regulations. In spite of the strength of the taboo, incest is not rare, even in the United States. Father-daughter and brother-sister incest occur at all levels of society, although mother-son incest is much less common.

Homosexuality

In terms of age, social class, education, occupation, and interests, the homosexual is represented in every segment of society. Since 1929 surveys in the United States, Great Britain, and Europe have indicated that 10 to 15 percent of the population is overtly homosexual for a period of three or more years in adult life. Homosexuals do not usually act, speak, or dress differently from heterosexuals. Most prefer to conceal their inclinations and activities because of the ridicule, alienation, and legal punishments that they would possibly face if their activities became known.

Male and female homosexuals who have not "come out" and declared to the world at large that they are homosexual often suffer stress and anxiety from living double lives. Should their activities become known or even suspected, they may lose their jobs. They may also be rejected by family and "straight" friends. If they are not able to find companionship and support in a homosexual "community" or with homosexual friends, they are liable to feel lonely and depressed. Men more often than women may face imprisonment,

blackmail, or physical abuse.

What characterizes an act as homosexual is not the act itself but the fact that the partners are of the same sex. Typical homosexual behavior includes kissing, mutual masturbation, and oral-genital contact. Males may also engage in anal intercourse. A common belief is that lesbians use phallic substitutes to simulate heterosexual intercourse. In fact, they seldom do this, relying instead on clitoral stimulation to achieve orgasm. Another common misconception is that homosexuals assume and maintain either an active or a passive role in their sexual activities. To the contrary, most partners alternate between active and passive in any given act or from one relationship to another.

Numerous biological and psychological theories have been put forth to explain the causes of homosexuality, but no single theory is conclusive.

Homosexuality may be encouraged, some researchers feel, by negative experiences with members of the opposite sex. Negative attitudes may also be developed if children are told by their parents that sex-play with members of the

opposite sex is evil and dirty. Rejection, ridicule, and humiliation experienced in initial attempts to relate to the opposite sex may also influence later attitudes and behavior. If early homosexual experiences prove to be sexually satisfying and emotionally fulfilling, homosexual behavior may be reinforced as a preferred activity.

In situational homosexuality, as in prisons, individuals may engage in homosexual acts because other outlets are not available. Such individuals do not regard themselves as homosexuals and usually return to heterosexual behavior when they can. In prisons particularly, homosexual acts, most often forced anal intercourse, may also be used to establish dominance and masculinity.

Opinion differs as to whether or not homosexuality is an illness. The more popular view among therapists today is that a homosexual seeking therapy should be helped to adjust to his or her homosexuality. In the relatively few cases where the homosexual wishes to adopt a heterosexual life-style, behavior modification therapy has had some success.

Pedophilia   *Pedophilia* (literally "child love") is strongly prohibited in this society. None of our sexual taboos is stronger than those involved in the effort to isolate children from sex. For a child all possible sex partners are excluded by taboos. When sex does occur between an adult and a child, the assumption—both legally and culturally—is that all sexual content was brought to the encounter by the adult. And an adult accused of child molestation may not use the child's consent as a defense because the child does not have the legal right to consent. There are societies in which sex between a child and an adult is not taboo.

Excessive Sexual Behavior   An increase in the amount of sexual activity beyond society's norms is called *nym-*

phomania when it occurs in the female and *satyriasis* when it occurs in the male. These people seem to have high-level, insatiable, uncontrolled sex drives that bear no relation to emotional involvement. The causes of this type of variance differ from person to person. In most, psychological reasons for the behavior can be discovered, while in a few, a disorder of the hypothalamus has been suspected.

Change is the one most universal quality of sexual attitudes and perceptions in America today. We are not one culture but many, and the range of diversity can be staggering. We have a world in which one person's kinkiness is the next person's everyday sex, and in which today's kinkiness may be tomorrow's everyday sex.

Sexual Responsiveness Scale

Read the following statements carefully. Choose the one in each section
that best describes you at this
moment and record its score at the
right. (For example, "satisfied sexually" has a score of 4.) When you
have identified five statements, total
your score and find your position on
the scale.

5   very satisfied sexually
4   satisfied sexually
3   somewhat satisfied sexually
2   rarely satisfied sexually
1   frustrated sexually

Score _____

5   considers partner's needs before
       own
4   is sensitive to partner's needs
3   is sensitive to partner's needs
       most of the time
2   is rarely sensitive to partner's
       needs
1   is insensitive to partner's needs

Score _____

5   openly discusses sexual needs
4   discusses sexual problems with
       partner
3   is embarrassed by frank sexual
       discussions
2   is reluctant to discuss sexual
       problems
1   is unable to discuss sexual
       problems

Score _____

5   enjoys sex as part of a total rela-
       tionship
4   prefers intimacy to an exclusively
       sexual relationship
3   is affectionate with sexual partner
2   has frequent sexual encounters
1   has unsatisfactory sexual en-
       counters

Score _____

5   communicates sexual pleasures
       to partner
4   reveals sexual preferences to
       partner
3   is easily aroused
2   seeks immediate sexual grat-
       ification
1   views self as sexually inadequate

Score _____

Total score _____

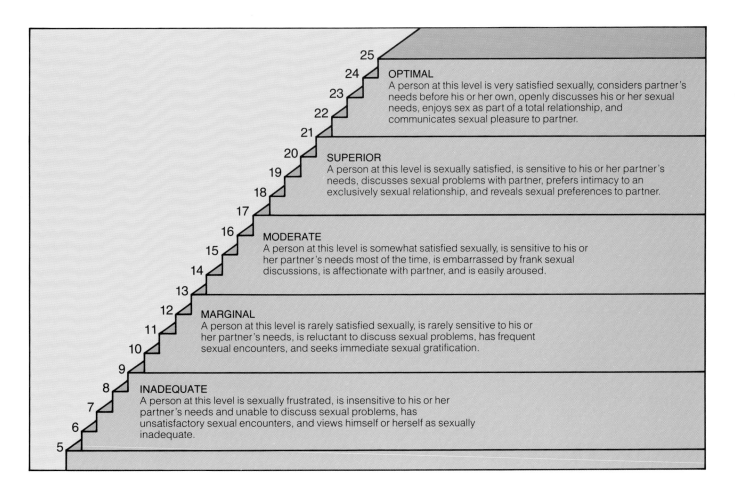

25
24   OPTIMAL
23   A person at this level is very satisfied sexually, considers partner's
22   needs before his or her own, openly discusses his or her sexual
21   needs, enjoys sex as part of a total relationship, and
         communicates sexual pleasure to partner.

20   SUPERIOR
19   A person at this level is sexually satisfied, is sensitive to his or her partner's
18   needs, discusses sexual problems with partner, prefers intimacy to an
17   exclusively sexual relationship, and reveals sexual preferences to partner.

16   MODERATE
15   A person at this level is somewhat satisfied sexually, is sensitive to his or
14   her partner's needs most of the time, is embarrassed by frank sexual
13   discussions, is affectionate with partner, and is easily aroused.

12   MARGINAL
11   A person at this level is rarely satisfied sexually, is rarely sensitive to his or
10   her partner's needs, is reluctant to discuss sexual problems, has frequent
9   sexual encounters, and seeks immediate sexual gratification.

8   INADEQUATE
7   A person at this level is sexually frustrated, is insensitive to his or her
6   partner's needs and unable to discuss sexual problems, has
5   unsatisfactory sexual encounters, and views himself or herself as sexually
         inadequate.

Take Action

Your answers to Probing Your Emotions at the beginning of this chapter and your placement level on the Sexual Responsiveness Scale will, we hope, encourage you to begin a process of self-discovery that you will continue. Reflect on the entire chapter's content and ask yourself how each point relates to your own life. Then take action:

1. In your Take Action notebook, list the behaviors or attitudes that you see as most positive in fulfilling your sexual needs and that give you the most satisfaction. How can you strengthen these behaviors or attitudes? Now list behaviors or attitudes that you see as barriers or blocks to achieving sexual maturity. Reread Chapter 1 to review some general techniques for accomplishing changes that will improve your sex life. Discuss them in class or with a close friend.

2. Ask an intimate to choose five items from the Sexual Responsiveness Scale that best describe your sexual maturity. Compare his or her rating with your own. Discuss with him or her any discrepancies (in a nondefensive way).

3. Complete the Sexual Anxiety Inventory on page 113. How does your level of anxiety compare to that of other college students? What steps can you take to reduce your anxiety? Consider discussing this question with a friend who has also completed the inventory.

Before you leave this chapter, review the questions that open the chapter. Have your feelings or values changed? Are you now better equipped to handle the complex and very human problems associated with human sexual response?

Chapter Six

Birth Control

Probing Your Emotions

1. You are a parent of a 14-year-old girl who tells you that she would like to take oral contraceptives. How would you feel about this? What would you say to her?

2. A woman with nine children comes before a judge for child neglect. The judge says he will let her off if she agrees to be sterilized. How do you feel about this? How would you feel if the woman had two children?

3. After a stimulating evening you return to your apartment with your date with the intention of having sexual intercourse. After getting into bed you both realize that neither has any contraceptive device. What do you do?

4. How do you feel about discussing contraception with your partner? How can you get the conversation started?

Chapter Contents

CONTRACEPTION
Oral contraception—the pill
The "morning-after" pill
Intrauterine devices (IUDs)
Condoms
Diaphragms and jelly
Cervical cap
The sponge
Vaginal spermicides
Some other methods of contraception
Factors that contribute to failure rates

STERILIZATION
Male sterilization or vasectomy
Female sterilization

NEW METHODS OF CONTRACEPTION
Menstruation-inducing pill
Long-acting injectables
Implants under the skin
Vaginal ring
Chemical contraceptives for men
Contraceptive immunization
Reversible sterilization
Prostaglandins
Luteinizing hormone-releasing hormone

ABORTION METHODS
Vacuum aspiration
Dilatation and curettage
The saline method
Prostaglandins
Hysterotomy

ABORTION COMPLICATIONS

Boxes

Attitudes toward birth control
Planned parenthood
Assessing risks
What are the costs of having children?
Study refutes claim that vasectomy is
    health hazard
Abortion—the hard question

Conception
The formation of a zygote (fertilized egg), the cell resulting from the fusion of ovum and sperm and, in normal conditions, capable of survival and maturation.

Contraceptive
Any agent that can prevent conception. Condoms, diaphragms, intrauterine devices, and contraceptive pills are examples.

Ovulation
The release of the egg (ovum) from the ovaries.

Corpus luteum
A gland in the ovary that forms after ovulation; secretes progesterone. If the ovum is not fertilized, the corpus luteum degenerates.

Progesterone
A hormone used in birth control pills to prevent ovulation.

Estrogen
A female hormone that is produced in the ovaries and is an active ingredient in birth control pills.

Synthetic
Produced by chemical synthesis rather than originating in nature.

Oral contraceptive
Any of various hormone compounds in pill form taken by mouth. Oral contraceptives prevent conception by preventing ovulation.

6 Coitus without the risk of *conception,* a dream people have pursued for more than two thousand years, has only recently come close to being a reality. As long ago as 850 B.C., women inserted a cervical plug made of crocodile dung and honey before intercourse. Sponges, douches, and crude methods of abortion were mentioned in the writings of Plato and Aristotle and the physician Hippocrates. The lengthy list of materials that have been used for birth control includes seaweed, lemon juice, parsley, camphor, opium, olive oil, copper sulfate, and foam from the camel's mouth. American Indian women chewed certain roots as oral *contraceptives.* People also used condoms and diaphragms made from animal substances for several centuries.

Most of these methods of contraception either did not work or were dangerous, or both. Birth control did not begin to be practical until rubber condoms and diaphragms were introduced in the nineteenth century, and a high level of effectiveness did not become possible until modern oral contraceptives and intrauterine devices appeared in the 1950s and 1960s.

The consequences have been staggering. For many "the pill" has meant a new freedom. It has been credited with reducing the number of unwanted pregnancies in all age groups, including those among teenagers. It almost certainly has played a major role in recent changes in sexual consciousness. It also appears to have halted, at least in the United States, a potentially disastrous runaway growth in population.

In this chapter we will examine the most widely used forms of reversible contraception, as well as sterilization, abortion, and new methods of contraception.

Contraception

Modern contraception did not become possible until advances were made in endocrinology, steroid chemistry, gynecology, and plastics technology. From this accumulation of knowledge came the development of the contraceptive pill and the IUD (intrauterine device).

Oral Contraception—The Pill   A century ago or more a key observation was made: *Ovulation does not occur*

during pregnancy. Further research showed that ovulation is controlled by the *corpus luteum,* a gland that appears and disappears with each new menstrual cycle. It forms in the ovary after ovulation and then degenerates at the end of the cycle and is absorbed into the system. In pregnant women, however, the corpus luteum remains and continues to secrete a hormone called *progesterone.*

To test the theory that progesterone prevents ovulation, extracts of progesterone were given to animals that were not pregnant. Ovulation did not occur. Researchers later found that a second hormone produced in the ovaries, *estrogen,* also prevents ovulation. Estrogen, progesterone, and certain closely related *synthetic* compounds are the active ingredients in birth control pills.

In addition to preventing ovulation, the birth control pill also has other backup contraceptive effects. It hampers the movement of sperm by the thickening of cervical mucus, alters the rate of ovum transport by means of its hormonal effects on the Fallopian tubes, and may inhibit implantation by changing the lining of the uterus, in the unlikely event that a fertilized ovum reaches that area.

One kind of *oral contraceptive* is in common use today: the combination pill. A one-month series of the combination pill consists of 21 identical tablets, each containing estrogen and progesterone. A second, much less common, type of oral contraceptive is the "minipill," a small dose of a synthetic progesterone taken every day of the month. The minipill has fewer side effects, but it also carries a higher risk of pregnancy and irregular bleeding.

Schedules   In taking the combination pill, pill 1 is usually taken on day 5 of the menstrual cycle, the first day of the menstrual period being counted as day 1. Another pill is taken each day until all 21 pills (the usual number) in the package have been taken. A menstrual period will usually begin from two to four days after the last pill in a series.

In most cases, women with a typical menstrual cycle of 28 to 30 days are protected against pregnancy as soon as they take the first pill. The few women who have cycles of 21 or fewer days and who may ovulate early in the first cycle of use run a greater risk of pregnancy

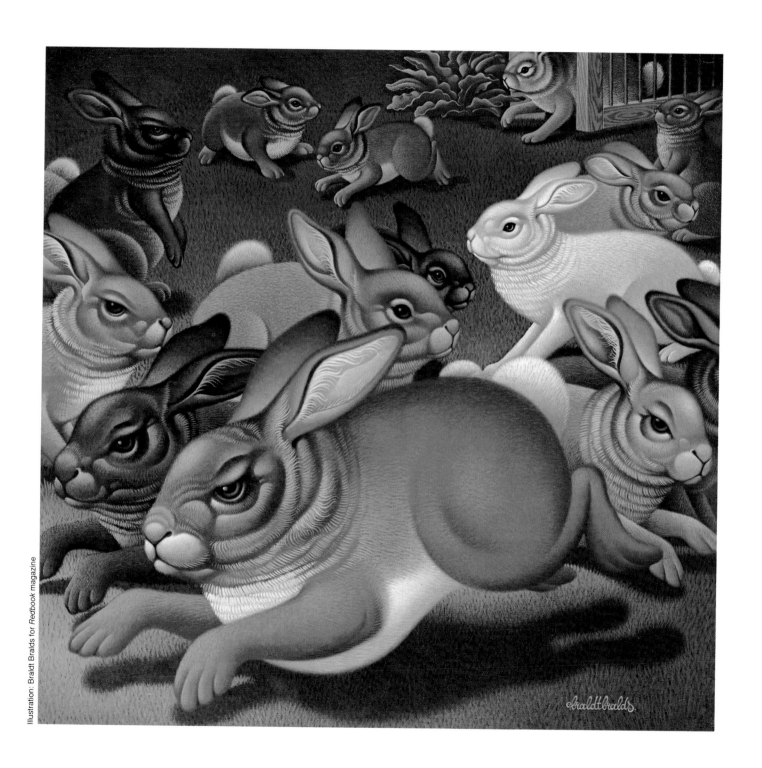

Illustration: Braldt Braids for *Redbook* magazine

Attitudes Toward Birth Control

Here are some of the personal reasons why we sometimes have trouble using birth control or don't even use it at all:

■ We are embarrassed by, ashamed of, confused about our own sexuality.

■ We cannot admit we might have or are having intercourse because we feel (or someone told us) it is wrong.

■ We are romantic about sex—sex has to be a passionate, spontaneous sharing, and birth control seems too premeditated, too clinical, and often too messy.

■ We hesitate to inconvenience our sex partner.

■ If we are using natural birth control we sometimes have a hard time abstaining during our fertile days because we fear our partner will get angry and find sex elsewhere.

■ We feel, "It can't happen to me. I won't get pregnant."

■ We have questions about birth control and sex and don't know whom to talk with.

■ We hesitate to go to a doctor or clinic and face the hurried, impersonal care or, if we are young or unmarried, the moralizing and disapproval that we feel likely to receive.

■ We don't recognize our deep dissatisfactions with the method we are using and begin to use it haphazardly.

■ We want a baby and can't admit it to ourselves. Or we feel tempted to get pregnant just to prove to ourselves that we are fertile, or to try to improve a shaky relationship.

What Can We Do?

Facing these many obstacles to our using birth control effectively, what can we do? First, we can learn for ourselves and teach one another about the available methods. By speaking openly and by carefully comparing experiences and knowledge, we can guide each other to competent doctors and reasonable methods. We can learn to recognize when a doctor is not sufficiently thorough in examinations or explanations, and support each other to

ask for the attention we need. By talking together we can also get a better handle on the more subtle personal hassles we have with birth control. We can begin the long but worthwhile process of talking with men about birth control, so that they can no longer comfortably ignore their share in the responsibility. We can learn to be more accepting of our sexuality and join proudly together to insist that legislatures, courts, high schools, churches, doctors, research projects, clinics and drug companies change their attitudes and practices so that we can enjoy our sexuality without becoming pregnant. We can work to create self-help clinics and other alternative health care institutions where our needs for information, discussion and personal support in the difficult choice of birth control will be better met.

The Boston Women's Health Book
   Collective
Our Bodies, Ourselves

and should always use another method of contraception besides the pill during the first two to four weeks of the first pill cycle. Some clinicians recommend a backup method for *all* women in the first two to four weeks. A woman changing from one type of pill to another should also use an additional contraceptive, especially if she is changing to a pill that contains a lower hormone dosage.

The pill should be taken at about the same time every day. If one pill is forgotten, it should be taken as soon as remembered, and the next pill should be taken at its scheduled time. If two pills are forgotten, two should be taken on each of the next two days, and an additional contraceptive used for the rest of the cycle.

The pill-taking schedule should be continued as directed even if *spotting* occurs between periods. If spotting lasts longer than two monthly cycles, the doctor who prescribed the pills should be told.

If menstruation does not occur when it is expected, a new series of pills should be started one week after the end of the last series. Pregnancy is practically impossible if a pill has been taken every day for 21 days. If a pill was not taken every day in the last series and no period occurs, or if periods fail to occur more than one time, a doctor should be consulted.

Pill use in the United States reached an all-time high in the mid-1970s and then declined rather rapidly between 1975 and 1977, following the intense publicity regarding possible health risks. In recent years, however, many of those risks have been reduced through use of lower-dosage pills and through clarification of the personal factors that place a specific woman in a high-risk category. Currently, use of the pill is increasing slightly; in 1982, of all U.S. women aged 15 to 44 who were at risk of unintended pregnancy, an estimated 27 percent were relying on the pill. The overall decline in

Spotting
Losing a slight amount of menstrual blood from the uterus between periods.

Fertility
The state or condition of being able to reproduce.

Ovarian hormone
A chemical substance in the body that controls the menstrual cycle and the functions of pregnancy and promotes the development of sex characteristics. Estrogens and progesterone are the major female hormones.

Side effect
Any effect of a drug accompanying its intended effect.

---

pill use is most marked among women who have been married more than ten years, with the main challenge coming from the increasingly popular method of surgical sterilization. Among couples in whom neither partner has been sterilized, however, no other birth control method comes close to the birth control pill in popularity.

Advantages   Oral contraceptives are:

1. Almost completely effective in preventing pregnancy; nearly all unplanned pregnancies result because the user has not followed the schedule.
2. Relatively simple to use.
3. Not a hindrance to sexual spontaneity. No mood-destroying interruptions are required.
4. Not irreversible. *Fertility* returns after the pill is discontinued, although not always immediately.
5. Known to decrease the incidence of the following conditions: benign breast disease, iron-deficiency anemia, pelvic inflammatory disease, rheumatoid arthritis, ectopic pregnancy, uterine cancer, and ovarian cancer. (Women who have never used the pill are twice as likely as users to develop uterine or ovarian cancer.)

Disadvantages   *Ovarian hormones* influence all tissues of the body, and they can lead to a variety of minor disturbances, some temporary and some not, and for some women, to serious *side effects*. Symptoms of early pregnancy—morning nausea, weight gain, and swollen breasts, for example—may appear during the first few months of oral contraception. They usually disappear by the fourth cycle. Other complaints include depression, nervousness, alterations in the sex drive, dizziness, generalized headaches, migraine headaches, bleeding between periods, and changes in the lining of the walls of the vagina, with an increase in clear or white discharge from the vagina. Chloasma, or "mask of pregnancy," occurs occasionally, causing brown "giant freckles" to appear on the face. Acne may develop or worsen, but in most women the use of the pill causes acne to clear up, and is sometimes prescribed for young women for that purpose.

Yeast fungus infections are more common among women who are taking the pill. These infections are not serious, but the itchiness and increased discharge in the vagina that accompany them are often extremely uncomfortable. Medical treatment, usually in the form of vaginal creams, gives prompt relief most of the time.

Serious side effects of pill use have been reported in a small number of women. These include thrombosis and thromboembolism, conditions in which a clot obstructs a blood vessel and damages tissues, and the formation of benign tumors of the liver that may bleed and rupture. Pill users also show a slight increase in the incidence of high blood pressure, which is usually quickly reversed upon discontinuation of the pill, and of gall bladder disease. Studies completed on oral contraceptives and their possible association with cancer of the breast and the cervix have resulted in conflicting conclusions, and thus far the evidence on both sides is considered tentative.

Oral contraceptives should not be prescribed for women who have or have had blood clots in any part of the body, stroke, heart disease or defect, severe endocrine disorder, recurrent jaundice of pregnancy, markedly impaired liver function, any form of cancer, or abnormal genital bleeding from unknown causes. Also, the pill is not recommended for women over 35 years old, especially if they are smokers.

Many health care professionals also advise women with present or previous high blood pressure not to use oral contraceptives. Physicians usually give more frequent follow-up appointments when oral contraceptives are prescribed for women who have present or previous high blood pressure, varicose veins, migraine headaches, diabetes, asthma, epilepsy, fibroids of the uterus, excessive smoking, significant psychiatric problems, gall bladder disease, sickle-cell disease, non-malignant breast disease, or irregular menstrual cycles. When women with any of these conditions or with a family history of cancer, high blood pressure, or diabetes do choose to use the pill, preliminary tests and careful follow-up examinations are important. Women who have or have had liver disease, kidney disease, or mild endocrine disorders must be successfully treated for those conditions before they start to use oral contraception.

In trying to decide whether to use oral contraception, an attempt must be made to weigh the benefits against

Theoretical effectiveness
Failure rate of contraceptives when "taken as directed."

Use effectiveness
Failure rate of contraceptives when adherence to prescribed instructions is unknown.

Continuation rate
The percentage of women who continue to use a particular contraceptive after a specified period of time.

Diethylstilbestrol (DES)
A synthetic hormone that produces the effects of natural estrogen. Currently, the safety of DES is highly questionable.

Uterus
The hollow, thick-walled, muscular organ in which the egg develops into a fetus; the womb. It is located directly above the vagina.

Intrauterine device (IUD)
A plastic device inserted into the uterus as a contraceptive.

---

the risks for each individual woman. For most women, the known, directly associated risk of death from use of the pill is much lower than the risk of death from pregnancy. However, many long-term effects are still not completely understood and thereby complicate the decision-making process. Nevertheless, there are many important actions that the potential user can take to make the most informed decision possible. She can discuss and evaluate the risk variables that *are known* and that apply to her with a health care professional; request a low-dosage pill (50 micrograms or less of estrogen); stop or decrease smoking if she currently smokes; carefully and consistently follow the pill-taking instructions; be alert to preliminary danger signals (severe headaches, problems with vision, severe pain in the abdomen, chest, or legs); have regular checkups of her blood pressure, weight, and urine, and an annual examination of the thyroid, breasts, abdomen, and pelvis. By following these measures, women can better evaluate and actively affect the benefit-risk ratio of pill use.

Effectiveness   Contraceptives can be evaluated according to either of two standards: theoretical effectiveness or use effectiveness. *Theoretical effectiveness* is the failure rate of a contraceptive when it is "taken as directed." It cannot be accurately measured, but it is inferred from studying the most successful users. For the combination pill, the theoretical effectiveness is one pregnancy per 1,000 women during one year of use.

Use effectiveness is the failure rate of a contraceptive when it is used under average conditions by average people. This measurement includes pregnancies that result from an erratic schedule of pill taking, as well as those that occur when a woman discontinues her pill, fails to use another method of contraception, and then has unprotected intercourse. When these pregnancies have been taken into account, the use effectiveness of the combination pill has been reported to be as low as 10 pregnancies per 1,000 women during one year of use. This figure will differ markedly, as it depends on numerous patient and program variables. Again, it is critical that the woman become throughly informed in regard to all aspects of pill use and that she follow all guidelines carefully.

Effectiveness is also measured by the *continuation rate*—the percentage of women who continue to use the method after a specified period of time. The continuation rate for oral contraceptives has also varied considerably from one group of users to another, with the range being 50 to 75 percent after one year.

The "Morning-After" Pill   The term *"morning-after" pill* actually refers to pills containing large doses of estrogen. These pills are taken during the five days immediately following unprotected coitus, and they reduce the occurrence of pregnancy to a very low level. The usual dose is 25 to 50 milligrams per day of *diethylstilbestrol* (*DES*), a synthetic preparation that mimics all the effects of natural estrogen.

Nausea, vomiting, and other undesirable changes in metabolism commonly accompany large doses of estrogen. There is also some controversy over the safety of DES. Claims that it causes cancer have led the governments of Australia and New Zealand to ban its use. In the United States, the FDA recommends that DES be used for emergency situations only and emphasizes that when DES is used and fails, a therapeutic abortion should be considered because of the possibility that DES will damage the fetus.

Intrauterine Devices (IUDs)   Placing objects inside the *uterus* is one of the oldest methods of birth control. Over two thousand years ago, Hippocrates, the Greek physician, described various devices, including one that was inserted into the uterus through a piece of lead tubing. Another example, perhaps more familiar, is the method used by camel owners who insert small stones into the uterus of the camel before a long desert trip. The possibility of intrauterine methods of birth control was almost ignored in modern times until E. Gräfenberg, a German physician, reported his use of an intrauterine coil of silkworm gut and silver in 1930. Gräfenberg's coil did not work because of flaws in design and insertion techniques. Since then, improvements in materials, design, and insertion techniques have greatly increased the acceptability of the *intrauterine device* (*IUD*). In the United States there was a sharp increase in IUD use between 1965 and 1973.

By 1976, however, there was a slight decline, which

Cervix
The neck of the uterus, that is, the lower
and narrow end, which opens into the
vagina.

was probably related to the publicity about the dangers of the widely used Dalkon Shield and its subsequent withdrawal from the market. In recent years IUD use has leveled off, and in 1982 an estimated 6 percent of all U.S. women aged 15 to 44 who were at risk of unintended pregnancy were relying on the IUD for contraception. The four remaining types most commonly used today are the Lippes loop, the saf-t-coil, copper 7 and copper T, and the progestasert.

No one knows exactly how the IUD works. It may interfere with the movement of eggs or sperm; it may cause the production of egg- or sperm-killing cells and biochemical products; or it may interfere with the implantation of eggs in the uterus. All have been suggested.

Insertion and Removal   Before an IUD is inserted, a medical history and a gynecological examination should be completed to rule out the presence of pregnancy, infection, anatomical abnormalities, or other potentially complicating conditions. If none of these complications exist, the IUD is threaded into a sterile inserter, which is then introduced into the cervical canal until it reaches the lowermost portion of the uterus. The plunger pushes the IUD into the uterus, and the inserter is withdrawn. The threads protruding from the *cervix* are trimmed so that only 1 to 1½ inches remain in the upper vagina. These are unnoticeable during coitus. (See Figure 6–1.)

The best time for insertion (and removal) of the IUD is during the menstrual period because the cervical canal is most open during that time and there is the least possibility of an unsuspected pregnancy.

IUDs with nylon threads can usually be removed by pulling on the threads. Only a trained professional should undertake this process, however, because the cervix might have to be expanded, or dilated. IUDs without threads are pulled out with a small blunt hook. Timing of removal can be crucial; some unwanted pregnancies have resulted when sperm have survived from intercourse that took place a couple of days before the IUD was removed.

Advantages   Intrauterine devices:

1. Are highly reliable (second only to the pill).
2. Are relatively safe, although long-term effects are not known.

3. Can be used indefinitely. (Some types, e.g., the copper IUDs and the progestasert, must be replaced periodically.)
4. Are simple to use, requiring no attention except periodic self-examination.
5. Have only localized side effects.
6. Do not require anticipation or interruption of sexual activity.
7. Are a fully reversible method. Fertility is restored as soon as the IUD is removed.
8. Have a low long-term cost.

Disadvantages   Most side effects of IUD use are limited to the genital tract. By far the most common complaint is abnormal menstrual bleeding. The menstrual flow tends to appear sooner, last longer, and become heavier after insertion of an IUD. Bleeding and spotting between periods may also occur. Another common complaint is pain, particularly uterine cramps and backache, side effects that seem to occur most often in women who have never been pregnant. Uterine cramps that accompany insertion usually disappear after a few days, but in some cases they are severe enough to require the removal of the device.

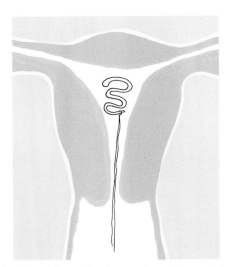

Figure 6-1   An IUD (Lippes loop) properly positioned in the uterus. The attached threads that protrude from the cervix into the upper vagina allow the woman to check to see that the IUD is in place.

Planned Parenthood

"Every child a wanted child": Since its stormy beginnings over 60 years ago, Planned Parenthood Federation of America has sought to end compulsory parenthood by making birth control devices accessible to all who want them. Taking up their cause in local communities and courtrooms throughout the nation, Planned Parenthood has committed itself to making all Americans aware of the problems caused by unrestrained population growth, both here and abroad.

Serving more than 250 communities in 43 states and the District of Columbia, Planned Parenthood provides medical services to more than 1 million persons a year. In 1975 alone, 1.1 million women received pelvic examinations, 1.25 million people received blood pressure tests, 890,000 people were screened for venereal disease, 870,000 received Pap smears to check for cervical cancer, and 180,000 women received pregnancy tests.

Planned Parenthood's educational goals are equally far-reaching. In the offices of all of its affiliates, basic birth control information is provided through films, group discussions, and individual counseling sessions. In addition, many affiliates offer special discussion groups for young people, where participants can talk about their anxieties, ask their questions, and share their problems in a supportive environment.

All the agency's affiliates also provide educational services within the community. Its trainers prepare teachers, social workers, nurses, and clergy to educate others in matters related to human sexuality and birth control.

Since Margaret Sanger, the agency's founder, began her courageous fight for voluntary parenthood, Planned Parenthood has actively opposed state and federal laws that interfere with parenthood by choice. In 1969, the agency published the nation's first county-by-county study of birth control needs and services among low-income women. This study was probably the single most important piece of research leading to the Family Planning Services and Population Research Act of 1970. With the passage of this act, the federal government for the first time authorized funds ($225 million) for birth control research, expanded family planning services, and the creation of the Office of Population Affairs within the Department of Health, Education, and Welfare.

Planned Parenthood's activities literally span the globe. The International Planned Parenthood Federation (IPPF) is the world's largest voluntary family planning organization. Dedicated to the formation and support of national family planning associations throughout the world, it assists in developing programs to educate people about the personal, social, and economic benefits of family planning. IPPF also provides technical information to several agencies of the United Nations and gives national associations financial support and technical assistance.

Spontaneous expulsion of the IUD happens in 5 to 15 percent of all users within the first year after insertion, and if a woman does not notice that she has lost it, an unwanted pregnancy may result. Most expulsions occur during the first months after insertion, usually but not always during the menstrual period, so checking menstrual pads for the device is a wise precaution. It is also a good idea to check occasionally that the device is in place by locating the threads. Expulsion after the first year is uncommon. If one IUD is expelled, the risk of expulsion becomes two to three times greater, although about one-half of all women who experience a first expulsion eventually retain the device. The older the woman is and the more children she has had, the less likely she is to expel the device.

From 5 to 20 percent of women who have had IUDs inserted have them removed during the first year of use, usually because they experience bleeding and cramping.

Over the long term, IUDs are removed far more often than they are expelled.

A serious complication sometimes associated with IUD use is *pelvic inflammatory disease* (*PID*). Many research studies indicate that this condition occurs most commonly during the first two weeks following insertion, with an incidence of 1 to 5 percent during the first year of use. However, the actual incidence of PID may be higher because pain and bleeding are often reported as the chief reasons for removal rather than the infection, which also may have been present. Most pelvic infections among IUD users are relatively mild and can be treated successfully with antibiotics. However, early and adequate treatment is critical, for a smoldering infection can lead to tubal scarring and subsequent infertility.

In about one out of 2,000 insertions, the IUD punctures the wall of the uterus and migrates into the abdominal cavity.

Pelvic inflammatory disease (PID)
An infection that progresses from the vagina and cervix and eventually moves into the pelvic cavity.

Spontaneous abortion
A miscarriage; the premature expulsion of a nonliving fetus.

Condom
A sheath usually made of thin rubber designed to cover the penis during sexual intercourse. The condom is used for contraception and to prevent disease.

Sexually transmitted disease
Any of several contagious diseases such as syphilis and gonorrhea contracted through intimate contact.

Ejaculation
An abrupt discharge of fluid, especially of semen, from the penis.

Circumcise
To remove the foreskin of the penis.

No evidence has been found that IUDs cause cancer in women, but the long-term effects are not well known.

Because of the risk of infection, use of IUDs is not recommended for women who have pelvic infection, suspected pregnancy, large tumors of the uterus or other anatomical abnormalities, irregular or unexplained bleeding, history of ectopic pregnancy, rheumatic heart disease, or diabetes. Many doctors also recommend against the use of IUDs by young women who have never been pregnant because of the increased incidence of side effects and the risk of infection with the possiblilty of subsequent infertility. The risk of infection is higher for women who have multiple sex partners.

Early IUD danger signals that the user should be alert for are abdominal pain, fever, chills, foul vaginal discharge, irregular menstrual period, and other unusual vaginal bleeding. An annual checkup is recommended. This should include a Pap smear and a blood check for anemia if menstrual flow has increased.

Effectiveness The use effectiveness rate of IUDs is about 50 pregnancies per 1,000 women during the first year of use. Many of these pregnancies are due to undetected partial or complete expulsion of the device. For all types the failure rate tends to decline rapidly after the first year. Because most pregnancies occur in the first few months after IUD insertion, some doctors advise using an additional method of contraception during that time. Regular checking of the cervix to verify the presence of thread and absence of the IUD stem is also recommended.

Pregnancy may occur with the device in place. If the patient wishes to maintain the pregnancy, the IUD should be removed. Following removal, there is a 25 percent chance of a *spontaneous abortion*. Birth defects are no more common among babies born of such pregnancies than among other babies. Pregnancy with an IUD left in place may lead to infection, bleeding, and/or premature labor.

The continuation rate of IUDs of the open type commonly used is 70 to 85 percent after one year of use.

Condoms Italians and Chinese used *condoms*, sheaths worn over the penis, in the sixteenth and seventeenth

centuries as a protection against *sexually transmitted diseases*. By the eighteenth century the contraceptive function of the condom had been recognized, and the French and English used condoms made of sheep gut or the amniotic membrane of newborn lambs. Sheaths of skin were too expensive for most people, but the vulcanization of rubber in 1844 made a less expensive condom possible. Since the early 1900s "rubbers" have, by and large, replaced skin condoms.

The condom is still one of the most popular contraceptives in North America; 800 million to a billion are sold every year in Canada and the United States. In 1982 an estimated 12 percent of all U.S. women aged 15 to 44 exposed to unintended pregnancy were relying on the use of condoms for birth control, making this method the third most popular, exceeded only by the pill and sterilization. (See Figure 6-2.)

The user or his partner must put on the condom before the penis is inserted into the vagina, as the small amounts of fluid secreted prior to *ejaculation* often contain sperm capable of causing pregnancy. The rolled-up condom is placed over the head of the erect penis and unrolled down to the base of the penis, leaving a half-inch space at the tip to collect semen. If the user has not been *circumcised,* he must first pull back the foreskin of the penis. He and his partner must be careful not to damage the condom with fingernails, rings, or other rough objects.

Some condoms are sold already lubricated. If the users wish, they can lubricate their own condoms with vaginal foam, cream, or jelly, or other nongreasy jellies. Vaseline or any other kind of petroleum jelly or oil should never be applied to rubber condoms: Rubber dissolves in petroleum.

When the male loses his erection after ejaculation, the condom loses its tight fit. To avoid spilling semen, the condom must be held around the base of the penis as the penis is withdrawn. If any semen is spilled on the vulva, the sperm may easily find their way to the uterus.

A new type of condom that is already popular in England and several European countries has recently been introduced in the United States. The lubricant of this condom contains the same spermicidal agent found in many of the contraceptive foams and creams that women use. Since this agent kills many of the sperm

Spermicide
An agent destructive to sperm.

soon after ejaculation, its addition may significantly decrease contraceptive failure associated with breakage and the spilling of semen and may be used to replace the recommended combination of foam and condom use.

Advantages   Condoms are:

1. Easy to purchase.
2. Simple to use.
3. Available without prescription or medical supervision.
4. Virtually free of medical side effects.
5. Helpful in protecting against sexually transmitted diseases, which in turn may diminish the likelihood of cervical cancer in some women.

Disadvantages   The two most nearly universal complaints about condoms are that they diminish sensation and interfere with spontaneity. While some people find these to be serious drawbacks, others consider them to be only minor disadvantages. It is hard to think of a human activity in which losing sensation would be less welcome than it would be in coitus. And more than one couple

has reached a mellow place only to have contact broken and the spell shattered as the woman waits for her partner to fumble with a foil wrapper. Many couples, however, learn to creatively integrate condom use into their sexual activities.

Effectiveness   Condoms, when used exactly as directed during each act of intercourse, have a theoretical effectiveness of 30 pregnancies per 1,000 women during one year of use. In actual use, however, the failure rate is considerably higher, reaching approximately 100 pregnancies per 1,000 women during one year of use. At least some of these pregnancies happen because the condom is carelessly removed after ejaculation. Some may also happen because of a break or a tear, which is estimated to occur once in every 150 to 200 instances. If either type of accident occurs, the risk of pregnancy can be reduced somewhat by the prompt use of a vaginal *spermicide* (a preparation for killing sperm). The use effectiveness of the condom can be greatly improved, to approach that of the pill, by using a spermicidal foam, inserted just *before* intercourse, along with a condom.

The most common cause of pregnancy with condom users is "taking a chance"—that is, not using a

Figure 6-2   A sample of condoms presently available. The elongated tip on the unrolled condom (*bottom*) is a reservoir to collect semen.

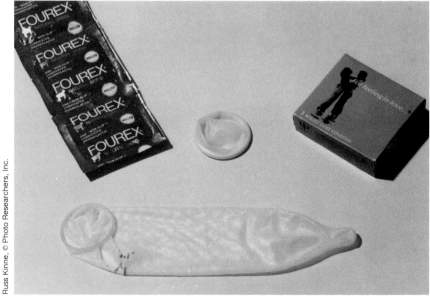

Russ Kinne, © Photo Researchers, Inc.

Diaphragm
A contraceptive consisting of a flexible,
sombrero-shaped disk that covers the
cervix. The diaphragm prevents sperm
from entering the uterus.

---

condom at all. The aforementioned objections to using a condom make taking a chance very tempting in the heat of passion.

Diaphragms and Jelly   Before oral contraceptives were introduced, about one-fourth of all couples in the United States who used any form of contraception relied on the *diaphragm.* Many former diaphragm users have been won over to the pill or to IUDs, but the diaphragm is still the choice for some couples.

Wilhelm Mensinga, a German physician, invented a rubber diaphragm in the late 1800s, and there have been few changes in design since. The diaphragm is a dome-shaped cup of thin rubber stretched over a collapsible metal ring. When the diaphragm is correctly used with spermicidal cream or jelly, it covers the mouth of the cervix, preventing sperm from entering the uterus.

Diaphragms can be obtained only by prescription. Because of individual differences in women, a diaphragm must be carefully fitted to ensure that it will be both effective and comfortable, and only a trained person can make these adjustments. The fitting should be checked with each routine annual examination, as well as after childbirth, abortion, or a weight change of more than ten pounds.

Before inserting the diaphragm, the woman should spread about a tablespoon of spermicidal jelly or cream over the surface of the dome that will be against the cervix. The diaphragm is easiest to insert if the user squats, lies down, or stands with one foot raised. The user squeezes the diaphragm into a long narrow shape with one hand. She holds the labia apart with the other hand and pushes the diaphragm up along the back wall of the vagina as far as it will go, keeping it behind the cervix. She then tucks the front rim up behind the pubic bone. (See Figure 6-3.) Because the vagina has a backward tilt, a user who inserts the diaphragm while she is standing up must insert it almost horizontally. Plastic or metal inserters can be helpful to women who are excessively fat, who have short fingers, or who dislike touching their genitals.

After the diaphragm is inserted, its position should be checked. The cervix should be located and felt through the dome of the diaphragm to make sure that it is completely covered and that the front rim of the diaphragm is pushed up behind the pubic bone.

The diaphragm must not be inserted more than two hours before intercourse. If the time between insertion and coitus is longer than two hours, an applicator-full of spermicide should be inserted into the vagina, or the diaphragm should be taken out and spermicide freshly applied before it is reinserted. Additional cream or jelly should also be inserted into the vagina before any additional act of coitus. The diaphragm must be left in place for at least six hours after the last act of coitus to give the spermicide enough time to kill all the sperm.

To remove the diaphragm, the user simply hooks the front rim down from behind the pubic bone with one finger. After the diaphragm is removed, it should be washed with mild soap and water, rinsed, and patted dry. It should then be examined for holes or cracks. Defects are most likely to develop near the rim, and they can usually be spotted by looking at the diaphragm in front of a bright light. After the diaphragm is inspected, it can be dusted with cornstarch and put away.

Advantages   Diaphragms are:

1. Virtually free of medical side effects.
2. Slightly less destructive of spontaneity than the condom because one can be inserted up to two hours before intercourse.
3. Relatively reliable.

Disadvantages   Some women find that the need to plan ahead for coitus dampens their spontaneity. Even after the diaphragm is in place, it cannot be forgotten, since it only works for two hours. The alternative, waiting until coitus is about to happen before inserting the diaphragm, may also be seen as disruptive. However, many couples discover ways to diminish this potentially negative effect by incorporating insertion into foreplay activity. Some women cannot wear a diaphragm because of their anatomies. And using a diaphragm is not a suitable method of contraception for women who are unwilling to insert it before each act of coitus or for those who feel fear or disgust when they touch their genitals.

Effectiveness   When used consistently, the diaphragm has a theoretical effectiveness of 20 to 30 pregnancies per 1,000 women during one year. In actual practice, women rarely use the diaphragm correctly every time

Sponge
A contraceptive device about 2 inches in diameter that fits over the cervix and acts as a barrier, spermicide, and seminal fluid absorbent.

Toxic shock syndrome
A disease whose major symptoms include high fever, vomiting, diarrhea, headache, sore throat, and rash. Although primarily associated with menstruating women who use tampons, the disease has also been reported in men. It is thought to be caused by the bacterium *Staphylococcus aureus,* for which there is no effective antibiotic; most patients recover in 7 to 10 days; mortality rate is 10 to 15 percent.

they have intercourse, and the use effectiveness of the diaphragm is 130 pregnancies for 1,000 women during one year. The main causes of failures are inaccurate fitting and incorrect insertion. Sometimes too, the vaginal walls expand during sexual stimulation, causing the diaphragm to be dislodged. This displacement seems to happen most commonly with the woman-on-top position. It is recommended that placement be checked before ejaculation.

Cervical Cap   The cervical cap is a thimble-shaped rubber or plastic cup that fits snugly over the cervix and is held in place by suction. It is used in a manner similar to the diaphragm and offers effectiveness within the same range. Use of the cervical cap in the United States remains limited. Its chief advantage is that it can be used as an alternative for women who have anatomical features that preclude diaphragm use. The cap's disadvantages include difficulties with insertion and removal and the very unpleasant odor that may result if it is left in place for more than one day.

The Sponge   The *sponge,* a new addition to the barrier methods, is a pillow-shaped device about 2 inches in diameter with a polyester loop on one side (for removal) and a concave dimple on the other side, which helps

it to fit snuggly over the cervix. Most sponges are made of polyurethane and presaturated with the same spermicide found in contraceptive creams and foams. The sponge acts as a barrier, spermicide, and seminal fluid absorbent and has an effectiveness rate similar to that of the diaphragm. Its advantages are that it requires no professional fitting because one size fits all women and that it may be left in place for 24 hours for repeated intercourse without the addition of spermicide. Reported disadvantages thus far include odor if left in place for more than 18 hours and difficulty of removal. The major safety concern with sponge use is the possible risk of *toxic shock syndrome,* an occasionally fatal disease often related to tampon use. Although no direct relationship has been established between the sponge and this syndrome, it is recommended that during menstruation, when risk is highest, the sponge be inserted just before coitus and be removed within six hours after coitus. Also unknown at this time is the amount of spermicide absorbed through the vaginal walls with this device and the possible effects of recurring, extended exposure.

Vaginal Spermicides   For thousands of years people have tried to prevent pregnancy by putting various gooey substances into the vagina to act as a barrier to sperm travel. In recent years spermicidal compounds devel-

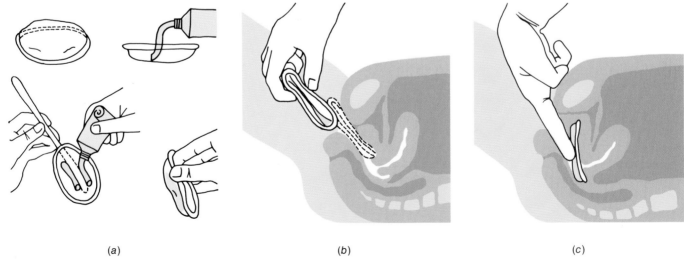

(a)   (b)   (c)

Figure 6-3   Use of the diaphragm: (*a*) spermicidal jelly is placed in the concave side of the diaphragm, and the diaphragm is pressed firmly between the thumb and forefinger; (*b*) diaphragm is inserted in the vagina; (*c*) diaphragm is checked for correct position against the cervix.

oped for use with a diaphragm have been adapted for use without a diaphragm by combining them with a bulky base.

Foams, creams, jellies, foaming tablets, and suppositories are all available. In recent years the spermicidal suppository has become widely marketed and publicized in the United States. It is small and easily inserted like a tampon. Because body heat is needed to activate effervescence barrier formation over the cervix, it is important to wait at least ten minutes after insertion before having sex. Because the suppository's spermicidal effects are limited in time, intercourse should take place within one hour of insertion. An additional suppository is required for each additional act of intercourse.

Of the various types of spermicides, foam has the greatest advantage. It is more effective in preventing pregnancy because its effervescent mass forms a more dense and evenly distributed barrier to the cervical opening. Tablets and suppositories are less effective than foams, creams, and jellies and are not generally recommended. Foam is sold in an aerosol bottle or a metal container with an applicator that fits on the nozzle. Creams and jellies are sold in tubes with an applicator that can be screwed onto the opening of the tube. (See Figure 6-4.)

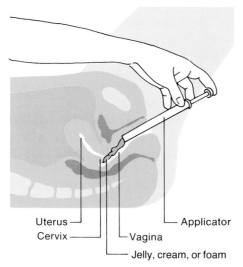

Figure 6-4   Application of spermicidal jelly, cream, or foam.

Assessing Risks

Activity	Chance of Death in a Year
Motorcycling	1 in 50
Smoking, 1 pack per day	1 in 200
Horse racing	1 in 750
Automobile driving	1 in 6,000
Power boating	1 in 6,000
Rock climbing	1 in 7,500
Playing football	1 in 25,000
Canoeing	1 in 100,000
Using tampons	1 in 350,000
Using Rely tampons	1 in 50,000
Using birth control pills (nonsmoker)	1 in 63,000
Using birth control pills (smoker)	1 in 16,000
Using IUDs	1 in 100,000
Using diaphragm, condom, or spermicide	None
Using fertility awareness methods	None
Undergoing sterilization:	
laparoscopic tubal ligation	1 in 10,000
hysterectomy	1 in 1,600
vasectomy	None
Pregnancy:	
continuing pregnancy	1 in 10,000
illegal abortion	1 in 3,000
legal abortion:	
before 9 weeks	1 in 400,000
before 9–12 weeks	1 in 100,000
before 13–16 weeks	1 in 25,000
after 16 weeks	1 in 10,000

Robert Hatcher et al.
It's Your Choice

Abstinence
Avoidance of sexual intercourse. This is one method of birth control.

Rhythm method
A method of preventing conception based on avoiding coitus during the fertile phase of a woman's cycle.

Foams, creams, and jellies must not be applied more than one-half hour before intercourse. After an hour, their effectiveness is drastically reduced, and a new applicator-full must be inserted. Another application is also required before each repeated act of coitus. If the woman wants to douche, she should wait for at least six hours after the last coitus to make sure that there has been time for the spermicide to kill all the sperm.

Advantages   Vaginal spermicides:

1. Are relatively simple to use.
2. Are readily available in most drugstores.
3. Do not require a prescription or a pelvic examination.

Disadvantages   Occasionally a man or a woman may develop an allergic irritation after coitus in which a vaginal spermicide was used. When this condition occurs, a doctor should be consulted. The physician may recommend another brand of spermicide or method of contraception.

Some recent studies have indicated that spermicide use around the time of conception may be associated with a higher rate of miscarriage, low birth weight, and certain birth defects. Other investigations have not found any such relationship, and no definitive conclusion can be made at this time. Similarly, the effects on the user herself of extended exposure to relatively high doses of spermicide are unknown at present.

Effectiveness   The reported failure rates of vaginal spermicides cover a wide range, again depending partly on how consistently and carefully instructions are followed. The actual failure rate is estimated to be 150 pregnancies per 1,000 women during one year of use. Vaginal spermicides are used by many couples in combination with condoms or as a backup with other birth control methods.

Some Other Methods of Contraception   Millions of people throughout the world do not use any of the methods we have described. Either they will not because of religious conviction or cultural prohibitions or they cannot because of poverty or ignorance. If they use any method at all, they are likely to use one of the following.

Abstinence   *Abstinence,* the decision not to engage in sexual intercourse for a chosen period of time, has been followed by human beings throughout history for a variety of reasons. Until relatively recently, many people abstained because of a lack of other birth control measures. Today, abstinence is being selected by individuals who have access to other means of pregnancy prevention, as well as by those who have limited alternatives. To some people all other methods simply seem unsuitable for a specified period of time in their life cycle. Concern regarding possible side effects and/or unwanted pregnancy may be factors. In some situations, intercourse may be temporarily avoided because of medical reasons such as recent illness or surgery. In other cases, abstinence may be seen as the wisest choice in terms of personal emotional needs. A delay or temporary moratorium of sexual intercourse may be chosen as a time to focus energies on other aspects of interpersonal growth or other facets of personal growth. Religious and cultural beliefs are sometimes motivating factors. For a variety of reasons, what may seem "right" and highly desirable for one person may be unacceptable for another. External pressure alone, either from individuals or from society at large, is being recognized as an unsatisfactory reason to engage in intercourse.

Many couples who do choose to abstain from sexual intercourse in the traditional penis-in-vagina sense turn to other mutually satisfying alternatives. When open communication between partners exists, many new avenues may be explored. These may include dancing, massage, hugging, kissing, petting, masturbation, and oral-genital sex. Sexual feelings may be expressed and satisfied through a wide range of activities and intimacy, in diverse interactions.

Rhythm   The *rhythm method* is based on avoiding coitus during the fertile phase of a woman's cycle. Ordinarily only one egg is released by the ovaries per month, and it lives about 24 hours unless it is fertilized. Sperm deposited in the vagina are apparently on the average capable of fertilizing an egg for about 48 to 72 hours; so conception theoretically can only occur during four days of any cycle. Predicting which four days these are is what is difficult. It is done either by the calendar method or by the temperature method. Recent informa-

What Are the Costs of Having Children?

Social scientists and psychotherapists have spent a lot of time studying the effects of parents on children, but very little studying the effects of children on parents. Even so, the effects are many, and the costs of having children emotionally and physically—as well as financially—are very great, even when people want the child.

Straining the Husband-Wife Relationship

As soon as the first child arrives, the focus of the marriage switches from the husband-wife relationship to the child. One study shows that the amount of time husband and wife spend talking to each other is cut in half with the coming of the first child. And when they do talk, they talk about the child rather than about themselves and their relationship, their inner feelings, and sex.

The parents are unable to go as many places as they did before or see as many people, so there is less to talk about. In fact, there is less emotionally charged interaction of any kind when young children are around. Couples may laugh less often together, have fewer stimulating exchanges of ideas, fight less, and be less likely to work on some activity or project together or to discuss things. Essentially, when there are three or more children, marriages sacrifice the husband-wife relationship for the parent-child relationship. Communication, intimacy, romance, and satisfaction with some aspects of the marriage seem impaired.

Effects of Children on Parent's Sexual Relations

In the United States, many people stop coitus one month before the woman is to deliver, often on advice from a doctor. Some couples, for fear of disturbing the well-being of the fetus, abstain the entire nine months. One-half of a sample of pregnant women reported no change in sexual desires during pregnancy; one-fourth, less desire; one-sixth, more desire.

After the baby's arrival, parents are sometimes too exhausted from work and loss of sleep to want sex. They sometimes feel themselves or their spouses to be less attractive. Or children may make the home seem less appealing as a place for sex relations.

Children as Competitors for Love and Care

With every new member of the family, each person is likely to have a thinner slice of attention. The husband is usually more likely to feel neglected than the wife, because she is most actively involved in caring for the child. With the arrival of the first child, the family's schedule usually begins to revolve around the child rather than the father. Because of this change, fathers may feel rivalry with the child, directly expressing hostility toward it or otherwise showing displeasure by being excessively demanding or punitive to the child. The father may also be jealous of the attention the child pays to the mother. Perhaps with men taking a more active role in child care, mothers can look forward to feeling neglected.

Anxiety and Conflict Between Parents over How to Raise Children

In one fairly large study, conflict over how to raise children ranked second only to problems with sexual adjustment. There is no agreement on how a child should be raised—theories range from applying very strict discipline to being very permissive—so a parent can be sure of criticism and blame if the child does not turn out right. Parents are often not sure whether what they are doing is right or wrong and this uncertainty brings its own stress.

When parents are asked to note the main problems in caring for children, they list:

1. Difficulties in discipline and obedience
2. Difficulty in being tolerant with the child
3. Extensive guilt over failures as parents
4. Embarrassment over what others think of their children

Children often do not turn out as well as their parents think they should. It is possible that some parents have an additional child so that they can atone for mistakes with earlier ones and try to turn out a better model.

Strain of Interaction and Parent-Child Conflict

Children's struggles for independence begin before they leave home, and when ideas of parents and children differ, there is often a battle of wills. Parents are likely to alternate between permissiveness and irritated punitiveness, and they must pay a price in either case: They feel guilty for being punitive, and they are afraid that children will not be able to make the right decisions. Parents also experience conflicts of conscience when children do things they cannot approve of; and they may be hostile toward children who dare to oppose them.

(continued on next page)

What Are the Costs of Having Children? (continued)

Mess, Noise, Confusion, Congestion

No one who has ever lived with several children needs reminding of the chaos that can reign when a couple of them are hungry or excited or fighting with each other. And even when things are flowing smoothly, there are the thousands of toys in the passageways and the clothes that never seem to be in the closet. Some people are bothered more than others by such congestion, and "crowded" living is a matter of perception. People who are thinking of having children would probably be wise to consider how they respond to the lack of privacy that comes with them.

Time, Confinement, Hard Work

Studies in Great Britain, France, and the United States show that women with no children and no job outside the home average about 60 hours of work in the house per week. The coming of the first child actually about doubles the housework required. The time it takes to care for the child is phenomenal: diapers, baths, messes to clean up, baby-sitters to look for, stories to read. It is estimated that a family of four needs 3,500 dishes washed every month.

Effects on the Mother

In the United States the price of having children falls most heavily on the mother. She may have to give up or postpone further education or a career that she would like to pursue—both things that potentially can bring her some interaction with other people, ego-fulfillment, financial income, and confidence in herself. Many young mothers are isolated. They find they have no close friends while they are deeply involved in just coping with and looking after small children. Their freedom is greatly restricted and their outside interests very much curtailed. And there is a physical toll for childbearing and for always "having to be there" for small children.

---

tion on cyclical changes of the cervical mucus has also been helpful in determining the time of ovulation. The calendar method is based on the knowledge that the average woman releases an egg 14 to 16 days before her next period begins. Few women menstruate with complete regularity, so a record of the menstrual cycle must be kept for 12 months, during which time some other method of birth control must be used. The first day of each period is counted as day 1. To determine the first fertile, or "unsafe" day of the cycle, 18 is subtracted from the number of days in the shortest cycle. To determine the last unsafe day of the cycle, 11 is subtracted from the number of days in the longest cycle. The calendar method is illustrated in Figure 6-5.

A woman's body temperature drops slightly just before ovulation and rises slightly after ovulation. This fluctuation is the basis for the temperature method. A woman using the temperature method records her BBT (basal, or resting, body temperature) every morning before getting out of bed and before eating or drinking anything. Once the temperature pattern can be seen (usually after about three months), the period unsafe for coitus can be calculated as the interval from day 5 (day 1 is the first day of the period) until three days after the rise in BBT. To arrive at a shorter unsafe period, some women use a combination of the calendar method and the temperature method, calculating the first unsafe day from the shortest cycle of the calendar chart and the last unsafe day as the third day after a rise in the BBT.

Also useful in predicting the fertile period are changes in the cervical secretions throughout the menstrual cycle. During the preovulatory phase cervical mucus increases and is clear and slippery. At the time of ovulation some women can detect a slight change in the texture of the mucus and find that it is more likely to form an elastic-like thread when stretched between thumb and finger. Following ovulation these secretions become cloudy and sticky and decrease in quantity. Infertile, safe days are likely to occur during the relatively dry days just before and after menstruation. See Figure 6-6. This is called the *Billings, or mucus, method.* These additional clues have been found helpful by some couples who rely on the rhythm method. One possible problem that may interfere with this method is that vaginal infections or the use of vaginal products or medication can alter changes in cervical mucus.

The rhythm method is not recommended for women who have very irregular cycles—about 15 percent of all menstruating women. Any woman for whom pregnancy would be a serious problem should not rely on the rhythm method alone, since the failure rate is high—150 to 300 pregnancies in 1,000 women during one year.

Coitus Interruptus   Probably the oldest known method of contraception, *coitus interruptus,* is mentioned in the Book of Genesis. In this method, the male withdraws his penis just before he ejaculates. Coitus interruptus has three advantages: It is free; it requires no preparation;

Billings, or mucus, method
A method of predicting the fertile period in a woman's cycle by means of the texture, color, and amount of cervical mucus.

Coitus interruptus
Sexual intercourse purposely interrupted by withdrawal of the penis prior to ejaculation (to avoid conception).

Length of shortest cycle	First "unsafe" day after start of any menstrual period	Length of longest cycle	Last "unsafe" day after start of any menstrual period
20 days	2nd day	20 days	9th day
21 days	3rd day	21 days	10th day
22 days	4th day	22 days	11th day
23 days	5th day	23 days	12th day
24 days	6th day	24 days	13th day
25 days	7th day	25 days	14th day
26 days	8th day	26 days	15th day
27 days	9th day	27 days	16th day
28 days	10th day	28 days	17th day
29 days	11th day	29 days	18th day
30 days	12th day	30 days	19th day
31 days	13th day	31 days	20th day
32 days	14th day	32 days	21st day
33 days	15th day	33 days	22nd day
34 days	16th day	34 days	23rd day
35 days	17th day	35 days	24th day
36 days	18th day	36 days	25th day
37 days	19th day	37 days	26th day
38 days	20th day	38 days	27th day
39 days	21st day	39 days	28th day
40 days	22nd day	40 days	29th day

Figure 6-5   The rhythm method of contraception—how to calculate the "safe" and "unsafe" days for coitus.

Prediction of "safe" and "unsafe" days for a woman whose menstrual cycle varies from 25 to 31 days over a 12-month period.

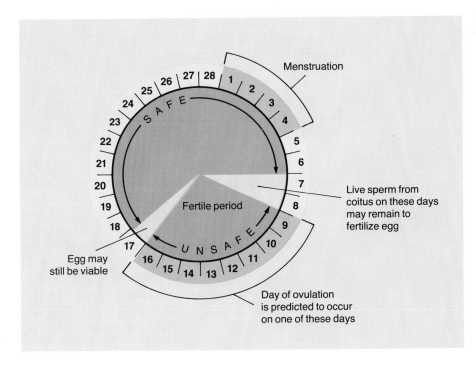

Douche
To cleanse or treat by applying a stream
of water or other solutions to a part or
cavity of the body such as the vagina; not
a contraceptive technique.

and it is always available. For many people, these advantages are far outweighed by the disadvantage: The male has to overcome a powerful biological urge that is also his heart's desire. The fear that withdrawal may be too late can wreck sexual pleasure for both partners. And finally, since in many societies a woman takes longer than a male does to reach orgasm, withdrawal before the woman's orgasm is likely and can leave the woman frustrated if she relies on coitus for satisfaction. The failure rate for coitus interruptus is 200 to 300 pregnancies per 1,000 women during one year. One key factor in this high failure rate is the demanding degree of self-control that is necessary to this method. In addition, pre-ejaculatory fluid, which often contains

viable sperm, is commonly secreted before actual ejaculation occurs.

Douches   Douching with water, vinegar, or any of various other substances after coitus has long been a popular method of birth control, but its use is now decreasing because its ineffectiveness is becoming more widely recognized. Sperm can move so rapidly that the douche is not likely to reach all of them in time. In some cases the douching fluid may actually help the sperm move upward into the cervical canal rather than remove them. Besides being an extremely ineffective contraceptive method, douching frequently can cause a bacterial imbalance in the vagina.

Prolonged Breast Feeding   Breast feeding delays the renewal of fertility, although for how long cannot be predicted. As a method of contraception, it is extremely unreliable.

Factors That Contribute to Failure Rates   About half of the pregnancies that occur in the United States are unintended. Of all U.S. women aged 15 to 44 who are at risk of unintended pregnancy, approximately 8 percent use no contraception of any type. The percentage of those using no method is highest among the young—18 percent of all teenagers who are sexually active—and then decreases with age to 6 percent of women aged 25 to 44 (see Table 6-1). Also important, however, is the fact that many couples who do practice contraception do not use the most effective methods or use them inconsistently (see Figure 6-7).

Causes of failure to prevent unintended pregnancy seem to fall into two groups. The causes in the first group are related to what the user knows about the method, how he or she feels about it, the strength of motivation, and religious belief. (Causes related to the product, such as cost and availability, are also in this group.) The second group consists of more subtle psychological causes. People who say they do not want pregnancy often act in ways that seem designed to produce "accidents." Some teenagers may be motivated by a wish to use pregnancy and marriage as a springboard out of unpleasant home situations. Some people equate love with

Figure 6-6   The cervical mucus method relies solely on the presence and quality of cervical mucus to indicate fertile and infertile periods of the menstrual cycle. The beginning of the fertile period is indicated by the onset of mucus flow. The day of the 'peak mucus symptom' is the last day of wet, slippery mucus, after which mucus thickens and disappears. The fertile period is presumed to last until four days after the peak symptom.

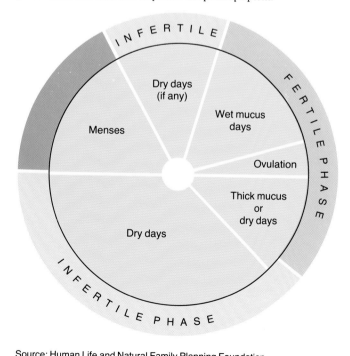

Source: Human Life and Natural Family Planning Foundation.

Table 6-1 Estimated Number and Percentage Distribution of U.S. Women Aged 15-44 Who Are Exposed to the Risk of Unintended Pregnancy, by Method of Contraception Currently Used, According to Age Group

Method	Number (in 000s)							Percent						
	Total	15–19	20–24	25–29	30–34	35–39	40–44	15–19	20–24	25–29	30–34	35–39	40–44	Total
Total	36,478	3,563	7,848	7,853	7,144	5,795	4,263	10	22	21	20	16	12	100
Sterilization	11,643	*	468	1,942	3,039	3,578	2,616	*	4	17	26	31	22	100
Tubal	(6,783)	(*)	(278)	(1,135)	(1,809)	(2,063)	(1,498)	(*)	(4)	(17)	(27)	(30)	(22)	100
Vasectomy	(4,860)	(*)	(190)	(807)	(1,230)	(1,515)	(1,118)	(*)	(4)	(17)	(25)	(31)	(23)	100
Pill	9,996	1,539	3,958	2,664	1,191	446	199	15	40	27	12	5	2	100
IUD	2,307	102	479	602	632	334	158	4	21	26	27	15	7	100
Condom	4,475	726	986	962	876	469	456	16	22	22	20	10	10	100
Spermicides	1,463	260	267	270	279	178	211	18	18	18	19	12	14	100
Diaphragm	1,908	39	546	573	471	168	112	2	29	30	25	9	6	100
Withdrawal	930	176	258	225	113	95	63	19	28	24	12	10	7	100
Rhythm	553	13	74	114	104	167	83	2	13	21	19	30	15	100
Other	150	66	7	11	47	10	9	†	†	†	†	†	†	100
None	3,053	642	823	490	392	350	356	21	27	16	13	11	12	100

*Less than 500 or less than 0.5 percent.

†Total N too small to distribute.

Source: *Family Planning Perspectives* 15(4), July–August 1983.

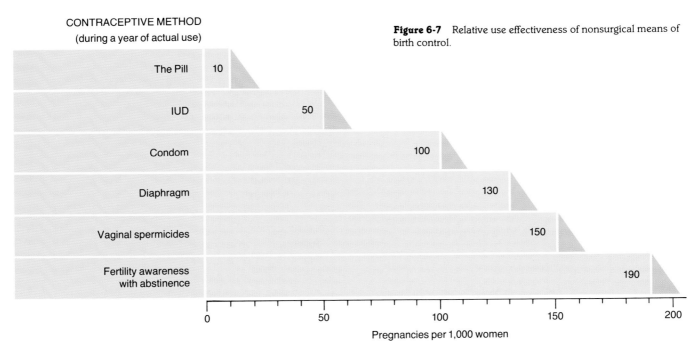

CONTRACEPTIVE METHOD
(during a year of actual use)

Figure 6-7 Relative use effectiveness of nonsurgical means of birth control.

The Pill   10

IUD   50

Condom   100

Diaphragm   130

Vaginal spermicides   150

Fertility awareness with abstinence   190

0   50   100   150   200

Pregnancies per 1,000 women

Source: Planned Parenthood.

Sterilization
Surgically altering the reproductive system so as to prevent pregnancy. Vasectomy is the procedure in males, tubal sterilization or hysterectomy in females.

Vasectomy
Surgical severing of the vasa deferentia, the ducts that carry the sperm to the ejaculatory duct.

Vasa deferentia
(Vas deferens, singular form) The two ducts that carry sperm to the ejaculatory duct.

Table 6-2 What the User Can Do to Improve Contraception Effectiveness Rates

Combination oral contraceptive	Follow pill-taking instructions carefully and consistently. Use a backup method such as foam or condoms during the first month.
IUD	Have IUD inserted by experienced clinician. Frequently check for IUD's position during the first few months. (User should feel thread in cervical opening but not the stem of the IUD.) Use a backup method such as foam or condoms during the first three months and, if desired, at mid-cycle thereafter.
Condom	Use with every act of intercourse. Put condom on penis before *any* penis-vagina contact. Leave space in tip of condom for semen. Remove carefully to avoid spillage. Avoid damage to condom; handle carefully. Avoid heat and use of Vaseline. Do not use after two years. Buy a good brand. Use foam along with condom.
Diaphragm and jelly	Use with every act of intercourse. Ask for thorough instruction with initial fitting. Have diaphragm fit checked every one to two years by an experienced clinician. Always use ample amounts of jelly or cream; add as necessary. Check position after insertion. Front rim must be behind pubic bone, and dome must cover cervix. Inspect regularly for defects or holes. Avoid use of Vaseline or perfumed powders, as they can damage the latex.
Vaginal spermicides	Use with every act of intercourse. Follow instructions regarding time limits of effectiveness. Use ample amounts. When using foam, shake vigorously before use. Use condoms along with spermicide.
Rhythm	Combine calendar, temperature, and mucus methods.
Coitus interruptus	Avoid penis-vagina contact during secretion of pre-ejaculatory lubricating fluid (very difficult to detect). Use foam along with coitus interruptus.

self-sacrifice and risk taking. For some people, fertility is a symbol of virility or femininity. For others, getting pregnant is a way of acting out unconscious hostility toward oneself or toward others. The wish to conceive sometimes seems to be part of the sex drive itself. A few people just plain want children but may not be aware of that feeling. Refusing to believe that pregnancy is possible is a common mechanism among the unconscious self-saboteurs. Failures to prevent pregnancy offer ample testimony that people often do act out of motives unknown to themselves.

Sterilization

Surgical attempts to control human fertility have a long history. Most were mutilating, dangerous, and ineffective until aseptic surgery (surgery without the danger of infection) and anesthetics became available in the late nineteenth century.

Sterilization is permanent, and it provides complete protection, with no further action needed at any time. For these reasons, it is becoming an increasingly popular method of birth control. At present it is the most commonly used method in the United States. It is especially popular among couples who have been married ten or more years, as well as among couples who have had all the children they intend. In 1982 an estimated 32 percent of all U.S. women aged 15 to 44 and at risk of unintended pregnancy were relying on sterilization for birth control; 19 percent had had tubal sterilization, and 13 percent had partners who had had vasectomies.

An important consideration in choosing sterilization is that, in most cases, it cannot be reversed. It should not be done without serious thought, and both partners must recognize it as a final decision to end childbearing.

Although some doctors will perform surgery for sterilization "on request," most require a thorough discussion with both partners before the operation. Most doctors also recommend that people who have religious conflicts, psychiatric problems related to sex, or unstable marriages not be sterilized. Young couples with one or two children, who might later change their minds and

Study Refutes Claim That Vasectomy Is Health Hazard

A new government-funded study has branded as unfounded fears that vasectomy may cause long-term health problems ranging from arthritis to heart disease—concerns believed to underlie a worldwide decline in popularity of vasectomy that began in 1977 and 1978, when the first negative health reports emerged.

New worldwide popularity for the procedure may result from dissemination of what doctors perceive as good news about vasectomy. Such a trend would reverse a process in which the number of vasectomies performed in the United States fell from 507,000 in 1976 to 424,000 in 1981.

Incidence of Disease Among Men

The incidence of death and a total of 54 different diseases was tabulated for 10,590 pairs of men matched statistically so the only significant difference between members of each pair was that one man had had a vasectomy and the other had not. Deaths and reports of any of the 54 disorders were rare, primarily because the vast majority of research subjects are under 50 and most are under 40. Among the most significant pairings were these:

	Vasectomized Men	Nonvasectomized Men
Death	212	326
Asthma	71	71
Heart attack	244	321
Angina pectoris	325	400
Stroke	37	40
Hepatitis	82	70
Diabetes	141	200
Rheumatoid arthritis	32	43
Cancer	133	181
Impotence	162	155

Allan Parachini

---

want more, are also frequently advised not to undergo sterilization.

Male Sterilization or Vasectomy   *Vasectomy* involves severing the *vasa deferentia*, two minute ducts that transport sperm from the testicles to the seminal vesicles. The testicles continue to produce sperm, but the sperm are absorbed into the body. Since the testicles contribute only about one-tenth of the total seminal fluid, the actual quantity of ejaculate is only slightly reduced. Hormone output from the testicles apparently continues with very little change.

Vasectomy is ordinarily done in the doctor's office and takes about 30 minutes. The patient is instructed to present himself with all pubic hair shaved. After the scrotal region is washed with a surgical cleanser, a local anesthetic is injected into the skin of the scrotum and about the vasa. Small incisions are made at the upper end of the scrotum where it joins the body, and the vas deferens on each side is exposed, severed, and closed off. The incisions are then closed with sutures, and a small dressing is applied. (See Figure 6-8.)

As the local anesthetic wears off, the patient feels a dull ache in the surgical area and often in the lower abdomen. Pain and swelling are usually slight and can be relieved with an ice bag, aspirin, and use of a scrotal support. Bleeding and infection occasionally develop but are in most cases easily treated. Most men are ready to return to work in two days.

Men can have sex again as soon as they feel no further discomfort; for most men this means after about a week. Another method of contraception must be used for the first few weeks after vasectomy, however, because sperm produced before the operation may still be

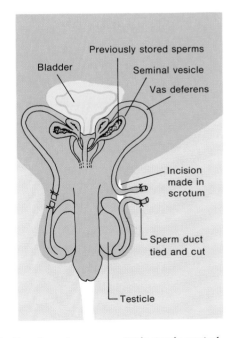

Figure 6-8   Vasectomy is a comparatively simple surgical procedure.

Tubal sterilization
The process of severing or in some manner blocking the oviducts. This prevents conception by preventing ova (eggs) from reaching the uterus.

Laparoscopy
A method of examining the internal organs by inserting a tube containing a small light through an abdominal incision.

present in the semen. To make sure that sperm are no longer in the ejaculate and that another method of contraception is no longer necessary, a semen specimen should be examined under a microscope.

We do not know much about long-range complications. Recent studies do not support an earlier hypothesis that a vasectomy may accelerate atherosclerosis (the formation of fat deposits that clog arteries).

In about 1 percent of vasectomies, a severed vas rejoins itself, and sperm can again travel up through the duct and be ejaculated in the semen. Because of this possibility, some doctors advise that a semen specimen be examined yearly.

So far, attempts to restore fertility have failed more than half the time.

Female Sterilization   The most common method of female sterilization involves severing or in some manner blocking the Fallopian tubes, thereby preventing the egg from reaching the uterus and the sperm from entering the tubes. Ovulation and menstruation continue, but the unfertilized eggs are released into the abdominal cavity and absorbed.

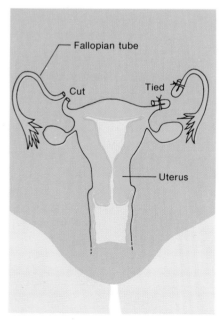

Figure 6-9   Compared to vasectomy, tubal sterilization is somewhat more complex.

One method of *tubal sterilization* is accomplished by making a small incision in the abdominal wall, locating each Fallopian tube, bringing it into view, severing it, removing a small section, and tying or stapling shut the two ends. (See Figure 6-9.) Another method involves making the incision through the vaginal wall, an approach that leaves no visible scar and requires a shorter hospitalization. Some conditions, however, such as obesity or recent pregnancy, make this method difficult or impossible. As a rule, a general anesthetic is used in either type of tubal sterilization, and the operation takes about 30 minutes. The usual hospital stay is two to three days. The operation can be performed shortly after a normal delivery, or in the case of Caesarian section immediately after the incision in the uterus is repaired.

Female sterilization by the standard abdominal or vaginal procedure is riskier than male sterilization. About 7 percent of the patients experience problems after the operation. Such problems arise mainly from wound or urinary infection. Serious complications, among them bowel obstruction, phlebitis, pulmonary embolism, or hemorrhage, are rare. The death rate is an estimated 25 per one million operations. Most of these deaths occur in patients with underlying medical conditions that would also make pregnancy more risky.

An increasing number of tubal sterilizations are being done by a method called *laparoscopy*. A laparoscope, which is a tube containing a small light, is inserted through a small abdominal incision and the surgeon looks through it to locate the Fallopian tubes. Instruments are passed either through the laparoscope or through a second small incision, and the two Fallopian tubes are coagulated (sealed off) by electrocautery. Either a regional or general anesthetic can be used, but a general anesthetic is more common. The operation takes 15 minutes and can be done without overnight hospitalisation. Most women leave the hospital two to four hours after surgery. Complications, such as bowel trauma, hemorrhage, and pelvic variocosities, occur in approximately 0.4 percent of laparoscopic sterilizations. This figure varies widely, however, depending on the experience of the surgeon and type of equipment available. The mortality rate is 10 to 20 per one million procedures.

Laparoscopy has approximately the same failure rate

Hysterectomy
Total or partial surgical removal of the uterus.

Progesterone
A hormone that prepares the uterus for a fertilized ovum (egg) and maintains pregnancy.

---

as standard tubal ligations, about 3 out of every 1,000 cases. Reversibility varies with the method used: The standard abdominal tubal sterilization has the higher incidence of fertility restoration (about 50 percent reversibility when micro surgical techniques are available); laparoscopy has a considerably lower rate because of the wider destruction of tubal tissue.

Complaints of long-term abdominal discomfort and menstrual irregularity have been reported following female sterilization, but these have been difficult to interpret. No clear connection has been found between these complaints and sterilization. Most women are satisfied. The number of women who feel regret varies in follow-up studies, and this fact, too, is difficult to interpret. Regret, when it does appear, seems to be related to previous difficulties, initial doubts and reservations, feelings of being pressured by the spouse, or changes in marital and family circumstances.

Hysterectomy, removal of the uterus, is the preferred method of sterilization for only a small number of women, usually women with preexisting menstrual problems. Because of the risks involved, hysterectomy is not recommended unless the patient has serious gynecologic problems such as disease or damage of the uterus and future surgery appears inevitable.

New Methods of Contraception

Even with all the improvements of recent years, the best of the present methods of birth control have drawbacks. The search still continues for the ideal method, the one that will be more effective, safer, cheaper, easier to use, more readily available, and acceptable to more people.

An increase specifically in the male contraceptive alternatives is viewed by many as a high priority. Throughout history, the responsibility for birth control has been assumed predominantly by women, partly because of the greater personal investment women have in the prevention of pregnancy with its many risks and the greater child-rearing demands that are placed upon them. Complete control has been seen as crucial by some women in some settings. In addition, more birth control options have been available for female use, one

factor being the more numerous points of intervention in the female reproductive system. Another factor in the paucity of male methods of birth control may be the long history of underrepresentation of women in medicine, scientific research, pharmaceutical management, the FDA, and other political forces. Participation by women and the expression of their needs vis-á-vis birth control has been minimized in these areas.

Following are some of the new methods currently considered most promising. Although no major breakthroughs are likely to be widely applicable for several years, small signs of progress may be found. Many of the methods resulting from this research have reached the stage of testing on humans in clinical settings.

Menstruation-Inducing Pill   A menstruation-inducing steroid pill is taken for four days of the month, starting two days before the expected beginning of menstruation. The pill prevents the cells of the uterus from absorbing *progesterone,* a hormone necessary to sustain pregnancy. With the progesterone blocked, the uterus sheds its lining as it would with a normal period, and the fertilized egg, if present, is expelled along with the menstrual flow.

Long-Acting Injectables   Injections of 150 milligrams of progestin every 90 days are almost 100 percent effective in preventing pregnancy. This method still has disadvantages, however, including irregular menstrual bleeding patterns in the uterus and long delays (12 to 21 months) in the return of ovulatory cycles after injections are stopped. Injections of 500 milligrams twice a year are also being tested.

Implants Under the Skin   An inch-long, spaghetti-width capsule filled with progestin and inserted under the skin of the inner arm or thigh can provide protection for five years or longer. Side effects are similar to those of long-acting injectable progestins.

Vaginal Ring   The vaginal ring resembles the rim of a diaphragm and is molded of a mixture of progestin and a silicone polymer. The woman inserts the ring herself and wears it for three weeks, during which time progestin is absorbed into her bloodstream preventing

Testosterone
A male hormone that is produced in the testes and affects secondary sex characteristics.

Prostaglandins
Naturally occurring chemicals, two of which induce abortion of the embryo or fetus when injected into the amniotic sac or inserted into the uterus.

ovulation. Menstruation follows removal, and then a new ring is inserted.

Chemical Contraceptives for Men   Male and female hormones can interfere with sperm production and development in the male in a way similar to ovulation suppression in the female. However, effectiveness of these hormones is often unpredictable and side effects may include both the loss of libido (sex drive) and the development of female secondary sex characteristics, for example, enlarged breasts.

Gossypol, a derivative of cottonseed oil used extensively for several years in China, also results in very low sperm counts and temporary infertility. Reported side effects include disturbances in potassium metabolism and general weakness. *Testosterone* levels are apparently not affected, and decreased libido, noted in a small percentage of men, tends to return to normal with ongoing use. Further studies are currently underway in many countries.

Contraceptive Immunization   Theoretically, immunity to fertility can be produced by sensitizing a man to his own sperm cells so that he produces antibodies that inactivate them as if they were a disease. Similarly, a woman could be sensitized against her own egg cells or against her partner's sperm cells. Experimentally, at least, the theory works, but widespread human testing cannot begin until several questions have been answered. How long the immunity lasts and how to control it are not yet known, and serious allergic reactions could be a life-threatening problem.

Reversible Sterilization   Present methods of sterilization of both men and women are permanent more than 50 percent of the time. Several new techniques of sterilization are being studied in the hope that restoring fertility can be made easier and more predictable.

Female sterilization has been attempted by injecting liquid silicone into the Fallopian tubes, where it solidifies and forms a plug. In animal experiments, however, such plugs have been readily dislodged by normal muscle activity, so this method is not likely to be very effective.

Reversible male sterilization has been tried by several methods. One of these methods involves inserting a thread into the vas. The thread is then anchored to the skin so that it can be easily found and removed. The thread partially blocks the vas, causing a low sperm count. The effectiveness of this technique has not been proved.

Totally blocking sperm flow with removable clips and with various plugs has been tried, but both clips and plugs damaged the vasa, making restoration of fertility less likely. Recanalization of the vas, a phenomenon in which the sperm make a new path around the plug, has also occurred with plugs. Some of the plugs tested contain a tiny valve that can be opened manually or magnetically.

Even when tissue damage and recanalization can be prevented, researchers face another problem: Some vasectomized men develop antibodies to their sperm, which might persist after vasectomy reversal.

Prostaglandins   *Prostaglandins* are currently being used to initiate second trimester abortions. However, a new and promising use of prostaglandins is their application to tampons, which are inserted to bring on menstruation shortly after a period is missed. Prostaglandins tampons used regularly at the end of each cycle could induce menstruation each time whether or not the cycle had been fertile.

Lutenizing Hormone-Releasing Hormone (LHRH)   LHRH, a naturally occurring compound in both men and women, acts on the pituitary gland, triggering the release of its hormones, which in turn play an essential role in sperm formation and ovulation. Manmade analogs of LHRH, which are over 100 times as powerful as natural LHRH, are currently available. After these analogs are administered, there is a sharp rise in the levels of pituitary hormones, followed by a drop to subnormal levels, probably the result of overstimulation and exhaustion of the pituitary gland. Once the low levels are established, it appears that in women, on whom most of the studies thus far have been completed, the pituitary-ovary cycle is effectively disrupted, and temporary cessation of ovulation and menstruation results. No immediate side effects have been detected. However, many questions regarding this complex interaction and its long-term effects remain, and any possible clinical application is undoubtedly several years away.

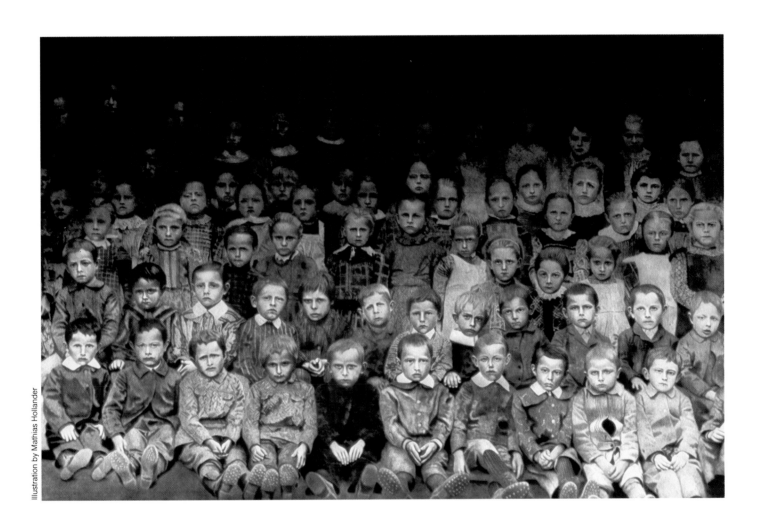

Illustration by Mathias Hollander

Abortion
The premature expulsion or removal of an embryo or fetus from the uterus.

Vacuum aspiration
Also called suction curettage, this procedure involves removal of the fetus by means of suction.

Abortion Methods

During the 1970s changes in the United States in attitudes toward *abortion* led to a sociomedical revolution. With liberalization of the abortion laws, the number of legal abortions dramatically increased, more women applied for abortion early in pregnancy, hospital admissions for incomplete (presumably illegal) abortions decreased, and there was a drop in deaths related to abortion. In 1980, however, governmental funding for abortions was decreased markedly, and controversy between "pro-choice" and "pro-life" groups was again raging. Therefore, whether or not the recent trend toward fewer abortion complications and deaths will continue largely depends on the political and legal decisions of the rest of this decade.

Five methods of abortion are currently in use: vacuum aspiration, dilatation and curettage, saline, prostaglandin, and hysterotomy.

Vacuum Aspiration   *Vacuum aspiration* (also called suction curettage), first developed in China in 1958, has rapidly become the preferred method for abortions up to the fifteenth week of pregnancy. It can be done

quickly, and the risk of hemorrhage or other complications is small. It is usually done on an outpatient basis and in most cases requires only a local anesthetic.

A sedative may be given, along with a local anesthetic. A speculum, which is a device used to open the vaginal entrance, is inserted into the vagina and the cervix is cleansed with a surgical solution. The cervix is dilated with instruments (or other materials that expand slowly when left in place), and a suction curette—a specially designed hollow tube—is then inserted into the uterus. The curette is attached to the rubber tubing of an electric pump, and suction is applied to the uterine cavity. (See Figure 6-10.) In about 20 to 30 seconds the uterus is emptied. Moderate cramping is common during evacuation. To ensure that no fragments of tissue are left in the uterus, the doctor will usually scrape the uterine lining with a metal curette, an instrument with a spoonlike tip. The entire operation takes only five to ten minutes.

After a few hours in a recovering area, the woman is allowed to return home. She is usually instructed not to douche, have coitus, or use tampons for the first week or two after the abortion, and to return for a two-week postabortion examination. This examination is impor-

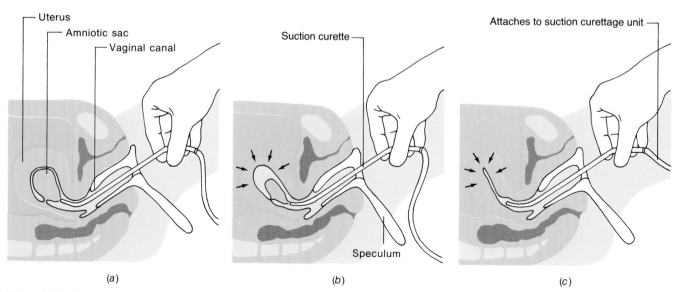

Uterus
Amniotic sac
Vaginal canal

Suction curette

Attaches to suction curettage unit

Speculum

(a)   (b)   (c)

Figure 6-10   Vacuum aspiration takes only five to ten minutes and can be performed up to the twelfth week of pregnancy.

Abortion–The Hard Question

An NBC News poll found that 58 percent of the people questioned (and 46 percent of the Roman Catholics) approved of laws permitting abortions during the first three months of pregnancy—or wanted them liberalized. But there was also a growing awareness that abortion poses some hard moral questions.

Some doctors and nurses who regularly perform abortions have been shaken by the sight of tiny arms and legs being sucked out of the womb. The surgical procedure called hysterotomy and generally employed only as a last resort in late-term abortions can be profoundly disturbing when a fetus emerges with some sign of life. "It's terrible," says one San Francisco obstetrician, recalling one episode. "You cut a hole in the uterus and take the baby out and put it in a basin. It's a little kid. It wiggles and lets out some squeaks. Somebody covers it up. Sometimes it lives for an hour or two." Dr. Bernard Nathanson, an early leader of the campaign to make abortion legal in New York, eventually resigned as a director of a large abortion clinic there after concluding that "human life exists within the womb from the very onset of pregnancy." And that problem is bound to become even more complicated as science improves its capacity to sustain fetuses at ever-earlier points of emergence from the womb.

There are no universally accepted ethical standards for the preservation of new life—born or unborn. The ancient Spartans, among others, left sickly infants on exposed mountainsides to die. In the U.S., most states did not even pass anti-abortion laws until the mid-nineteenth century, and then the motive was mainly to protect women from serious injury or death in a highly risky procedure, Similarly, it was to protect women from the butchery of illegal abortionists that contemporary reformers sought to have anti-abortion laws overturned.

In 1973, the Supreme Court explicitly legalized abortion in the U.S. for all practical purposes. The procedures for abortion during the first three months of pregnancy were so safe, wrote Harry Blackmun, that a woman, in concert with her doctor, had the clear right to choose an abortion during that period if she wished. Dangers during the second trimester, however, gave the state a "legitimate interest in preserving and protecting the health of the woman"—and a consequent right to regulate abortions, requiring, for example, that they be performed in fully equipped hospitals rather than a doctor's office. Only in the last twelve weeks of pregnancy did the Court recognize that an "important and legitimate interest in potential life" might actually outweigh the mother's right and wishes. At that point, said Blackmun, a state "may go so far as to proscribe abortion except when necessary to preserve the life or health of the mother."

Ironically, the increasing acceptance of abortion and the growing number of women who have resorted to it (up by a third from 1972) have prompted some second thoughts among many Americans. The late-term hysterotomy is a particularly emotional experience, and nurses in a Bakersfield, Calif., hospital actually disobeyed doctors' orders by trying to save the aborted fetus.

Even those who continue to believe that abortions are necessary have been touched by the palpable reality of life's termination. Former abortion-clinic director Nathanson writes: "I am deeply troubled by my own increasing certainty that I presided over 60,000 deaths." He argues not for changing the law but for cultivating the "pervasive sense of loss that should accompany the abortion."

On a purely practical level, fostering an atmosphere in which abortions are even more widely accepted—and quickly obtained— would avoid the late-term procedures that involve the most viable fetuses. Still, as science becomes more sophisticated in its ability to sustain fetal life, that argument loses some of its moral weight. One religious answer is that society must enforce a stricter sense of personal responsibility in this era of sexual freedom—although Dr. [Kenneth J.] Ryan notes, "people forget that there used to be plenty of anger over teaching children about reproduction. Well, if you don't want abortion, you have to put some more effort into family planning."

Right-to-life advocates have been generally silent on the question of abortion in cases where the fetus is determined to be genetically defective, but even then some argue that birth should proceed. "Abortion replaces the Hippocratic oath with a utilitarian ethic," says Dr. Mildred F. Jefferson, an assistant professor of surgery at Boston University Medical School and chairman of the board of the National Right to Life Committee. Another view is that abortion involves not only life but the quality of life. What is the unwanted— perhaps defective—child being saved for? "I try to see [the pro-life] point of view, but have they ever stopped to think of the socioeconomic problems involved in unwanted children?" asks Dr. Edgar N. Jackson, medical director of the Hillcrest Clinic and Counseling Service

(continued on next page)

Abortion—The Hard Question (continued)

of Atlanta. Says Dr. Theodore Howard, the black director of Friendship Medical Center in Chicago: "We end up with people who are poorly fed, poorly housed, and poorly clothed. My years in the Mississippi Delta have convinced me that abortion is really a blessing in disguise for black people."

Any society that can spend millions on moon rockets and atom bombs ought to be able to care for unwanted children, the right-to-lifers reply. And seven states have adopted laws that make a public

ward of any fetus that survives an abortion. "You must eliminate the problems people have," says John Short of the Long Island Coalition for Life, "not the people themselves." But even many religious opponents of abortion will countenance other forms of killing—war, for example—in order to preserve a particular quality of life: democracy, liberty, the American Way.

The point that bothers most doctors is that if abortion is significantly restricted or made illegal again, women—and especially poor

women—will be forced back to the butchers. "You don't have to see too many women with their guts hanging out before you realize that we must do what we are doing now," says Dr. William Little, chief of obstetrics and gynecology at Jackson Memorial Hospital in Miami. So the controversy resolves itself into a calculus of life-for-life. And no matter how it is resolved, the answer can never be totally satisfying to any but the most doctrinaire.

David M. Alpern
Newsweek

---

tant to verify that the abortion was complete and that no signs of infection are present.

Dilatation and Curettage In *dilatation and curettage* (commonly called D and C) the embryo and placenta are removed by surgical instruments rather than by suction. A curette is used to scrape the tissues from the wall of the uterus; an ovum forceps, a long grasping instrument, is also used. Because a D and C takes longer, causes a greater loss of blood, and requires a longer recovery period, it has been largely replaced by vacuum aspiration.

The Saline Method After the fifteenth week of pregnancy, the saline method is usually used, because suction becomes more difficult, and D and C so late in pregnancy leads to greater complications than if it is performed earlier. A local anesthetic is given, and a long needle is inserted through the abdominal and uterine walls into the *amniotic sac. Amniotic fluid* is drained from the sac and replaced with an equal amount of 20-percent salt solution. The injection must be made slowly and with great care to avoid introducing the solution into the woman's circulation. The woman must be fully awake to report pain or other symptoms.

The death of the fetus, enclosed in the amniotic sac, occurs immediately, followed by a miniature labor and delivery within a day or two. The uterus is scraped to reduce chances of infection or hemorrhage. The recovery period is slightly longer than for suction curettage, and complications are more frequent. The saline method is not advisable for women with heart

or kidney disease, a history of toxemia, or a previous delivery by *Caesarean section.*

Prostaglandins Two of the prostaglandins, a group of naturally occurring chemicals, bring on abortion, apparently by stimulating contractions of the uterus. They can be injected into the amniotic sac or inserted through the cervical canal into the uterus. Their major shortcoming is their effect on the muscles of the digestive tract, which produces nausea, vomiting, and diarrhea. Refined prostaglandins have fewer side effects than natural ones.

Hysterotomy Abortion by *hysterotomy* is a major surgical procedure (a modified Caesarean section) usually performed under a general anesthetic, although a spinal anesthetic may be effective. Incisions are made in the walls of the abdomen and the uterus: The fetus and placenta are removed; and then the incisions are repaired. After a woman has had a hysterotomy, many doctors insist that Caesarean section be used for all deliveries to avoid the risk that the uterus will rupture during labor contractions. The saline and prostaglandin methods have largely replaced hysterotomy.

Abortion Complications

The incidence of immediate problems following abortion (incomplete abortion requiring repeat curettage, perforation of the uterus, hemorrhage, and infection) varies widely. It is significantly reduced with early

Dilatation and curettage (D and C)
Dilatation of the cervix and scraping of the uterus to remove the fetus—or for other medical purposes.

Amniotic sac/Amniotic fluid
The bag of watery fluid lining the uterus, which envelops and protects the fetus.

Caesarean section
A surgical incision through the abdominal wall and uterus; performed to extract a fetus.

Hysterotomy
A modified Caesarean section in which the fetus is removed and the incisions are afterward repaired.

---

abortion, use of the suction method, performance by a well-trained clinician, and availability and use of prompt follow-up care. Reports on long-term complications (subsequent infertility, spontaneous second abortions, premature delivery, and low-birth-weight babies) have been inconsistent. No conclusions are as yet clearly established. The actual death-to-case rate varies from 0.6 per 100,000 abortions for under 8 weeks gestation to 7.8 per 100,000 for 13 to 15 weeks gestation.

Complications occur least often with the suction method, followed by D and C, saline, and hysterotomy, in that order.

Psychological side effects of abortion are less clearly defined. Responses vary, depending on the individual woman's psychological makeup, emotional health, family background, and many other factors. Feelings women experience after abortion cover the range from guilt and depression to great relief. A temporary mild-to-moderate depression similar to "postpartum blues" (depression following childbirth) may be quite common. For many, the chief feeling is relief from the acute distress associated with unwanted pregnancy.

The woman who is considering abortion may be able to diminish her fears and the possible psychological side effects of the operation if she explores and evaluates her feelings about it with a woman who has herself had an abortion. If she is uncertain or if someone else is pressuring her to get an abortion, a "cooling off" period of a week or two may help her to crystallize her feelings. Sometimes alternatives to abortion, such as offering the baby for adoption or finding ways to keep the baby, may be more suitable.

Birth Control Behavior Scale

Read the following statements carefully. Choose the one in each section that best describes you at this moment and record its score at the right. (For example, "well educated about birth control" has a score of 5.) When you have identified five statements, total your score and find your position on the scale.

5 well educated about birth control
4 knowledgeable about birth control
3 familiar with birth control methods
2 unfamiliar with many birth control methods
1 ignorant of birth control methods

Score _____

5 openly discusses birth control methods
4 discusses birth control methods with partner
3 resists discussions of birth control
2 avoids discussions of birth control
1 resents discussion of birth control

Score _____

5 takes responsibility for contraception
4 shares responsibility for contraception
3 shares costs of contraception
2 resists responsibility for contraception
1 takes no responsibility for contraception

Score _____

5 prefers inconvenience of contraception to risk of pregnancy
4 sacrifices convenience to avoid an unwanted pregnancy
3 if contraception is inconvenient, will sometimes risk pregnancy
2 believes the female should be responsible for birth control
1 risks unwanted pregnancy for the sake of convenience

Score _____

5 educates others about birth control
4 discusses contraceptives with pharmacist
3 is uncomfortable buying contraceptives
2 avoids buying contraceptives
1 refuses to buy contraceptives

Score _____

Total score _____

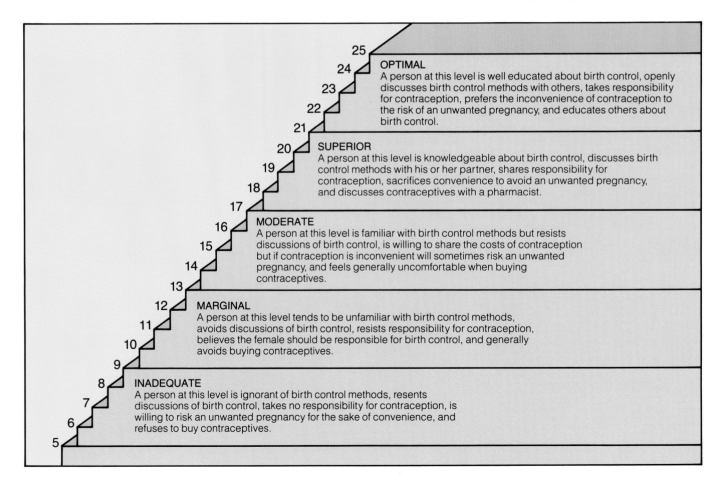

25
24
23
22
21 OPTIMAL
A person at this level is well educated about birth control, openly discusses birth control methods with others, takes responsibility for contraception, prefers the inconvenience of contraception to the risk of an unwanted pregnancy, and educates others about birth control.

20
19
18
17 SUPERIOR
A person at this level is knowledgeable about birth control, discusses birth control methods with his or her partner, shares responsibility for contraception, sacrifices convenience to avoid an unwanted pregnancy, and discusses contraceptives with a pharmacist.

16
15
14
13 MODERATE
A person at this level is familiar with birth control methods but resists discussions of birth control, is willing to share the costs of contraception but if contraception is inconvenient will sometimes risk an unwanted pregnancy, and feels generally uncomfortable when buying contraceptives.

12
11
10
9 MARGINAL
A person at this level tends to be unfamiliar with birth control methods, avoids discussions of birth control, resists responsibility for contraception, believes the female should be responsible for birth control, and generally avoids buying contraceptives.

8
7
6
5 INADEQUATE
A person at this level is ignorant of birth control methods, resents discussions of birth control, takes no responsibility for contraception, is willing to risk an unwanted pregnancy for the sake of convenience, and refuses to buy contraceptives.

Take Action

Your answers to Probing Your Emotions at the beginning of this chapter and your placement level on the Birth Control Behavior Scale will, we hope, encourage you to begin a process of self-exploration and self-discovery that you will continue. Reflect on the entire chapter's content and ask yourself how each point relates to your own life. Then take action:

1. Consider the different methods of contraception. In your Take Action notebook rank the methods according to how they best suit your particular life-style. Take into account such considerations as how often you have sexual intercourse, cost requirements, and convenience.

2. Consider what health risks you or your partner takes (or would take) by using a particular form of birth control. For example, if you are a smoking female and are taking the pill, you have an increased risk of a future heart attack or stroke. Make a list of the different birth control methods and indicate whether they carry any additional risk for you or your partner. Don't forget to include the risk of pregnancy. Compare this list with your list in item 1.

3. List the positive behaviors and attitudes that help you adhere to your beliefs about birth control. How can you strengthen those behaviors? Also list behaviors and attitudes that block your beliefs and actions. Consider each of these behaviors and attitudes

and decide which ones you can change in order to improve.

4. Where do you stand on the issue of abortion? Are you "pro-choice" or "pro-life"? If you are unsure, go to the library and read at least two recent articles on each side of the issue. In your notebook draw up a list of the pros and cons of abortion and try to come to a conclusion. Write a letter to your senator or representative briefly defending your view and asking him or her to consider your view when voting on any upcoming abortion legislation.

Before leaving this chapter, review the questions that open the chapter. Have your feelings or values changed?

Are you now better equipped to handle the complex and very human problems associated with birth control?

Chapter Seven

Pregnancy, Childbirth, and Parenting

Probing Your Emotions

1. Does it frighten you to think a tiny child may (or does) depend on you for food, clothing, a home, emotional support, and almost constant attention, at least for a few years of your life? Can you support a child emotionally? If so, how? If not, why not?

2. Your sister is seven months pregnant. She has not visited a doctor because she does not consider pregnancy an illness. She wants to deliver her child at home but has not found a physician or midwife willing to attend. How do you feel about her position? What would you counsel her to do?

3. What did your parents know about raising children? What do you know about parenting? Did you learn what you know from your parents? Can you learn anything about disciplining, encouraging, loving, teaching, and tolerating children from courses and textbooks? From observing and thinking about other families?

4. Will or do you treat your children differently from the way your parents treated you? Will you require more work of them? Teach them more things? Spend more time with them? Let them find out that experience is the best teacher?

Chapter Contents

THE REPRODUCTIVE PROCESS

FETAL DEVELOPMENT
First trimester
Second trimester
Third trimester

CHANGES IN THE MOTHER'S
BODY DURING PREGNANCY
The signs and symptoms of pregnancy
Changes that continue throughout pregnancy
Changes and complications in
   the later stages of pregnancy

THE IMPORTANCE OF EARLY
PRENATAL CARE

EXERCISE AND WORK DURING PREGNANCY

LABOR AND DELIVERY
First stage of labor
Second stage of labor
Third stage of labor
Prepared childbirth

THE PUERPERIUM
Postpartum depression
Breast feeding and rooming-in
Uterine shrinkage
Return of menstruation

PROSPECTIVE PARENTS AS CONSUMERS
IN THE MEDICAL MARKETPLACE
Informed decisions about birth procedures
The alternatives

PARENTING

Boxes

Rh negative blood
Routine delivery procedures some parents
   would like to change
Sudden (unexplained) infant death syndrome
Am I parent material?
How to win without losing

Ovary
One of the two female sexual glands in which the ova (eggs) and hormones are formed. Each ovary contains a mass of vascular fibrous tissue that contains a number of follicles, each enclosing an ovum.

Follicles
The thousands of protecting, enclosing spherical bubbles in the ovaries in which the ova mature. Each follicle contains a liquid supplied with estrogen.

Oviducts (Fallopian tubes)
The two passages through which ova leave the ovaries and pass to the uterus.

Uterus
The hollow, thick-walled, muscular organ in which the egg develops into a child; the womb. It is located directly above the vagina.

Fertilized egg
The egg after it has been penetrated by a sperm.

Sperm cell
A mature male germ cell that serves to impregnate the ovum.

Fertilization
The initiation of biological reproduction, as, for example, when the sperm and ovum unite to form a zygote (fertilized egg).

---

7 Our changing attitudes toward nature are nowhere more apparent than in our changing attitudes toward birth. Only a few years ago most of us had an unqualified faith that technology could do anything and that whatever nature could do, science could do better.

That faith has begun to fade, and people in the medical profession, like many other people, are having second thoughts. Natural childbirth may not be the answer for every mother, but more and more women are requesting it. At the same time, some doctors are pointing to possible harmful effects of drugged childbirth, for both the baby and the mother. Breast feeding is increasingly viewed as beneficial in all ways to both mother and baby. The practice of forcing labor is being challenged, as is routine circumcision of male babies. The father, once virtually ignored during the birth process, is now often brought into the labor and delivery rooms to take part.

More and more parents are insisting on their right to decide how their children will be born. Some mothers want to be unconscious or numb. Others want to be aware, to experience giving birth. The current emphasis on awareness reflects a basic change in cultural values. The pendulum of change is swinging in both directions at once. For example, bottle feeding first became popular in the upper economic classes. Its popularity is still growing, especially in the South and Southwest, formerly strongholds of breast feeding, and in the lower economic classes. At the same time breast feeding is becoming the most widespread method in the upper economic classes, especially among college-educated women.

Still another change in attitudes is reflected by a greater understanding on the part of many people that a baby's growth and development are strongly influenced by events early in its life. Very young babies whose mothers spend most of their waking hours singing to them and positioning them to ensure the greatest possible eye contact with them are less afraid of strangers. And the more their fathers care for them and play with them, the more they relate to their fathers in a close and satisfying way. Babies who do not crawl enough to sufficiently develop hand-eye coordination appear to have difficulty developing verbal skills when they go to school. Babies who do not receive a lot of touching and other forms of sensory stimulation are more likely to develop severe psychological problems. Stimulation seems to be the one most necessary ingredient of growth.

The Reproductive Process

Every month during a woman's fertile years, her body prepares itself for childbearing. In one of her *ovaries* an egg ripens and is released. It bursts from its *follicle*. The egg is then drawn into the *oviduct*, through which it travels to the uterus. The journey takes three to four days. The lining of the *uterus* has already puffed out to accept the implanting of a *fertilized egg*. An unfertilized egg lives about 24 hours, and then it disintegrates. It is expelled along with the uterine lining during menstruation.

Each egg is about the size of a pinpoint, 1/250 inch in a diameter, and there are about a half million eggs in a girl's ovaries when she is born. At most, only about 500 of these eggs will ripen and be released during her lifetime.

Sperm cells are smaller than egg cells—about 1/32 the size of an egg cell (or 1/8,000 inch in diameter). They are also much more plentiful; an average ejaculation contains about 400 million sperm cells. During ejaculation, sperm cells travel from the testicles, where they develop, through two ducts (vasa deferentia) and the seminal vesicles, pouches where they are temporarily stored. At the prostate gland they enter the uretha, through which they are propelled with great force into the partner's vagina. The life span of a sperm cell—unless it fertilizes an egg—is at most about 48 to 72 hours. Many of the sperm cells do not survive the acidic environment of the vagina. Those that do quickly migrate to the cervix, the neck of the uterus, where secretions are more alkaline and thus more hospitable. Once through the cervix and into the uterus, many are diverted to the wrong oviduct or get lost in a wrinkle. Those that enter the tube that harbors the traveling egg face one more obstacle: The egg is surrounded by a tough skin tissue, or membrane. However, each sperm cell that touches the egg cell deposits a small amount of an enzyme that breaks down this tough membrane, causing parts of it to dissolve. The first sperm cell that bumps into a bare spot on the egg cell can swim into the cell to merge with the nucleus, and *fertilization* occurs. The

Genetic code
The message in genetic material. The chemically active ingredient in the chromosomes is DNA (deoxyribonucleic acid), a very complex molecule structured like a coiled ladder. Hereditary specifications are thought to be coded in DNA's structure.

Embryo
The developing cluster of cells from the end of the first week to the end of the eighth week following conception.

Trimester
One of the 13-week periods of pregnancy.

Fetus
The name given to the embryo from the end of the eighth week after conception to the moment of birth.

---

sperm's tail (its means of locomotion) gets stuck in the outer membrane and drops off, leaving the sperm head inside the egg. No more sperm can enter the egg, possibly because once it has been fertilized, it releases a chemical that makes it impregnable.

The ovum (egg) carries the hereditary characteristics of the mother and her ancestors; sperm cells carry the hereditary characteristics of the father. Together they contain what can be called the *genetic code*. The parent cells (the egg and the sperm cell) each contain 23 chromosomes, each of which in turn contains at least 1,000 genes, so small that they cannot be seen through a microscope. These genes are packages of chemical instructions for the design of every part of a new baby. They specify that the infant will be human, what its sex will be, whether it will tend to be (depending also on its environment) short, tall, thin or fat, healthy or sickly, and how intelligent it will be.

About 30 hours after the egg is fertilized, the cell inside the membrane reproduces itself by dividing in half, both cells then dividing again about 10 hours later. This process repeats many times, the cells growing smaller with each division. They are held together by a clear membrane and resemble the facets of a mulberry. This floating cluster continues to move through the oviduct. By the time it reaches the uterus (three to four days), it has multiplied to about 36 cells. It attaches itself to the lining of the uterus and remains attached until birth. One week after conception the cells number over 100, and the cluster becomes an *embryo*.

Fetal Development

The period of fetal development is usually divided into three periods of 13 weeks each, called *trimesters*.

First Trimester   During the first trimester the embryo develops into a *fetus* about 4 inches long and weighing 1 ounce. All its parts are developed; its sexual organs are well formed and it has a whole range of nerve and muscle responses. In fact, the timetable for the formation

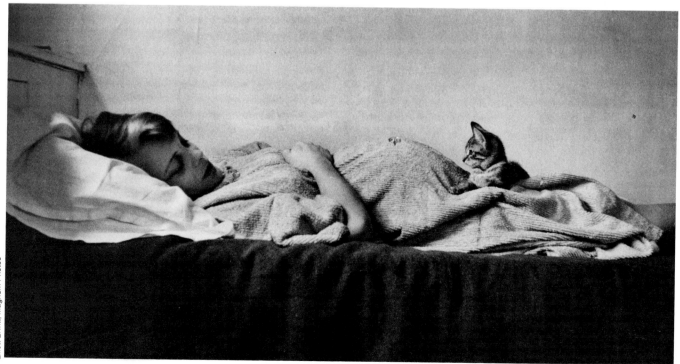

Conception
The formation of a zygote (fertilized egg), the cell resulting from the fusion of ovum and sperm and, in normal conditions, capable of survival and maturation.

Endometrium
The mucus membrane that lines the cavity of the uterus.

Placenta
The organ connected to the fetus by the umbilical cord and attached to the wall of the uterus. The placenta is the organ through which the fetus receives nourishment and empties waste into the circulatory system of the mother. Following birth, the placenta is expelled.

Amniotic sac
The bag of watery fluid that lines the uterus and envelops and protects the fetus.

Specialized cells
Cells have particular and special functions to perform, such as blood cells, bone cells, or muscle cells.

Umbilical cord
The cord that connects the fetus with the placenta.

---

of the body is so consistent that at any time during the first 48 days of life an embryologist can look at an embryo and tell its exact age from its body formation.

First Month As the cluster of cells drifts down the oviduct after *conception,* some cells divide faster than others, and several different kinds of cells emerge. The entire genetic code is passed to every cell, but new cells do not follow the entire instruction or there would be no different organs or parts of the body. For example, all cells carry genes for hair color and eye color, but only the cells of the hair follicles and irises respond to that information.

On about the fourth day of its journey the cluster arrives in the uterus; there are at that time about 36 cells. The cluster becomes hollow at its center; in this form it is called a blastocyst.

The outermost shell of cells eventually becomes the placenta, umbilical cord, and amniotic sac. The inner cells separate into three layers. One layer becomes inner body parts, the digestive and respiratory systems; another layer becomes the skin, hair, and nervous tissue; and the middle layer becomes muscle, bone, marrow, blood, kidneys, and sex glands.

On the sixth or seventh day the blastocyst implants itself in the lining of the uterus, usually along the upper curvature. The cells begin to draw nourishment from the *endometrium* (the uterine lining). A network of roots called chorionic villi sprouts from the blastocyst, tapping the small blood vessels in the endometrium and firmly planting the cell cluster. These villi, and a membrane called the chorion, eventually form the *placenta,* the outermost membrane that surrounds the embryo. The villi remain, drawing nourishment from the mother's blood through a thick, spongy layer, into the embryo's blood. Waste products are removed through the same route.

Inside the placenta is the *amniotic sac,* or bag of waters. The embryo floats in this, cushioned against physical injury and insulated against temperature change.

By the third week the embryo is 1/10 inch long, and the brain has two lobes. Young blood cells, the first *specialized cells,* appear by the seventeenth day. Soon afterward, blood vessels begin to form, and blood flows through them. By the fourth week the embryo is almost

1/2 inch long, is about one-third head, and has a trunk and visible arm buds. The nervous system appears as a hollow tube by the twenty-fourth day, the same day the tubular heart begins to beat, slowly and regularly at first. After a few days of practice it pumps 65 times a minute to circulate newly formed blood.

By the end of the first month the embryo also has simple kidneys, a liver, and a digestive tract, and there is a primitive umbilical cord. The embryo is 10,000 times as large as the fertilized egg was and is a finely structured although incomplete body. See Figure 7–1 and Figure 7–2(a).

Second Month During the second month the embryo becomes a well-proportioned, small-scale baby. In the fifth week the arm buds subdivide into hand, arm, and shoulder. By the sixth week the eyes appear as black circles; they are partly closed. The internal hearing apparatus is nearly complete, and the outer ear is starting to form. The nose is fully formed with two separated air passages. The embryo has a reptilelike head and tail and complete skeleton of cartilage. See Figure 7–2 (b).

By the seventh week the embryo has a human face with eyes, ears, nose, lips, tongue, and even milk-teeth buds in the gums. The body is nicely rounded, padded with muscles and covered by a thin skin. The arms have hands with fingers and thumbs already budding. The legs, which develop more slowly than the arms until after two years, have recognizable knees, ankles and toes. The tail has begun to be absorbed, and bone has begun to replace cartilage in the skeleton.

In the eighth week the embryo is about 1¼ inches long and weighs 1/30 ounce. Almost all internal organs have begun to develop. The brain sends out impulses that coordinate the functioning of the other organs. The heart beats steadily, and blood circulates. The stomach produces some digestive juices. Blood cells are manufactured by the liver. The kidneys extract some uric acid from the blood. The *umbilical cord* joins the circulatory system of the embryo to the placenta, where nutrients and wastes are exchanged with the mother's circulatory system. Oxygen comes to the embryo through the mother's lungs, and waste from the embryo goes out through the mother's kidneys.

The embryo now has a complete body. It has become

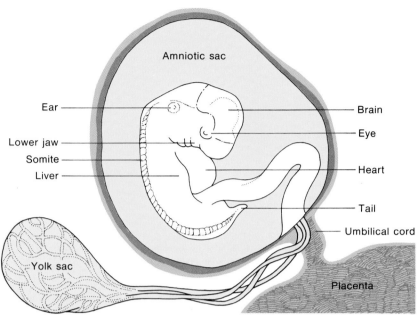

Figure 7-1 The early embryo (about 28 days) in the amniotic sac. At this stage the yolk sac aids in nourishing the embryo, but later it degenerates as the placenta takes on the nourishment function.

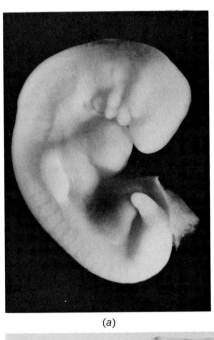
(a)

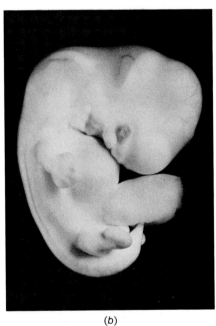
(b)

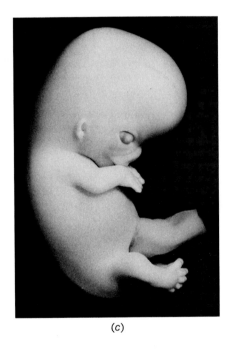
(c)

Figure 7-2 Stages in fetal development: (a) about 4 weeks; (b) about 6 weeks; (c) about 9 weeks; (d) 24 to 26 weeks.

(d)

Sucking reflex
Involuntary sucking behavior of a fetus exhibited before and after birth.

Viral infection
An infection caused by a virus.

Congenital malformation
A physical defect existing at the time of birth, either inherited or caused during gestation.

a fetus, and all further changes in the body will be in size and refinement of working parts. See Figure 7–2(c).

Third Month   The fetus, now 3 inches long and weighing 1 ounce, begins to be quite active. By the end of the month it can kick its legs, turn its feet, and curl and fan its toes, make a fist, move its thumb, bend its wrist, turn its head, squint, frown, open its mouth, and press its lips tightly together.

The twelfth week brings a whole new range of reponses. The thumb can move in opposition to the fingers. The *sucking reflex* begins to appear. The fetus swallows and may even breathe. It does not drown because its oxygen supply still comes through the umbilical cord. The eyes are sensitive to light, although they have closed now and will stay closed until the sixth month. The fetus hears the mother's heartbeat and voice, as well as outside noises.

Internal organs have begun to function. The halves of the roof of the mouth fuse, making it possible to eat and breathe at the same time. Taste buds and salivary glands appear. Amniotic fluid that is swallowed is digested in the stomach. Bile is produced in the liver, and sterile drops are urinated, to be carried away in the regular exchange and freshening of the amniotic waters.

Around the eighth or ninth week, female and male embryos have the same sex gland and the same genital—a vertical slit with a swelling on either side and a small rounded bud at the top of the slit. In the female the bud becomes the clitoris, and the swellings become the labia. In the male the bud grows into a penis. The slit closes underneath around the urethra, and the swellings fuse into the scrotum. The testicles descend from the abdomen into the scrotum at about the seventh month. During this time the internal reproductive organs become well formed and already contain some egg or sperm cells.

In the first trimester the fetus is extremely vulnerable to *viral infections* and radiation. Either can cause malformations. The most susceptible parts of the body are the parts growing most rapidly at the time. German measles, for example, can easily cause a *congenital malformation* of a delicate system such as the eyes or ears. Another danger is fever in the mother, which could cause premature labor.

Second Trimester   During the second trimester the fetus grows to about 14 inches and 2 pounds. The body grows faster than the head. The skin on the hands and feet forms distinctive patterns, which are different in each individual.

Fourth Month   In this month the fetus grows to half its height at birth (an increase of about 6 inches to a height of 10 inches) and increases its weight to 6 ounces. To achieve this growth the fetus must have large amounts of food, oxygen, and water, which come from the mother through the placenta. (See Figure 7–3.) The placental system is so efficient that within an hour or two the fetus receives any substance entering the mother's bloodstream, including not only nutrients but also all drugs.

Fifth Month   The fetus grows to be 1 foot long and weighs 1 pound. Much of the skeleton hardens; hard nails form first on fingers and then on toes. Girls and boys both develop nipples and mammary glands with milk ducts. The skin is now covered by a cheesy wax made up of cells and secretions from the sebaceous and sweat glands.

The heartbeat may be loud enough to be heard with a stethoscope. The digestive organs are formed, but they are not ready to take in food. Muscles are much stronger, and the fetus begins definite kicking and turning. It can move freely within the amniotic sac, surrounded by a quart of fluid that is changed at the rate of 6 gallons per day. The fetus may suck its thumb. It can be startled by noises.

Sixth Month   The fetus grows to 14 inches and 2 pounds. It grows eyelashes and can open or close eyelids. Most important, it can breathe regularly for 24 hours if it is born prematurely, which means that it may be able to survive premature birth. See Figure 7-2(d).

Third Trimester In the last three months, the third trimester, the fetus grows to 20 inches and gains most of its birth weight: about 1 pound in the seventh month and 2 pounds in each of the eighth and nine months. Some of this weight is fatty tissue under the skin that serves as insulation and food supply and gives the baby its characteristic chubbiness. The baby may be too fat, however, if the mother overeats during this time.

The fetus must obtain large amounts of calcium, iron, and nitrogen from the food the mother eats. Some 85 percent of the calcium and iron she consumes goes into the fetal bloodstream.

Although the fetus is able to live if it is born during the seventh month, it needs the fat layer acquired in the eighth month and time for the organs, especially the respiratory and digestive organs, to develop. It also needs the immunities the mother supplies in the last three months. Her blood provides protection to the fetus against all the diseases to which she has acquired immunity. These immunities wear off within six months after birth, but they can be replenished by the mother's milk if the baby is breast-fed.

Changes in the Mother's Body During Pregnancy

During the first trimester the mother's uterus enlarges about three times the size it was when she was not pregnant, but it still cannot be felt in the abdomen. The mother experiences relatively few bodily changes. Most symptoms are fairly common.

The second trimester is generally the most peaceful time of pregnancy, with the fewest complications. If the mother experienced nausea and morning sickness, these

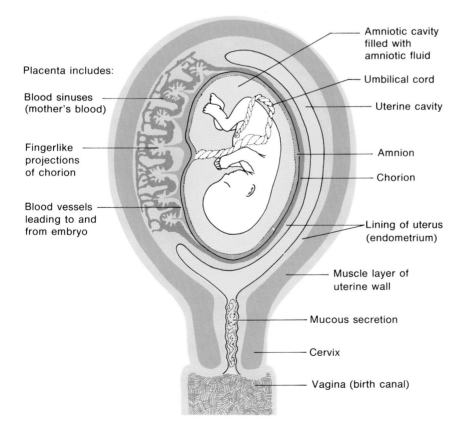

Placenta includes:

Blood sinuses (mother's blood)

Fingerlike projections of chorion

Blood vessels leading to and from embryo

Amniotic cavity filled with amniotic fluid

Umbilical cord

Uterine cavity

Amnion

Chorion

Lining of uterus (endometrium)

Muscle layer of uterine wall

Mucous secretion

Cervix

Vagina (birth canal)

Figure 7-3 A cross section of the uterus in pregnancy.

Amenorrhea
The absence or abnormal stoppage of
menstrual periods.

Hormones
Chemical substances secreted into the
body fluids by the endocrine glands.

---

begin to subside, and she gains weight. Some women report feeling unusually healthy and energetic and having a sense of well-being. Some feel prettier. These feelings are governed by the physical changes as well as the mother's feelings toward having a child.

The third trimester is the hardest for the mother. She must breathe, digest, excrete, and circulate blood for two people. The weight of the fetus, its pressure on her own body organs, and its increased demands on her own system cause discomfort and fatigue. As a result, the mother may become increasingly lethargic both physically and emotionally. During the last weeks fears for the safety and well-being of herself and her child sometimes appear and she may worry that the child will be abnormal.

The Signs and Symptoms of Pregnancy   Early recognition of pregnancy is very important. The pregnancy symptoms described here are not absolute indications of pregnancy as such. Other, far more reliable methods of determining pregnancy are available through the medical professionals. It is best for a woman to visit a gynecologist after missing two menstrual periods.

Amenorrhea   If the uterine lining is retained, then, of course, no menstrual period occurs. This condition, called *amenorrhea,* is one of the first signals of pregnancy.

Slight Bleeding   During early pregnancy, some women bleed lightly, but this is nothing to worry about. It is caused by the implanting of the fertilized egg in the uterine wall; because it happens at about the time of a normally expected period, it is sometimes mistaken for a menstrual flow. The bleeding usually lasts only a few days.

Nausea   One of the first noticeable symptoms of pregnancy is nausea, although about one-third of the women who become pregnant never experience it. It occurs in most women in the morning, which is the reason it is called "morning sickness." Nausea is probably a reaction to greater amounts of progesterone and related *hormones* that are produced during pregnancy. Nausea usually disappears of its own accord by the twelfth week.

Sleepiness, Fatigue, and Increased Frequency of Urination   Sleepiness and fatigue also result from hormonal changes. The pressure of the expanding uterus against the bladder causes the need to urinate more often. After the twelfth week the uterus rises higher in the abdomen, away from the bladder, and the rate of urination returns to normal. In the third trimester urination again becomes more frequent.

Dietary Cravings   About the third month some women crave strange foods or other substances, including coal, chalk, laundry starch, and highly flavored foods and fruits. The sense of taste is dulled during pregnancy, which may account for the desire for salted and spiced foods. Only women who have nutritional deficiencies seem to suffer from these unusual cravings, and no harm comes from *not* giving in to them.

General Weepiness   Women are likely to experience rapid and unpredictable emotional changes when there are major variations in their hormone levels—at puberty, menopause, during the premenstrual phase of each cycle, and most of all during pregnancy and immediately after birth. Many women during the first trimester have mixed feelings toward the fetus. Even a mother who has planned the pregnancy and wants the child may be delighted one moment and upset the next.

Need for Affection and Support   So much of the pregnancy experience is beyond the mother's total control—her energy level, her changing appearance, her variable emotions—that she must absorb and adjust to many new feelings and ideas. She usually needs extra encouragement, moral support, and especially affection during pregnancy.

Change in Sexual Activity   Sexual activity often changes in quantity and style during pregnancy. Varying levels of circulating hormones affect the mother's libido. Some women report less interest in sexual intercourse. Others experience increased interest, especially during the fourth to sixth month when the pelvic area is newly swollen and sensitive but not so large as to make close physical contact awkward.

Both responses are common and are influenced by

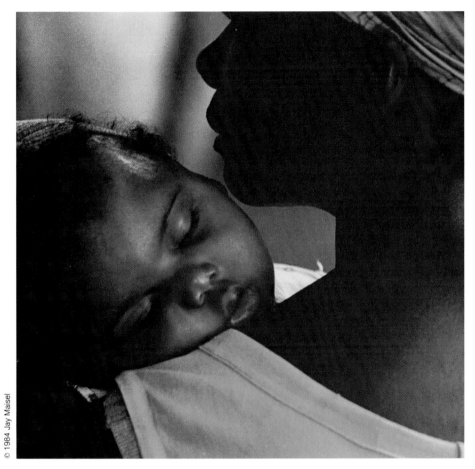

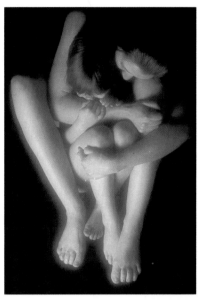

161

Metabolism
The processes by which the body uses food.

Corpus luteum
A gland in the ovary that forms after ovulation; secretes progesterone. If the ovum is not fertilized, the corpus luteum degenerates.

Cervix
The neck of the uterus, that is, the lower and narrow end, which opens into the vagina.

Colostrum
The thin milky fluid secreted by the mammary glands around the time of childbirth until milk comes in, about the third day.

---

both partners' attitudes toward sexuality during pregnancy. If an overprotective partner fears that intercourse is harmful, the woman may infer that he does not find her attractive. If he is insensitive to her fears or shows hesitance or lack of interest in intercourse, she may feel he does not consider her feelings important. Communicating freely with each other and even with a counselor can help. Late in pregnancy intercourse becomes physically awkward, but new positions can be tried to the satisfaction of both people.

Changes That Continue Throughout Pregnancy The mother's body continually prepares the way for the fetus. The ribs flare out long before the uterus needs the room to expand. The uterus and the amniotic sac expand long before the fetus needs room. The *metabolism* of the mother becomes more efficient than usual, providing a positive nutritional balance for both mother and fetus. The following specific changes occur in the mother's body during pregnancy.

Bone and Muscle Structure Beginning early in pregnancy, the muscles and ligaments attached to bones such as the pelvis begin to soften and stretch. The joints between the pelvic bones, which are normally solid, loosen and spread, and become movable by the tenth to twelfth week. This change is possibly caused by the hormone relaxin, which is produced by the *corpus luteum*. It makes having a baby easier, walking more difficult.

Reproductive Organs By the sixth week the *cervix* softens and turns a bluish color. During the first three months the uterus enlarges to three times its nonpregnant size. By the fourth month the uterus becomes large enough to make the abdomen protrude. By the seventh or eighth month the uterus pushes up into the rib cage, which makes breathing slightly more difficult. The breasts enlarge and are sensitive by the eighth week, and they may tingle or throb. The pigmented area around the nipple, the areola, darkens and becomes broader. After the tenth week *colostrum*, a thin milky fluid, may be squeezed from the mother's nipples, but actual secretion of milk is prevented by high levels of estrogen and progesterone.

Circulatory System During pregnancy the mother's blood takes up more oxygen in the lungs, and nutrients are held longer in the bloodstream. Both oxygen and nutrition can then be more readily given to the fetus through the placenta. The increased efficiency of the mother's circulatory system results from about a 50 percent increase in blood plasma and an 18 percent increase in blood cells. Heart output increases by midpregnancy from 9 pints to 12 pints per minute. Circulation is also more rapid. Most of the increased blood flow goes to the uterus and placenta and to the kidneys.

Lungs Because the mother needs more oxygen during pregnancy, she takes in up to 40 percent more air. It is not faster breathing but the widening of her rib cage that permits the greater intake.

Kidneys During pregnancy kidneys must become highly efficient. Waste products from fetal circulation are passed into the mother's bloodstream through the placenta and then are removed by her kidneys. Hormonal changes cause a pregnant woman to retain more water, and by midpregnancy the kidneys can produce prodigious amounts of urine. In late pregnancy, however, this capacity drops below normal level.

Skin When skin is stretched, as it is in pregnancy or sometimes even with moderate weight gain, small breaks occur in the elastic fibers of the lower layer of skin, which does not stretch well. The result is "stretch marks," narrow, linear streaks.

Increased production of hormones causes the skin to darken in 90 percent of pregnant women. The darkening is especially noticeable in places that have stretched, as well as in the nipples, the vulva, moles and scars, and in the *linea nigra*, a dark line that develops during pregnancy and runs from the pubic bone up to above the navel. Ultraviolet radiation also stimulates pigment production, and women who do not want their skin to darken should avoid exposure to sunlight.

Figure 7–4 indicates some of the physiological changes that occur during pregnancy.

Changes and Complications in the Later Stages of Pregnancy By the sixth month the increased needs of the fetus for oxygen, nutrition, and excretion increase the burden on the mother's lungs, heart, and kidneys. Her legs swell, and the activity of the fetus sometimes makes it hard for her to sleep. To maintain her balance while she is standing, she must throw her shoulders well back.

Figure 7–5 shows the position of the fetus and uterus at the seventh or eighth month of pregnancy.

Heartburn, constipation, and occasionally nausea occur, especially in the late months of pregnancy. These conditions make the mother feel as if her body is not functioning well. In spite of her impression, there is a strong possibility that both digestion and metabolism are unusually efficient.

The amount of water in the body increases. Even women who have no abnormal swelling retain up to 3 quarts of liquid. Some women also gain weight, with swelling in the face, hands, ankles, or feet resulting from increased absorption through the kidneys of water, sodium, and chlorides. This type of fluid retention causes a ring to be too tight for the finger.

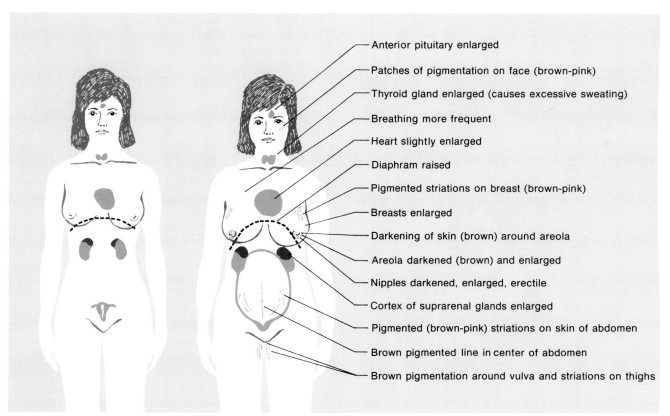

Figure 7-4 Physiological changes during pregnancy: (*left*) the female body at the time of conception; (*right*) development after 30 weeks of pregnancy.

Toxemia of pregnancy
A series of metabolic disturbances characterized at first by a rise in blood pressure, excess albumin in the urine, and fluid retention. More severe symptoms follow in the second stage and without appropriate medical attention cause death.

Diuretic
An agent that promotes the excretion of urine.

Lightening
A labor process in which the uterus sinks downward about 2 inches because the baby's presenting part settles far down into the pelvic area.

False labor
Rather intense and painful contractions of the uterus that do not actually thin the cervix or make obvious progress toward delivery.

Labor
The act or process of giving birth to a child, expelling it with the placenta from the mother's body by means of uterine contractions.

Contraction (uterine)
A shortening of the uterus that reduces its size and eventually forces expulsion of the fetus.

Toxemia of Pregnancy Sometimes swelling can be a symptom of *toxemia of pregnancy,* a potentially dangerous series of metabolic disturbances that occurs in three stages. In the first stage, blood pressure goes up, there is too much protein in the urine, and the face and extremities swell. In the second stage, vision is blurred, and there are continual headaches. The third stage can bring convulsions and coma. Because of this danger, it is critically important that any woman who notices swelling go immediately to a doctor. Malnutrition is strongly suspected of being a major factor in toxemia of pregnancy, and diet is absolutely crucial in controlling it. Salty foods and other sources of sodium are forbidden. Bed rest often helps, and *diuretics,* drugs to increase the flow of urine, are sometimes prescribed. Some nutritionists and obstetricians believe, however, that diuretics cause complications. Symptoms of toxemia usually appear after the twenty-fourth week.

Lightening In the ninth month the baby settles far down into the pelvic bones, its head (the part that will usually be born first) fitting snugly. This process is called

lightening, and it allows the uterus to sink downward about two inches and the abdomen to fall. Pelvic pressure is increased and pressure on the diaphragm reduced. Breathing becomes easier at the same time that the frequency of urination increases.

False Labor Throughout pregnancy the uterus practices contracting, and as the delivery date nears the contractions become more vigorous. Sometimes they are painful enough to be mistaken for true *labor* pains. They are usually irregular and short and stop within a few hours, however.

The Importance of Early Prenatal Care

While a baby's brain, bones, lungs, and eyes are forming, they are extremely vulnerable. If they don't receive exactly the right kind of building blocks through mother's diet, or if they receive harmful drugs, even drugs that normally are not harmful to adults (those found in some cough syrups and cold remedies, for example), the child's body system may be impaired for life. Special attention to the mother's health and diet during pregnancy is one of the best investments a person can make, since she reaps the benefits for the rest of her and her child's life.

Early advice from midwives, obstetricians, and teachers of childbirth and baby care can be invaluable. These professionals offer nutritional and physical fitness guidance and suggest which household medicines can be harmful. They usually have the latest information concerning the effects of smoking and alcohol and caffeine on the baby. Obstetricians can test for Rh incompatibilities, maternal infections harmful to the baby such as rubella (German measles), herpes, toxoplasmosis, syphilis, and gonorrhea. They can detect early signs of problems with the mother's health resulting from pregnancy, including toxemia and infections. Professional prenatal care lessens the chances of poor maternal health during pregnancy and increases the chances of a healthy baby born well.

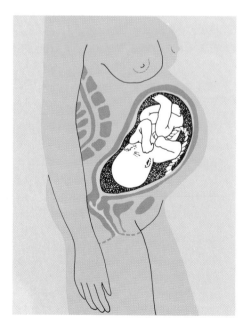

Figure 7-5   Position of the uterus and fetus after 32 weeks of pregnancy.

Rh Negative Blood

Women with Rh negative blood can build up an immunity to Rh positive blood. If such a woman bears a child who has Rh positive blood and the Rh positive blood enters her bloodstream during the delivery, the natural defense mechanism of her body produces antibodies in response. The Rh positive blood is a foreign substance, and the antibodies act to neutralize it exactly as if it were harmful bacteria. Such anti-bodies increase with each succeeding pregnancy, and they attack the blood of the fetus in subsequent pregnancies. The blood corpuscles of the fetus are destroyed, and the baby is born with various degrees of anemia and jaundice. If the child's life is to be saved, its blood must be exchanged. This change of blood used to be done after the child was born, but it is now possible to give the fetus transfusions.

An even more recent scientific advance is a vaccine that prevents antibodies from forming in some women. It must be administered within 72 hours (the sooner the better) of childbirth, miscarriage, or abortion, but it is beneficial only to those Rh negative women who show no evidence of having already formed antibodies.

Exercise and Work During Pregnancy

Physical activity is particularly valuable during pregnancy. The prospective mother should continue all reasonable exercising that she is accustomed to—tennis, swimming, golf, gardening, dancing—until her stomach inhibits movement. The amniotic sac protects the fetus so that normal activities will not harm it. Later in pregnancy, walking is probably the best exercise. More strenuous activities that could result in a fall—skiing or skating, for example—are best delayed till after birthing.

Exercising particular parts of the body such as the abdomen, back, and legs is helpful in increasing muscle tone. Classes in childbirth preparation often include exercises for the parts of the body involved in birth. Toned up muscles aid delivery and help the body readjust to its normal shape after birth.

Working often helps keep a prospective mother's mind off the symptoms and anxieties of pregnancy. Many women whose jobs are not too physically demanding work through their seventh or eighth month of pregnancy.

Labor and Delivery

Just before birth the uterus is stretched to its limits. The baby's head is about 4¼ inches in diameter, a tight fit for the opening in the pelvic bones through which it must pass. The baby's skull does have some "give" between its five separated bone plates, however.

Birth is never easy for the baby, and it may last many hours. Average duration of birth is 14 hours for a first baby, 8 hours for following ones. (See Figure 7–6.)

No one knows exactly what triggers birth, but the placenta and the muscles of the uterus seem to play a part. The uterus is the largest human muscle, and its size increases 50 to 60 times during pregnancy. Muscle fibers in the upper portion can contract and then relax to a shorter length than they were originally without a change in tension. The uterus becomes gradually smaller so that it can continue to supply the force necessary for completion of delivery. *Contraction* of the uterus also closes off each channel of blood flow during and after the third stage of labor, the expulsion of the placenta.

While the upper portion of the uterus thickens during labor, the lower portion—the cervix—must enlarge so that the baby's head can pass through. It thins out and lengthens, a process that is the result of labor contractions. Contractions are hard work (hence, "labor") for the mother. Each contraction normally supplies a 55-pound push against the baby, and "birthing" the baby's head requires a 100-pound push.

Contractions vary in intensity. They are slight to begin with, but as they travel downward from the top of the uterus, they become more intense. Over a cup of blood is expelled from the uterus under tremendous pressure. The mother feels pain—not from the contraction but from the grinding pressure of the baby's presenting part against the cervix and the pelvic structures. At their very worst, contractions cause an extremely intense grinding type of pain, lasting about 50 seconds to a minute at the most. This pain is considered an integral part of giving birth, signaling that all is well. However, the pain can be heightened needlessly by tensing and attempting to block it.

When birth is about to occur, the uterus repeatedly narrows, causing the baby's body to straighten so that its head or pressing part is pressed against the cervix.

First Stage of Labor   The first stage of labor lasts an average of 13 hours for the first birth, and at the end the cervix is fully dilated, opened to about four inches.

The uterus and vagina together form a curved passage along which the baby can pass, helped along by uterine contractions and additional pushes of the mother's abdominal muscles. At this point the head is usually midway down the mother's pelvis, and she is ready to go to the hospital. See Figure 7–6 (b).

During the first stage of labor the contractions usually

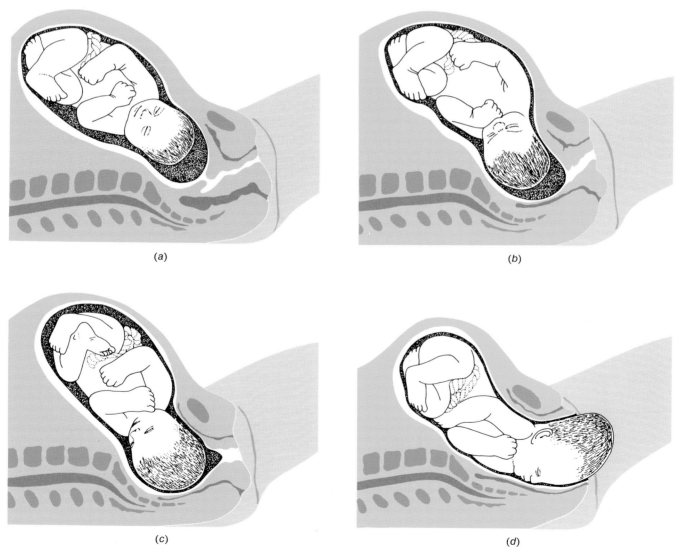

(a)   (b)

(c)   (d)

Figure 7-6   The birth process: (a) full-term fetus before labor begins; (b) early stages of labor; cervix begins to dilate; (c) second stage of labor; cervix completely dilated; baby's head begins turning toward mother's back; (d) late stage of labor; baby's head is completely turned; head begins to emerge.

Caesarean section
A surgical incision through the abdominal walls and uterus; performed to extract a fetus.

Episiotomy
A surgical incision in the vulva to widen the birth canal.

General anesthetic
An agent that usually produces unconsciousness to relieve pain.

last 25 to 35 seconds and come every 15 to 20 minutes at first, more often later. The mucous plug, which has closed off the cervical canal during the months of pregnancy, keeping out infection, is expelled. Its expulsion is a sure sign that labor has begun.

For first births, the obstetrician should be notified when pains occur about every 6 minutes and last for 30 seconds. The woman who is in labor should not eat or drink anything because food stays undigested in the stomach.

In about 20 percent of women the amniotic sac ruptures from the pressure of a contraction, and the fluid rushes or trickles out. This action speeds up labor, and usually indicates that the second stage is about to begin. If the sac has not ruptured by the time the cervix has dilated about 2 inches, the doctor will probably rupture it, improving the effectiveness of contractions and shortening labor.

Second Stage of Labor   The second stage of labor begins when the cervix is completely dilated and the baby's head is in the birth canal [Figure 7–6 (c)]; it ends with delivery of the baby. It lasts from about 30 minutes to 2 hours for a first baby and from 10 to 30 minutes in subsequent deliveries. If the mother is unable to supply the 100 pounds of force needed to birth the head, the doctor must help with forceps or deliver the baby by *Caesarean section,* a procedure that involves cutting the abdomen and uterus open and removing the baby by hand. In some deliveries, the position of the baby or the narrowness of the mother's pelvic opening makes a Caesarean necessary.

When the head appears, it stretches the tissue between the vagina and the rectum, called the perineum, and the tissue may tear. To avoid a jagged tear, the doctor often cuts the tissues into the margin of the vagina with scissors. The operation, called *episiotomy,* is usually done under local anesthesia.

Use of Anesthetics During Labor   Of the many controversies surrounding childbirth, the one over the use of anesthetics during labor is probably the most intense. Many advocates of natural childbirth claim that drugs given to the mother during childbirth are always harmful in some degree to the baby and are sometimes harmful to the mother. Because of differences in their body weights, the baby gets about 20 times the mother's dosage. In general, the more awake, alert, active, and vigorous the mother and baby are during birth, the more safely and competently they complete their task, and the more the experience tends to be joyful instead of horrifying. *General anesthesia* is not widely favored because it deprives the mother of all consciousness of the experience of birth. Such anesthetics also depress the mother's physiological functioning and permit less oxygen to reach the baby. The baby's respiratory functions can be depressed so much that it may have trouble taking its first breaths.

Many doctors believe that a woman who understands the mechanics of labor and is well prepared for the experience will need only minor amounts of pain-relieving drugs or possibly none at all (see the section on prepared childbirth, page 169).

Birth   A final push "crowns" the baby's head (pushes the widest part into the vulva). The doctor then assists in delivering the baby, telling the mother when to push and when to pant or breathe quietly as the baby slowly and gently emerges. The baby's head appears, face toward the mother's back usually, and the doctor helps rotate it to one side to avoid tearing the soft tissues of the vulva. (See Figure 7–6 (d).) As soon as the head is delivered, the doctor feels for a loop of umbilical cord around the neck, and if there is one he either disentangles it or cuts it if it cannot be disentangled. After the shoulder can be seen, the doctor waits about 30 seconds to give the uterus time to retract and get smaller. Another half-minute is allowed after the shoulder is delivered before the rest of the body is slowly pulled out by the shoulders. The cord is then stripped of blood toward the infant several times, adding about two and one-half ounces of blood to the baby's bloodstream. After the crowning of the head, birth is completed in two to three minutes. (See Figure 7–7.)

The cord is tied and cut. Nature seals it with a jellylike substance that swells up on exposure to air and squeezes the embedded blood vessels shut. The buildup of carbon dioxide in the baby's blood that results stimulates the respiratory center of the brain, and the baby takes its first breath and cries.

Suzanne Arms, © 1978 Jeroboam, Inc.

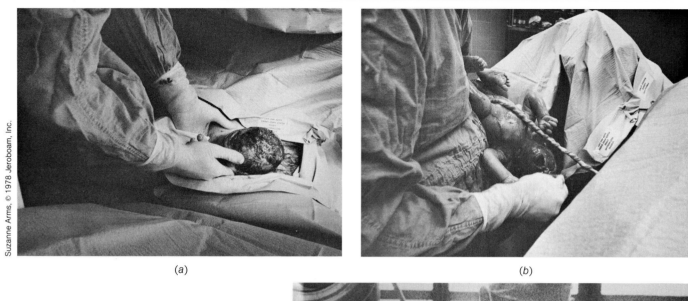

(a)   (b)

Figure 7-7 The sequence of birth after the baby's head emerges: (a) assistance from the doctor; (b) the newly born infant; (c) the mother's first sight of her baby.

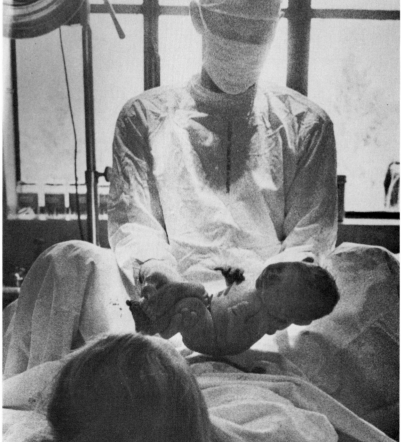

Eve Arnold, Magnum Photos

(c)

Gonorrheal infection
A sexually transmitted infection caused by a bacterium.

Natural childbirth
Childbirth without the use of painkillers for the mother or tools such as forceps to deliver the baby.

Lamaze method
A method of natural childbirth in which the father participates by helping the mother to relax and by providing moral support.

Psychoprophylaxis method
A method of childbirth that emphasizes relaxation by conditioning reflexes with self-induced signals during uterine contractions.

Puerperium
The period of about six to eight weeks after labor during which the mother's reproductive organs, particularly the uterus, return to the nonpregnant state.

The first breath requires five times as much effort as an ordinary breath because thousands of tiny uninflated air sacs of the lungs must be expanded—like blowing up thousands of little balloons. Breathing is irregular for the first couple of days; it takes that long for the air passages to clear of mucus. The early cries help to clear out obstructing fluids. Those cries may be a reflex response, or they may be an expression of the baby's discomfort.

The baby has much to cry about. He—or she—has just been forced through an incredibly narrow tunnel. He has lost the world that sustained him for his entire life, a world in which he had been suspended weightlessly in a warm, living, pulsating sea, and in which all sounds were muffled and the light if any, was dim. The light is blinding. Every sound is sharp and terrifyingly loud. It is cold (20° F colder than in the uterus). Gravity pins him down. There is a sudden frightening freedom of movement, and those reassuring walls he has been tapping against for the last five months have disappeared.

For the first time ever he is in contact with matter that is not alive. He is put on a table, wiped off, examined, wrapped in cloth, put in a box, and left in a sterile room. If the baby is a boy, then perhaps no more than two hours later he may be strapped to a tray and circumcised.

In the course of the examination, the doctor weighs and measures the baby, and checks its heart rate, breathing, muscle tone, reflex irritability, skin, lungs, eyes, nose, palate, abdomen, and rectum. Its eyes are routinely treated with silver nitrate solution to prevent any possibility of *gonorrheal infection,* and vitamin K is injected to regulate blood-clotting time.

Third Stage of Labor   After the birth, continuing uterine contractions separate the placenta from the uterus and force it downward into the cervix and the vagina. Usually the doctor assists by applying pressure on the abdomen just above the pubic bone, gently pulling on the cut cord at the same time. Expulsion of the placenta ordinarily takes less than five minutes.

The episiotomy is sewn up, and the uterus is massaged as it becomes smaller. The mother relaxes and sleeps in the delivery room for about an hour after delivery and then returns to the lying-in ward.

Prepared Childbirth   In the 1920s Grantly Dick-Read, an English doctor, noticed that women in so-called primitive societies have a much less difficult time in childbirth than woman in highly civilized, technological societies. He concluded that fear, especially fear of the unknown, was responsible for much of the pain women in the latter group suffered. The more the woman tensed up to avoid or block the pain, the more unbearable the pain was, and the more she obstructed the natural process of birth. To make childbirth easier for his patients, Dick-Read devised a system of childbirth training called *natural childbirth,* which he described in the book *Childbirth Without Fear* (4th ed., 1972). Several methods of childbirth training are in use now, all designed to improve the mother's chances of an easier birth through knowledge, exercise, or a combination of the two. Two well-known methods are the Lamaze method and psychoprophylaxis.

The Lamaze Method   The *Lamaze method* as practiced in the United States emphasizes not so much how the mother performs, but rather how she thinks. A positive attitude is considered very important in childbirth. The mother is taught to regard her labor as a time of activity, work, concentration, and confidence rather than helplessness and suffering. The father, too, is encouraged to take part throughout the birth, reminding the mother to relax, massaging her, giving moral support, monitoring her breathing, and keeping her informed of her progress. It is an important time for the parents to be together.

Psychoprophylaxis   Developed in the 1940s by the Soviet scientists Pavlov and Nicoläiev, the *psychoprophylaxis* (literally a "mind-health preventive") *method* stresses relaxation by conditioning reflexes with self-induced signals during uterine contractions. The method has been popularized in the United States largely through a book by Irwin Chabon, *Awake and Aware: Participating in Childbirth Through Psychoprophylaxis* (1969).

The Puerperium

The *puerperium* is the time following childbirth during which the mother's sex organs, especially the uterus, slowly return to the nonpregnant state. This return takes

Postpartum depression
An emotional low experienced by the mother following childbirth.

Antibodies
Proteins in the blood that are generated in reaction to foreign proteins, producing immunity from them.

Lochia
A vaginal discharge occurring one or two weeks after childbirth

six to eight weeks. Most maternity patients stay three to five days in the hospital after delivery. The trend is toward shorter hospital stays, and women need not stay in bed if they do not feel fatigued.

Postpartum Depression   During the first week or so after childbirth some women are emotionally explosive. A few experience some degree of *postpartum depression,* which may be caused in large part by the great drop in hormone levels in the first days following birth. These women vacillate between highs and lows and seem to overreact. They also experience general bodily discomfort as well as discomfort from stitches and sore breasts. Frustration and boredom with the hospital stay are common reactions.

Breast Feeding and Rooming-In   After the child is born, the mother's pituitary gland releases the hormone prolactin, which stimulates the formation and secretion of milk. In most cases, the advantages of breast feeding far outweigh the disadvantages. No other food is quite so good for the child as the mother's milk. It is sterile and contains *antibodies* that help protect the child against diseases the mother has had. It is better for humans than cow's milk, parts of which are difficult for humans to digest. It has more milk sugar, more vitamins, and a better balance of minerals than cow's milk.

Breast feeding usually gives the baby a sense of security and is generally comforting to the mother as well. One study has shown that female animals experience a 50 percent reduction in stressful responses to situations when they are nursing their young. Infants are especially sensitive to their mother's emotional states, so any reduction in the mother's feelings of stress means a reduction in the infant's feelings of stress. Parents are also spared the bother of sterilizing bottles and preparing formulas. Bleeding stops sooner also, and the uterus and other tissues recover their normal state more rapidly if the mother is nursing.

On the other hand, a nursing mother is somewhat confined. She cannot leave the child for long periods of time, and if she has to return to work soon, she will probably not be able to continue breast feeding. A very few mothers do not have enough milk to feed the child. Breast size has nothing to do with the amount of milk

produced. Small breasts can produce as much milk as large ones. The nursing mother must also continue to eat as much as she did during the late pregnancy.

Breast feeding is more convenient if in the hospital the baby remains beside the mother's bed rather than in the nursery. It is generally better for both the mother and the baby if they are together during these first few days. The baby feels more secure, and the mother has a chance to develop confidence in handling the baby. Rooming-in also avoids the risk of cross infection that exists in the hospital nursery.

Uterine Shrinkage   After childbirth the uterus weighs about 2¼ pounds and can be felt as a firm, globular bulge extending up to the navel. By the end of the second week after birth, its weight shrinks to about 11 ounces, and it can no longer be felt in the abdomen. In four or five weeks, it returns to normal. For about three to six weeks there is a discharge called *lochia,* a mixture of blood from the site in the uterus where the placenta was attached and from the crumbling of the uterine lining. Exercise is helpful in restoring the abdomen to its original size, shape, and muscle tone.

Return of Menstruation   When a mother does not nurse, menstruation usually recurs within ten weeks. Breast feeding can prevent the menstrual period from returning for as long as six months. The hormone prolactin, which is involved in the production of milk, suppresses the hormones that are important to the development of the corpus luteum and mature eggs, and the ovaries produce less estrogen and progesterone. However, ovulation—and pregnancy—can occur before the return of menstruation. If the mother becomes pregnant during the nursing she should stop nursing.

Prospective Parents as Consumers in the Medical Marketplace

As consumers, prospective parents can demand satisfaction from hospitals and medical professionals or deprive them of business. Equipped with adequate information

Routine Delivery Procedures Some Parents Would Like to Change

Routine Prepping Prepping, shaving of the mother's pubic hair when she is ready to deliver, may contribute to a sterile environment for emergency surgery, but it appears unnecessary in the majority of births. Many women experience itching and discomfort while the hair is growing back and feel that routine prepping should be done away with except in cases where complications point toward possible Caesarean delivery.

Routine Enemas Enemas are given to the mother about to deliver to guarantee that the delivery bed will not be made unsterile just at the moment of birth, when she is pushing hard and cannot always control her bowels. However, an enema administered to a woman while she is in intense labor causes great physical and mental discomfort, distracting her just when she needs to concentrate hard on breathing and relaxing.

Routine Episiotomy Routine episiotomies are not necessary because the vagina can often stretch sufficiently during birth without tearing. Episiotomies are most necessary in cases in which a baby's head is so large or its birth position is such that it would tear the surrounding flesh badly. Usually an episiotomy is performed to ensure the birth of the baby as speedily as possible and to allow the quicker healing of a straight, neat incision rather than a ragged-edged tear. However, episiotomy stitches are uncomfortable, and they itch, and many women would prefer to deliver without an episiotomy unless complications indicate that it is necessary.

Routine Delivery in the Supine Position Hospital deliveries in the United States usually occur while the mother lies in a supine (on her back) position on the delivery bed. In other cultures and times women often have delivered sitting in a labor chair. Today many women in the United States also believe that an upright sitting position or a semi-sitting position is the most comfortable one for delivery and that it is the safest position, partially because it allows gravity to aid the mother in pushing out the baby.

It is inefficient to have to push a baby uphill during birth. Giving birth in the supine position stresses the respiratory and circulatory systems, both of which are already being taxed. When the woman lies supine, the uterus presses on the interior vena cava, impeding the blood supply to the uterus. This can cause both shocklike symptoms in the mother and fetal distress in the baby.

Researchers are now working to design adjustable labor beds that can double as delivery beds. Laboring and delivering in a semi-upright position would allow voluntary muscles to work with gravity to push the baby downward and outward.

Caesarean Sections Caesarean section is delivery of a child through an incision made in the abdominal wall and through the uterus. Usually the mother is given a regional anesthetic of the spinal type so that she will not experience pain and yet can be awake when the baby is delivered. Both incisions are stitched up after the baby and placenta have been removed. Caesarean sections are performed when hard labor accomplishes insufficient cervical opening or

when the mother's pelvic structure is too small to allow the baby to move through the birth canal. They are also performed if the placenta loosens and begins to prolapse, if the cord prolapses, or if excessive bleeding occurs.

The number of these operations is increasing. They should be performed to save the life of either the mother or the child, but, in fact, they are becoming more common with the increasing threat of malpractice suits. Caesarean delivery is not as safe for the mother or baby as is a normal delivery because it is a major abdominal operation and carries with it the risk that any major operation involves. But in case of complications during labor it may be the safest way to deliver the child.

All parents should consider the possibility of a Caesarean and hope they will never have to use it. The best way to avoid an unnecessary C-section is to choose a doctor carefully. Interview obstetricians to find out when and why they consider a Caesarean necessary, how many hours they consider an adequate test of labor, whether they use sonograms, amniocentesis and X rays to check a baby's progress before making a decision, and how long Caesarean patients stay in the hospital. Decide whether the doctor considers a Caesarean as primarily birth or primarily surgery. It is important to know beforehand if the doctor suspects there will be complications in the delivery, so that one can prepare psychologically for it. Unfortunately, doctors often keep that information from the parents for fear of scaring them.

Inducing Labor Inducing labor refers to a deliberate attempt to

(continued on next page)

Routine Delivery Procedures Some Parents Would Like to Change (continued)

start labor. This can be done by rupturing membranes or by using chemical substitutes for hormones present in natural labor. While it may make scheduling a birth more convenient, it presents risk to both child and mother. When induced, labor contractions are usually more painful and more intense than ordinary ones, and the intravenous oxytocin drip must be carefully and wisely monitored to avoid potentially fatal complications. Too heavy a dose can cause the uterus to rupture, maternal blood pressure to rise, and the umbilical cord to prolapse.

More important, if contractions are too intense and too frequent, as they often are during induction, the baby

registers a dangerous decrease in heart rate. It has insufficient time to recover enough oxygen between contractions, and the reduced heart rate indicates fetal distress. Consequently, fetal heart monitors are used almost routinely on women in labor. Sensors are placed on the mother's abdomen and a tape constantly records the heartbeat of the unborn infant. The continual monitoring reveals fetal distress that might not even be noticed if the mother were simply checked intermittently with a stethoscope. For women evidencing some abnormality, a more obtrusive monitor places a catheter inside the uterus (through already ruptured membranes)

alongside the fetal head and measures uterine contractions. Additionally, a small electrode is attached to the baby's scalp to record the electrocardiogram and heart rate. The intrauterine catheter can provide an entry for infection and should be used only when abnormalities are evident.

Use of both the oxytocin drip and the intrauterine catheter introduces new risks as well as possible advantages to the birth process. Some hospitals do not permit induction for convenience, but the practice of inducing labor is becoming more common nevertheless.

about the quality of obstetrical care they wish to pay for and the service they want, parents have the power to change hospital birth procedures.

Informed Decisions About Birth Procedures Parents have objected to routines performed to maintain the sterile environment necessary for surgery even though childbirth procedures do not usually require such rigor. Many doctors formerly insisted on routine enemas and prepping (shaving pubic hair) for the mother, kept the father out of the delivery room, and separated the baby from its parents immediately after birth. Some physicians routinely anesthetize the mother, induce labor, use forceps and fetal monitoring, deliver by Caesarian section, and generally manipulate the birth process for their own convenience, occasionally to the detriment of both mother and child.

All of these procedures may be necessary at certain times, but decisions to use them are controversial even among doctors. Some medical professionals and state governments are recognizing childbirth as the natural and healthy process it is. They are attempting to break down rigid hospital routines in the delivery room and to offer parents a variety of options. Fathers are often allowed in the delivery, there is more emphasis on keeping mother and child together, rooming-in is now routine, and in some hospitals fathers even spend the night.

Although parents may not have sufficient knowledge to decide the advisability of performing a Caesarian section or inducing labor, they can choose a doctor who will use such procedures in extraordinary rather than ordinary cases. They can choose a doctor who offers options for treatment—up to the limit of medical safety—to control their own pregnancy and childbirth.

The Alternatives Many families are turning to alternative settings and methods of childbirth to avoid the impersonal environment, imposing equipment, and technology of the hospital, even though the risk to life during emergencies is greater.

Home Births During the last decade an increasing number of Americans have chosen to have their children born at home. For example, about one of every ten California babies is born at home.

Midwives Home births create a demand for midwives to assist in pre- and postnatal care and delivery. The medical establishment, after several centuries of outlawing midwives, is finally allowing them a useful role complementary to their own. Some states are certifying nurses to become midwives, establishing programs to train them, and specifying the conditions under which they can practice. In California an extra 12 to 18 months of training for midwife certification is required in ad-

Alternative Birth Center (ABC)
A hospital-provided setting that is an alternative to home birth and traditional hospital birth. The ABC aims to foster emotional warmth and is reserved only for those expected to have an uncomplicated birth and to return home within 24 hours.

dition to the nursing degree. Usually midwives first work in conjunction with a physician and then move into obstetric clinics and private practice.

The procedure often follows this order: If a woman is classified as a low-risk patient at her initial pregnancy examination by a doctor, after considering her health and record of past births, the doctor may recommend that she be attended by a midwife. About three-fourths of all expectant mothers could be so categorized.

The nurse midwife administers all prenatal care and, barring complications, also performs the delivery and subsequent treatment. Ideally, this frees the obstetrician to concentrate on patients with potential problems. The

midwife can devote time to the psychosocial aspects of routine births, including mental and physical conditioning, long natural labors, and family counseling. It has been convincingly shown that women administered to by a midwife are more likely to adhere to pre- and postnatal treatment than are those who see a doctor.

Alternative Birth Centers In response to the increase in the number of home births, some hospitals are introducing *alternative birth centers* (*ABCs*) to alleviate some of the criticisms of traditional hospital routines. ABCs have evolved for prospective parents who train toward natural childbirth and who are expected to have

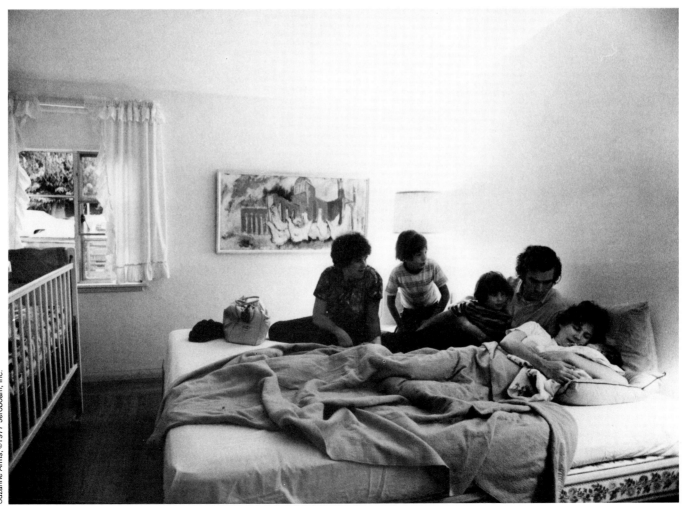

Sudden (Unexplained) Infant Death Syndrome

A mysterious disease commonly known as "crib death" is more accurately described as sudden infant death syndrome (SIDS). It cannot be predicted or anticipated, even by well-qualified physicians. An apparently healthy infant or, in about half the cases, a baby with a slight cold is put to bed at night and is found dead the next morning. The baby gives no warning or cry of pain and does not struggle. Routine autopsies do not reveal abnormalities serious enough to account for death.

Sudden infant death syndrome kills between 7,000 and 10,000 babies in the United States each year. It is the leading cause of death in infants from one month to one year old. Most deaths occur between the ages of one to six months, with peak frequency between the ages of two and four months. In areas where seasonal temperatures vary a great deal, SIDS occurs most commonly between the months of November and February. Boys appear to be slightly more susceptible than girls, as do premature and low birth-weight babies. In the United States, SIDS occurs most often in low-income families living in crowded conditions. Many of the victims have mild respiratory infections. But,

mysteriously, SIDS also strikes children with none of these conditions.

Many theories have been put forth to account for SIDS. Most of them have been disproved, but several promising lines of investigation are developing. The most promising SIDS research suggests that its cause is a defect in the mechanism of the lower brain stem that controls breathing. In high-risk children, insufficient neural development appears to cause frequent and prolonged apnea, periods of not breathing. These periods last as long as 15 to 20 seconds, contrasted with normal periods of 6 to 10 seconds. Incidents of irregular apnea may be triggered by mild respiratory infection. Low birth-weight infants also have more frequent and prolonged apnea, which eventually leads to severe oxygen deprivation and sometimes to heart failure.

The breathing control center in the central nervous system may be highly affected by respiratory disturbances. SIDS victims suffer a chronic lack of oxygen concentration in the blood. Evidence for this oxygen deficit is found throughout the body. Victims have abnormally large amounts of muscle in the small arteries and lungs and prolonged retention of birth fat around the adrenal glands. They also synthe-

size red blood cells in the liver instead of in the bone marrow alone.

Reduced respiratory drive may also contribute to the causes of SIDS and appears to be affected by anemia and low red blood cell concentration. Mothers in poor socioeconomic environments, where SIDS occurs most frequently, are less likely to get prenatal treatment for iron deficiency and are more likely to be anemic.

Viruses are also suspected as a factor contributing to SIDS. And another growing body of evidence indicates that SIDS victims are unable to synthesize glucose and therefore require frequent feedings to maintain adequate blood-sugar levels. Since most crib deaths occur at the age when babies begin to sleep through the night without feedings, it is suggested that the drop in blood sugar is too great. Combined with the stress of cold weather, the drop in concentration of blood sugar might be fatal.

Researchers are slowly sorting out the more fruitful theories. It is hoped that they will soon be able to establish conclusively the characteristics of high-risk infants. When that is accomplished, it should be possible to prevent the events that lead to SIDS.

low-risk, uncomplicated births. The centers are alternatives to both home birth, where emergencies might not be adequately handled, and to traditional hospital birth, where procedures sometimes seem too impersonal and technological. ABCs attempt to provide a supportive environment to meet emotional needs; since they are located in a hospital, scientific know-how and equipment are available.

Usually the ABC is decorated like an ordinary bedroom. The woman labors, gives birth, and rests afterward in an ordinary bed. Ordinarily no drugs are

administered, although in some cases a mild painkiller may be given. Friends and relatives may be invited, and in some instances children attend the birth. The father may spend the night, and the baby stays in the same room. Usually the stay is short for mother and child, 6 to 24 hours after birth, and an ABC nurse visits them several times during their first few days at home. The cost is substantially lower than that of a regular hospital birth. Though emergency equipment may be present in the room, any complications result in a transference to a regular maternity ward. Many women, around one-

Am I Parent Material?

These questions are posed to you as you consider the most important decision you will ever make—whether or not to have a child. The decision to have a child is one that you will have to live with for the rest of your life. The responsibility of a new life is awesome. These questions are designed to raise ideas that you may not have otherwise considered. There are no "right" answers and no "grades." You must decide for yourself what your answers reveal about your aptitude for parenthood.

You *do* have a choice. Exercise that choice with knowledge and careful thought. And then do what seems right for you.

Is My Life-Style Conducive to Parenting?

1. Would a child interfere with my educational plans? Would I have the energy to go to school and raise a child at the same time?

2. Would a child restrict my individual growth and development?

3. Could I handle children and a career well? Am I tired when I come home from work or do I have lots of energy left?

4. Does my job or my partner's job require a lot of traveling?

5. Am I financially able to support a child? Am I prepared to spend almost $100 a week to rear my child to age 18? Or over $80,000, not including one partner's income loss if he/she would choose to remain at home?

6. Do I live in a neighborhood conducive to raising a child? Would I be willing to move?

7. Would I be willing to give up the freedom to do what I want to do, when I want to do it?

8. Would I be willing to restrict

my social life? Would I miss lost leisure time and privacy?

9. Would my partner and I be prepared to spend more time at home? Would we have enough time to spend with a child?

10. Would I be willing to devote a great part of my life, at *least* 18 years, to being responsible for a child? And spend my entire life being concerned about my child's welfare?

11. Would I be prepared to be a single parent if my partner left or died?

Am I Ready to Raise a Child?

1. Do I like children? Have I had enough experiences with babies? Toddlers? Teenagers?

2. Do I enjoy teaching others?

3. Do I communicate easily with others?

4. Do I have enough love to give a child? Can I express affection easily?

5. Would I have the patience to raise a child? Can I tolerate noise and confusion? Can I deal with disrupted schedules?

6. How do I handle anger? Would I abuse my child if I lost my temper?

7. What do I know about discipline and freedom? About setting limits and giving space? Would I be too strict? Too lenient? Am I a perfectionist? How do I deal with change?

8. Do I know my own values and goals yet? Could I help my child develop constructive values?

9. What kind of relationship did I have with my parents? Would I repeat the same mistakes my parents made or would I over-indulge or restrict my child in an attempt not to repeat my parents' mistakes?

10. How much would I worry about

my child's health and safety? Would I be able to take care of a hurt or sick child?

11. What if my decision to have a child turns out to have been wrong for me?

What Do I Expect to Gain from the Parenting Experience?

1. Do I enjoy child-centered activities?

2. Would having a child show others I am a mature person?

3. Would I want my child to be a miniature version of me? Would I be willing to adopt a child?

4. Would I feel comfortable if my child had ideas different from mine? How different?

5. Would I expect my child to make contributions I wish I had made in the world?

6. Would I expect my child to keep me from being lonely in my old age?

7. Would I be prepared emotionally to let my child leave when he/she grows up?

8. Would I expect my child to fulfill my relationship with my partner?

9. Do I need parenthood to fulfill my role as a man or woman?

10. Do I need a child to make my life meaningful?

11. Would I feel strongly about wanting my child to be a boy/girl? What if I didn't get the one I wanted?

Have I Adequately Discussed the Parenting Question with My Partner?

1. Does my partner want to have a child? Is he/she willing to ask these questions of himself/herself? Have we adequately discussed our reasons for wanting a child?

(*continued on next page*)

Am I Parent Material? (continued)

2. Do my partner and I understand each other's feelings about religion, work, family, child raising, future goals? Are our feelings compatible? Are they conducive to good parenting?

3. Would both my partner and I contribute our fair shares in raising the child?

4. Could we provide a child with a really good home environment? Is our relationship stable? Do we have a good sexual relationship?

5. After having a child, would my partner and I be able to separate if we should have unsolvable problems? Or would we feel obligated to remain together for the sake of the child?

6. Would we be able to share each other with a child without jealousy?

7. Do we want to bring a child into today's overpopulated world to face the social problems of our times?

8. Does my partner or do I have a hereditary abnormality we might pass on to a child? Could I emotionally and financially deal with having a physically or mentally handicapped child?

9. Suppose one of us wants a child and the other doesn't. Who wins?

10. Which of the questions in this [questionnaire] do we really need to discuss before making a decision?

Carole Goldman

---

third of those who preregister in ABCs, do not give birth there. Some have last-minute complications, such as breech presentations, and others are transferred during labor.

Parenting

When the anticipation and anxiety of pregnancy and delivery are over, the joy and anxiety of parenting begin. Many attitudes of parents toward their children are related to how the parents accept and react towards themselves. People who can rejoice in themselves and tolerate their own foibles find it much easier to appreciate the uniqueness and understand the weaknesses of others.

One of the most important but difficult things for parents to realize is that their children are separate and potentially independent beings. Parents who have insights into their own needs and desires and who have a healthy respect for the rights of their children develop long-term positive relationships with them. How do such parents behave toward their children? They first recognize the difference between nurturing and domineering. They tend to use praise and attention to reinforce their children's appropriate behavior. They teach them personal hygiene skills, value orientations, personal responsi-

bility. They recognize that parents tend to be models for their children and try to act accordingly. They pay attention to their children and are patient with them.

Too often parents see their children as extensions of themselves. Such parents attempt to "achieve" through their children, foisting on them their own desires and goals. An early possessive behavior on the part of parents encourages an unhealthy dependence on the part of a child. In later years, usually during adolescence, the dependent child often must turn away from the parents—reject or rebel against them—just to find out who he or she is. For both the parents and the child, this is a painful situation, and the rift that results may never be healed.

Parenting well does not come automatically. Good parents are not just born; they work at it. And it is hard work. Educating ourselves about the best methods of behavior and care during pregnancy and childbirth reduces pain and increases the safety and pleasure of those important events. The same careful preparation toward parenting will yield similar results. Parents can learn much about what to expect from children and from themselves as parents. Observing other children, comparing ideas with other parents, reading about childhood development and behavior, and attending classes on parenting can all contribute to the joys of parenting and reduce the frustrations and anxieties.

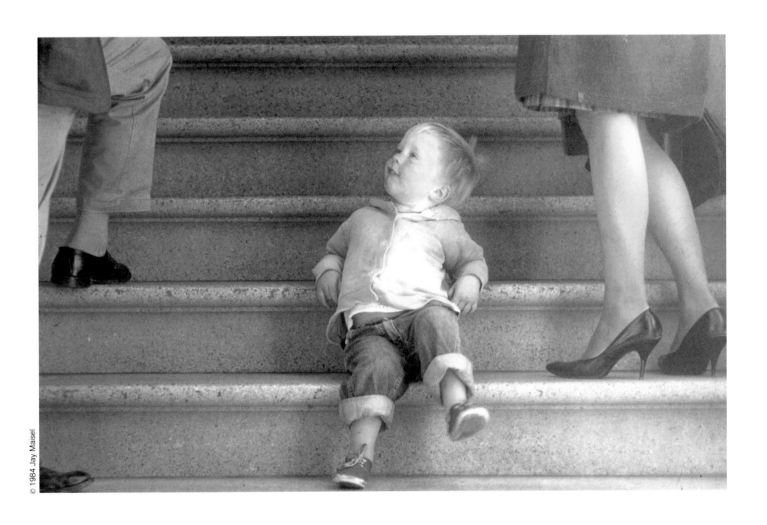

How to Win Without Losing

Parents who are in the midst of a declared or undeclared war with their children over chores and responsibilities should recognize the fact that this war cannot be won. Children have more time and energy to resist us than we have to coerce them. Even if we win a battle and succeed in enforcing our will, they may retaliate by becoming spiritless and neurotic, or rebellious and delinquent.

There is only one way in which we can win: by winning the children over. This task may seem impossible: it is merely difficult, and we have the capacity to accomplish it. Even if we do not presently have friendly relations with a child, such relations can be built in the near future.

Parents can initiate favorable changes in their child by:

1. Listening with sensitivity. Children experience frustration and resentment when parents seem uninterested in their feelings and thoughts. As a result, they conclude that their own ideas are stupid and unworthy of attention and that they themselves are neither lovable nor loved.

A parent who listens with attentiveness conveys to his child that his ideas are valued and that he is respected. Such respect gives the child a sense of self-worth. The feeling of personal worth enables the child to deal more effectively with the world of events and people.

2. Preventing "grapes of wrath." Parents should consciously avoid words and comments that create hate and resentment.

Insults: You are a disgrace to your school and no credit to your family.

Name calling: Bum, big shot, shrimp, idiot.

Prophesying: You will end up in a federal penitentiary, that's where you'll end up.

Threats: If you don't settle down you can forget about your allowance.

Accusations: You are always the first to start trouble.

Bossing: Shut up, and let me tell you a thing or two.

3. Stating feelings and thoughts without attacking. In troublesome situations, parents are more effective when they state their own feelings and thoughts without attacking their child's personality and dignity.

When parents listen with sensitivity, suspend cutting comments, and state their feelings and requirements without insult, a process of change is initiated in the child. The sympathetic atmosphere draws the child nearer to the parents; their attitudes of fairness, consideration, and civility are noticed and emulated. These changes will ultimately be rewarded.

In adopting these new attitudes and practices, a parent will accomplish a large part of educating his child for responsibility. And yet, example alone is not enough. A sense of responsibility is attained by each child through his own efforts and experience. While the parent's example creates the favorable attitude and climate for learning, specific experiences consolidate the learning to make it part of the child's character. Therefore, it is important to determine what specific responsibilities to give to children at different levels of maturity.

Haim Ginott
Between Parent and Child

Family Planning Potential Scale

Read the following statements carefully. Choose the one in each section that best describes you at this moment and record its score at the right. (For example, "enjoys children" has a score of 5.) When you have identified five statements, total your score and find your position on the scale.

5 enjoys children
4 feels comfortable around children
3 doesn't mind looking after children
2 feels uncomfortable around children
1 dislikes children

   Score _____

5 knows how to plan for pregnancy
4 knows about hereditary factors
3 is familiar with the nutritional requirements of pregnancy
2 is unfamiliar with nutritional requirements of pregnancy
1 is ignorant about planning a pregnancy

   Score _____

5 knows how to plan for childbirth
4 is familiar with routine delivery procedures
3 is willing to learn about childbirth
2 is uninterested in childbirth information
1 is ignorant about childbirth procedures

   Score _____

5 understands the benefits of breast feeding
4 favors breast feeding
3 is unfamiliar with the benefits of breast feeding
2 dislikes breast feeding
1 disapproves of breast feeding

   Score _____

5 recognizes that parents are models for children's behavior
4 respects the rights of children
3 views children as extensions of parents
2 has little respect for children's rights
1 dominates children

   Score _____

   Total score _____

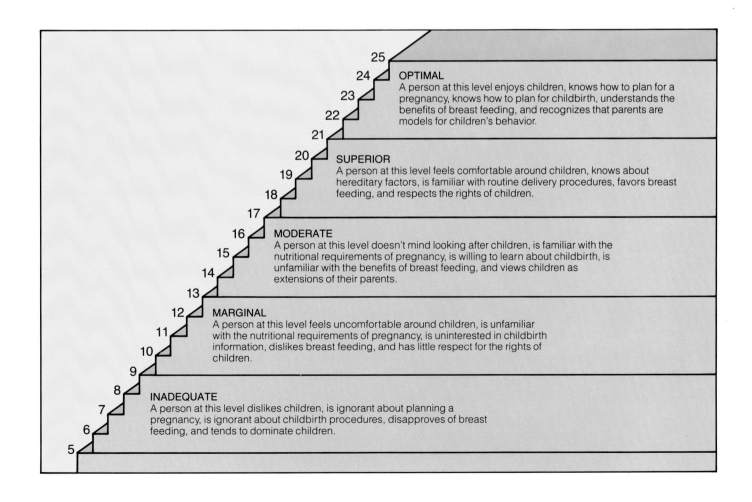

OPTIMAL
A person at this level enjoys children, knows how to plan for a pregnancy, knows how to plan for childbirth, understands the benefits of breast feeding, and recognizes that parents are models for children's behavior.

SUPERIOR
A person at this level feels comfortable around children, knows about hereditary factors, is familiar with routine delivery procedures, favors breast feeding, and respects the rights of children.

MODERATE
A person at this level doesn't mind looking after children, is familiar with the nutritional requirements of pregnancy, is willing to learn about childbirth, is unfamiliar with the benefits of breast feeding, and views children as extensions of their parents.

MARGINAL
A person at this level feels uncomfortable around children, is unfamiliar with the nutritional requirements of pregnancy, is uninterested in childbirth information, dislikes breast feeding, and has little respect for the rights of children.

INADEQUATE
A person at this level dislikes children, is ignorant about planning a pregnancy, is ignorant about childbirth procedures, disapproves of breast feeding, and tends to dominate children.

Take Action

Your answers to Probing Your Emotions at the beginning of this chapter and your placement level on the Family Planning Potential Scale will, we hope, encourage you to begin a process of self-exploration and self-discovery that you will continue. Reflect on the entire chapter's content and ask yourself how each point relates to your own life. Then take action:

1. Volunteer to baby-sit for friends or relatives. Take along a copy of the Family Planning Potential Scale and rate yourself during the evening. If you are feeling venturesome baby-sit with a child who is under two years of age.

2. Visit a hospital and ask to observe the delivery of a baby as part of a health class project. Alternatively, interview an expectant mother and an expectant father. What emotions or attitudes do they share? Which are clearly different?

3. Visit a Lamaze class. Observe the participants and imagine yourself in their place.

4. Carry with you an uncooked egg in its shell for 24 hours. Keep it warm. Never leave it alone except for two one-hour naps. If you must leave it for a time, arrange for an egg sitter.

5. Answer the questions on page 175. Are you parent material? What do your answers reveal about your aptitude for parenthood?

Before leaving this chapter, review the questions that open the chapter. Have your feelings or values changed? Are you now better equipped to handle the complex and very human problems associated with pregnancy, childbirth, and parenting?

Part Three

Substance Use and Abuse

Chapter Eight

Tobacco

Probing Your Emotions

1. You have just met a very attractive person who becomes more and more interesting as your conversation continues. You finally part but agree to get together again for lunch. During the second meeting you discover that your new friend is a heavy smoker. Does learning about this habit change your feelings toward the friend?

2. If you are currently smoking, do you like yourself better for being a smoker or are you disappointed in yourself for not being able to stop the habit?

3. If you are not currently smoking, how would you feel if you discovered that your child, brother, or sister had just started smoking? What responsibility, if any, would you have to intervene? What would you do?

4. Do smokers make you angry? When you are in an elevator or restaurant and someone lights a cigar, what do you do about it?

Chapter Contents

THE HISTORY OF TOBACCO
TOBACCO SMOKE
IMMEDIATE EFFECTS OF SMOKING
THE SMOKING HABIT
BEHAVIORAL ASPECTS OF SMOKING
HEALTH HAZARDS OF SMOKING
Lung cancer
Emphysema
Other respiratory diseases
Cardiovascular disease
Other health hazards
Cumulative effects
SMOKERS' EFFECTS ON NONSMOKERS
OTHER FORMS OF TOBACCO USE
OTHER OPINIONS ABOUT THE HEALTH HAZARDS OF TOBACCO
WHAT CAN BE DONE?
BENEFITS FROM QUITTING

Boxes

Trends in U.S. cigarette use, 1965–1980
"Light" cigarettes: deadly as ever
Smoking and life expectancy
Smoking used to be good for me
The secondhand smoke issue
The strength of commitment
Gum to help you stop smoking

Psychoactive
Affecting the mind; specifically said of
drugs that affect the brain or nervous
system.

8 According to the 1983 surgeon general's report on smoking, many studies have documented higher rates of disease and earlier death in cigarette smokers than in nonsmokers. This report indicates that up to 30 percent of all deaths from coronary heart disease can be attributed to cigarette smoking. Cigarette smoking is also a primary cause of chronic obstructive lung disease and a variety of cancers. Smoking remains the largest avoidable cause of illness and death in the United States. These findings are consistent with the U.S. Public Health Service's position that tobacco use is the number one drug problem in America today.

Many people have heard the story about the man who was so upset after reading a report about smoking and lung cancer that he immediately gave up reading. Other smokers have been known to react to news about the health hazards of smoking in much the same way.

Giving up smoking can be extremely difficult. Most smokers have filled their daily activities with cues that continue to say "time to light up." And when smokers feel the urge to light up, they can think of a thousand reasons to do so, no matter how strong their resolve to quit. Smokers may not know their real reasons for smoking—reasons that might include calming their nerves, relieving boredom, keeping their hands occupied, or satisfying basic oral needs. Like alcoholics and heroin addicts, smokers who stop experience withdrawal symptoms. Also like alcoholics and heroin addicts, smokers now have the equivalent of Alcoholics Anonymous and other self-help organizations to turn to for help.

Many smokers believe that if only they had enough of some magical thing called "willpower," the willpower would do the job for them. But smokers who quit last year seem to have no more "willpower" than those who are sure they will quit next year. Psychologists have not yet learned enough about the psychological factors in dependence on tobacco to predict and control them, but physiologists and biochemists know full well the consequences of failing to do so.

The History of Tobacco

Nicotiana tabacum, the tobacco plant, was first cultivated by American Indians, who smoked it during some of their ceremonies. European explorers acquired the habit from the Indians and soon spread it around the world. For a time tobacco was called *herba panacea*—a cure for all ills—and its use was promoted for a variety of medical purposes. After that, most Europeans came to consider tobacco smoking to be nothing more than an expensive but harmless habit. More than 300 years elapsed between the first widespread use of tobacco and the recognition of its harmful effects: a higher incidence of lung cancer, emphysema, coronary heart disease, fetal abnormalities, and many other health hazards.

For aesthetic, religious, and health reasons, using tobacco has been outlawed in many countries at different times. In 1633 in Constantinople the sultan Murad IV decreed the death penalty for smoking tobacco, and he personally executed soldiers unfortunate enough to be discovered in this criminal act. As is true with most pleasurable and addicting drugs, however, even severe punishment did not prevent the continued spread of tobacco smoking.

Attempts to prevent people from smoking have continued into the twentieth century. These attempts have been based on religious and moral considerations rather than on the threat of death, but they have not been successful either. Following the prohibition of alcohol, 14 states passed laws aimed at prohibiting cigarettes, and many other state legislatures considered anti-cigarette bills at the same time. These laws also did not work. By 1927 the last of them had been repealed, leaving in effect only restrictions against the sale of cigarettes to minors. The history of tobacco clearly shows that once a *psychoactive* agent without apparent ill effects has been widely accepted by the public, neither religious nor political prohibitions can curb its use.

Tobacco Smoke

Tobacco smoke is a mixture of gases, vapors, and small particles. How much of each depends on the type of tobacco, the way it is smoked, and the temperature at which it burns. Smoke from a typical nonfiltered cigarette contains about 5 billion particles per cubic millimeter—50,000 times as many as are found in an equal volume of polluted urban atmosphere. The particles in tobacco smoke are made up of several hundred

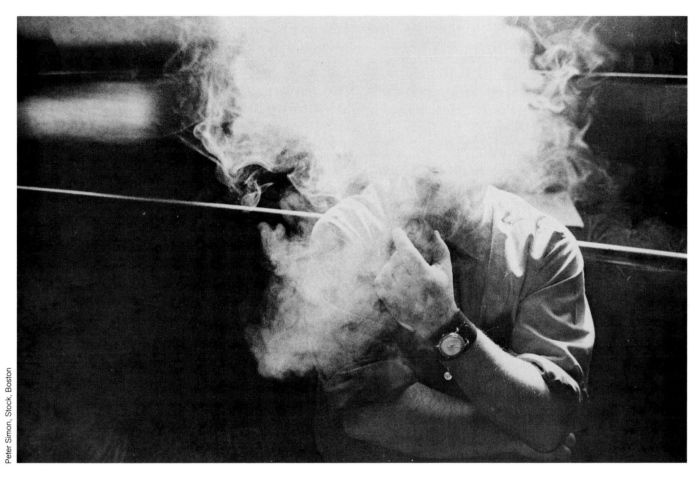

Tar
A thick, sticky, dark fluid produced when tobacco is burned.

Carcinogen
Any cancer-causing agent.

Cancer
A malignant growth of cells; disease caused by the uncontrolled growth of body, lymph, or blood cells; can occur in nearly all portions of the body.

Cocarcinogen
The material that works with a carcinogen to produce a cancer.

Respiratory system
The structures by which the body takes oxygen from the air, uses it, and gives off the by-products (carbon dioxide and water vapor). The nose, mouth, trachea (windpipe), and lungs are parts of the respiratory system.

Smoker's bronchitis
An inflammation of the lining of the tubes (bronchioles) that carry air in and out of the lungs.

Nicotine
A poisonous substance found in tobacco and responsible for many of the effects of tobacco.

Inhale
To breathe a substance into the lungs.

different chemicals, many of them toxic. These particles, when condensed, form the brown, sticky mass called cigarette *tar.*

Some chemicals in tobacco tar are *carcinogenic;* that is, they produce *cancer.*

Other chemicals in tobacco tar are *cocarcinogens.* Cocarcinogens are substances that do not themselves cause cancer but combine with other chemicals to stimulate the growth of certain cancers, at least in laboratory animals. For example, the phenols present in tar, although not particularly carcinogenic themselves, greatly increase the carcinogenic potency of benzopyrene, a substance also in the tar. Still other compounds, although probably not promoters of cancer, directly irritate the tissues of the *respiratory system* and damage the respiratory cilia, which normally operate to keep the air passages free of mucus and dust.

It is well known that smoking interferes with the functioning of the respiratory system and often leads rapidly to smoker's throat, smoker's cough, and *smoker's bronchitis.* Table 8–1 shows some of the physical complaints of smokers and nonsmokers. These conditions usually disappear in people who stop smoking.

Nicotine, the predominant "drug" in tobacco, is one of the toxic chemicals. It is a colorless, oily compound contained in cigarettes in amounts varying from 0.5

milligram per cigarette in some brands to as much as 2.0 milligrams in others. When a smoker deeply *inhales,* over 60 percent of the nicotine in the smoke is absorbed through the mucus of the lungs into the bloodstream.

Of importance is that this blood travels by way of the heart directly to the brain. Thus, unlike drugs taken by mouth, sniffed through the nose, or injected into a vein in the forearm, nicotine absorbed by the lungs reaches the brain more quickly—about 7 seconds after the smoke enters the lungs as compared with 12 seconds or more with intravenous administration and as long as 30 minutes with oral ingestion. Furthermore, the nicotine is not extensively diluted before it reaches the brain along with blood from other organs. In this manner the brain of the smoker receives with each puff of the cigarette a transient, concentrated mass of nicotine. Nicotine appears to be the substance in the cigarette that causes addiction, as well as the cause of most of the *cardiovascular* damage resulting from smoking.

Cigarette smoking produces *carbon monoxide,* the lethal gas in automobile exhaust, in concentrations 400 times greater than what is considered safe in industry. Carbon monoxide combines with hemoglobin in red blood cells, displacing oxygen; the result is that cigarette smokers become short of breath when they exert themselves or when they are at high altitudes. In the

Table 8-1   Physical Complaints of Smokers and Nonsmokers

Complaint	Cigarette smokers (percent)	Nonsmokers (percent)	Ratio (smokers) to nonsmokers
Cough	33.2	5.6	5.9
Loss of appetite	3.3	0.9	3.7
Shortness of breath	16.3	4.7	3.5
Chest pains	7.0	3.7	1.9
Diarrhea	3.3	1.7	1.9
Easily fatigued	26.1	14.9	1.8
Abdominal pains	6.7	3.8	1.8
Hoarseness	4.8	2.6	1.8
Loss of weight	7.3	4.5	1.6
Stomach pains	6.0	3.8	1.6
Insomnia	10.2	6.8	1.5
Difficulty in swallowing	1.4	1.0	1.4

Source: E. Cuyler Hammond, "The Effects of Smoking," *Scientific American* (July 1962): 49. Copyright © 1962 by Scientific American, Inc. All rights reserved.

Cardiovascular
Having to do with the heart and blood vessels.

Carbon monoxide
A colorless, odorless, poisonous gas formed when carbon is burned in a small amount of air. Carbon monoxide can displace the oxygen in human blood, thus causing suffocation.

Tolerance
Raised-dose sensitivity so that a given dose no longer exerts the usual effect and larger doses are needed.

Cerebral cortex
The outer layer of the brain, which controls the complex behavior and mental activity of human beings; also called the new cortex.

Physical dependence (addiction)
A state in which withdrawal of a drug that has been taken repeatedly produces physical withdrawal symptoms.

---

blood of the average smoker, carbon monoxide inactivates 2 to 6 percent of the hemoglobin, making it unavailable to carry oxygen. In people who smoke more than a pack (20 cigarettes) a day, this figure may go up to 8 percent. Carbon monoxide also impairs visual acuity, especially at night. The assumption is that it directly affects the retina, the innermost layer of the eye. Hydrogen cyanide, a potent poison, is another gas found in cigarette smoke, but we do not know whether the concentrations are great enough to have an effect.

All smokers absorb some gases, tars, and nicotine from cigarette smoke, but those who inhale bring most of these substances into their bodies and keep them there. In one year, a typical one-pack-per-day smoker takes in 50,000 to 70,000 puffs. Smoke from a cigarette, pipe, or cigar is taken directly into the mouth, throat, and respiratory tract; the nose, which normally filters out about 75 percent of the foreign matter in the air we breathe, is completely bypassed.

In a cigarette the unburned tobacco itself acts as a filter. As a cigarette burns down, there is less and less filter, and several times more chemicals are taken into the body during the last third of a cigarette than during the first. A smoker can cut down on absorption of harmful chemicals by not smoking cigarettes down to short butts, but any gains made with this technique will be offset if he or she smokes more cigarettes, inhales more deeply, or puffs more frequently.

Immediate Effects of Smoking

Nicotine produces most of the immediate physical and behavioral changes associated with cigarette smoking. The beginning smoker often has symptoms of mild nicotine poisoning: dizziness, faintness, rapid pulse, cold, clammy skin, and sometimes nausea, vomiting, and diarrhea. The effects of nicotine on people who have been smoking for a while are complex. They depend greatly on the size of the nicotine dose and on how much *tolerance* has been built up by previous smoking. Depending on dosage, nicotine can either excite or tranquilize the nervous system. Generally, the smoker feels stimulated first, but this stimulation gives way to persistent tranquilization.

Nicotine has many other effects. It stimulates the part of the brain called the *cerebral cortex*. It also stimulates the adrenal glands to discharge adrenaline. It inhibits the formation of urine, constricts the blood vessels, especially in the skin, increases the heart rate, and elevates blood pressure. Higher blood pressure, faster heart rate, and constricted blood vessels require the heart to pump more blood. In healthy individuals, the heart can usually meet this demand, but in people whose coronary arteries are damaged so as to interfere with the flow of blood, the heart muscle may be strained.

Frequently, people who smoke do not feel as hungry as people who do not. There are several reasons for this occurrence. Smoking depresses hunger contractions. It also causes the liver to release glycogen, which results in a small increase in the level of sugar in the blood. Smoking also dulls the taste buds, and food does not taste as good as it would otherwise. People who quit smoking usually notice how much better food tastes.

The Smoking Habit

There is firm scientific evidence that regular cigarette smoking is not just a psychological habit but a classic case of *physical dependence* (*addiction*) to nicotine. Smokers gradually develop a tolerance for nicotine, so they need to smoke more and more to get the same physiological reaction. The body also demands that certain amounts of nicotine periodically reach the brain. Experimental subjects were given cigarettes that tasted and looked exactly the same but varied widely in how much nicotine they contained. Without knowing how much nicotine they were getting, the subjects automatically adjusted their rate of smoking and depth of inhalation so as to assure that the usual amount of nicotine was absorbed. In other studies heavy smokers were given nicotine without their knowing it, and they cut down on their smoking.

The automatic and unconscious adjustments made by many heavy smokers may have implications for the current popularity of low-tar and low-nicotine cigarettes. Using these cigarettes, many smokers will merely puff more frequently, inhale more deeply, smoke down to a shorter butt, or smoke more cigarettes and in the

Withdrawal symptoms
Unpleasant physical and mental sensations experienced when abstaining from a drug to which one is addicted.

Secondary reinforcers
Stimuli that are rewarding not because they are pleasurable in themselves, but because they have been associated with other stimuli that are pleasurable

Psychometric
Relating to mental measurement.

process expose themselves (and those around them) to a greater total amount of smoke.

Like all true addicts, chronic smokers who stop suffer physiological *withdrawal symptoms*. Sudden abstinence produces changes in brain waves, heart rate, blood pressure, and levels of certain body chemicals. These people are irritable and complain of insomnia, muscular pains, headache, nausea, and other discomforts. During withdrawal many chronic smokers are easily distracted and perform poorly on objective tests that require sustained attention. Some investigators claim that most heavy smokers continue their addiction not for any pleasure that it adds to their lives, but because they are unwilling to go through the many discomforts of the withdrawal process.

Behavioral Aspects of Smoking

Various psychological and social forces combine with physiological addiction to perpetuate the tobacco habit. Many people, for example, have established habit patterns of smoking while they are doing something else—smoking while talking, smoking while working, smoking while drinking, and so on. It is more difficult for these people to quit smoking because the activity that has become associated with it continues to trigger the desire for a cigarette. Behavioristic psychologists call such activities *secondary reinforcers*. These act in concert with the forces of physiological addiction to keep people dependent on tobacco.

Most people start to smoke as teenagers or young adults. Recent studies have identified certain behavioral characteristics in these people. Smoking at an early age is commonly linked to curiosity, low self-esteem, and status seeking. The imitation of close friends, older siblings, and parents is a very important force. Most teenage regular smokers report that their best friends and parents are smokers. For many teenagers, the choice to smoke or not revolves around the issue of conformity to a particular group or a similar social factor. "Everybody smokes and so do I" is a common explanation. Older teenagers and young adults are somewhat more likely to report their involvement in smoking in more

personal terms—stimulation, pleasure, or alleviation of unpleasant moods such as anxiety or depression. Most of these people are well aware of the health hazards associated with smoking but have developed rationalizations, often along the line that most health hazards are being overemphasized these days.

It is clear that different people smoke (and use alcohol, drink coffee, and so forth) for different reasons. Of interest is that people who are heavy smokers are also more likely to be users of a wide variety of other psychoactive drugs, including coffee and alcohol. Some studies have indicated that over 90 percent of heroin addicts and 80 percent of alcoholics are heavy cigarette smokers. These findings suggest that there might be a few specific underlying psychological or physiological processes associated with general tendencies toward drug dependence. Yet efforts to identify characteristics have not been especially successful. No single factor has been found highly predictive by itself of smoking versus nonsmoking or of quitting versus not quitting. Efforts to use *psychometric* tests and personality measures to identify which people respond to stop-smoking treatment programs have also been generally unsuccessful. Some demographic variables are correlated with smoking behavior. People from higher socioeconomic classes are less likely to start smoking and are somewhat more successful in their efforts to stop. Since the surgeon general's initial report on the health hazards of smoking, physicians and other health professionals have stopped smoking at a higher rate than most other professionals. However, these statistics are not very useful in predicting the behavior of a given individual.

Some people do not quit smoking even in the face of serious illness and the threat of death. Sigmund Freud, for example, had a bad heart and cancer of the oral cavity. He was in constant pain and frequently unable to talk or to swallow, yet he continued to smoke up to 20 cigars a day. When he tried to stop he suffered from unbearable depression, which he described as "an oppression of mood in which the images of dying and farewell scenes replaced the more usual fantasies."

Sufferers from Buerger's disease provide one example—perhaps the most extreme one there is—of the strength of tobacco addiction. In Buerger's disease, nico-

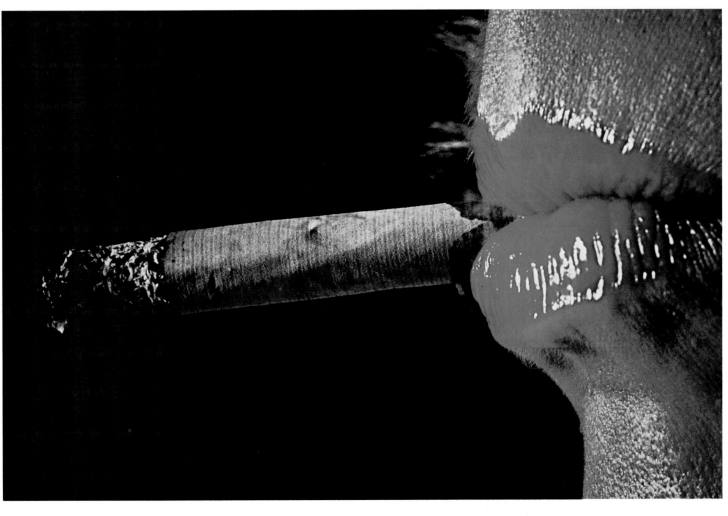

Trends in U.S. Cigarette Use, 1965–1980

1. The proportion of current regular smokers declined steadily between 1966 and 1980 (from 42.8 percent to 33 percent). The decline was steeper among males than among females, particularly among older males.

2. The proportion of never smokers increased steadily from 1966 to 1980 among males (24.8 to 34.6 percent), except those 65 years old and older. Among females, only 21- to 34-year-olds showed an increase in proportion of never smokers.

3. The mean number of cigarettes smoked per day by current smokers increased slightly from 1970 to 1980 (from 20 to 21.7 cigarettes).

4. Males smoked the highest mean number of cigarettes throughout the period 1970–1980, but the number for males and females increased about the same amount.

5. Heaviest daily consumption was in the middle-aged group (35–65 years). The greatest mean increase was observed among women aged 35 to 44.

6. The proportion of current smokers who smoked fewer than 20 cigarettes per day decreased between 1970 and 1980 (39.8 to 29.6 percent); the proportion smoking one pack (20 cigarettes) remained constant (34.9 to 34.2 percent); the proportion smoking from 21 to 39 cigarettes increased slightly (13.7 to 15.3 percent); and the proportion smoking two packs or more per day increased dramatically (11.4 to 30.8 percent).

7. The proportion of current smokers who attempted to quit three or more times decreased slightly from 1966 to 1980 (41.2 to 38.7 percent).

8. The proportion of former smokers having made three or more attempts to quit increased sharply (36 to 53.2 percent) from 1966 to 1975.

9. The proportion of current smokers who had attempted to quit during the past year increased from 1966 to 1980 (26.0 to 36.7 percent).

10. Among current smokers, younger persons and females were more likely than older persons and males to have attempted to quit during the previous 12 months.

11. The proportion of former smokers who had attempted to quit during the previous 12 months decreased from 1966 to 1975 (13.8 to 9.8 percent).

12. Among former smokers, younger persons and females were more likely than older persons and males to have quit during the previous 12 months.

13. The proportion of current smokers who resumed smoking within 6 months after a quit attempt decreased between 1966 and 1980 (80.1 to 72.2 percent).

U.S. Public Health Service
Health Consequences of Smoking: A Report of the Surgeon General, 1983

---

tine seriously damages circulation, especially in the legs. If the patient continues to smoke, gangrene may set in, starting at the toes. As long as the patient continues to smoke, gangrene will repeatedly set in at the extremity, progressing—amputation after amputation—to the hips. Whenever the patient stops smoking, the gangrene stops appearing. Yet surgeons who have been involved with these cases say it is not unusual to find a patient still smoking even after the third or fourth amputation.

Health Hazards of Smoking

In the monumental 1964 report *Smoking and Health* and in later reports, the surgeon general's team evaluated three major types of evidence linking tobacco smoking to disease.

The first type of evidence was drawn from animal studies: Nicotine and the other chemicals contained in tobacco smoke were given to animals, and the resultant damage to their tissues was measured.

The second type of evidence was gathered from clinical and autopsy studies of tissue damage occurring most often in smokers.

The third type of evidence came from two kinds of population studies: (1) studies of the past smoking habits of individuals with a particular disease and (2) studies that followed groups of smokers and nonsmokers over a period of years to record the occurrence and progress of certain diseases, including chronic cough and sputum production, sure signs of bronchitis. These studies also compared death rates and causes of death for the two groups.

A great deal of scientific evidence now indicates that the total amount of tobacco smoke inhaled is a key factor contributing to disease. Individuals who smoke more cigarettes per day, inhale deeply, puff frequently, smoke cigarettes down to small butts, or begin smoking at an early age run a greater risk of disease than do those who

"Light" Cigarettes: Deadly as Ever

The massive switch from high- to low-tar and nicotine cigarettes has done nothing to reduce the incidence of lung cancer among smokers, according to a recent study by the National Academy of Sciences. In fact, the report indicates that the 20-year trend toward presumably safer cigarettes has been accompanied by a "substantial and unexpected increase" in lung cancer among older smokers, perhaps because habituated smokers unconsciously alter their behavior to maintain the level of nicotine to which they are accustomed.

The study, which was directed by University of Rochester pharmacologist Louis C. Lasagna, concludes that only outright quitting can guarantee any health benefits to smokers. Combining existing data on lifetime cigarette consumption and death rates due to cancer of the respiratory system, the NAS panel found that men over 35 died more often, pack for pack, in 1975 than in 1955 (comparable data were not available for women). During the same time, the average tar and nicotine in cigarettes dropped by half. The report offers two "plausible" explanations for these findings. It may be that even the recent lung cancer deaths are a consequence of the protracted process of carcinogenesis—a

process that actually began with early exposure to high levels of tar and nicotine. Or, the report suggests, it may be that low-tar, low-nicotine cigarettes are actually more hazardous, especially for people who are accustomed to a more potent cigarette.

If the newer brands of cigarettes do indeed contribute to more deaths, it is probably—at least in part—because of the way people smoke them, the report suggests. Laboratory measurements of tar and nicotine are made by a smoking machine that is incapable of simulating complex human smoking behavior; if smokers light up more often, take more puffs from each cigarette, or inhale more deeply when they switch brands, the report says, then the laboratory results will not have much value predicting human consequences. And most research indicates that smokers do tend to "compensate"—though incompletely—for the decreased potency of their cigarettes, the report says.

The NAS panel's conclusion is different from that of Lawrence Garfinkle, who in the 1960s studied the health effects of filtered and unfiltered cigarettes for the American Cancer Society. Garfinkle found that, when he controlled for the number of cigarettes smoked, filtered cigarettes were safer; he also

found that people did not compensate significantly by smoking more. But the cigarettes he studied were very different from the "light" cigarettes of today. It is quite possible that people alter their smoking behavior when they switch to these brands, he says.

Garfinkle emphazises, however, that although there may be some behavioral compensation, there is no evidence that smokers compensate fully—that they will smoke twice as many cigarettes when tar and nicotine are cut in half. If the newer brands are more hazardous, the explanation must go beyond human behavior; the explanation may, according to the NAS report, involve the thousands of chemicals contained in cigarettes that—unlike tar and nicotine—are not routinely measured in government laboratories. Research indicates, for example, that reducing the tar and nicotine in cigarettes does not necessarily reduce the exposure to carbon monoxide and other gases—and may actually increase such exposure. In addition, the report notes, "flavorings" in cigarettes are protected as trade secrets, and the toxicity of such additives is therefore unknown.

W. Herbert
Science News

---

are moderate in any of these aspects or who do not smoke at all. Many diseases have been linked to smoking. Among them are diseases of the respiratory system, including lung cancer, various others cancers, and cardiovascular diseases. These, as well as others, are discussed on the following pages.

Lung Cancer   Cigarette smoking is the main cause of lung cancer in humans. The risks of developing lung cancer increase according to the number of cigarettes

smoked each day, the number of years the person has been smoking, and the age at which the person started smoking.

Cigar and pipe smokers run a higher risk of lung cancer than nonsmokers but a lower risk than cigarette smokers. Smoking filter-tipped cigarettes reduces health hazards a bit, unless the smoker compensates by smoking more of them.

Evidence indicates that beginning one year after a person stops smoking the risk of lung cancer decreases

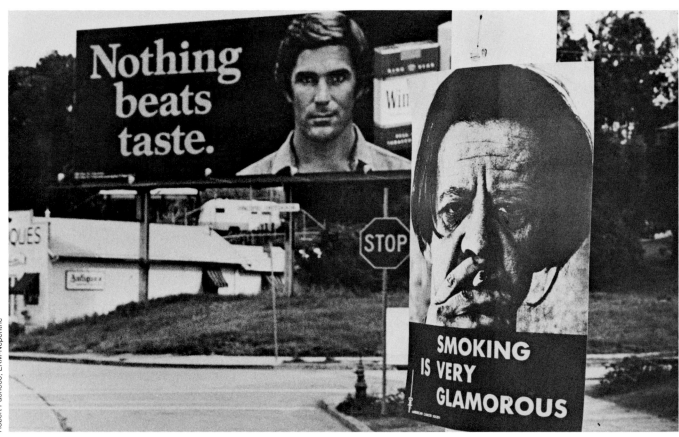

Larynx
The organ that produces the voice. It is located at the upper end of the windpipe.

Emphysema
Loss of lung tissue elasticity and breakup of the many small air sacs in the lungs so that fewer, larger, and less elastic air sacs are formed. The progressive accumulation of air causes difficulty in breathing.

Chronic bronchitis
An inflammation of the lining of the bronchial tubes that lasts over a period of years.

Congestion
An abnormally large amount of blood or other bodily substance collected in one part of the body.

Cilia
Hairlike appendages on certain cells that are capable of motion.

---

steadily. After 10 years the incidence of lung cancer is only slightly higher for those who had been heavy smokers before they quit than for those who never smoked. If smoking is stopped before cancer has started, lung tissue tends to repair itself, even if changes leading to cancer are already present.

Smoking is also associated with other cancers of the respiratory system. Cancer of the *larynx*, which occurs most often in men 55 to 70 years old, is much more common among smokers than among non-smokers. Experimental work with animals indicates that tobacco extracts and tobacco smoke contain chemicals that both initiate and promote cancerous change in the oral cavity. In addition, pipe smoking, alone or together with other tobacco use, is related in part to cancer of the lip.

Emphysema   *Emphysema* is a particularly disabling lung disease caused by smoking. The walls of the air sacs in the lungs lose elasticity and are gradually destroyed. The lungs' ability to obtain oxygen and remove carbon dioxide is impaired. A person with emphysema becomes breathless and feels like he or she is drowning. The heart must pump harder and may become enlarged. Death from a damaged heart frequently occurs. There is no known way to reverse the damage caused by emphysema. In its advanced stage the victim is bedridden and severely disabled.

Other Respiratory Diseases   Cigarette smoking is linked to other diseases of the respiratory system, especially chronic bronchitis. *Chronic bronchitis* is a persistent, recurrent inflammation of the bronchial tubes. When the cell lining of the bronchial tubes is irritated, it secretes an excess amount of mucus. Bronchial *congestion* is followed by a chronic cough, which makes breathing more and more difficult.

Cigarette smokers are up to 18 times more likely to die from pulmonary emphysema and chronic bronchitis than nonsmokers. If smokers have chronic bronchitis, they face a greater risk of lung cancer, no matter how old they are or how many (or few) cigarettes they smoke. Chronic bronchitis seems to be a shortcut to lung cancer. Smokers with chronic bronchitis are also much more likely to suffer from chronic cough, excess phlegm production, and breathlessness. They also do not have much tolerance for exercise.

Smoking and Life Expectancy

A 25-year-old, two-pack-a-day smoker of cigarettes . . . has a life expectancy 8.3 years shorter than his nonsmoking counterpart. For groups of men smoking fewer than 10 cigarettes per day, the loss of years of life expectancy is 4.6 years; smoking 10 to 19 cigarettes a day shortens the life expectancy by 5.5 years; and smoking 20 to 39 cigarettes a day, by 6.2 years.

E. C. Hammond
Life Expectancy of American Men in Relation to Their Smoking Habits

Even smokers of high school age show impairments in functioning of the respiratory system as compared with nonsmokers of the same age. Pipe and cigar smokers are more likely to die from chronic smoking and respiratory disease than nonsmokers, but they face a smaller risk than cigarette smokers. The risk of developing respiratory diseases goes up with the number of cigarettes smoked and becomes less if smoking is stopped.

Cigarette smoking is a much more important cause of respiratory disease than atmospheric pollution, at least for most people in the United States. But exposure to both atmospheric pollution and cigarette smoking is more dangerous than exposure to either by itself.

Even when there are no signs of respiratory impairment and no symptoms of respiratory disease, cigarette smoking damages the respiratory system. Normally, the cells lining the bronchial tubes secrete mucus, a sticky fluid that collects particles of soot, dust, and other substances in inhaled air. Mucus is carried up to the mouth by the continuous motion of the *cilia*, little hairlike structures that protrude from the inner surface of the bronchial tubes. If the cilia are destroyed or do not work, or if the pollution of inhaled air is more than the system can remove, this protection is lost.

Cigarette smoke first slows, then stops the action of

Macrophages
Large cells in the body that absorb dead tissue and dead cells.

Coronary heart disease (CHD)
Heart disease caused by hardening of the arteries that supply oxygen to the heart muscle.

Atherosclerosis
Heart disease caused by the deposit of fatty substances in the walls of the arteries.

Plaque
A deposit on the inner wall of blood vessels. Blood can coagulate around a plaque and form a clot.

Angina pectoris
Severe chest pain.

Myocardium
The muscles of the heart.

Aorta
The largest artery of the body. It carries blood from the left ventricle of the heart.

Immunity systems
Systems involving the resistance to disease.

---

the cilia. Eventually it destroys them, leaving delicate membranes exposed to injury from substances inhaled in cigarette smoke or from the polluted air in which the individual lives or works. Special cells of the body, the *macrophages* (literally "big eaters") also work to remove foreign particles from the respiratory tract, which they do by engulfing them. Cigarette smoking appears to make macrophages work less efficiently.

Although cigarette smoking can cause many disorders and diseases of the respiratory system, the damage is not always permanent. Once a person stops smoking, he or she can usually look for steady improvement in overall respiratory function. Chronic coughing subsides, phlegm production returns to normal, and breathing becomes easier. The likelihood of respiratory disease is greatly reduced. Individuals of all ages, even those who have been smoking heavily for decades, improve after they stop smoking. If given a chance, the human body has remarkable powers to restore itself.

Cardiovascular Disease   Cigarette smoking is related to various types of cardiovascular disorders, that is, disorders involving the heart and blood vessels. One type of cardiovascular disorder is *coronary heart disease* (*CHD*). CHD often results from a disease called *atherosclerosis*, in which fatty deposits called *plaques* form on the inner walls of heart arteries causing them to narrow and stiffen. The crushing chest pain of *angina pectoris*, a major symptom of CHD, results when the *myocardium* does not get enough blood. Sometimes a plaque will form at a narrow point in a main coronary artery. If the plaque completely blocks the flow of blood to a portion of the heart, that portion may die. This condition is called myocardial infarction. CHD can also interfere with the normal electrical activity of the heart, resulting in disturbances of the normal rhythm of heartbeats. Sudden and unexpected death is a common result of CHD. See the more extensive description of cardiovascular disease in Chapter 17.

The most widespread single cause of death for cigarette smokers is CHD. Studies have been done in which some factors related to CHD—high serum cholesterol, high blood pressure, physical inactivity, obesity, and irregularities in the rhythm of heartbeats—were controlled. The incidence of coronary heart disease was

still higher among cigarette smokers than among nonsmokers. Deaths from CHD associated with cigarette smoking are most common in people 40 to 50 years old. This age bracket is almost 20 years earlier than the age at which people have the greatest risk of dying from lung cancer caused by smoking. Cigar and pipe smokers have a much lower risk than cigarette smokers.

We do not understand how cigarette smoking increases the risk of CHD. It may promote the formation of plaques and speed the blood-clotting process. It may also increase tension in the myocardial walls, speed up the rate of muscular contraction, and increase the heart rate. The work load of the heart is thus greater, as is its need for oxygen and other nutrients. Carbon monoxide, which is produced by cigarette smoking, combines with hemoglobin in the red blood cells, displacing oxygen. This process means that less oxygen is available to the myocardium. Carbon monoxide in the system may also contribute to the development of atherosclerosis.

It is important to note again that the risks of CHD in cigarette smokers decrease when smoking is stopped. This decrease in risk for CHD occurs quite promptly after a person quits. The decrease is apparently most marked in younger ex-smokers. Cigarette smoking has also been found to be linked to several other cardiovascular diseases, including:

1. *Stroke*—sudden interference with the circulation of blood in a part of the brain.
2. *Aortic aneurism*—a bulge in the *aorta* due to a weakening in its walls.
3. *Pulmonary heart disease*—a disorder of the right side of the heart caused by changes in the blood vessels of the lungs

Cigarette smoking is a likely contributor in the development of atherosclerosis of the aorta. Besides possibly contributing to the formation of plaques in small blood vessels throughout the body, it also seems to make already existing diseases of the blood vessels worse. It definitely alters the circulation in the small blood vessels that carry blood from the arteries to the veins and actually bathe body tissue.

Other Health Hazards   Cigarette smoking is associated with many other health hazards, and the list keeps

Smoking Used to Be Good for Me

"I smoke for my health," I proclaimed in an essay in the *New York Times* in 1979. Since I am a physician, this medical advice attracted amused attention. I reasoned that smoking made me cough and thus prevented pneumonia. Smoking made my heart go faster and eliminated the need for additional exercise. Smoking curbed my appetite and kept me from getting fat.

I no longer smoke for my health.

My health can't stand the help. At 51, I had a heart attack. I squandered my inheritance. Risk factors for early heart attacks include hypertension, diabetes, a family history of heart disease, abnormal blood lipid patterns, and smoking. All the risk factors that I had no control over were in my favor. I chose to smoke.

Strange how the evidence that linked smoking to heart disease appeared equivocal to me last month, and now the same data appear overwhelmingly convincing.

Why stop now? Smokers who stop after their first heart attack have an 80 percent chance of living 10 more years—if they don't, a 60 percent chance.

As a smoker, I always resented the fact that we, as a group, received no gratitude, only scorn, from nonsmokers. How could nonsmokers know that smoking was bad for health if there were no smokers to prove it? Being a member of the experimental group, rather than the control group, deserves a certain measure of societal appreciation. I've done my time—I'm now ready to be a control.

Will I miss the late-night trips to find a store still open and selling cigarettes? Will I miss rummaging through ashtrays to find the longest butt that is still smokeable? Only time will tell. Not smoking may give me the time to find out.

Was it easy to stop? Sure. Here is all you have to do:

First, experience a severe crushing pain under your breastbone as you finish a cigarette. Next, have yourself admitted to a coronary-care unit and stripped of your clothing and other belongings. Finally, remain in the unit at absolute bed rest for four days while smoking is prohibited.

This broke my habit. See if it works for you.

Frank A. Oski
New York Times

---

getting longer. Most of these associations have only recently been discovered, however, so we still do not know whether there is a causal relationship between them or whether they merely exist together. Further research may link cigarette smoking to still other disorders.

Disorders of the mouth and gums are associated with cigarette smoking, as is tobacco amblyopia, a rare disorder of vision. About 19 percent of all people are allergic to tobacco smoke, tobacco pollen, and tobacco leaf. Tobacco also has harmful effects on the *immunity systems* of some people.

Cancer We have already noted the link between tobacco use and cancer of the lungs, oral cavity, and larynx. Pipe smoking has been identified as a cause of lip cancer. People who continue to smoke after the discovery of a mouth or throat cancer run a greater risk of developing a second independent mouth or throat cancer. Alcohol use also contributes to mouth and throat cancers, and people who both smoke and drink run a greater risk of mouth or throat cancer than do those who use only one of the drugs. Cigarette smoking has also been linked to cancers of the bladder and the pancreas.

Smoking and Pregnancy In recent years evidence has accumulated indicating that smoking during pregnancy has many more harmful effects than was formerly thought. This is especially true for mothers who are very young or very old or who have poor nutrition, are anemic, or have other health problems. These harmful effects include increased risk of spontaneous abortion, miscarriage, and stillbirths. If the baby is born alive, it is at increased risk for congenital abnormalities and its birth weight is likely to be lower. Lower birth weights are associated with increased mortality and a variety of diseases, especially infections. If the smoking mother has twins, the risk of at least one perinatal death (death just before, during or shortly after birth) is more than twice what it would be if she had stopped smoking during her pregnancy.

In addition to these established hazards, preliminary evidence suggests that infants born to smoking mothers are more likely to die from sudden infant death syndrome (see Chapter 7) and are more likely to show long-term impairments in physical growth and intellectual development. As if these problems were not enough, animal research evidence suggests that certain cancers may be more common in animals that were

Peptic ulcers
Open sores on the lining of the stomach or duodenum.

Acute disease
A severe disease of short duration.

Chronic disease
A disease that lasts a long time or recurs frequently.

Sinusitis
An inflammation of the linings of the air cavities that open into the nasal passages.

---

exposed as fetuses to cigarette smoke. Although there is no reason to think humans would be any less vulnerable, more investigation is clearly needed.

Ulcers Men who smoke cigarettes are more likely to have *peptic ulcers* than men who do not smoke, and they are more likely to die from them, especially from ulcers of the stomach. It is recommended that people who have ulcers stop smoking because smoking slows the rate of ulcer healing.

Cumulative Effects Statistical data has shown the cumulative effects of smoking.

Reduced Life Expectancy A boy who takes up smoking before age 15 and continues to smoke is only half as likely to live to age 75 as a boy who never smokes. If he inhales deeply, he risks losing one minute of life for every minute of smoking. Women who have similar smoking habits also have a reduced life expectancy.

Frequent Illness A National Health Survey begun in 1964 has produced some interesting findings. Smokers spend one-third again as much time away from their jobs as nonsmokers. Women smokers spend 17 percent more days sick in bed than women nonsmokers (including both women who work inside the home and women who work outside). Lost workdays associated

with cigarette smoking number 77 million. Days lost from work correspond to the intensity of smoking: Those who smoke half a pack a day lose nine-tenths of a day more per year than those who do not smoke, and those who smoke two packs a day lose three more workdays per year than nonsmokers.

Both men and women cigarette smokers show a greater rate of *acute* and *chronic disease* than those who have never smoked, and, as we have seen, certain diseases are more frequent among smokers. The U.S. Public Health Service estimates that if all people had the same rate of disease as those who never smoked, there would be 1 million fewer cases of chronic bronchitis, 1.8 million fewer cases of *sinusitis*, and 1 million fewer cases of peptic ulcers in this country every year. See Table 8–2.

There are also, of course, many areas in which the effects of smoking cannot be reduced to statistics. General health and well-being are not easy to measure.

Smokers' Effects on Nonsmokers

Smoke from the burning end of a cigarette differs from the smoke inhaled by the smoker in that it is not filtered by the remaining tobacco in the cigarette. Thus this unfiltered "sidestream" smoke contains twice as much tar and nicotine, five times as much carbon monoxide,

Table 8-2   Some Additive and Synergistic Effects* of Smoking

Smoking plus . . .	Enhances the risk of . . .
1. Hypertension	Coronary heart disease
2. Elevated cholesterol	Coronary heart disease
3. Diabetes	Peripheral vascular disease
4. Oral contraceptives containing estrogen	Heart attack (by tenfold)
5. Exposure to asbestos, rubber fumes, or uranium mining	Lung cancer
6. Exposure to coal dust, cotton dust, chlorine, or radiation	Chronic obstructive lung disease

*An *additive effect* means that if one behavior increases the risk of disease by 10 percent and a second behavior also increases the risk by 10 percent, then the combined risk to the person who demonstrates both of these behaviors is 20 percent. A *synergistic effect* means that the combined risk factor is greater than the sum of its parts.

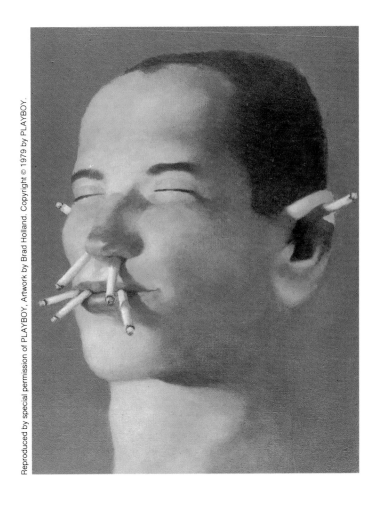

Statistical correlation
The amount of correspondence between
two sets of data.

and as much as 46 times as much ammonia as exists in inhaled smoke. Added to this concentrated source of air pollution is the 20 percent of smoke that the smoker inhales but does not absorb. Cigarette smoke from these two sources constitutes the most frequent and severe form of air pollution that most Americans experience. The most frequent violations of national air-quality standards take place in rooms where there is smoking. In some instances the concentration of nicotine and tar is so high that the nonsmoker is inhaling in an hour the equivalent of four to five cigarettes. It should not be surprising that nonsmokers exposed to such concentrations begin to develop many of the problems of smokers. After an hour or so in such an environment the nonsmoker has the same difficulties as the smoker in performing difficult perceptual tasks. Nonsmoking adults who regularly work in the same air space as smokers have objectively measured reductions in their breathing capacities. Similarly, nonsmoking children of smoking parents have a greater than average rate of breathing difficulties; infants of mothers who smoke require hospitalization for bronchitis and pneumonia significantly more often than infants whose mothers do not smoke. The higher incidence of these diseases in those exposed to smoke increases with the increasing number of cigarettes smoked by the mothers.

As more nonsmokers become aware of the health hazards being inflicted on them by smokers, they are becoming more militant in insisting on their rights to breathe clean air. An increasingly common assertion is that the smoker's right to smoke stops when his or her smoke reaches a nonsmoker's nose. In most scientifically advanced countries, the movement to protect people from tobacco smoke is gaining strength.

Other Forms of Tobacco Use

Snuff—powdered tobacco that the user sniffs—has never been very popular in America, although recently there has been an upsurge in its use. Chewing tobacco—tobacco leaves that have been mixed with molasses to be chewed—was the most popular form of tobacco use at the turn of the century, but it declined in popularity as cigarette smoking became more prevalent. Now it is

again coming into vogue in some parts of the country. Cigars also lost popularity, especially with the sharp increase in cigarette smoking that came about after World War I. Pipe smoking remained popular until the 1940s, but it is less so now. Some smokers have switched from cigarettes to pipes, cigars, or small cigars on the theory that they are less likely to inhale the smoke and therefore less likely to expose themselves to harm. This technique often does not work and is especially suspect when applied to small cigars. With these, the smoker may be changing only the color of the wrapping around the tobacco, not the degree of risk.

Other Opinions About the Health Hazards of Tobacco

Spokesmen for the tobacco industry and a few physicians have objected to studies that identify smoking as a cause of disease. A common argument is that these studies merely show a *statistical correlation* between smoking and health problems and cannot be taken as conclusive evidence of a causal relationship between the two. This argument ignores the fact that modern methods of scientific analysis and statistical assessment have resulted in predictions of great accuracy.

Another line of reasoning put forth by tobacco apologists goes like this: Cancer is evidently caused by a virus. How then can smoking be called a cause of cancer? The most likely explanation is that smoking upsets an equilibrium between the virus and the body cells, thus allowing the cancer to grow. Disease organisms and parasites, for example, often exist in the body but do not damage health until the body's internal ecology is disturbed.

Still another objection comes in the form of a question: "If smoking causes these diseases, why don't all smokers have them?" It is normal and expected that some smokers will not have these diseases because individuals differ so widely in their resistance to disease. Many diseases, including measles, smallpox, and the flu, are not contracted by everyone exposed to them.

Although the tobacco industry spokesmen claim there is no scientific proof that smoking causes any disease, the evidence—as summarized by H. S. Diehl in *Tobacco*

The Secondhand Smoke Issue

If you are a nonsmoker you need to be concerned about being exposed to tobacco smoke. It is an unnecessary hazard to your health. Compared to the smoke inhaled, there is twice as much tar and nicotine from the burning end of a cigarette, five times as much carbon monoxide, and 46 times as much ammonia. There are about 4,000 compounds generated by burning tobacco. Studies have shown that newborn children of smoking parents are twice as likely to develop pneumonia or bronchitis in the first year of life. Studies of the respirable suspended particulates (RSP) in indoor and outdoor environments in relation to smoking by the Environmental Protection Agency showed that "under the practical range of ventilation conditions and building occupation densities, the RSP levels generated by smokers overwhelm the effects of ventilation and inflict significant air pollution burdens on the public (*Science, 208:464, 1980*)." In an independent investigation from the University of California reported in the *New England Journal of Medicine* (March 27, 1980), Drs. J. R. White and H. F. Froeb wrote, "We conclude that chronic exposure to tobacco smoke in the world environment is deleterious to the non-smoker and significantly reduces small-airways function." The investigators demonstrated conclusively that "passive smoking," being forced to inhale the air polluted by smokers, does significantly affect the lung function, and the decreased lung function can be measured.

Many of the studies of the harmful effects of passive smoking are based on studying healthy people. The harmful effects of secondhand tobacco smoke can be much greater on those who have some illness. Dr. W. S. Aronow of the Long Beach Veterans Administration Hospital has studied the influence of passive smoking on men who have coronary artery disease and develop angina pain during exertion. He had men sit in a room with smokers and then tested them to determine how much exercise they were able to do before developing heart pain. Exposure to a room with smokers significantly decreased the amount of exercise the men could do before the pain started (*New England J. of Medicine*, July 6, 1978). He also noted an increase in blood pressure and irregular heart beats after the patients were exposed. The irregular heart beats could be serious, as such beats in heart patients may be the beginning of a serious and sometimes fatal irregularity.

Obviously the patient who has a pulmonary disease such as asthma or chronic bronchitis should not have the added burden of exposure to air polluted with tobacco smoke.

The Health Letter

---

and Your Health: The Smoking Controversy (1969)— is substantial:

> The diseases attributable to smoking are more frequent in smokers than in nonsmokers. They increase with dosage, that is, with the number of cigarettes smoked daily, with the degree of inhalation, and with the age at which smoking was begun; and the risk of developing these diseases decreases with the discontinuance of smoking. The tars in cigarette smoke produce skin cancer in animals; the nicotine affects the cardiovascular system; and cigarette smoke has produced lung cancer in mice and produces emphysema in dogs. Furthermore, there is no explanation other than one of cause and effect for the consistent . . . association of these diseases with cigarette smoking.

Furthermore, studies of large numbers of individuals born during the same period of time indicate that for each decade since 1890 there has been a progressive increase in smoking-related disorders among men. A similar increase did not show up for women until smoking became popular among women. Overall assessment of all these independent lines of investigation leads overwhelmingly to the conclusion that there is a direct cause-and-effect relationship between smoking and many health hazards.

What Can Be Done?

What can be done about the enormous health hazards associated with cigarette smoking? Much of what can be done on a political level has already been started. Advertising of cigarettes on radio and television has been eliminated. Cigarette packages and ads are required to carry the words "Warning: The Surgeon General Has Determined That Cigarette Smoking Is Dangerous to Your Health." More and more restrictions are being placed on smoking in public buildings, on airliners, and in other public places.

These efforts have been somewhat successful in reducing cigarette smoking in some age groups, but they are opposed by an impressive concentration of economic, social, and political power. Perpetuating tobac-

The Strength of Commitment

People strive to be right, and values and beliefs become internalized when they appear to be correct. It is this striving to be right that motivates people to pay close attention to what other people are doing and to heed the advice of expert, trustworthy communicators. This is extremely rational behavior. There are forces, however, that can work against this rational behavior. The theory of cognitive dissonance does not picture man as a rational animal; rather, it pictures man as a rationalizing animal. According to the underlying assumptions of the theory, man is motivated not so much to be right—rather, he is motivated to believe that he is right (and wise, and decent, and good). Sometimes, a person's motivation to

be right and his motivation to believe that he is right are working in the same direction. This is what is happening with the young lady who doesn't smoke and, therefore, finds it easy to accept the notion that smoking causes lung cancer. This would also be true for a smoker who encounters the evidence linking cigarette smoking to cancer and does succeed in giving up cigarettes. Occasionally, however, the need to reduce dissonance (the need to convince oneself that one is right) leads to behavior that is maladaptive and therefore irrational. For example, psychologists who have tried to help people give up smoking have reported the incidental finding that people who try to give up smoking and *fail*

come, in time, to develop a less intense attitude toward the dangers of smoking than those who have not yet made a concerted effort to give it up. The key to this apparent paradox is a person's degree of commitment to a particular action. The more a person is committed to an action or belief, the more resistant he will be to information that threatens that belief, and the more he will attempt to bolster his action or belief. If he has tried to quit smoking and has failed, he is committed to smoke. Thus, he becomes less intense in his belief that smoking is dangerous.

Elliot Aronson
The Social Animal

co use is a matter of some interest to these forces. The United States government has placed itself in the ironic position of paying for an aggressive anti-tobacco campaign at the same time that it subsidizes tobacco interests to the tune of about $30 million each year.

Our national epidemic of tobacco-related disease and death will not be reversed until each individual begins to take responsibility for his or her own health and well-being. To help in the process, a number of stop-smoking programs have become popular in the last few years. So far there is no convincing evidence that one particular method is more useful than others, particularly when the follow-up periods are a year or longer.

Most programs to stop smoking emphasize either a health-education approach or a pharmacological one. The traditional health-education programs often implicitly assume that if an individual has learned the facts about smoking he or she will make the rational decision to stop smoking and will quit. Since human behavior is not that simple and not that rational, the failure rate of these clinics tends to be quite high. For one reason, nicotine's powerful addicting qualities often overwhelm the smoker's conscious desire to stop smoking.

Most smoking clinics treat stopping as an event and assume that when the program is over, the smoking problem will also have stopped. These clinics provide

a social environment with psychological supports that no longer function for the smoker when the program ends. The behavioral reinforcers that maintained abstinence are no longer present. Learning theory suggests that when the reinforcers disappear, so does the behavior. Giving up smoking (or other drug dependencies) is invariably a long-term, intricate process. Heavy smokers who say they have stopped "cold turkey" do not reveal the thinking and struggling and other mental processes that contributed to the final overt behavior. The naïve assumption that smoking is an event rather than a process probably accounts for the unspectacular results of most programs. These programs stand in contrast to Alcoholics Anonymous, an apparently successful intervention group (although scientific evidence is lacking) that manages to provide a supportive social environment for long periods of time. It is interesting to note that when people drop out of Alcoholics Anonymous they frequently resume drinking.

Contemporary pharmacological programs usually emphasize the substitution of nicotine-containing chewing gum or other substances for cigarette smoking. These programs seem to be effective with a small number of smokers, usually fewer than 25 percent, especially if combined with other forms of psychological and social reinforcement. However, their major draw-

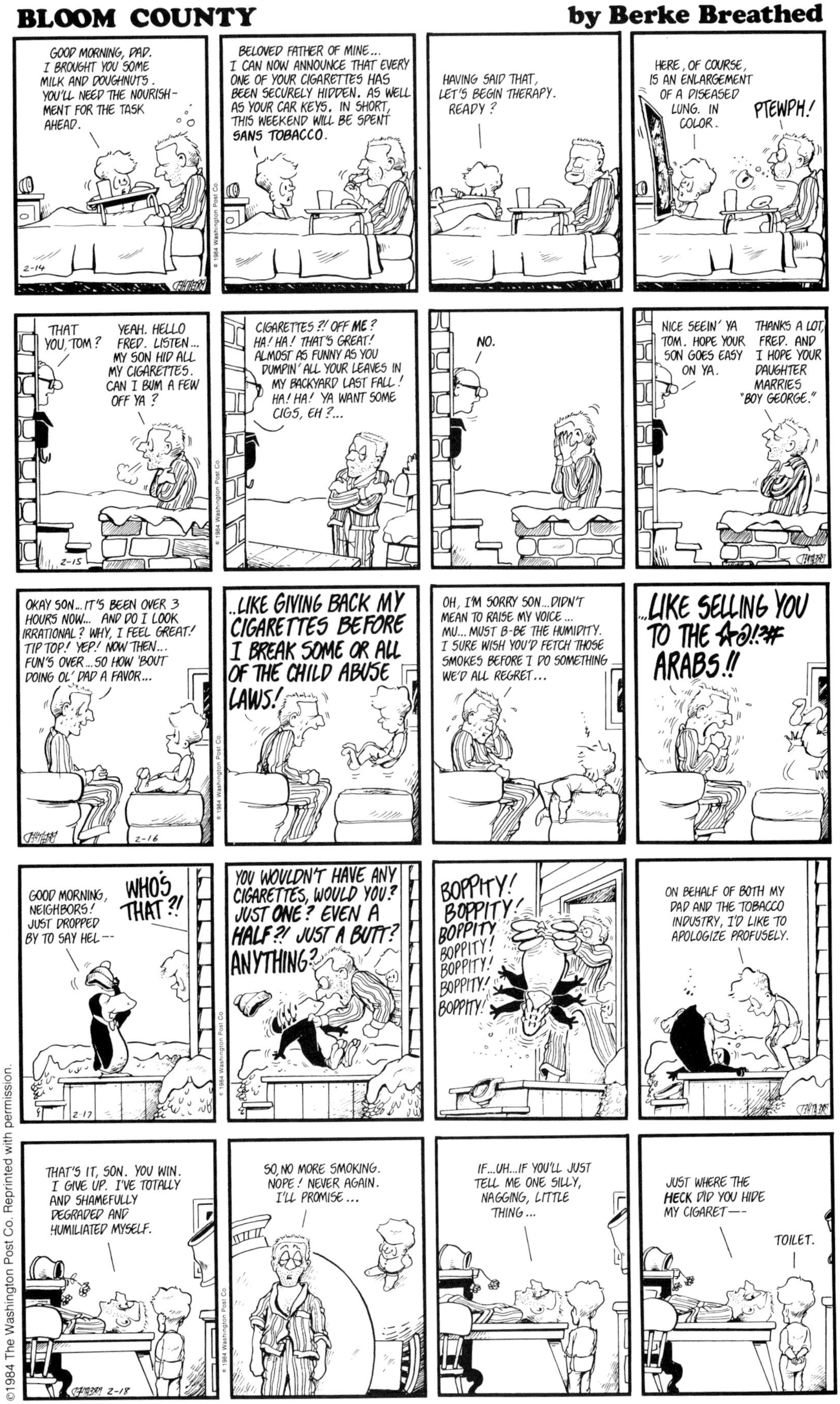
BLOOM COUNTY
by Berke Breathed
GOOD MORNING, DAD. I BROUGHT YOU SOME MILK AND DOUGHNUTS. YOU'LL NEED THE NOURISHMENT FOR THE TASK AHEAD.
BELOVED FATHER OF MINE... I CAN NOW ANNOUNCE THAT EVERY ONE OF YOUR CIGARETTES HAS BEEN SECURELY HIDDEN. AS WELL AS YOUR CAR KEYS. IN SHORT, THIS WEEKEND WILL BE SPENT SANS TOBACCO.
HAVING SAID THAT, LET'S BEGIN THERAPY. READY?
HERE, OF COURSE, IS AN ENLARGEMENT OF A DISEASED LUNG. IN COLOR.
PTEWPH!
2-14
THAT YOU, TOM?
YEAH. HELLO FRED. LISTEN... MY SON HID ALL MY CIGARETTES. CAN I BUM A FEW OFF YA?
CIGARETTES?! OFF ME? HA! HA! THAT'S GREAT! ALMOST AS FUNNY AS YOU DUMPIN' ALL YOUR LEAVES IN MY BACKYARD LAST FALL! HA! HA! YA WANT SOME CIGS, EH?...
NO.
NICE SEEIN' YA TOM. HOPE YOUR SON GOES EASY ON YA.
THANKS A LOT, FRED. AND I HOPE YOUR DAUGHTER MARRIES "BOY GEORGE."
2-15
OKAY SON... IT'S BEEN OVER 3 HOURS NOW... AND DO I LOOK IRRATIONAL? WHY, I FEEL GREAT! TIP TOP! YEP! NOW THEN... FUN'S OVER... SO HOW 'BOUT DOING OL' DAD A FAVOR...
..LIKE GIVING BACK MY CIGARETTES BEFORE I BREAK SOME OR ALL OF THE CHILD ABUSE LAWS!
OH, I'M SORRY SON... DIDN'T MEAN TO RAISE MY VOICE... MU... MUST B-BE THE HUMIDITY. I SURE WISH YOU'D FETCH THOSE SMOKES BEFORE I DO SOMETHING WE'D ALL REGRET...
..LIKE SELLING YOU TO THE @!?# ARABS!!
2-16
GOOD MORNING, NEIGHBORS! JUST DROPPED BY TO SAY HEL--
WHO'S THAT?!
YOU WOULDN'T HAVE ANY CIGARETTES, WOULD YOU? JUST ONE? EVEN A HALF?! JUST A BUTT? ANYTHING?
BOPPITY! BOPPITY! BOPPITY BOPPITY! BOPPITY! BOPPITY! BOPPITY!
ON BEHALF OF BOTH MY DAD AND THE TOBACCO INDUSTRY, I'D LIKE TO APOLOGIZE PROFUSELY.
2-17
THAT'S IT, SON. YOU WIN. I GIVE UP. I'VE TOTALLY AND SHAMEFULLY DEGRADED AND HUMILIATED MYSELF.
SO, NO MORE SMOKING. NOPE! NEVER AGAIN. I'LL PROMISE...
IF... UH... IF YOU'LL JUST TELL ME ONE SILLY, NAGGING, LITTLE THING...
JUST WHERE THE HECK DID YOU HIDE MY CIGARET--
TOILET.
2-18
© 1984 Washington Post Co.

Gum to Help You Stop Smoking

Mark Twain once noted, ironically, that it was quite easy to stop smoking: "I've done it a thousand times."

Most smokers—especially cigarette smokers—know exactly what Twain meant. National surveys indicate that nearly one-third of the cigarette smokers in the U.S. attempt to quit each year, but less than 20 percent of those who try remain abstinent for even a few months.

Millions of Americans have become ex-smokers since 1964, the year the first surgeon general's report on smoking was issued. But there are still some 55 million cigarette smokers in the U.S.—2 million more than in the year following that landmark report. At a conference last January commemorating the 20th anniversary of the report, Dr. Luther Terry, the surgeon general in 1964, attempted to explain why.

In the initial weeks following the report's release, said Terry, "millions of people gave up smoking. Sales dropped—in some stores, to literally no sales at all. And we were jubilant." He and his colleagues thought they might have "conquered" cigarette smoking, "which would have meant that we had conquered lung cancer," he said, "or at the very least, most cases of lung cancer."

"We were wrong," Terry continued. "Not altogether wrong, but mostly wrong. In a very few days people were back smoking again." In hindsight, he explained, "we vastly underestimated the dependency factor involved in cigarette smoking." For most smokers, what was commonly called a "habit" was actually a classic form of addiction, involving the drug nicotine.

In recent years, that new perception has spurred research on ways to deal with the addictive nature of smoking. One result has been the development of a product intended to help smokers quit. Early in [1984], the Food and Drug Administration approved a nicotine chewing gum, *Nicorette,* for marketing in the U.S. Described as a "nicotine resin complex" by its U.S. distributor, Merrell Dow Pharmaceuticals Inc., *Nicorette* is a prescription drug in chewing-gum form. The patented formulation is made in Denmark by A. B. Leo, a Swedish company. It is the only brand currently on the world market. The gum is marketed as a temporary aid for smokers trying to quit, especially in physician-supervised programs or in smoking-cessation groups or clinics.

Nicorette comes in a packet containing 96 individual squares of gum, each supplying a two-milligram dose of nicotine (roughly the yield of two *Winstons* or *Marlboros*). The gum is chewed slowly for 20 to 30 minutes, releasing nicotine gradually. This serves to relieve the withdrawal symptoms—such as irritability, restlessness, difficulty in concentration, and the like—that most smokers experience on quitting. . . .

A Stubborn Addiction

. . . While all forms of tobacco use can be addictive, cigarette smoking is especially so. Most cigarette smokers inhale the smoke into their lungs, where a high concentration of nicotine passes into the pulmonary veins and travels to the brain within seven seconds. By comparison, heroin injected into a vein in the arm requires about 14 seconds to reach the brain. Thus, with each puff, the cigarette smoker administers a rapid, concentrated dose of nicotine to the brain, achieving a measure of gratification that may be stimulating, relaxing, or satisfying in some way. And this act is repeated hundreds of times a day, more frequently than any other form of drug-taking.

Over the years, researchers have sought ways of administering nicotine without the accompanying smoke. Nicotine isn't benign, of course (a large dose can be lethal, and the small doses in tobacco smoke may have adverse effects on the cardiovascular system and the fetus). However, other substances in tobacco smoke, such as the chemicals collectively called "tar," are the ones implicated in causing cancer. So, if the nicotine craving could be satisfied by nicotine administered alone, the risk of cancer would be reduced or avoided.

Nicotine in pills or capsules doesn't serve the purpose because ingested nicotine is broken down by the liver before it ever reaches the brain. Injections of nicotine bypass the liver; they will reduce both cigarette consumption and the craving to smoke. But too many injections are needed for the approach to be practical.

An alternative method—the one exemplified by *Nicorette*—is to combine nicotine into a chewing gum. The nicotine is absorbed through the lining of the mouth directly into the bloodstream. The user controls the release of nicotine by the rate of chewing.

Nicorette can produce overall blood levels of nicotine similar to those obtained from cigarettes. What it can't do, however, is deliver the rapid, concentrated doses of nicotine that inhaling on a cigarette does.

Consequently, while *Nicorette* may ease the physical craving for nicotine, it doesn't offer the nicotine "rush" a cigarette smoker experiences. The effect is practical rather than pleasurable. The aim is to relieve withdrawal symptoms, which may last for days or months. The smoker still has to adjust to living without the gratification that was obtained from cigarettes.

Does It Work?

In promotional literature, Merrell Dow emphasizes that *Nicorette* is not a panacea. And indeed it isn't, as its track record in clinical trials reveals. But those trials also indicate that *Nicorette* is significantly better than a placebo.

At the Addiction Research Unit of Maudsley Hospital in London, for example, 116 cigarette smokers participated in a well-controlled trial of *Nicorette*. Half of the participants received the actual nicotine gum, while the rest received a placebo gum identical in appearance and taste. Both the treatment and control subjects received support and counseling, including instructions on the use of the gum, several weekly group meetings, and follow-up visits to the addiction center.

The results of the study, reported in the *British Medical Journal* in August, 1982, indicated that *Nicorette* had a decided effect. Forty-seven percent of those who used the active gum were not smoking at the end of one year, compared with 21 percent of those who chewed the placebo.

A more recent study conducted in California also produced results favoring *Nicorette*. Sixty participants receiving similar counseling and support were divided at random into equal treatment and control groups. Both groups were composed of long-term, heavy smokers who had repeatedly tried to quit. At the end of one year, 30 percent of the *Nicorette* group were still not smoking, while only 20 percent of the control group remained abstinent. Although the difference wasn't as pronounced as in the London study, it was still statistically significant.

The study, which was conducted jointly by researchers at UCLA and the Veterans Administration Medical Center in Brentwood, also included a separate "dispensary" group of 36 subjects. The participants received no counseling or other support. They were merely given supplies of *Nicorette* or an identically contrived placebo. Under these conditions, only about 10 percent were not smoking after one year, and the difference in success rates between *Nicorette* and the placebo gum was insignificant.

Overall, the researchers in London and California drew several conclusions from the studies. Among the most important was that *Nicorette* had its main effect during the early phase of quitting. It enabled more smokers to quit initially and remain abstinent during the first several weeks, the period when withdrawal symptoms are likely to be most intense.

Careful instructions and professional support, including both information and encouragement, were found to be highly important. For example, nicotine gum produces a mild burning sensation or "peppery" taste that is slightly unpleasant. It also causes transient side effects, such as mild indigestion and hiccups, especially if the gum is chewed too vigorously. Being prepared for such drawbacks can make it easier to tolerate them.

In the London study, the people using *Nicorette* found their gum more distasteful initially than did the people using placebos. By the second week, however, the situation was reversed. The *Nicorette* users had adjusted to the gum and were finding it more satisfying than the placebo users found theirs, which wasn't easing withdrawal pangs.

If you're hoping to give up smoking, don't settle for a doctor who simply writes a prescription for *Nicorette* and leaves it at that. As one expert remarked, that's like "handing a diabetic patient some insulin and syringes and saying 'Good luck.'" Ask the doctor to refer you to a program or to another professional familiar with the use of the gum.

Meanwhile, two other points are worth considering—one suggested by the studies and one suggested by virtually all experts in the field of smoking cessation. First, bear in mind that the participants in the trials were all highly motivated to quit. If you're not eager to give up smoking, *Nicorette* is unlikely to be of much help. Second, and more important, is that few smokers succeed in quitting permanently on the first try—or even on the first few attempts. It can take several efforts to achieve long-term success. If you've tried and failed before but still want to quit, *Nicorette* offers another opportunity. It's nothing like a sure-fire cure, but it is the first product to come along that just might increase your chances of succeeding.

Consumer Reports

back is that the addiction to nicotine remains untreated. When these nicotine-containing substitutes for cigarettes are discontinued, many people begin to smoke again. In addition, many people do not find these substitutes very satisfying, and unpleasant side effects are common.

Since giving up smoking is usually a lengthy process that is influenced by many factors, not one of which is by itself highly predictive of success in quitting, it is reasonable to consider smoking cessation programs that combine a number of different approaches. These programs, which sometimes operate in industrial settings, may be attractive to people who would not participate in a smoking clinic. They often include such components as altering the social environment by setting up demands and expectations against smoking. Peer support is often an extremely important influence on behavior, as is shown by experiences with Alcoholics Anonymous. The persistent encouragement of colleagues, family, and friends can be critical in giving up drug dependencies. Providing individual or group incentives is another intervention that can be usefully combined with other techniques. Determining an individual's cardiac and respiratory status can be a compelling method of inducing an individual to stop smoking. And documenting improvement in vital functions after the cessation of smoking can continue to provide positive reinforcement.

Benefits from Quitting

Studies in the last few years have shown that when smokers stop, a number of changes start to occur. Food is absorbed more efficiently, the appetite increases, and the senses of taste and smell are improved. In some people these changes lead to unwanted weight gain—but they are signs of health. Cardiovascular changes include increased circulation—in the extremities especially—a reduction in heart rate, decreased blood pressure, and increased heart efficiency during rest and exercise.

Many ex-smokers report more energy, increased alertness, and need for less sleep. Because of the increase in microcirculation to the skin, some people report improvements in their facial complexion.

As one might expect, changes in the respiratory system are often pronounced. There is an immediate improvement in the efficiency of oxygen exchange between the lungs and the circulatory system, the maximal breath capacity increases, and the breathing rate decreases. Gradually there is a reduction in the cigarette-induced "smoker's cough" and improvement in long-term respiratory conditions such as bronchitis, emphysema, and asthma.

The younger people are when they stop smoking, the more pronounced the health improvements. And these improvements invariably increase as the period of nonsmoking increases.

Smoking Attitude and Behavior Scale

Read the following statements carefully. Choose the one in each section that best describes you at this moment and record its score at the right. (For example, "never smoked" has a score of 5.) When you have identified five statements, total your score and find your position on the scale.

5 never smoked
4 quit smoking over one year ago
3 quit smoking recently
2 smokes occasionally
1 smokes regularly

Score _____

5 objects to smoking environments
4 avoids smoking environments
3 tolerates smoking environments
2 is sensitive to nonsmokers' complaints
1 ignores no-smoking signs

Score _____

5 discourages smoking in others
4 discourages teenagers from smoking
3 complains about smoking around children
2 defends smoking habit
1 denies any health consequences of smoking

Score _____

5 views smoking as a serious health problem
4 views smoking as unattractive
3 finds cigarette ads distasteful
2 is somewhat influenced by cigarette ads
1 is strongly influenced by cigarette ads

5 supports no-smoking ordinances
4 would vote for no-smoking ordinances
3 occasionally complains to friends about their smoking
2 talks about quitting
1 has smoker's cough

Score _____

Total score _____

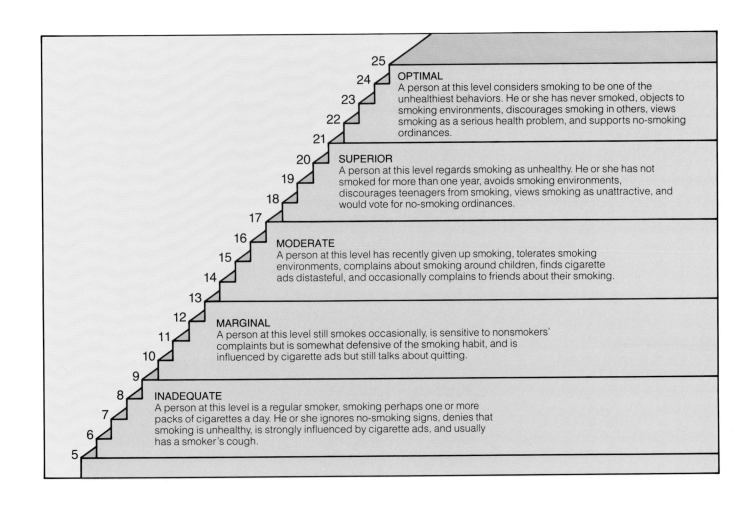

25
24 23 **OPTIMAL**
22 A person at this level considers smoking to be one of the unhealthiest behaviors. He or she has never smoked, objects to smoking environments, discourages smoking in others, views smoking as a serious health problem, and supports no-smoking ordinances.
21

20 19 **SUPERIOR**
18 A person at this level regards smoking as unhealthy. He or she has not smoked for more than one year, avoids smoking environments, discourages teenagers from smoking, views smoking as unattractive, and would vote for no-smoking ordinances.
17

16 15 **MODERATE**
14 A person at this level has recently given up smoking, tolerates smoking environments, complains about smoking around children, finds cigarette ads distasteful, and occasionally complains to friends about their smoking.
13

12 11 **MARGINAL**
10 A person at this level still smokes occasionally, is sensitive to nonsmokers' complaints but is somewhat defensive of the smoking habit, and is influenced by cigarette ads but still talks about quitting.
9

8 7 **INADEQUATE**
6 A person at this level is a regular smoker, smoking perhaps one or more packs of cigarettes a day. He or she ignores no-smoking signs, denies that smoking is unhealthy, is strongly influenced by cigarette ads, and usually has a smoker's cough.
5

Take Action

Your answers to Probing Your Emotions at the beginning of this chapter and your placement level on the Smoking Attitude and Behavior Scale will, we hope, encourage you to begin a process of self-exploration and self-discovery that you will continue. Reflect on the entire chapter's content and ask yourself how each point relates to your own life. Then take action:

1. In your notebook list the positive behaviors that help you avoid smoking or a smoker's environment.

Consider how you can strengthen those positive behaviors. Then list the behaviors that block your achieving wellness. Consider each behavior and decide which you can change. Begin with the easiest ones first. Reread Chapter 1 to review some general techniques for accomplishing these changes. Discuss them in class or with a close friend.

2. If you are a smoker, turn back to the personal contract for quitting smoking on page 10. Fill out and sign the contract and give it to a close friend. Ask him or her to return

it to you after the target date on the contract.

3. If you are a smoker, go to the student health clinic and ask to take a lung function test. Take along a friend who doesn't smoke and ask that he or she be allowed to take the test, too. Compare the results. If you don't smoke, recruit a smoking friend.

4. Read the following Behavior Change Strategy, and take the appropriate action.

Behavior Change Strategy

Quitting Smoking

There are relatively few bright lights on the horizon of smoking research. Many very intriguing, well-intentioned, and soundly based programs have failed to show any effectiveness. Most of the available research is based on people who have attended smoking cessation clinics even though the vast majority of smokers try to quit without such "hands-on" assistance.

The following program has demonstrated relatively greater therapeutic benefits than alternative approaches. You are urged to approach quitting smoking as a significant problem-solving challenge.

Any program, no matter how detailed, cannot possibly address all of the facets of the smoking habit in a way that will make it work for everyone. Yet there are some strategies and steps than can improve personal chances—your probability of lasting success—if they are modified by means of the feedback of experience.

There are three phases to quitting smoking: (1) preparation, (2) quitting, (3) and maintaining success. Each of

these stages will be discussed in order.

Preparation for Quitting   Preparation for quitting involves the collection of personal smoking information through the use of a detailed smoking diary. The format and a representative diary appear in Chapter 1, page 7. It is important to notice that the diary enables the smoker to collect two major types of information—cigarettes smoked and smoking urges. Part of the job of collecting this information is to identify patterns of smoking that are connected with routine situations (for example, the coffee-break smoke, the after-dinner cigarette, the tension-reduction cigarette, and so on).

The second major task of this preparation phase is to learn how to use nonsmoking relaxation methods. Many smokers find that they use cigarettes to help them unwind in tense situations or to relax at other times. Because smoking performs this useful function, it will be difficult to eliminate from your repertoire of behaviors unless you find effective substitutes. Since it takes time to become proficient at using progres-

sive relaxation, initial practice of this procedure is recommended early in the process of preparation. Refer to the more detailed discussion of progressive relaxation found on page 45 in Chapter 2.

Quitting   Quitting smoking is the goal that most smokers want to reach, but in this program it represents a necessary but insufficient accomplishment—staying off cigarettes is the ultimate objective. Quitting involves establishing a personal Quit Contract that specifies the day and time when you will stop smoking as well as possible rewards that can provide you with some immediate incentive for quitting. In this regard, it might be useful to identify the amount of money that you will save by not smoking a pack or so of cigarettes a day. You might set this money aside as a nonsmoking "salary."

In regard to the personal contract, smokers are usually torn between quitting abruptly (the so-called "cold turkey" approach) or through gradual reduction (one step at a time). Research favors the abrupt approach but with enough time set aside to learn and practice effective quitting skills. One useful approach to quitting helps the smoker appreciate the natural unpleasantness of his or her smoking. The procedure that can assist in the reawakening of this unpleasant side of smoking is called *aversive smoking* or, as we will refer to it here, *focused smoking.*

In focused smoking, the smoker stops all normal smoking and smokes only in unusual circumstances and in a manner that helps him or her concentrate only upon the negative aspects of normal smoking. Here is a suggested schedule for this practice. Note that there are "yes" days and "no" days; these refer to whether smoking is permitted in the special smoking sessions. All normal smoking is automatically prohibited. (It is simply too hard to establish unpleasant associations if one continues normal smoking.)

Many people may choose not to follow this focused smoking approach because they think that it is the same thing as self-punishment. In fact, the procedure serves several useful functions in that it avoids the withdrawal problems that might be encountered if you were to quit smoking abruptly; it solidifies a personal commitment to change; and it can help revive vivid images of the unpleasant impact of smoking on your immediate physical sensations (burning eyes, throat, mouth, and so on).

Maintaining Nonsmoking   Maintaining nonsmoking over time is the ultimate goal of any stop-smoking program, and it is the third phase of this program. The lingering smoking urges that remain once you have quit are the targets of work and planning because they will cause relapse if left unattended. Just as there are patterns to smoking, there are also patterns to lingering smoking urges that

Typical focused smoking schedule		Typical focused smoking session	
Monday:	YES	Step 1:	Smoke at regular pace with total concentration upon unpleasant aspects of the experience
Tuesday:	YES		
Wednesday:	YES		
Thursday:	No Smoking		
Friday:	YES	Step 2:	Five-minute rest period for reflection
Saturday:	No Smoking		
Sunday:	YES		
Monday:	YES (Quit Day)	Step 3:	Smoke one cigarette at normal pace with total concentration on the unpleasant features of that experience

Source: Adapted from B. G. Danaher and E. Lichtenstein, *Become an Ex-Smoker.* Englewood Cliffs, N.J.: Prentice-Hall, 1978.

can be identified through the use of an Urge Diary that looks very much like the smoking diary that appears on page 7. Patterns are often linked to situations in what seem like simple and innocuous ways. If you always used to sit the same way every evening to read the paper and watch the evening news—and have a cigarette—then even after you have quit smoking you may have smoking urges that are linked to that situation. By changing something in the situation—sitting in another chair or reading in another room—you may be able to break the strength of past associations. In the same way you will have to practice a new repertoire of nonsmoking skills if stress or boredom is a strong smoking-urge "signal" for you. It is very helpful to practice the relaxation procedures (which you should have been using since the preparation phase) to deal effectively with boredom or stress.

Cognitions, too, can be a source of considerable trouble during the maintenance phase of becoming an ex-smoker. Testing yourself ("I can prove that I'm stronger than that nicotine-filled product; let me smoke just one to prove my personal strength") and remembering

cigarettes as long-lost friends or part of a better, more enriched time in your life ("the good old days") can erode your sense of resolve and your skills in resisting lingering smoking urges. Identifying and listing personal pro-smoking self-statements can be exceedingly helpful in alerting you to the ways in which you can unwittingly undermine your own progress. Of course, it is essential to go beyond merely listing these thoughts; it is critical to *attack them* and *reduce their frequency* of occurrence.

Finally, in conjunction with the self-reward approach noted earlier (the nonsmoking "salary" idea), keep track of the emerging benefits that come from having quit smoking. Items that might appear on such a list include improved stamina, an increased sense of pride at having kicked a personally troublesome problem, improved sense of taste and smell, and so on.

There is no available cookbook of stop-smoking recipes that can be used word for word. This section has outlined some of the strategies that have helped others to quit smoking. Reread Chapter 1 to review the notion of personal problem solving and adaptation of these suggestions.

Chapter Nine

Alcohol

Probing Your Emotions

1. You have just come back from a football game and settled into a booth at a local tavern with some friends. Everyone orders a beer and begins to talk about the game. After you have been there for ten minutes another friend, Bill, comes into the room, and you call over to invite him to join your group. The waitress comes over and everyone orders another round. Bill orders a ginger ale. What goes through your mind about Bill when you hear his order? Do you feel negative, neutral, or positive about him?

2. Last Saturday you and three friends drove to a local roadhouse four miles from your college and spent the evening drinking and dancing. When you drove home you knew that alcohol was affecting your driving, but somehow you made it back without incident. The next day you don't remember precisely where you parked the car. In the Tuesday morning paper you read of a drunk driver who lost control of his car, careened through a road guard, and killed a pedestrian. You realize that accident could have been caused by you. How do you feel about the incident reported in the newspaper? How would you feel if the driver had been you?

3. You have just spent the evening enjoying a party you held at your home. In the early morning you are saying goodnight to a group that is leaving. One person in the group is staggering drunk. You realize that he should not drive home. You suggest he leave his car and ride home with someone else. He shakes off your suggestion and weaves out to his car. How do you feel about this risk? If you feel responsible, what should you do? What *would* you do?

Chapter Contents

ALCOHOL AND BEHAVIOR
Dose-response relationship
Time-action function
THE METABOLISM OF ALCOHOL
IMMEDIATE EFFECTS OF ALCOHOL
MEDICAL USES OF ALCOHOL
ALCOHOL ABUSE AND ALCOHOLISM
Complications of alcoholism
Treatment
THE RESPONSIBLE USE OF ALCOHOL

Boxes

The discovery of alcohol
Early indications of alcohol abuse
Alcohol-related social problems in the United States
College students' ten most common reasons for drinking alcohol
The autobiography of an alcoholic

Alcohol
The intoxicating ingredient in fermented liquors. A colorless, pungent liquid.

Intoxication
The stage of being mentally affected by a drug.

Distillation
The process of heating a mixture and recondensing the vapor. This process intensifies the mixture's properties and eliminates impurities. Distillation is used in manufacturing whiskey and brandy.

Psychoactive
Affecting the mind; specifically said of drugs that affect the brain or nervous system.

Intoxicant
Something that intoxicates; any drug that can affect one mentally.

Table wines
Beverages made from the fermented juice of grapes or other fruits with no extra alcohol added.

Fortified wines
Wines strengthened with additional alcohol. Sherry is an example of a fortified wine. Brandy is added to make it stronger.

Fermented
Describes a substance in which complex molecules have been broken down by the action of yeast or bacteria. Fermentation of certain substances produces alcohol.

Proof value
Two times the percentage of alcohol

9 People long ago recognized a power in alcoholic beverages: The "spirit" changed feelings and behavior. Ever since, *alcohol* has had a somewhat contradictory role in human life. It has been associated with good times, cheerfulness, and conviviality, but it is also associated with escape, with blotting out the world, with inch-by-inch suicide, and with general self-destructiveness. Many of our slang expressions for *intoxication* reflect its less positive aspects—"getting stoned," "smashed," "bombed," "blind drunk."

Alcohol is probably the oldest drug in the world; we have evidence that beer and berry wine were used at least by 6400 B.C. and probably even earlier. Alcohol has been used in religious ceremonies, in feasts and celebrations, and as a medicine for thousands of years.

Once the *distillation* process was developed (about A.D. 800), the spirit could be concentrated in a purer and more potent form. It was called *al-kuhl,* an Arabic word meaning "finely divided spirit." Throughout history alcohol has been more popular than any other drug, in spite of a great variety and number of prohibitions against it. In fact, forbidding the use of alcohol seems only to make it more popular. Even the newer *psychoactive* drugs have not diminished that popularity.

Ethyl alcohol, in various concentrations, is the common psychoactive ingredient in wine, in beer, in what are called hard liquors, and in liqueurs. Beer, a mild *intoxicant* brewed from a mixture of grains, usually contains from 3 to 9 percent of ethyl alcohol. Wines are made by fermenting the juices of grapes or other fruits.

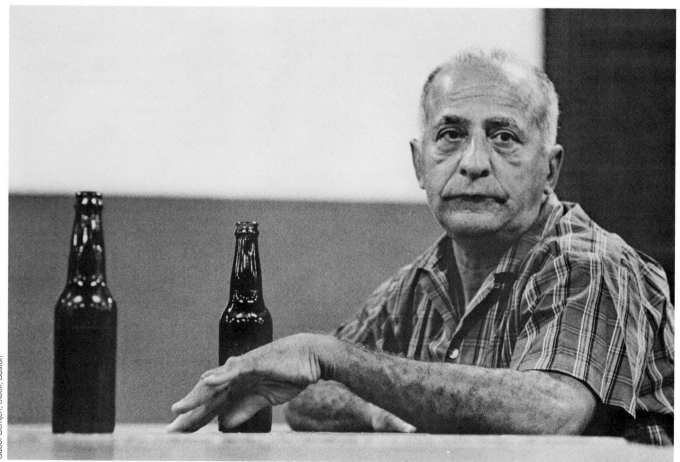

Gabor Demjen, Stock, Boston

Central nervous system
The brain and spinal cord.

Depressant
Something that decreases nervous or muscular activity.

Stimulant
Something that increases nervous or muscular activity.

Dose-response relationship
The relationship between the amount of a drug taken and the intensity or type of drug effect.

Blood alcohol concentration (BAC)
The amount of alcohol in the blood in terms of weight per unit volume.

Sedate
To calm by the use of a drug that quiets the activity of the nerves.

Stupor
A state of dulled mind and senses in which an individual has little or no appreciation of his or her surroundings.

Inhibition
The slowing down or suppression of a function.

The concentration of alcohol in *table wines* is about 9 to 14 percent. Other wines such as sherry, port, and madeira contain about 20 percent alcohol. These types are called *fortified wines* because distilled alcohol has been added to them. The stronger alcoholic beverages, such as gin, whiskey, brandy, and rum and liqueurs, are made by distilling brewed or *fermented* grains or other products. These beverages contain (usually) from 35 to 50 percent alcohol, a concentration about ten times that of beer.

Alcohol concentration in a beverage is indicated by the *proof value*, which is two times the percentage concentration. If a beverage is 100 proof, it contains 50 percent alcohol. Two ounces of 100 proof whiskey contain one ounce of pure alcohol. The proof value of the stronger alcoholic beverages can usually be found on the bottle labels. A convenient way of remembering alcohol concentrations is that the usual 12-ounce bottle of beer, 5-ounce glass of table wine, and cocktail with 1½ ounces of liquor all contain the same amount of alcohol—about 0.6 ounces.

Alcohol and Behavior

Alcohol is classified as a *central nervous system depressant*. When people drink in social settings, alcohol often seems to act as a *stimulant*, encouraging conversation and friendliness. This response probably occurs, however, because alcohol acts on people to make them lose their inhibitions, not because it stimulates the nervous system.

Dose-Response Relationship We do not know exactly how alcohol acts to influence individual behavior, but we can measure its effects according to relationships and factors that apply to most drugs. One important relationship in understanding the action of alcohol is the *dose-response relationship*. This term simply means that the influence of alcohol on behavior is likely to depend on how much the person takes in. The concentration of alcohol in the blood, called the *blood alcohol concentration (BAC)*, is a major determinant of drug effects. Alcohol at low concentrations makes people feel

relaxed, jovial, and euphoric, but at higher concentrations people are much more likely to feel angry, *sedated*, or sleepy. Subjects in experiments have been able to do simple motor tasks at low dose levels of alcohol better than otherwise. They do worse in the same tasks when they have had moderate higher doses. Very high BACs can cause *stupor* and sometimes death.

The effects of alcohol are first recognized at BACs of about 0.03 to 0.05 percent. These effects may include light-headedness, relaxation, and release of *inhibitions*. When the BAC reaches 0.1 percent, a major reduction in most sensory and motor functioning occurs. At 0.2 percent the drinker is totally unable to function, either physically or psychologically. Usually coma accompanies a BAC of 0.35 percent, and any higher level can kill a person. Figure 9–1 shows the results of a study of the relationship between drinking and driving. How much a person drinks (the dose) has an effect on how he or she drives (the response).

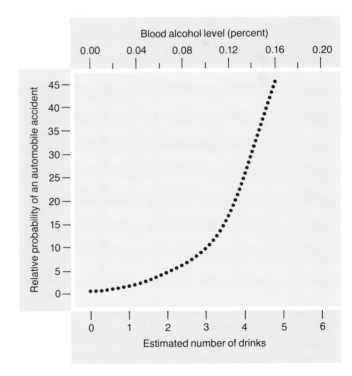

Figure 9-1 The dose-response relationship of alcohol levels and automobile accidents.

The Discovery of Alcohol

Man's first alcoholic beverage of which we have any historical record is beer. Clay tablets unearthed from the ruins of ancient Babylon show that the Babylonians were familiar with beer back in 5000 B.C. They considered it a gift from the gods and brewed it in their temples as part of their religious ceremonies. The brewers, all women, were priestesses.

The most avid beer drinkers of the ancient world were the Egyptians. Like the Babylonians, they regarded brewing as a divinely imparted secret, a gift from their goddess of nature, Isis. Every year Egypt's pharaohs consecrated a large quantity of beer in her honor and distributed it to the workers and peasants. The usual allotment was two jugs a day. The rest of the Egyptians bought their beer. For

their protection, there was an official superintendent of breweries who made sure that beer sellers offered only the best and purest brews.

Egyptian beer was called *hek*. It was made from barley bread that was crumbled into jars, covered with water, and allowed to ferment. The liquid was then strained off and drunk. For long journeys across the desert, only the fermented bread crumbs were carried. When the travelers reached an oasis, water was added to the jars; the result: instant beer.

At some point in history, brewing was also discovered by the tribes of Northern Europe. There, too, it was involved with religion. The Allemanni, a German tribe, had their beer brewed under the supervision of their priests, who also blessed it

before it was consumed. The Vikings not only drank beer in great quantities, they also believed that the spirits of their dead warriors were taken to an enormous banquet hall, Valhalla, where they feasted every night on copious supplies of ale.

The art of brewing probably developed soon after man took up farming. His first crop was grain, from which he made bread. From there it was only a short step to the discovery of fermented grain, from which he made beer. In countries where grapes grew more abundantly than grain, however, the favorite drink was invariably wine.

Alice Fleming
Alcohol: The Delightful Poison

The estimated number of drinks is shown on the bottom axis. This representation is a rough guide in which one drink can be one cocktail, a 5-ounce glass of table wine, or one bottle of beer. The drinker is assumed to be a person of average weight (150 pounds). It takes more drinks to achieve a given BAC if the person weighs more, if he or she has eaten recently, or if the drinking is done more slowly. The vertical axis represents how likely the drinker is to have an automobile accident. Clearly, low doses of alcohol do not greatly increase risk, but as the dose increases, the risk of an automobile accident increases at a spectacular rate.

Time-Action Function   Over time, the body absorbs and *metabolizes* alcohol, causing a change in the BAC and, in turn, changes in behavior. The relationship between the time elapsed after taking a drug and its effects is referred to as the *time-action function* of a drug. For the same dosage, for example, the effects of alcohol are usually greater when the BAC is rising than when it is stable or decreasing.

The time-action function of alcohol is different in different individuals, depending on how quickly they absorb alcohol, how quickly they metabolize it, and how

much they weigh. How much people have already had to drink, their motivations for drinking, and expectations of it are also factors. A *syndrome* known as pathological intoxication is an example of individual variation in response to alcohol. Enough alcohol to make most people feel relaxed and mildly euphoric causes wild agitation, extreme mood swings, violent behavior, and amnesia in people with this syndrome.

How much experience people have had with alcohol greatly influences their response. When alcohol is used frequently, every day or so, and in large quantities, many people develop a *tolerance* and show fewer changes in behavior than one would expect for a given dose. *Chronic* users of alcohol may experience increased discomfort rather than reduced anxiety and feel worse rather than better. They may not get the positive effects from drinking that they look for.

The Metabolism of Alcohol

Alcohol is absorbed into the bloodstream from the stomach, small intestine, and colon. How long *absorp-*

Metabolize
To chemically transform food and other substances in the body into energy and wastes.

Time-action function
The relationship between the time elapsed since a drug was taken and the intensity of a drug effect.

Syndrome
The various characteristics of a condition or disease.

Tolerance
Lower sensitivity to a drug so that a given dose no longer exerts the usual effect and larger doses are needed.

Chronic
Describes a condition or disease that lasts a long time or recurs frequently.

Absorption
The passage of substances through the skin, lungs, and gastrointestinal tract into the blood.

---

tion from the stomach takes depends on the amount, type, and proof of the beverage, the time taken to drink it, individual differences in such factors as weight and metabolic rate, and whether or not there is food in the stomach. Food in the stomach generally slows the absorption process. Absorption from the small intestine, however, is rapid and complete. It is not affected by either the BAC or the presence of food.

After alcohol is absorbed, it is distributed throughout the tissues of the body. In general, the greater the blood supply of a part of the body, the higher the concentration of alcohol. Since women usually have a higher percentage of fat at any given body weight than men do and since less alcohol is distributed in fatty tissues, women will have a higher BAC with the same amount of alcohol than will a man of the same weight (see Table 9–1). From 90 to 98 percent of alcohol is completely metabolized

in the liver at a rate that stays about the same in each individual. A person who weighs 150 pounds and has normal liver function metabolizes on the average about 0.3 ounce of alcohol per hour.

If an individual drinks slightly less alcohol each hour than the amount he or she can metabolize in an hour—about half a bottle of beer or half of an ordinary-size drink—the BAC remains low. People can drink large amounts of alcohol this way over long periods of time without becoming noticeably intoxicated.

If this same individual drinks just a little bit more than he or she can metabolize, his or her BAC will steadily increase, and he or she will become more and more drunk (see Table 9–2). Despite popular myths, there is no way that people can significantly speed up their metabolism of alcohol. The rate of alcohol metabolism is the same whether the person is asleep or awake.

Table 9-1   Drinking and Blood Alcohol Concentrations

Alcoholic beverage consumed in one hour	Blood alcohol levels (mg/100 ml-%w/v)					
	100 lb		*150 lb*		*200 lb*	
	Female	*Male*	*Female*	*Male*	*Female*	*Male*
One can or bottle of beer (12 ounces of 5% beer) *or* One glass of wine (5 ounces of 12% table wine) *or* One cocktail or mixed drink (1½-ounce jigger or shot of 80-proof spirit)	0.05	0.04	0.03	0.027	0.024	0.020
Two cans/bottles of beer *or* Two glasses of wine *or* Two cocktails/mixed drinks	0.10	0.08	0.06	0.05	0.05	0.04
Four cans/bottles of beer *or* Four glasses of wine *or* Four cocktails/mixed drinks	0.20	0.16	0.12	0.10	0.09	0.08

Immediate Effects of Alcohol

Alcohol acts as a depressant on the central nervous system. This fact is the overall reason for the changes that result from drinking. Physiologically, it first depresses a part of the brain that is involved in coordinating various parts of the nervous system. It also interferes with the processes that control inhibitions and depresses the function of nerves, muscles, including the heart muscle, and many other body tissues. We do not know precisely how alcohol exerts these effects.

Most people are familiar with the usual immediate effects of alcohol on behavior. These effects include anxiety reduction, mild euphoria, muscle incoordination, slurring of speech, and enhanced conviviality or assertiveness. As we have noted, low doses of alcohol sometimes make people better able to perform simple tasks, but complex behavior, such as driving, is impaired. Moderate doses markedly interfere with coordination, intellectual functions, and verbal performance.

At higher doses the individual may be easily angered or given to crying. Drinkers who take very high doses risk pronounced depression of the central nervous system, with stupor, unconsciousness, even death.

Shakespeare described the effects of alcohol on sexual performance. He said (in *Macbeth*) that it "provokes, and unprovokes; it stirs up desire, but it takes away the performance." His description was accurate. Small doses may improve sexual performance for individuals who are especially anxious or self-conscious, but higher doses usually make it worse. Excessive alcohol use on either an acute or chronic basis can result in reduced capacity for an erection response in the sexually aroused man and in reduced capacity for vaginal lubrication in the sexually excited woman.

Alcohol, particularly in large amounts, definitely changes sleep patterns. Even after the habitual drinker stops drinking, his or her sleep patterns may be altered for weeks or months.

Alcohol even in relatively small amounts can alter liver

Table 9-2   Alcohol Metabolism

Blood alcohol levels (percent)	Behavioral effects	Hours required for alcohol to be metabolized
0.00–0.05	Slight change in feelings—usually relaxation and euphoria. Decreased alertness.	2–3
0.05–0.10	Emotional lability with exaggerated feelings and behavior. Reduced social inhibitions. Impairment of reaction time and fine motor coordination. Increasingly impaired during driving. Legally drunk at 0.08 in Utah and 0.10 in many other states.	4–6
0.10–0.15	Unsteadiness in standing and walking. Loss of peripheral vision. Driving is extremely dangerous. Legally drunk at 0.15 in all states.	6–10
0.15–0.30	Staggering gait. Slurred speech. Pain and other sensory perceptions greatly impaired.	10–24
More than 0.30	Stuperous or unconscious. Anesthesia. Death possible at 0.35% and above.	More than 24

Cardiovascular system
The heart and blood vessels.

Alcoholic
A person addicted to drinking alcoholic beverages.

High-density lipoprotein (HDL)
Chemical in the blood thought to be protective against heart disease.

Fetal alcohol syndrome
Birth defects caused by excessive alcohol consumption by the mother.

Coagulant
A substance that causes or speeds blood clotting.

Angina pectoris
Severe chest pain.

---

function and can irritate and inflame the pancreas, a condition that can mean nausea, vomiting, abnormal digestion, and severe pains in the abdomen. It may harm the kidneys over longer periods of time, but such harm does not happen often. It also increases production of urine.

Alcohol affects the *cardiovascular system* in numerous ways. Although some *alcoholics* develop cardiovascular diseases, it is not clear that these conditions develop as a direct result of sustained alcohol use. Since alcoholics derive most of their caloric requirements from alcohol, the malnutrition and vitamin deficiencies that many of them experience in combination with alcohol use may cause certain types of heart disease. In addition, most heavy drinkers also are heavy smokers. On the other hand, recent studies suggest that moderate amounts of alcohol increase blood levels of certain *high-density lipoproteins (HDLs)*, substances that are thought to offer some protection against heart attacks. However, the relationship between cardiovascular disease and alcohol use remains unclear.

Alcohol causes blood vessels near the skin to dilate, and drinkers often feel warm; their skin flushes, and they may sweat more. Flushing and sweating contribute to loss of heat from the body, and so the internal body temperature falls. High doses of alcohol may affect the body's ability to regulate temperature, causing it to drop sharply, especially if the surrounding temperature is low. Drinking alcoholic beverages to keep warm in cold weather does not work, and it can even be dangerous.

Alcohol use has been linked to certain cancers of the upper digestive and respiratory tracts. It is difficult to get a clear picture of the relationship, however, because most heavy drinkers also smoke cigarettes, a practice that definitely increases the risk of several types of cancer. It is possible that alcohol is the main factor in certain cancers. It may also increase the risk already present from tobacco use.

Recent studies of animals and humans indicate that alcohol ingested during pregnancy can have harmful effects on the fetus. Women who drink, especially in excessive amounts, are at increased risk of giving birth to children who have a collection of birth defects known as the *fetal alcohol syndrome*. These children are small

at birth, are likely to have heart defects, and often have abnormal anatomical features including small, wide-set eyes. Even with the best of care, their physical and mental growth rate is slower during childhood than normal. In adolescence they sometimes catch up with their age mates in terms of physical size but not usually in mental abilities. Most remain mentally retarded with IQs in the 40 to 80 range. Although it was initially thought that the fetal alcohol syndrome was caused by poor nutrition associated with the alcoholism of the mother, subsequent research indicates that it results directly from excessive alcohol intake. We should remember that alcohol is distributed evenly throughout all water-containing tissues; when the mother has a blood level of 0.03 so does her fetus, and when a father has a blood alcohol level so does his sperm. There is no precise blood alcohol threshold level above which damage occurs and below which there is no danger. Instead the frequency and severity of defects progressively increase as the amount of drinking increases. As is the case with other drugs, the fetus seems especially vulnerable to alcohol during the first trimester of pregnancy. The safest course of action is abstinence.

Medical Uses of Alcohol

The value traditionally placed on alcohol "for medical purposes" is based more on imagination than fact. Alcohol sponges are commonly used to reduce fever because alcohol cools the skin by evaporation. In concentrations of 70 percent by weight, alcohol kills bacteria. It is used as an astringent and skin cleanser in treating skin disorders. Contrary to a popular myth, however, alcohol is not a good antiseptic for open wounds. It injures exposed tissues and may form a *coagulant* that protects rather than destroys bacteria. People who associate alcohol with dining pleasure may feel hungrier and digest their food better if they take a small amount of alcohol—a bottle of beer, a glass of wine—with their meals. Drinking alcohol has been thought by some to be useful in treating *angina pectoris,* a disorder in which the heart is unable to get enough

Alcohol abuse
The use of alcohol to a degree that causes physical damage, impairs functioning, or results in behavior harmful to others.

Alcohol dependence
Either pathological use of alcohol or functioning impairment due to alcohol and tolerance or withdrawal; also known as alcoholism.

Alcoholism
Chronic psychological and nutritional disorder from excessive and compulsive drinking; another name for alcohol dependence.

Cirrhosis
A disease of the liver caused by excessive and chronic drinking. Contrary to earlier medical belief, cirrhosis occurs even when nutrition is adequate.

---

oxygen. This remedy is doubtful. If the sufferer feels better, it is probably because he or she has been sedated rather than because his or her circulation is better.

Alcohol Abuse and Alcoholism

Recent definitions make a distinction between alcohol abuse and alcohol dependence, or alcoholism. According to the third edition of the *Diagnostic and Statistical Manual of Mental Disorders* (1980) of the American Psychiatric Association, "The essential feature of *alcohol abuse* is a pattern of pathological use for at least a month that causes impairment in social or occupational functioning. The essential features of *alcohol dependence*, which is also called *alcoholism*, are either a pattern of pathological alcohol use or impairment in social or occupational functioning due to alcohol, and either tolerance or withdrawal."

Other authorities use different definitions to describe problems associated with drinking. The important point is that one does not have to be an alcoholic to have problems with alcohol. The person who only drinks once a month, perhaps on payday or after an exam, but then drives while intoxicated is an alcohol abuser.

People of all social and economic classes use alcohol excessively, not just people who are considered to be skid row bums. Skid row bums account for only a small percentage of the total alcoholic population and usually represent the final stage of a drinking career that began years before. Among white American men, excessive drinking usually begins in the teens or twenties and gradually progresses through the thirties until the person is clearly identified as alcoholic by the time he is in his late thirties or early forties. It is relatively uncommon for alcoholism to begin in men after the age of 45 unless there are concomitant psychiatric problems such as depression. One should realize that there are different patterns of alcohol abuse. Here are four common patterns:

1. *Regular daily intake of large amounts.* This continuous pattern is the most common adult pattern of excessive consumption in most countries.

2. *Regular heavy drinking limited to weekends.* This continuous pattern is commonly followed by individuals in their teens.

3. *Long periods of sobriety interspersed with binges of daily heavy drinking lasting for weeks or months.* This episodic or "bender" pattern is common in the United States but quite uncommon in France, although the per capita consumption of alcohol is higher in France.

4. *Heavy drinking limited to periods of stress.* This "reactive" pattern is associated with periods of anxiety or depression, for example, examination or other performance fears, interpersonal difficulties, school or work pressures.

The "natural history" of alcoholism in women differs from that of men. Women tend to become alcoholic at a later age and fewer years of heavy drinking. It is not unusual for women in their forties or fifties to become alcoholic after years of controlled drinking, whereas this occurs infrequently in men. Women alcoholics also develop *cirrhosis* and other medical complications somewhat more often than men.

There are notable differences in patterns of alcoholic drinking among various racial and ethnic groups. For example, urban black males commonly start excessive drinking at a younger age than do urban white males, develop serious medical and neurological illnesses at an earlier age, and have a higher rate of alcoholism-related suicides. Excessive drinking among Indians varies from tribe to tribe and does not follow a consistent pattern. There is a very low rate of alcoholism in the Orient, and a high rate among the Irish.

Estimating the prevalence of alcoholism is complicated by disagreement about definition and other methodological problems. Although the figure of 9 or 10 million American alcoholics has often been cited, it is not based on scientific studies. More systematic studies of smaller geographic areas such as counties or states suggest that about 3 percent of all men are alcoholic and perhaps 0.1 to 1 percent of all women. It is somewhat easier to determine the quantity of drinking done by a given population. Studies show that about 20 percent of American men are heavy drinkers, meaning they drink daily and drink six or more drinks several times a month.

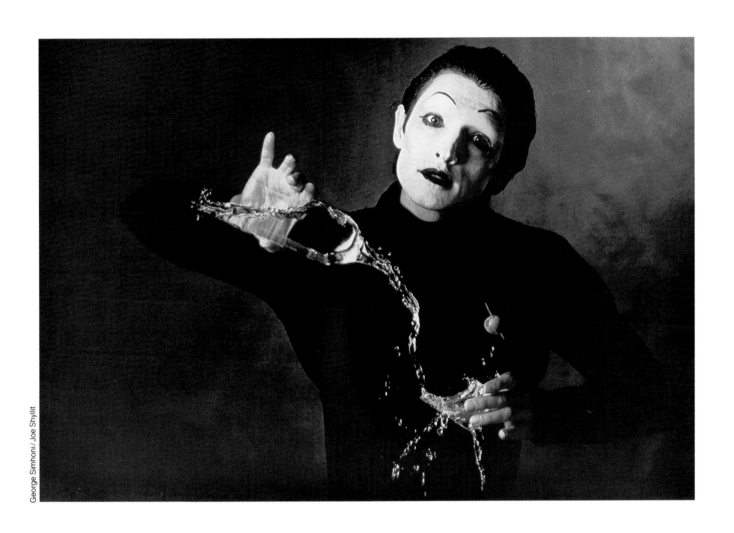

217

Withdrawal symptoms
Unpleasant physical and mental sensations experienced when abstaining from a drug to which one is addicted.

DTs (delirium tremens)
A state of confusion brought on by reduction of alcohol intake in a person addicted to alcohol. Other symptoms are sweating, trembling, anxiety, and hallucinations.

Hallucinations
False perceptions that do not correspond to external reality. A person who hears voices that are not there or sees visions is having hallucinations.

Early Indications of Alcohol Abuse

1. Drinking alone or secretively.
2. Using alcohol deliberately and repeatedly to perform or get through difficult situations.
3. Feeling uncomfortable on certain occasions when alcohol is not available.
4. Escalating alcohol consumption beyond an already established drinking pattern.
5. Consuming alcohol heavily in risky situations; for example, before driving.
6. Getting "drunk" regularly or more frequently than in the past.
7. Drinking in the morning or at other unusual times.

We do not know exactly what causes alcoholism. Probably a variety of factors are involved, all of which vary from individual to individual. Recent reliable studies have compared individuals who were adopted when they were young and individuals who lived with their biological parents. These studies showed that people are more likely to be alcoholics if their biological parents are alcoholics. Alcoholism in adopted parents, however, does not make individuals either more or less likely to become alcoholics. In other words, there apparently is a genetic contribution to susceptibility to alcoholism. Not all children of alcoholics become alcoholics, however, and it is clear that many other factors are involved. Personality disorders, being subjected as a child to destructive child-rearing practices, and imitating parents' and other important people's abuse of alcohol may all play a part. People who begin drinking excessively during their teenage years are especially prone to alcoholism later in life. Common psychological features of individuals who excessively use alcohol are denial—I don't have a problem—and rationalization—I drink because I need to socialize with my customers. The ten most common reasons given by college students for using alcohol are noted on page 220.

Certain social factors have been linked with alcoholism. These include urbanization, disappearance of the extended family and general loosening of kinship ties,

increased mobility, and changing religious and philosophical values.

Complications of Alcoholism   The consequences of alcoholism are well known. People definitely develop a tolerance to alcohol after repeated use. They require greater and greater amounts to produce the same psychological effect. Tolerance, however, develops at different rates to different effects of alcohol. For example, alcohol-induced depression of the respiratory system develops slowly and only to a small extent. Thus alcoholics are only slightly less susceptible to lethal respiratory depression from overdose than are moderate users. The same is true for users of barbiturates and most other sedating drugs.

When people continue to abuse alcohol for long periods of time, their tolerance may begin to decrease. Some chronic alcoholics have very little tolerance for alcohol, in part because their livers are so damaged that they no longer have adequate amounts of the enzymes necessary to metabolize alcohol.

When alcoholics stop drinking or cut their intake way down, they will have *withdrawal symptoms*. These can vary from merely unpleasant feelings to serious, even life-threatening, disorders. The jitters, or "shakes," are the most common withdrawal symptom and may last as long as two weeks. Seizures are less common, but they are more serious. Still less common is the severe withdrawal reaction known as the *DTs (delirium tremens)*, a dramatic state characterized by disorientation, confusion, and vivid *hallucination*, often of vermin and small animals.

Since alcohol is water soluble and distributed throughout most of the body, it can exert toxic effects on many different organs and tissues. Damage to the liver in the form of cirrhosis is just one well-known example. Asthma, gout, diabetes, and recurrent infections are more common in heavy drinkers than in people who drink moderately or not at all. Inflammations of the stomach, intestines, kidneys, bronchi, and peripheral nerves also occur more frequently in alcohol abusers. Other medical and psychiatric complications are associated with excessive alcohol use. Some of these alcohol-related medical problems are made worse by nutritional deficiencies that often accompany alcohol

Paranoia
A mental disorder characterized by false
beliefs that one is being persecuted, often
beliefs of a grandiose and logically systematic nature. There are no hallucinations,
and intelligence is not impaired.

abuse. Disorders of the liver, stomach, and intestine are
especially common, as are diseases of the nervous
system, but all vary among users. One individual may
primarily have defects of the central nervous system,
serious damage to the memory, and no liver or gastrointestinal damage. Another individual, with a similar
drinking and nutrition history, may have advanced liver
disease and no memory defects.

An alcoholic's medical and psychiatric problems often
respond rapidly to hospitalization, tranquilizers, and the
elimination of alcohol from the diet. These problems are
likely to return, however, if the person starts drinking
again. Some people have what is called *paranoid*
personalities. If they use alcohol excessively, they may
suffer delusions, jealousy, suspicion, and mistrust—the
so-called alcoholic paranoia.

Alcohol use causes more serious social problems than
all other forms of drug abuse combined. In a national
survey of drinking practices in the late 1960s, 31
percent of the people in the survey had had some
drinking problem during the previous three years. Of that
group, 40 percent of the men and 15 percent of the
women were psychologically dependent on alcohol; 12
percent of the men and 8 percent of the women had
health problems associated with drinking.

We cannot measure human suffering, but the toll from
alcohol must be staggering. Alcohol is involved more
often than any other drug in serious violent and sexual
crimes. In many violent crimes, both the offender and
the victim are found to have been drinking.

Alcohol abusers are also more likely to die in all types
of accidents. As we have already noted, the likelihood
of a serious or fatal automobile crash increases as the
BAC increases. Drinking even small amounts of alcohol
increases a person's chance of having an accident during
times of heavy traffic. When traffic is light, the effect of
small amounts of alcohol on driving usually is not great,
but the effect of large amounts is. Apparently, drivers
can make up for slight impairment in performance
caused by alcohol, but they cannot make the more
complex judgments demanded by heavy traffic. Visual
functioning is one specific aspect of driving that is
adversely affected by alcohol. In contrast to people who
are sober, intoxicated people blink more frequently and
have their eyes closed for longer periods of time; they

Alcohol-Related Social Problems in the United States

1. Alcohol-precipitated cirrhosis is the sixth leading
cause of death in the United States.
2. Alcohol abusers shorten their life spans by 10 to
12 years.
3. One-half of all traffic fatalities are associated with
alcohol use.
4. One-third of all homicides are associated with
alcohol use.
5. One-third to one-half of all fatal accidents (other
than traffic) are associated with alcohol use.
6. One-third to one-half of all crimes committed are
associated with alcohol use.
7. One-third of all arrests are for public intoxication.
8. Alcohol abuse and alcoholism drain the economy
of an estimated $15 billion per year. Of this total:
$10 billion is attributable to lost work time; $2
billion is spent for health and welfare services
provided to alcoholics and their families; and
property damage, medical expenses, and other
overhead costs account for another $3 billion.
9. One in every five persons is closely related to
someone who suffers from alcohol abuse.

also are unable to rapidly process as much information
when their eyes are open. The drinking driver is prone
to focus his or her gaze on one object such as a flashing
light or the center line and totally ignore other relevant
stimuli.

Unfortunately many individuals who have been drinking believe that their driving has improved, not gotten
worse. In fact, both their judgment and their coordination have been affected. When London bus drivers were
tested on their ability to drive a bus between two posts,
they showed little impairment in driving performance
despite drinking considerable amounts of alcohol. When
the experimenters moved the posts closer together
and reduced the distance between them to a few inches
less than the width of the buses, the sober drivers rec-

College Students' Ten Most Common Reasons for Drinking Alcohol

1. Increases my feelings of sociability.
2. Relieves anxiety or tension.
3. Makes me feel elated or euphoric.
4. Makes me less inhibited in thinking, saying, or doing certain things.
5. Enables me to go along with my friends.
6. Enables me to experience a different state of consciousness.
7. Makes me less inhibited sexually.
8. Enables me to stop worrying.
9. Alleviates depression.
10. Makes me less self-conscious.

ognized at once that the task was impossible, but the drunk ones did not and tried to drive between the posts anyway.

Treatment It is important to realize that some alcoholics recover without professional help. It is unknown how often this occurs, but perhaps as many as 25 percent of alcoholics "spontaneously" stop drinking or reduce their drinking to the point where problems do not occur. In a recent study of "problem drinkers," 9 percent of American adults were currently experiencing drinking problems. Another 9 percent had had drinking problems in the past but no longer did. One of the great debates in the field is whether "true" alcoholics can become controlled or social drinkers. Studies indicate this may occur, but it is the exception rather than the rule.

In any event, the majority of alcoholics do not stop their chronic excessive use of alcohol on their own. For these people treatment is difficult.

Many different kinds of treatment programs exist. Some, such as Alcoholics Anonymous, emphasize group and "buddy" support as well as personal testimonies. By contrast, the Raleigh Hills system includes

the use of aversion therapy in which the subject is conditioned to associate drinking alcohol with negative consequences such as medically produced nausea. The best treatment programs often involve a combination of a variety of techniques, such as Alcoholics Anonymous, psychotherapy (individual, group, and especially family or couple), and chemical therapies. None of these has been successful for all patients. As with the treatment of other drug dependencies, one major problem in treating alcoholics is predicting ahead of time which treatment will be most useful for a particular individual. Another major treatment problem has to do with long-term effectiveness. For example, one chemical treatment involves the use of disulfiram (trade name: Antabuse). Disulfiram causes patients to become violently ill whenever they drink. What usually happens is that after taking the drug for a while, the patient declares himself or herself to be "cured" and decides that he or she no longer needs the drug. The effect of the drug does not wear off for about four days, so the patient is able to avoid impulse drinking and may even gain enough momentum to stay "cured"—for a time. After weeks or perhaps months of not taking the drug, many patients start drinking again. We have yet to come up with satisfactory ways to treat people who have alcohol problems. That we do so is an urgent public health need.

Prescribing chemical substitutes such as diazepam (Valium) or chlordiazepoxide (Librium) for alcohol is a controversial treatment. Proponents argue that at least the more toxic alcohol is being replaced by a less toxic drug and thus the health hazard is reduced. Others claim that one drug dependency is merely being exchanged for another and many of the behavioral problems associated with the chemical abuse are unchanged. Like many controversies in the field of alcoholism and drug abuse, this one is unlikely to be resolved since value judgments are involved.

The Responsible Use of Alcohol

The responsible use of alcohol means drinking in such a way as to keep your blood alcohol level low so that your behavior is always under your control. Here are some tips.

The Autobiography of an Alcoholic

I took my first drink during my freshman year at college, the night I was initiated into my fraternity. One of the boys sold me on the idea that it was the thing to do in order to show I was a good sport. That first drink wasn't especially memorable. After all, one doesn't become a drunk overnight. I was a social drinker all during my college days. I've had many good times and suffered to some extent on the mornings after. In those days it never occurred to me to drink in the morning. I couldn't bear the sight of the stuff. I don't think it affected my scholarship much. In any event, I graduated—not brilliantly, but I did get my degree.

After college I began to drink more seriously. It was about two years after my school days that I took my first drink in the morning. I can see now that that morning was the beginning of the end. By then I was married and the father of a young son, but this added responsibility didn't seem to make any difference. Drinking was no longer a minor sport for me—I was becoming a pro. Now I drank every morning if I had had anything the night before—and I usually had.

Mysteriously enough, I managed to hold my first job for eleven years, but finally my boss reached the end of his endurance, and at almost the same time, so did my wife. Why go into all the details? Happy moments, yes, but terrible hours, too. Unbearable embarrassments, loss of friends, even jail. By this time, of course, I was really trying my damnedest to quit drinking. I spent hundreds of dollars on psychiatrists, and when I lost my job I went away to a private sanitarium for a month. This was an impressive experience, but it did me no good. I had the idea that this was a chance to build myself up physically, and when I got out I'd be able to start all over again—and this time I could handle it. I would never under any circumstances get drunk again.

From there I went to New York City and got a new job without much trouble. I started drinking again, but not the same way I had before. I'd have a couple of drinks, and then the next day it would be three, and the next day maybe four. This would go on for four or five weeks, and all this time I'd be going to work every day and managing not to make too many mistakes. Then the morning would come when I just couldn't make it to the office. For three or four days I'd stay in my apartment and drink. I wouldn't go out at all except to lay in another supply of the sauce.

Eventually the time would come when I'd be so weak and jittery that I knew I'd have to quit or die—and so I'd quit. Because when I was drinking I wasn't eating, I knew I ought to eat at least a little during these jags, and I'd fix a sandwich or something, but then I'd look at it and the thought of actually eating it was enough to make me sick. I was living alone and I didn't know anyone in New York well enough to ask for help, so the upshot was that I generally went to a hospital for a few days. Then I'd come out sober and repentant, and I'd be all right for a month or so, and then I'd start the whole thing over again.

Finally after losing my job again, I decided that the first thing I had to do was to go somewhere where I wouldn't be able to get a drink for a long time. And I did. The particular details aren't important, but what I've discovered about this whole business is: first, we problem drinkers must realize that we can never become moderate drinkers. The "reformed drunk" who becomes a moderate drinker never was a drunk in the true sense of the word. The real reformed alcoholic becomes a teetotaler. Second, and most important of all, we must decide that we don't *want* to become moderate drinkers. So long as the alcoholic persists in admiring the moderate drinker, so long as he wants to be a moderate drinker himself, sooner or later he's going to try it, and the only possible result is disaster.

Adapted from "Can the Alcoholic Become a Moderate Drinker?"
Mental Hygiene

---

1. *Drink slowly.* Learn to sip your drinks rather than gulp them. It helps to develop the habit of deliberately tasting and smelling the nuances of alcoholic beverages so that you can describe their similarities and differences. Learn to compare and contrast the different kinds of wines and beers.
2. *Space your drinks.* Learn to drink nonalcoholic drinks at parties—juices or tonic water without the alcohol, for example—and intersperse these with alcoholic drinks. Learn to refuse a round—"I've had enough for right now." It is easier for some people if they hold a glass of anything nonalcoholic that has ice and a twist of lime floating in it so that it looks like they are drinking alcohol. The time-worn trick of covertly watering house plants with drinks you didn't refuse still works.
3. *Eat before and while drinking.* Avoid drinking on an empty stomach. Food in your stomach will not

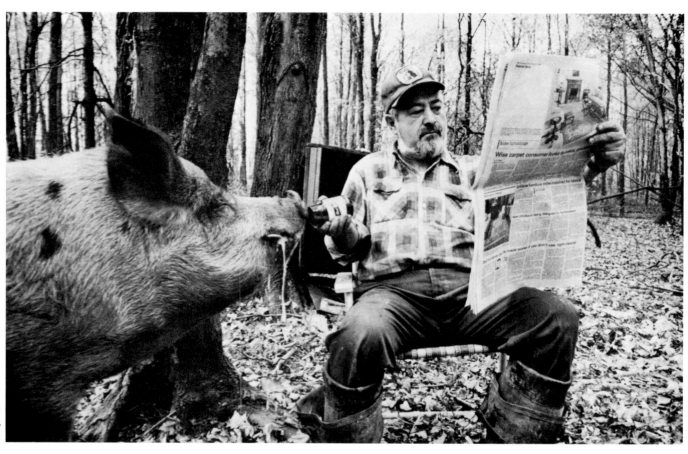

prevent the alcohol from eventually being absorbed, but it will slow down the rate somewhat, and thus the peak blood alcohol level will usually be lower.

4. *Know your limits and your drinks.* Learn how different blood alcohol concentrations affect you. In a safe setting such as your home, with your parents or roommate, see how a set amount—say, two drinks an hour—affects you. A good test is walking heel to toe in a straight line with your eyes closed or standing with your feet crossed and trying to touch your finger to your nose with your eyes closed. However, be aware that in different settings your performance, and especially your ability to judge your behavior, may change. At a given blood alcohol concentration you will perform less well when surrounded by activity and boisterous companions than you will in a quiet test setting with just one or two other people. This impairment results partially because alcohol reduces your ability to perform when your brain is bombarded by multiple stimuli. It is useful to establish the rate at which you can drink without increasing your BAC. Be able to calculate the approximate amount a given drink will increase your BAC.

5. *Determine what your reasons are for drinking.* How do they compare with those of most college students (see page 220)? In what other ways can you learn to fulfill the underlying needs as expressed by your reasons? It is often helpful to keep a diary of your drinking. Include in the diary not only times, settings, and amounts, but what you were feeling and thinking before you started drinking.

6. *Cultivate and model responsible attitudes toward alcohol.* Our society teaches us attitudes toward

drinking that increase the chances for alcohol-related problems, if not for ourselves, for others. Many of us have difficulty expressing disapproval to someone who has drunk too much. We are amused by the antics of the funny drunk. We accept the alcohol industry's linking of drinking and virility or sexuality. We treat abstainers as odd. These attitudes are not healthy.

7. *Learn to be a responsible host/hostess regarding alcohol.* In medieval England an important legal precedent, the dramskeeper's principle, was established. This principle put the responsibility for alcohol-related injuries or untoward results of the guest's drunken behavior on the innkeeper or tavern owner. Although the legal force of this principle has been muted over the centuries, it is a useful guide for our obligations to our guests. Acquire the habit of serving nonalcoholic beverages as well as alcohol and not asking guests if you can get them another drink. Always serve food along with alcohol, and offer tea or coffee for the road. Be able to insist that your guest who had too much take a taxi, ride with someone else, or stay at your house rather than drive.

8. *Develop alternatives to alcohol.* There are many pleasant alternatives to drinking. For example, many people who have adopted programs of vigorous physical exercise—aerobic dancing, jogging, exercycling—find that their alcohol consumption correspondingly drops. Other people have learned to spend evenings and weekends without drinking by changing their usual routine and deliberately excluding alcohol—taking a walk before or after dinner instead of having drinks, for example.

Alcohol Behavior Scale

Read the following statements carefully. Choose the one in each section that best describes you at this moment and record its score at the right. (For instance, "rarely drinks alcohol" has a score of 5.) When you have identified five statements, total your score and find your position on the scale.

5 rarely drinks alcohol
4 rarely drinks alcohol except with meals
3 has a drink at least once a day
2 sometimes drinks in the morning
1 usually drinks in the morning and evening

Score _____

5 drinks to be sociable
4 drinks to reduce tension
3 drinks to reduce inhibitions
2 drinks because others are drinking
1 drinks to avoid thinking about troubles

Score _____

5 never drives after having two or more drinks
4 rarely drives after having two drinks
3 often drives after having two drinks
2 often drives after having more than two drinks
1 drives regardless of amount of alcohol consumed

Score _____

5 is well informed about the effects of alcohol
4 knows a good deal about the effects of alcohol
3 knows something about the effects of alcohol
2 knows little about the effects of alcohol
is ignorant about the effects of
1 alcohol

Score _____

5 avoids drinking on an empty stomach
4 usually sips rather than gulps alcoholic beverages
3 knows how much alcohol is enough
2 gets intoxicated without realizing it
1 drinks without regard to amount or effect

Score _____

Total score _____

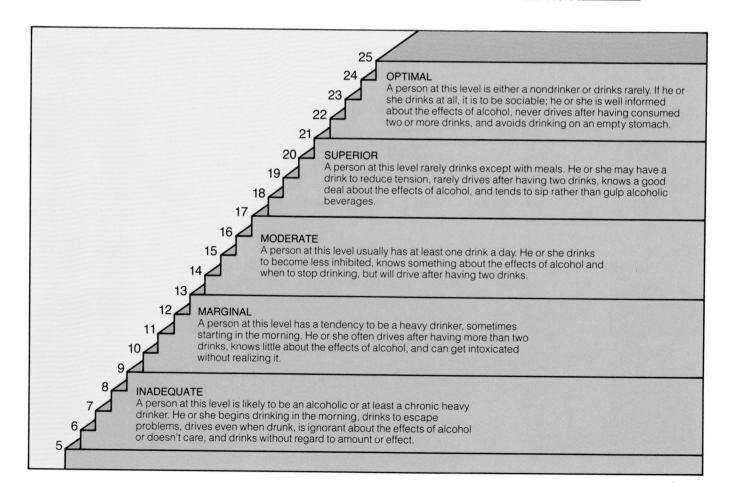

25
24 **OPTIMAL**
23 A person at this level is either a nondrinker or drinks rarely. If he or
22 she drinks at all, it is to be sociable; he or she is well informed
21 about the effects of alcohol, never drives after having consumed
    two or more drinks, and avoids drinking on an empty stomach.

20 **SUPERIOR**
19 A person at this level rarely drinks except with meals. He or she may have a
18 drink to reduce tension, rarely drives after having two drinks, knows a good
17 deal about the effects of alcohol, and tends to sip rather than gulp alcoholic
    beverages.

16 **MODERATE**
15 A person at this level usually has at least one drink a day. He or she drinks
14 to become less inhibited, knows something about the effects of alcohol and
13 when to stop drinking, but will drive after having two drinks.

12 **MARGINAL**
11 A person at this level has a tendency to be a heavy drinker, sometimes
10 starting in the morning. He or she often drives after having more than two
9   drinks, knows little about the effects of alcohol, and can get intoxicated
    without realizing it.

8   **INADEQUATE**
7   A person at this level is likely to be an alcoholic or at least a chronic heavy
6   drinker. He or she begins drinking in the morning, drinks to escape
5   problems, drives even when drunk, is ignorant about the effects of alcohol
    or doesn't care, and drinks without regard to amount or effect.

Take Action

Your answers to Probing Your Emotions at the beginning of this chapter and your placement level on the Alcohol Behavior Scale will, we hope, encourage you to begin a process of self-exploration and self-discovery that you will continue. Reflect on the entire chapter's content and ask yourself how each point relates to your own life. Then take action:

1. Attend an Alcoholics Anonymous meeting. What behavioral techniques are used to help people to stop drinking? How effective do you feel AA is?

2. Record or note advertisements for alcoholic beverages. What psychological techniques are used to sell the products? What are the hidden messages?

3. Drink a glass of wine at least one hour before dinner. Note both the physical effects and the behavioral effects. Do you feel warmer, cooler, dizzy, nauseated, excited, relaxed? Note the effects every 15 minutes for one hour.

4. List the positive behaviors that help you avoid alcohol entirely or keep your consumption to a minimum. Consider how you can strengthen your existing behavior. Also list the behaviors that block your achieving optimal health. Which ones can you change to improve your health?

Before leaving this chapter, review the questions that open the chapter. Have your feelings or values changed? Are you now better equipped to handle the complex and very human problems associated with alcohol consumption?

Chapter Ten

Other Psychoactive Drugs

Probing Your Emotions

1. How do you feel about people's using drugs that alter their consciousness? Most people feel strongly one way or the other about such habits. Why should passions be so strong regarding these psychoactive drugs? In what ways do people feel threatened by such patterns? Obviously, you would feel threatened if you were driving down the highway and knew that the approaching driver was high on LSD; however, statistically, it is more likely that the approaching driver would be under the influence of alcohol or Valium. Many people either forget about or tolerate traditional drug abuses, but they feel threatened by psychoactive drugs. Why?

2. You are at a party with college friends. Everyone is having a good time. Then someone in the group pulls out a bag of "grass" and begins rolling a marijuana cigarette. You are offered a smoke. What do you do? What do you say? What changes would you expect in your relationships with your friends if you accepted or declined the offered joint?

3. Can you think of any legitimate recreational use of drugs? If so, where do you draw the line between legitimate and illegitimate use?

4. If you were able to eliminate all nonmedical use of psychoactive drugs, would you do so? Why or why not?

Chapter Contents

FACTORS INFLUENCING DRUG EFFECTS
Drug factors
Physical differences in individual users
Psychological and social factors
MAJOR PSYCHOACTIVE DRUGS
Opioids
Central nervous system depressants with barbiturate-like effects
Central nervous system stimulants with amphetamine-like effects
Psychedelics
Marijuana and other cannabis products
DRUGS AND DELIRIUM
PSYCHIATRIC USE OF DRUGS

Boxes

Why people use drugs
Nonmedical drug use
Caffeine
Cocaine survey points to widespread anguish
The marijuana problem

Psychoactive drug
Any substance that when taken into the body can alter the user's consciousness.

Drug abuse
Taking drugs to a degree that causes physical damage, impairs functioning, or results in behavior harmful to others.

Central nervous system
The brain and spinal cord.

Dose-response function
The relationship between the amount of a drug taken and the intensity or type of drug effect.

Time-action function
The relationship between the time elapsed since a drug was taken and the intensity of a drug effect.

10 A few years ago the so-called generation gap was defined partly according to which drugs people chose to use or abuse: a martini or a Miltown on one side, a joint or a tab on the other. However clear this picture may have been then, it has become thoroughly clouded since. The "oregano" jar filled with marijuana has now moved into the middle-class household where it has become a standing joke, and more and more of the young and the rebellious are getting stoned on gin or Johnny Walker instead of acid or Acapulco gold.

The old lines that divided the generations have blurred, but overall there has been a tremendous increase in drug use among young and old, rich and poor, throughout the world. Only controlled, closed societies or remote countries isolated from mass transportation and communication are relatively untouched by the spread of drug use. Now, as in the past, the greatest controversies may grow out of the misuse of available information about drugs and their effects. People on all sides of the drug question tend to distort information about drugs to suit their own prejudices, no matter whether they are for or against drugs.

In this chapter we shall define a *psychoactive drug* as any substance that when taken into the body can alter a person's experience or consciousness—his or her sensations, feelings, thoughts, or the functions of the nervous system. We have arbitrarily divided psychoactive drugs into five categories: (1) opioids; (2) central nervous system depressants with barbiturate-like effects; (3) central nervous system stimulants with amphetamine-like effects; (4) psychedelics; and (5) marijuana and other cannabis products. We shall discuss each of these categories in turn.

Most of these drugs are used, or have been used in the past, to treat pain or other symptoms. Sometimes the abuse of a drug came about unexpectedly as a by-product of its medical use. To distinguish between drug use and drug abuse, we define *drug abuse* as drug taking to the extent that it causes physical damage to the user, impairment of the user's ability to function in social situations or on the job, or behavior that is harmful to others.

Factors Influencing Drug Effects

Drug effects are extremely complex and highly variable. The same drug may affect different users differently or the same user in different ways under different circumstances. The effects of a single dose also do not stay the same. The effects change as the body absorbs and metabolizes the drug. When the same drug has different effects, those differences must be due to factors not related to the drug itself—physical differences in individual users and psychological and social factors.

Drug Factors When different drugs or changes in dosage produce different effects, the differences are usually caused by drug factors—pharmacological properties of the drug, dose-response, time action function, cumulative effects, and method of use.

Pharmacological Properties So far we know relatively little about drugs and about the human nervous system, so it is not possible to say precisely how a certain drug acts on a human organism. We can, however, describe the general properties of some drugs. For example, some drugs are classified according to which part of the body they affect. Drugs that stimulate the *central nervous system* are called CNS (central nervous system) stimulants. Other drugs are classified by their chemical makeup as, for example, opioids or cannabis products.

Dose-Response Function Increasing the dose of a drug changes the way a drug affects people. This property is called the *dose-response function*. It is wrong to think, however, that increasing the dose simply intensifies the first effect, as in the familiar case of the person who becomes friendly after one cocktail and belligerent and hostile after six.

Time-Action Function The effects of a drug are greatest when tissue concentrations of the drug are changing the fastest, especially if they are increasing. A constant drug level, even if it is high, is less likely to change the user's experience or behavior. We can use

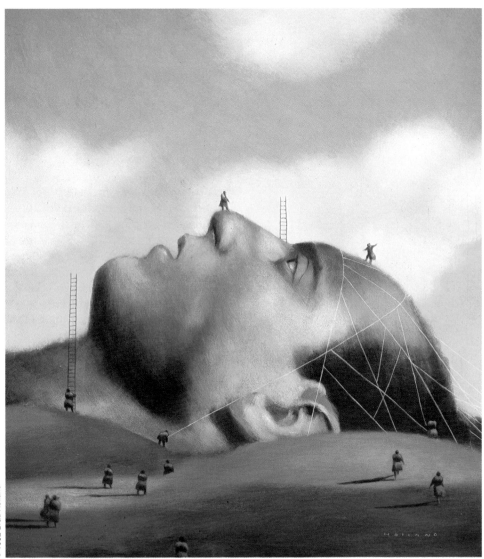

Metabolize
To chemically transform food and other substances into energy and waste.

Biochemical
Describes the branch of chemistry that deals with the life processes of plants and animals.

Pharmacological factors
The properties and reactions of drugs.

Setting
The environment in which something is done.

Set
A person's expectations or preconceptions in a given situation.

"High"
The subjectively pleasing effects of a drug; usually felt quite soon after the drug is taken.

Depressant
Something that decreases nervous or muscular activity.

Stimulant
Something that increases nervous or muscular activity.

Why People Use Drugs

In our society many people have come to expect that drugs will be a part of almost every aspect of daily living. Some believe that chemicals should be used to cure every discomfort and to enhance every pleasure. Through the powerful influence of peers, parents, and advertising, we are taught to seek solutions to many problems of living by using drugs rather than by other means. Common factors influencing drug use include

   peer pressure and need to conform

   the desire to alter one's mood and physiological state

   the need to cope with difficulties

   alienation and poor self-image

   simple boredom

   depression or anxiety

   curiosity

   ready availability of drugs

   the desire to enhance performance or obtain certain kinds of pleasure

alcohol, one kind of drug, as an example. Immediately after a person takes a drink, the alcohol begins to be absorbed into the digestive tract, and the level of alcohol in the blood begins to rise rapidly. As the alcohol is *metabolized*, the blood alcohol level gradually falls. Intoxication is usually greater when the level is rising than when it is falling, even though there may actually be somewhat less alcohol in the blood.

Cumulative Effects   Psychoactive drugs may over time cause physiological alterations in the body that change the effects of a drug. When habitual and occasional alcohol users take the same amount of alcohol, the habitual user is generally less affected.

Method of Use   When a drug is taken by a method that allows its rapid entry into the bloodstream and the brain, stronger effects are usually produced than when the method of use involves slower absorption. For example, injecting a drug generally produces stronger effects than swallowing the same drug. Inhaling (smoking) marijuana produces about three times the effects of the same dose ingested.

Physical Differences in Individual Users   Even when the drug factors are the same for two individuals, they may respond quite differently. Weight can make a difference. For example, the effects of a drug on a 100-pound person will be twice as great as the effect of the same amount on a 200-pound person. Other causes of differing responses include general health and various subtle *biochemical* states. Interactions between drugs, including many prescriptions drugs and over-the-counter drugs, can also have unpredictable effects.

Psychological and Social Factors   With large drug doses, *pharmacological factors,* the chemical properties of the drug itself, tend to have the strongest influence on the user's response. With small doses, psychological and social factors seem more important. These factors, or variables, are called the setting. The *setting* means the physical and social environment surrounding drug use. The *set* refers to how the user expects to react. Experiments have been conducted in which some subjects smoked small quantities of marijuana, while others (unknowingly) smoked a substance that smelled and tasted like marijuana but was not. The intensity of the *high* the subjects experienced was not related to whether or not they had actually smoked marijuana. Clearly, the setting and the set had greater effects on the smokers than the drug itself.

Major Psychoactive Drugs

We have classified psychoactive drugs into five groups—opioids, barbiturates and other central nervous system *depressants,* central nervous system *stimulants,* psychedelics, and marijuana and other cannabis prod-

Absorption
The passage of substances through the skin, lungs, or gastrointestinal tract into the blood.

Endorphin
A chemical produced naturally in the brain that has pain-killing effects.

Euphoria
An exaggerated feeling of well-being.

Addiction syndrome
A behavior pattern of compulsive drug users. The pattern is characterized by preoccupation with acquiring the drug and using it.

Tolerance
Lower sensitivity to a drug so that a given dose no longer exerts the usual effect and larger doses are needed.

---

ucts. We have by no means included all psychoactive drugs in this classification; many drugs that we do not include also have great potency.

Opioids   The opioids, also called opiates or narcotic analgesics, are natural or synthetic drugs that act as morphine does in the body. Opium, morphine, heroin, meperidine, and methadone are examples of drugs in this class. The various opioids have similar effects, but they do differ in dose-response and time-action characteristics. They are sometimes injected under the skin, into the muscles, or directly into the veins. They may also be taken into the body by *absorption* from the stomach and intestine, the membranes of the nose, and from the lungs. How the drug is taken determines how quickly it enters body tissues. If it is injected, the tissue level will change rapidly, and behavioral changes will result. The same dose taken by mouth will be less effective immediately, but it may last longer. The reason for the more lasting effect is that the drug enters the tissues more slowly.

Recent studies have found that in humans there are naturally occurring opioids, called *endorphins*. The endorphins, which appear to control pain and regulate emotional states and sensory input, may be involved in the addictive process, and their specific role is currently the subject of much research activity.

Effects   The opioids reduce pain and produce drowsiness, changes in mood, and mental clouding. Opioid users are unable to concentrate; they have trouble thinking; they feel apathetic and lethargic and cut down on physical activity; they cannot see as well; they feel less anxious; and they are less responsive to frustration, hunger, and sexual stimulation.

Opioids also induce *euphoria*. This property becomes important in the development of drug abuse, but many individuals at first feel vaguely uneasy and have muscular aches and other unpleasant sensations. It is not clear why some individuals go on to develop strong dependency on these drugs, but undoubtedly they do so because of a combination of psychological, social, and pharmacological factors.

All opioids in common use have a high potential for making people dependent on them; indeed, the chronic use of opioids is the usual example given of the classic *addiction syndrome*.

A key feature of the classic addiction syndrome is *tolerance*. Users develop a tolerance for the drug and need larger and larger doses to achieve the same effect. Users often try to stay one step ahead in the game by using a technique called "chipping." (See Figure 10–1.) They take only low doses and those not very often in a futile attempt to avoid getting "hooked." But too often the time between doses shortens, the dose gets bigger, and tolerance develops. The usual starting dose of heroin is about 3 milligrams, but tolerance can lead within a few months to doses of 1,000 milligrams. Heroin can be a very expensive habit.

If the addict chooses to reduce the expense by giving

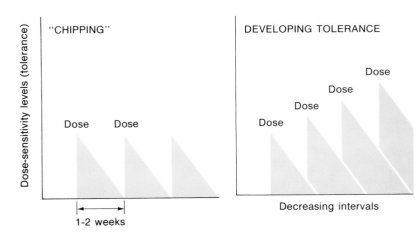

Figure 10-1   The key factor in avoiding developing a tolerance for a drug is to allow intervals between each dose.

Withdrawal
The process of abstaining from a drug to which one has been addicted.

Barbiturate
A type of sedative drug.

Sedative-hypnotics
Drugs that cause drowsiness or sleep.

up the habit or cutting way down on his dose, he faces yet another hazard of addiction. He will have to endure *withdrawal* symptoms. If a certain level of the drug is not maintained in the blood, flu-like symptoms result. These include running nose and eyes, yawning, and sweating. These symptoms develop into worse ones as the level of the drug in the bloodstream continues to drop: weakness, nausea, vomiting, stomach pains, and diarrhea. The user may have goose pimples, and back muscles, bones, and limbs may ache severely. With heroin these symptoms peak about 24 hours after the last dose and usually begin to fade in two to three days.

Treatment Most methods of treatment for opioid addiction have not worked very well. A fairly recent innovation is the substitution of methadone for heroin. Methadone maintenance eliminates the possibility of a severe withdrawal reaction and reduces the craving for heroin without interfering with the individual's ability to function normally in personal, social, and vocational spheres. However, methadone treatment should be viewed with some caution because it is basically substituting one drug addiction for another.

Central Nervous System Depressants with Barbiturate-like Effects   Central nervous system depressants slow down the overall activity of nerves, all muscles, including the heart, and many other body tissues. The result ranges from mild sedation to death, depending on which drug is used, how much is taken and in what way, the physical and emotional state of the user, and what his or her degree of tolerance is, if any.

The most common CNS (central nervous system) depressants are alcohol (discussed in Chapter 9), *barbiturates,* and other various *sedative-hypnotics* that are not barbiturates but have similar effects. During the last 20 years, many new drugs have been marketed as "safe" and "nonaddicting" sedative-hypnotics, but most of these have turned out to have the same side effects, disadvantages, and dangers as the barbiturates.

In most countries a variety of barbiturates are available. They are all similar in chemical composition and action, but they do differ in how quickly they act and how long their action lasts. Drug users call barbiturates "downers" and refer to specific brands by names that describe the color and design of the capsules: "reds" or

"red devils" for Seconal, "yellows" or "yellow jackets" for Nembutal, "blue heavens" for Amytal, and "rainbows" for Tuinal (a combination of secobarbital and amobarbital). People usually take barbiturates in capsules, but injecting them is also common.

Effects   Barbiturates as well as many other sedative-hypnotics have much the same effects on behavior as alcohol. They reduce anxiety (although how much varies); they cause mood changes, muscular incoordination, slurring of speech, and drowsiness or sleep. Cognitive and motor functioning are also affected, but the degree varies from person to person and also depends on the kind of task the person is trying to do.

Most people become drowsy with small doses, although a few become more active. However, when people take these drugs deliberately to alter their awareness or for social reasons, they can overcome most of the sedative effects and remain awake even with large doses. It is particularly easy for the user to overcome drowsiness if the user has developed tolerance or if the environment is stimulating and exciting.

Medical Uses   Barbiturates, methaqualone (*Quaalude* is the trade name of a common methaqualone compound), and other sedative-hypnotics are widely used for treating people with insomnia, as daytime sedatives, and for control of seizures. They are also used to modify the effects of other drugs (for example, to reduce the excessive physical activity often accompanying the use of CNS stimulants).

Patterns of Abuse   People who use CNS depressants for reasons other than medical ones use them in a variety of patterns. Some go on "sprees" from time to time; others take large doses every day for long periods. People usually have their first experience with barbiturates either by way of medical prescription or by way of friends in the drug subculture. Abuse for the medical patient may begin with repeated use for insomnia and progress to addiction through bigger and bigger doses at night coupled with a few capsules at stressful times during the day.

Most sedative-hypnotic drugs, including alcohol and the barbiturates, can lead to classical physical addiction, including pronounced tolerance and withdrawal

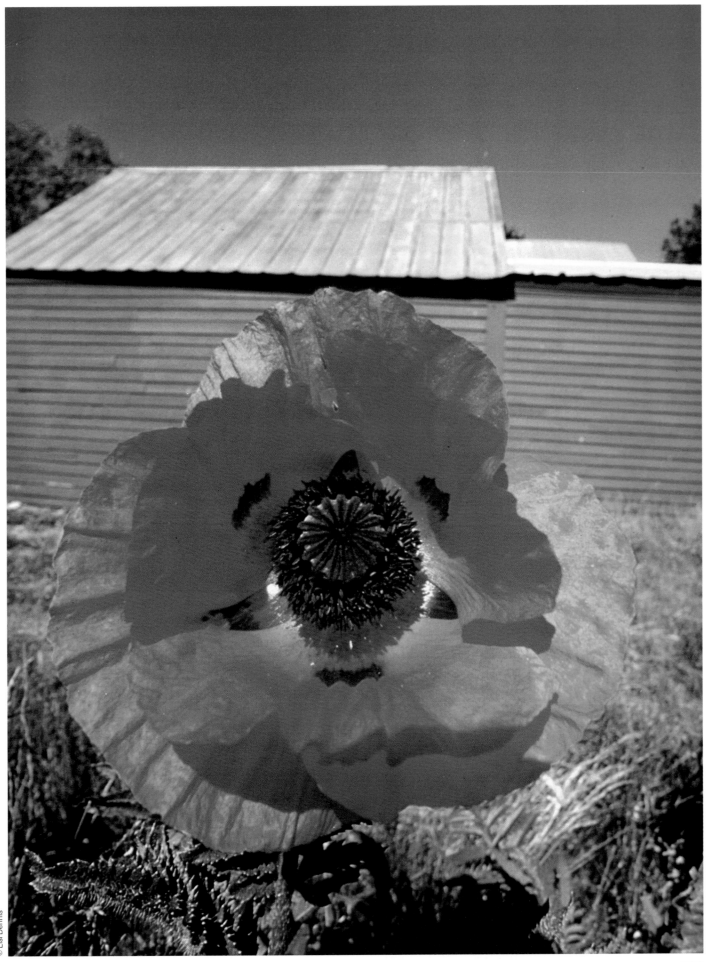

233

Nonmedical Drug Use

Following are projected estimates of the numbers of people who report having used drugs nonmedically. The two categories are young adults and the total population over the age of 12. Estimates are developed from the *National Survey on Drug Abuse: 1979*, by the National Institute on Drug Abuse.

	18-25 years (pop. 31,985,000)				Total (pop. 179,358,000)			
	%	Ever Used[a]	%	Current user[b]	%	Ever Used	%	Current User
Marijuana and Hashish	68	21,700,000	35	11,200,000	30	54,800,000	13	22,600,000
Inhalants	17	5,400,000	1	300,000	7	12,700,000	1	1,400,000
Hallucinogens	25	8,000,000	4	1,300,000	9	15,800,000	1	1,800,000
PCP	15	4,800,000	*	*	5	8,200,000	*	*
Cocaine	28	9,000,000	9	2,900,000	8	15,100,000	2	4,400,000
Heroin	4	1,300,000	—	—	1	2,600,000	—	—
Stimulants	18	5,800,000	4	1,300,000	6	13,900,000	1	2,100,000
Sedatives	17	5,400,000	3	1,000,000	6	13,900,000	1	2,100,000
Tranquilizers	16	5,100,000	2	600,000	5	9,800,000	—	—
Analgesics	12	3,800,000	1	300,000	5	8,200,000	—	—
Alcohol	95	30,400,000	76	24,300,000	90	160,800,000	61	108,600,000
Cigarettes	83	26,500,000	43	13,800,000	79	142,100,000	36	62,400,000

[a] one or more times in a person's life

[b] at least once in the 30 days prior to the survey

* not included in the survey

— amounts of less than .5% are not listed

symptoms. Tolerance, sometimes for up to 15 times the usual dose, can develop during a year or two of repeated use. Tolerance to the depression of the respiratory system caused by these drugs develops more slowly than tolerance to the behavioral effects of the dose. As with heroin and alcohol, the margin between a dose that does what the user wants and a lethal overdose narrows dangerously. Withdrawal symptoms are more severe than those accompanying opioid addiction and are similar to the DTs of alcoholism. They begin as anxiety, shaking, and weakness but may turn into convulsions and possible cardiovascular collapse, which may result in death.

Addiction to CNS depressants and severe alcoholism are alike in many ways. While intoxicated, addicts cannot function very well. They are mentally confused and are frequently obstinate, irritable, and abusive. Both the alcoholic and the person addicted to CNS depressants commonly have poor general health, and both may suffer from (sometimes permanent) brain damage with impairment of abilities to reason and make judgments. Furthermore, the incoordination caused by these drugs often results in injuries and accidents.

Barbiturates and other sedative-hypnotics are major agents of self-destruction. Barbiturate overdose is one of the most frequent methods of suicide among American women and accounts for over 3,000 known deaths

each year in the United States. Many accidental deaths result when people use barbiturates and alcohol together. Even if a single dose of either would not have been fatal, combined depressant effects of both can halt breathing. Alcohol and barbiturates are not unique in this respect; combinations of many depressants can exert more deleterious effects than a single depressant used alone. Barbiturate addicts, like alcoholics and opioid addicts, often become preoccupied with having enough of the drug and sometimes resort to criminal activities to make sure they do. Violent behavior has also been linked with barbiturate addiction and with the use of methaqualone.

Central Nervous System Stimulants with Amphetamine-like Effects The most commonly used CNS stimulants are nicotine (discussed in Chapter 8), caffeine and related compounds, amphetamine and amphetamine-like drugs, and cocaine.

Caffeine Caffeine is the main drug in coffee, tea, cocoa, and many cola drinks, and in some drugs sold over the counter for combating fatigue, such as No-Doz. In ordinary doses caffeine produces greater alertness and a sense of well-being. It also cuts down on feelings of fatigue or boredom, and using caffeine may enable a person to keep at physically exhausting or repetitive

Synthetic
Produced by chemical synthesis rather
than originating in nature.

Psychosis
A severe mental disorder in which there is
a distortion of reality. Symptoms might
include delusions or hallucinations.

---

tasks longer. Such use is usually followed, however, by a sudden letdown. Caffeine does not noticeably influence a person's ability to perform complex intellectual tasks unless fatigue, boredom, alcohol, or other factors have already affected normal performance.

Caffeine mildly stimulates the heart and respiratory system, it increases muscular tremor, and it enhances gastric secretion. Higher doses may cause nervousness, irritability, headache, disturbed sleep, and gastric irritation or peptic ulcers.

Drinks containing caffeine are rarely harmful for most individuals, but some tolerance develops and withdrawal symptoms of irritability and headaches do occur. Excessive caffeine consumption causes excessive anxiety in many people. People with certain psychiatric problems often feel better when they decrease or eliminate their intake of caffeine. (See "Caffeine," page 236).

Amphetamines Amphetamines are a group of *synthetic* chemicals that are potent CNS stimulants. Some common amphetamines are dextroamphetamine (trade name: Dexedrine), *d-l*-amphetamine (trade name: Benzedrine), and methamphetamine (trade name: Methedrine). Popular names for these drugs change often and are different in different parts of the country. Some of the more common ones are "uppers," "speed," "crank," "crystal," and "bennies." The properties of amphetamines are also shared by another group of synthetic chemicals, which include methylphenidate (trade name: Ritalin), phenmetrazine (trade name: Preludin), and diethylpropion (trade names: Tenuate and Apisate).

Small doses of amphetamines usually make people feel better, more alert and wide-awake, and less fatigued or bored. Small doses can produce some improvement in activities requiring extreme physical effort or endurance, such as certain athletic contests or military maneuvers. (See Chapter 13, "Exercise," for more information on the use of drugs and physical performance.) Amphetamines generally increase motor activity but do not measurably alter a normal, rested person's ability to perform tasks calling for complex motor skills or high-level thinking. Like caffeine, amphetamines do most to improve performance by counteracting fatigue and boredom.

Amphetamines in small doses also subdue the appe-
tite, increase the heart rate and blood pressure, and change sleep patterns.

Amphetamine-like drugs, such as Ritalin, have been used to control the behavior of so-called hyperactive children. Instead of stimulating these children to an even higher level of excitement, for some reason, still not known, the drug calms them. The controversy surrounding such use of drugs is heated.

Amphetamines are sometimes used to curb appetite, but after a few weeks the user develops tolerance, and higher doses are necessary. Sometimes, too, when people stop taking the drug, their appetites rebound, and they gain back the weight they lost. There has recently been a flood of over-the-counter diet drugs. However, all of these appetite-suppressant drugs have the intrinsic limitation of not permanently changing eating behavior. (See Chapter 12, "Overweight," for more information on this topic.) Amphetamines have other medical uses, but many physicians doubt their usefulness and consider other approaches more worthwhile and not as risky.

Much amphetamine abuse begins as an attempt to cope with a passing situation. A student cramming for exams or an exhausted long-haul truck driver, executive, or soldier can go a little longer by "popping a benny," but the results can be disastrous. The likelihood of making bad judgments significantly increases. An additional danger is that the stimulating effects may wear off suddenly, and the user may precipitously feel exhausted or fall asleep ("crash").

Repeated use of amphetamines, even in moderate doses, often leads to tolerance and the need for larger and larger doses. The result can be severe disturbances in behavior, including paranoid *psychosis* with illusions, hostility, delusions of persecution, and unprovoked violence. These behaviors make up what is called the "speed freak" syndrome. It is just like a nondrug psychosis except that it stops if the person stops taking the drug.

Some users inject large doses of amphetamines into their veins. Each injection immediately produces a feeling of intense pleasure, an orgasmic "flash," followed by sensations of vigor and euphoria that last for several hours. As these feelings wear off, they are replaced by feelings of irritability and vague uneasiness, along with physical aches. The discomfort strongly motivates the

Caffeine

Caffeine Content of Commonly Used Drugs

One Cup	Milligrams
Coffee (ordinary brewed or instant)	75–150
Coffee (decaffeinated)	2–5
Tea	25–150
Cocoa	10–50

One 12-ounce can	
Cola drink	40–50

One tablet	
Caffedrine	250
No-Doz	100

Criteria for Excessive Use of Caffeine

Have you recently consumed more than 250 milligrams of caffeine? Are you experiencing at least five of the following symptoms:

- restlessness
- nervousness
- excitement
- insomnia
- flushed face
- excessive sweating
- gastrointestinal problems
- muscle twitching
- rambling flow of thought and speech
- irregularities in rhythm of heartbeats
- periods of inexhaustibility
- excessive pacing or need to constantly move around

Ways of Decreasing the Consumption of Caffeine

1. Always keep some noncaffeine drink on hand, perhaps hot water or bouillon, to give a warm feeling to the hands and mouth.
2. Alternate between hot and very cold liquids.
3. Drink decaffeinated coffee or herbal teas.
4. Fill your coffee cup only half-way.
5. Avoid the office or school lunch-room or cafeteria and the chocolate area of the grocery store. (Many times people drink coffee or tea and eat chocolate simply because it is there.)

user to take another injection. The situation is somewhat similar to the injection of opioids. The result is a "run," a period of repeated injections of amphetamines. During a run, the individual often goes without sleep and without enough food or liquids. He or she is also likely to develop *paranoid behavior*.

A run ends when the user is too uncomfortable, too disorganized, or too paranoid to continue, or simply when the drug is all gone. The exhausted user will sleep for a day or two, then be lethargic or depressed. Injecting amphetamines instantly relieves the lethargy or depression, so the user is likely to begin another run.

Continued high-dose amphetamine use can develop into a dependency syndrome, with increasing tolerance and withdrawal symptoms (although these are less severe than with opioids). The individual is also likely to spend much of his or her time obsessively and compulsively seeking drugs.

People ending a run sometimes try to combat the stress and discomfort by using heroin or other CNS depressants. At least in this respect, amphetamines can be a stepping-stone to other drugs.

There is no evidence that certain personality traits make a person more likely to choose amphetamines or, for that matter, any one drug in preference to others. The main factors in choosing a drug are whether or not it is available and whether or not other people around are already using it.

Paranoia is only one of the hazards of amphetamine use. Others include malnutrition and loss of weight, damage to blood vessels, strokes, and other changes in the heart and blood vessels. The injection method brings an added danger, the risk of diseases caused by unsterile conditions.

Cocaine Cocaine, a potent CNS stimulant, can be made synthetically. It can also be obtained from the leaves of coca shrubs that grow high in the Andes Mountains in South America. For centuries natives of that region have chewed coca leaves both for pleasure and to increase their endurance. For a short time, Sigmund Freud was enthusiastic about the use of cocaine to cure morphine addiction and alcoholism. As is so often the case with new drug treatments, Freud's enthusiasm waned after he had more experience with the adverse side effects. At the beginning of the twentieth

Paranoid behavior
Behavior caused by the false belief that
one is being systematically persecuted.

Somatic changes
Changes in the body. For example, weight
loss is a somatic change.

Perceptual changes
Changes in sense awareness.

Synesthesia
A condition in which a stimulus evokes
not only the sensation appropriate to it
but also another sensation of a different
character. An example is when a color
evokes a specific smell.

Psychic changes
Changes in consciousness or mood.
Depression, euphoria, and anxiety are
examples of psychic changes.

Depersonalization
A state in which a person loses the sense
of his or her own reality or perceives his
or her own body as unreal.

Cross-tolerance
The capacity of one drug to prevent withdrawal symptoms when another drug is
abruptly discontinued.

Altered states of consciousness
Profound changes in mood, thinking, and
perception.

century, many patent medicines and nonalcoholic beverages such as Coca-Cola contained small amounts of
cocaine. Commercial considerations such as cost cutting
and later changes in drug control legislation ended this
practice. Today, Coca-Cola (for example) uses the flavor
from coca leaves, but all the cocaine has been extracted.

Cocaine produces a euphoria, which makes its illegal
use very popular. However, it is very expensive, costing
as much as $1,000 an ounce for high-quality supplies.
As you would expect for anything so expensive, cheaper
synthetic substitutes are now available. Vernacular
names for cocaine are "coke" and "snow." As with other
drugs, these names change over time and from place
to place. Often the same name is used for both cocaine
and substitutes.

Cocaine is usually snorted or sniffed instead of
swallowed because it is poorly absorbed into the
bloodstream from the stomach and intestine. Another
method of administration involves heating the cocaine
and then inhaling its alkaloid vapors.

The effects of cocaine are like those of amphetamines,
but they are more intense and do not last as long. Heavy
users who want to maintain the effects inject cocaine
intravenously every ten minutes. Cocaine also constricts
the blood vessels and acts as a local anesthetic. It is no
longer used for anesthesia, however, because synthetic
derivatives work better. Cocaine users, like amphetamine users, may develop paranoid and assaultive tendencies. The early stereotype of the crazed homicidal
"dope fiend" was the cocaine user, not the heroin
addict. However, even for the chronic cocaine user,
the "dope fiend" stereotype seldom applies.

Since cocaine (unlike the amphetamines) has a short
time-action function, tolerance and pronounced withdrawal reactions require very frequent usage. Chronic
use occurs anyway, probably because of psychological
factors such as craving. Also, when a steady cocaine user
stops taking the drug, he or she may feel pronounced
depression and lethargy. The depression is transiently
relieved by taking more cocaine, and thus continued use
is perpetuated.

Psychedelics   So much controversy surrounds *psychedelics* that people cannot even agree on what to call
them. Use of the term "psychedelic" emphasizes the

mind-expanding properties of these drugs; another
designation, "hallucinogenic," focuses on the perceptual
changes they bring about; and a third term, "psychoto-
mimetic," calls attention to their psychosis-mimicking
properties. We shall use the term "psychedelic" because
it is most widely recognized.

The psychedelics include LSD (lysergic acid diethylamide), mescaline, psilocybin, STP (dimethoxy-methyl-
amphetamine), DMT (dimethyl-tryptamine), and many
others. LSD is the most widely known of the psychedelics, and we shall discuss it as an example of the
entire group.

LSD is one of the most powerful psychoactive drugs. A
dose of 100 micrograms, an amount so small that it can
hardly be perceived, will produce noticeable effects in
most people. These effects are of three kinds: somatic,
perceptual, and psychic. *Somatic changes* include slight
dizziness, weakness, nausea, and dilation of the pupils.
Perceptual changes include disorders of vision, an improved sense of hearing, an altered sense of time, and a
phenomenon known as *synesthesia*. With synesthesia,
the sensory modes are blended, and people hear colors
and see sounds. *Psychic changes* include rapid changes
of mood, feelings of *depersonalization*, distortions in
how people see their bodies, and alterations in the relationship between self and external reality.

Many psychedelics induce biological tolerance so
quickly that after a few days' use their effects will be
reduced greatly. The user must stop taking the drug for
several days before his or her system can be receptive
to it again. These drugs cause little drug-seeking behavior and no physical dependence or withdrawal
symptoms. Switching from one psychedelic drug to
another does not change the tolerance because the
leading psychedelic drugs have *cross-tolerance*. An
individual who is tolerant to one psychedelic drug is
tolerant to all.

In smaller doses especially, the immediate effects of
psychedelics depend on psychological and social factors: the personality of the user and what he or she
expects, recent events in his or her life, and the setting.
Many effects of psychedelics are hard to describe
because they involve subjective and unfamiliar dimensions of awareness—the *altered states of consciousness*
for which psychedelics are famous.

Palinopia
Condition of experiencing prolonged visual
afterimages.

Chromosomes
Threadlike structures in the nuclei of cells.
They split as cells divide and carry the
genetic material that causes the new cells
to be like the original cell.

Psychedelics have acquired a certain aura not associated with other drugs. Some people have taken LSD
in search of a religious or mystical experience, or in the
hope of exploring new worlds, or as therapy, in an
attempt to solve their problems. LSD has been acclaimed
not only as a "mind blower" but also as an aid to
creativity and personal growth.

Scientific research does not support these claims.
People on LSD may make a greater number of original
responses, but they are less able to synthesize them, to
coordinate them into an appropriate pattern. Claims of
increased sensitivity and powers of insight are also not
supported by scientific evidence.

A severe panic reaction, which can be terrifying in the
extreme, is more common with a large dose of LSD, but
can sometimes happen even with a small dose; it is
impossible to predict when one will occur. Some LSD
users report having hundreds of pleasurable and ecstatic
experiences before an inexplicable "bad trip," or "bum-
mer." If the user is already in a serene mood and feels no
anger or hostility and if he or she is in secure surroundings with trusted companions, a bad trip may be less
likely, but a tranquil experience is not guaranteed.

Even after the drug's chemical effects have worn off,
spontaneous flashbacks and other psychological disturbances can occur. Flashbacks, or *palinopia,* are perceptual distortions and bizarre thoughts that occur after the
drug has been entirely eliminated from the body.
Flashbacks are relatively rare phenomena, but they can
be extremely distressing. They are often triggered by
specific psychological cues associated with the drug-
taking experience, such as certain mood states or even
types of music.

Many of the bad trips attributed to LSD may actually
be caused by impurities or other drugs and chemicals.
Purity of LSD bought on the street varies widely, and
it is a common practice to add other substances that
purportedly heighten one or another of the drug's effects.
Drug dealers often substitute less expensive psychoactive drugs (such as amphetamines or PCP) for more
expensive ones (such as cocaine or LSD) so they can
make more money. Chemical analyses of street LSD
have shown other dangerous chemicals, including
strychnine, also to be present.

Some researchers have claimed that LSD damages
chromosomes. Evidence so far indicates that LSD in
moderate doses does not damage chromosomes, at
least not in laboratory settings, that it does not cause
detectable genetic damage, and that it does not produce
birth defects. Laboratory LSD is pure. Street LSD is not.

It can be extremely risky for a pregnant woman to
use any drugs, illegal or otherwise, especially during the
first trimester when small chemical alterations in the
mother's body can have a large effect on the developing
embryo. Even later in pregnancy the fetus is usually
more susceptible than the mother to adverse effects of
any drug she takes.

Most other psychedelics have the same general effects
that LSD has, but there are some variations. As in LSD
use, the effects of small doses depend largely on
psychological and social factors, the set and the setting.
A DMT high does not last as long and is more intense
than an LSD high. An STP trip, in contrast, lasts longer
than an LSD trip. Ditran and related compounds cause
greater intellectual impairment and confusion than other
psychedelics.

Mescaline, the ceremonial drug of the Native North
American Church, supposedly produces a "mellower"
trip than LSD. Obtaining mescaline costs far more than
making LSD, however, so most street mescaline is
simply LSD that has been highly diluted. Psychedelic
effects can be obtained from certain mushrooms
(*Psilocybe mexicana*), some morning glory seeds,
nutmeg, jimsonweed, and other botanical products, but
unpleasant side effects—nausea and dizziness—have
limited the popularity of these products. Development
and use of new psychedelics will probably continue, at
least until they turn out to be less effective or to have
more unpleasant side effects than older drugs. A few will
probably have certain features that will make them
useful for some purposes. Research on therapeutic
applications of LSD practically stopped when LSD
became illegal. Before then LSD was being tried in the
treatment of alcoholism and, also under carefully controlled conditions, as an aid to psychotherapy. Many
experts feel this research should be resumed since
the therapeutic potential of psychedelics has not been
clearly determined.

Cocaine Survey Points to Widespread Anguish

An extensive new survey indicates that the use of cocaine continues to increase dramatically in the United States and that the problems associated with it are far worse than many people had believed.

These conclusions are drawn by researchers who have interviewed or talked briefly with thousands of callers on a "cocaine helpline," a telephone service set up to offer advice to the nation's five million cocaine users and to people asking quesions about cocaine-related problems.

The researchers now report receiving about 1,000 calls a day nationwide.

Medical and social difficulties appear to be particularly acute among people who take the drug intranasally—that is, by inhaling it through the nose. About half of the people interviewed who said they took the drug intranasally reported feelings of paranoia and panic, considered themselves to be addicted, and experienced withdrawal symptoms when they stopped using cocaine. . . .

Psychological Problems Linked to Cocaine Abuse

Incidence of cocaine-associated problems among 500 users who called the national cocaine "helpline," a telephone advisory service with headquarters at Fair Oaks Hospital, Summit, N.J.

Depression	83%
Anxiety	83%
Irritability	82%
Apathy	66%
Paranoia	65%
Difficulty concentrating	65%
Memory problems	57%
Loss of sex drive	53%
Panic attacks	50%
Attempted suicide	9%

Dr. Mark S. Gold of Fair Oaks Hospital in Summit, N.J., the medical director and founder of the telephone service, said the series of interviews was the largest ever compiled with American cocaine abusers. . . .

"The average caller was a white, 30-year-old employed male using 6.2 grams of cocaine per week," [Dr. Gold and his colleagues] reported. "Most rated themselves as addicts with multiple areas of drug-related dysfunction, irrespective of the route of cocaine administration."

Dr. Gold acknowledges that the callers interviewed were not a scientific sample; they were self-selected, they all knew the service's telephone number, and they were all in enough distress to call. All the same, he said: "What's devastating about the study is that we found that there is a huge chunk of nice, high-functioning people who are getting into something they don't understand. They have acquired through repeated use a life-long debilitating, chronic, relapsing illness for which there is treatment through remission and abstinence, but no known cure."

Dr. Gold and [his associate] Dr. Washton estimated that 5,000 Americans a day were trying cocaine for the first time, and that many would become dependent on the drug or addicted to it. . . .

According to Federal estimates, more than 20 million Americans have used cocaine, while about 5 million of them use it at least once a month.

Dr. [William] Pollin [director of the National Institute of Drug Abuse] contested the notion that the total number of Americans using cocaine is rising, if infrequent users are included in the count. "There are two contradictory trends taking

place," he said. "There is an overall trend that shows that since 1979 cocaine use either has leveled off or is even going down. This is based on two major national surveys. Yet while the number of users appears not to be going up, the percentage of users who are becoming heavy users of cocaine is increasing, and it is this trend that is causing a significantly increased number of medical problems."

The number of people who have lost control as a result of their use of cocaine increased dramatically, starting in 1976, Dr. Pollin said, adding, "The dangers of the widespread use of cocaine are very, very great, and potentially it can get worse. . . ."

It was partly in response to [a] lack of information that Dr. Gold and his colleagues set up the cocaine telephone service, whose other purpose is to provide information, advice and referral for treatment to cocaine users.

"Cocaine-related deaths and emergency room visits have increased over 200 percent since 1976 and cocaine related admissions to government treatment programs have increased over 500 percent," they wrote in a second, still unpublished report. "Despite these disturbing trends, the popular belief that cocaine is a relatively benign drug without significant hazards of addiction potential continues to be perpetuated."

The researchers interviewed 500 callers, asking them 21 questions dealing with their use of the drug.

Most callers were white, two-thirds were men, and three-quarters were employed, 40 percent of whom earned more than $25,000 a year. The group averaged 14 years of education. The average caller

(continued on next page)

Cocaine Survey Points to Widespread Anguish (continued)

had used cocaine for almost five years, and about half reported using it every day.

"At a street cost of $75 to $275 per gram, callers reported spending an average of $637 on cocaine during the week prior to calling the helpline," the report says of the 500 who were interviewed. "Callers reported numerous social, family, financial and employment problems associated with their cocaine use," including the loss of a spouse,

friends, a job and "all monetary assets."

"Callers also reported dealing cocaine and stealing from work, family or friends to support their cocaine habit," the report says. In addition, 12 percent said they had been arrested for a cocaine-related crime.

The new report also says the large volume of calls to the helpline suggests that cocaine abuse "is a massively escalating problem

that has been largely hidden from scientific or public analysis."

It continues, "If cocaine were more readily available and at a lower cost, or if social sanctions and scientific information failed to caution against the potential dangers, dysfunctional cocaine use might become more prevalent."

Richard D. Lyons
New York Times

Marijuana and Other Cannabis Products Marijuana is a crude preparation of various parts of the Indian hemp plant, *Cannabis sativa,* which grows in most parts of the world. THC (tetrahydrocannabinol) is the main active ingredient in marijuana. Concentrations of THC vary widely, depending on where the plant is grown and how it is cultivated, harvested, and cured. Hashish is a potent cannabis preparation derived mainly from the thick resinous materials of the flowering tops and upper leaves of the plant. It contains high concentrations of THC. THC can be synthesized, but it is a very expensive process. Because of the cost, pure THC is virtually never available on the illicit market. Drugs sold as THC are almost always something else.

Marijuana does not fit precisely into any of the established drug categories. In small doses it acts like the CNS stimulants, but these effects give way to sedation. In larger doses the effects of marijuana seem more like those of the psychedelics than those of any other drug category.

Effects of Marijuana As is true with most psychoactive drugs, what the user expects and what his or her previous experience with the drug has been strongly influence the effects of marijuana. At low doses, marijuana users typically experience euphoria, heightening of subjective sensory experiences, slowing down of the time sense, and a relaxed laissez-faire attitude. These pleasant effects are the reason why this drug is so widely used. With moderate doses these effects become stronger, and the user can also expect to have impaired memory function, disturbed thought patterns, lapses of attention, and subjective feelings of unfamiliarity.

The effects of marijuana with higher doses are determined mostly by the drug itself rather than by set

and setting. Very high doses produce feelings of depersonalization in which the mind seems to be separated from the body, as well as marked sensory distortion and changes in the body image (such as a feeling that the body is very light). People who have not had much experience with marijuana sometimes think these sensations mean that they are going crazy and become anxious or even panicky. Such reactions resemble an LSD bad trip, but they happen much less often, are less severe, and do not last long.

Physiologically, marijuana chiefly acts to cause increases in heart rate and dilatation of certain blood vessels in the eyes, which creates the characteristic bloodshot eyes. The user also feels less inclination for physical exertion.

Cannabis preparations were once medically prescribed for a variety of human illnesses, including insomnia, migraine, depression, and epilepsy. Now, however, none of these uses can be supported. Its medical use for sedative or euphoric effects is limited because of the perceptual and cognitive changes it brings about and also because individual reactions cannot be predicted. Somewhat more promising are current investigations into the use of THC to reduce nausea and improve appetite during cancer chemotherapy. In this situation, adverse side effects are less critical. THC and related compounds are also being studied for possible use in certain forms of glaucoma, the increased pressure within the eye sometimes leading to blindness.

We do not yet understand fully the long-term effects of cannabis use. We can predict, however, from experience with other drugs that the body systems and functions most affected in the beginning by marijuana are the ones most vulnerable to long-term injury. A small percentage of users will undoubtedly develop lung

The Marijuana Problem

The use of marijuana is such an emotional issue that facts are hard to establish. Those involved in its use refuse to accept demonstrated facts and those opposed to its use are often so strongly opposed that they look at information from a biased point of view. Add to this problem the certainty that many of the adverse effects that may occur will not be seen for years. . . . It took over 20 years to see that smoking cigarettes was associated with a rapidly increasing incidence of lung cancer. [In the same way,] it may be at least another 20 years before all of the effects of smoking marijuana are known. But some facts are already known. These were summarized in a report from the Council of Scientific Affairs of the American Medical Association (*JAMA* 246:1923, 1981). The highlights of the report are included here because of the universal nature of the problem related to health, particularly in our young people.

A national survey by the National Institute on Drug Abuse (NIDA) shows an increase in smoking marijuana among young people between 1971 and 1979. In 1971 only one in 10 adolescents ages 14 and 15 had used the drug, but by 1979 the figure had risen to one in three. In 16- and 17-year-olds the use had risen from 27 percent to 51 percent. And 22 percent of young adults from 18 to 25 years of age used marijuana five or more times during the previous month. This is especially important because marijuana has its greatest effects in young people who have not yet matured psychologically or physiologically.

Here are some of the interesting facts supported by recent research included in the Council's report:

1. Regular marijuana smoking may cause constrictive lung disease (fibrosis between the air sacs).

2. Because of poor combustion marijuana smoking produces 50% more polyaromatic hydrocarbons than tobacco smoke. (These are the chemicals associated with lung cancer.)

3. Rats inhaling marijuana smoke daily developed more severe lung disease than observed from tobacco cigarette smoke.

4. Smoking just one marijuana cigarette decreased the vital capacity (maximum air in and out with one breath) as much as smoking 16 tobacco cigarettes. This suggests that frequent marijuana smoking may cause far greater damage to the lungs than smoking tobacco cigarettes.

5. The effects of tobacco cigarette smoking and smoking marijuana are additive, further increasing the danger of severe lung damage in those who smoke both.

6. Smoking marijuana significantly reduces exercise tolerance in patients who have heart pain with exercise, suggesting that smoking marijuana should be avoided in people with heart disease.

7. Microscopic brain cell damage has been demonstrated in rhesus monkeys receiving the equivalent of one marijuana cigarette a day for six months. The Council notes that brain damage may not be visible (may be chemical) even when mental function is impaired.

8. Anecdotal reports suggest the need for more studies to establish the reports of lack of academic drive, the long-term sedative effects, and loss of attention in marijuana use. (Incidentally, marijuana active ingredients may be found in fat tissue for eight days after use, explaining that even infrequent use, more often than every eight days,

may lead to the accumulation of the active substances.)

9. Anything that requires a motor skill will be adversely affected by using marijuana. It impairs reaction time, motor coordination and visual perception. It is dangerous to drive and smoke marijuana. Driving after using any amount of marijuana should be avoided. Using alcohol and marijuana makes these problems worse and constitutes a highway safety problem.

10. In males marijuana smoking may reduce testosterone levels, reduce sperm counts and cause abnormalities in sperm cells.

11. In females long-term marijuana use may cause menstrual abnormalities, failure to ovulate and fetal damage. The possibility of abnormal fetal development as a result of the mother smoking marijuana during pregnancy cannot be ruled out.

12. Changes in chromosomes (genes) have been identified in association with marijuana smoking.

13. Immunity to disease may be decreased. Immune-globulin G was reduced in marijuana users.

14. Marijuana can produce panic reactions and flashbacks, and may precipitate schizophrenic reactions in patients who have a tendency to such problems. Individuals with emotional or psychiatric problems should avoid marijuana.

Having noted some of the adverse effects of marijuana, the report does discuss the possible medical uses of marijuana, mainly control of severe nausea during chemotherapy for cancer and to lower the intraocular pressure in patients with glaucoma. However, the beneficial uses of marijuana do not provide a basis for its use as a recreational drug any more than it would be safe and sensible to use morphine for fun.

The Health Letter

disorders. It is unlikely that all chronic cannabis users will suffer harmful effects. Individuals vary greatly in how susceptible they are to both immediate and long-term effects of drugs.

When we consider the long-term effects of marijuana (and of any other drugs), we should keep in mind the time-lag factor. A period of time must pass before long-term effects of a drug can be recognized. Tobacco, for example, was long thought to be a "harmless" drug.

Is marijuana addictive? Some tolerance can develop, but marijuana smoking irritates the throat and lungs. These unpleasant side effects make a steady increase in use of low-potency preparations unlikely. However, like all drugs that produce "good" feelings, marijuana can become the focus of the user's life to the exclusion of other activities. The chronic marijuana user will not necessarily limit his or her drug use to cannabis. Drug uses appear to be related, and the chronic marijuana user is more likely to be a heavy user of tobacco, alcohol, and other dangerous drugs.

Drugs and Delirium

Many drugs, and other substances not usually thought of as drugs, can bring on a form of abnormal behavior called delirium, or toxic psychosis. Delirium results from a temporary impairment of brain function. Different chemicals act on the brain in different ways, but the results are generally similar. They consist of changing levels of awareness to surrounding events, decreased ability to maintain attention to a task, and variable amounts of mental confusion. He or she may also experience hallucinations, especially visual ones.

Some drugs, such as belladonna alkaloid datura, or jimsonweed, produce a delirium that is characterized by profound memory impairments. Delirium can be produced by inhaling certain chemicals such as some glues, gases in aerosols, kerosene, gasoline, amylnitrite, and anesthetic agents such as laughing gas (nitrous oxide). Most inhaled chemicals interfere directly with brain function, but some do so indirectly by interfering with oxygen exchange in the lungs. Inhalants can be very dangerous to health; high concentrations of these sub-stances in the blood can cause brain, liver, and kidney damage or even asphyxiation.

Phencyclidine (trade name: Sernylan), also known as "angel dust," "PCP," "hog," and "peace pill," reduces and distorts sensory input, especially proprioception (awareness of the position of arms and legs, joints, and so forth), and creates a state of sensory deprivation. This drug was initially used as a human anesthetic, but was unsatisfactory because of the postoperative agitation, confusion, and delirium its use caused. However, it is still used in veterinary medicine as a large animal tranquilizer. Since the ingredients of PCP are readily obtainable and it can be easily made, it is often available on the illicit market and is sometimes used as a cheap adulterant for other psychoactive agents.

Following the faddish pattern of use of most psychedelics, PCP was extensively used in the mid-1960s. It declined in popularity when that generation became aware of the prevalence of adverse side effects including convulsions, memory impairments, coma, and occasionally death. In the mid-1970s PCP again became widely used and is currently a major drug problem. In some parts of the country, PCP is being replaced by a closely related drug, ketamine. Ketamine has most of the effects and associated risks of PCP.

Psychiatric Use of Drugs

Certain classes of psychoactive drugs can be useful in treating psychiatric problems. The antipsychotic drugs, also called neuroleptics or major tranquilizers, are helpful in some individuals who have schizophrenia. We do not know exactly why they work the way they do, but there is no question that in psychotic individuals they reduce bizarre motor activity, decrease responsiveness to external and internal stimuli, and check hallucinations and delusions. They accomplish these results without sedating individuals so much that they cannot continue their daily activities.

The antipsychotic agents apparently are not addictive. Almost all other potent psychoactive drugs can claim a few addicts, but no addicts have been reported with these drugs.

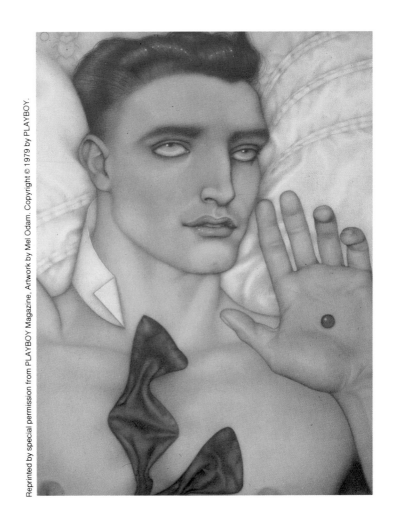

Anxiolytic
A term used to describe drugs that can reduce tension and anxiety without putting the user to sleep.

Psychoneurotic
A term used to describe the mental disorders characterized by symptoms such as anxiety, depression, compulsions, obsessions, and phobias. Unlike psychosis, a psychoneurotic reaction is usually free of gross distortion of reality.

Depression
A mild or severe emotional state characterized by dejection, low spirits, feelings of inadequacy, and inability to act.

Mania
An emotional disorder characterized by excessive enthusiasm, unstable attention, and exaggerated activity.

Some drugs are called *anxiolytic* drugs. Benzodiazepines such as Valium and Librium are examples of this group. They can reduce anxiety, relieve muscle tension, and cut down irritability in most people without putting them to sleep. Anxiolytic drugs are also used to treat other *psychoneurotic* reactions and many other conditions, but they are not effective in treating psychosis. They are extensively prescribed in contemporary medical practice. Patients demand them, and physicians often prescribe them for minor problems such as transient stresses that are an inevitable part of daily life. Virtually all such unpleasant stresses are better handled by learning appropriate psychological coping maneuvers. In addition, anxiolytic drugs can interfere with driving and do potentiate the effects of alcohol. All drugs, including anxiolytics, should be avoided during pregnancy, especially during the first three months. Because many women do not realize they are pregnant until the second month, obvious difficulties can occur.

As with other psychoactive drugs, distinctions between appropriate use of anxiolytic drugs and their abuse are often difficult to make. Most medical authorities would agree that ideally these drugs should be used primarily in time-limited situations where anxiety is so high the individual's usual coping abilities are completely overwhelmed. However, in our society these drugs are widely used where the situation is less clear-cut. Many people ingest anxiolytics on a frequent, often a daily, basis. The number of people who follow this pattern is far greater than the number of people who inject heroin, smoke opium, or inhale solvents. Is this pattern of consumption drug use or drug abuse? If we agree that any drug use resulting in impairment of functioning should be considered abuse, then the anxiolytics are commonly abused. When used daily or frequently, their anxiety-reducing effects tend to accumulate, alertness decreases, and various degrees of mental and behavioral impairment result.

Recent research has produced many drugs for treating mood disorders. Some of these drugs, called antidepressants, are used to treat long-lasting severe *depression*. Results vary, but in some individuals they cause significant elevations in mood and increased activity and drive. As with most psychoactive drugs, it is not known precisely how they achieve these results. It is difficult for doctors to tell which individuals will benefit most from antidepressants, but studies show that these drugs work best with individuals having "pure" severe depression with slowed body movements, reaction time, and speech pattern. The more the individual's depressed behavior is combined with anxiety, hostility, or disorders in thinking, the less effective the antidepressants seem to be.

Among the newest drugs for treating severe mood disorders are the lithium salts. Lithium salts are effective in reducing *mania*. This condition is marked by exaggerated euphoria, inappropriate self-confidence, and poorly controlled overactivity. Lithium salts are also useful in treating manic-depressive disorders, in which the individual swings back and forth between mania and depression. As with the antidepressants, lithium salts appear to work best with people whose mood disorders are not combined with disturbances in thinking or perception.

The study of the effects of drugs on the mind and behavior will undoubtedly see further development within the next few decades. We can especially expect to see refinements in people's abilities to predict which drug will be most useful for a given patient. New psychoactive drugs may present new possibilities for therapy or for social use. They also may present new possibilities for abuse. Making honest and unbiased information about drugs available to everyone, however, may cut down on their abuse. Lies about the dangers of drugs—"scare stories"—can lead some people to disbelieve *any* reports of drug dangers, no matter how soundly based and well documented they are.

Psychoactive Drug Behavior Scale

Read the following statements carefully. Choose the one in each section that best describes you at this moment and record its score at the right. (For example, "avoids addictive drugs" has a score of 5.) When you have identified five statements, total your score and find your position on the scale.

5   avoids addictive drugs
4   limits intake of caffeine
3   drinks coffee or tea regularly
2   uses marijuana
1   uses cocaine

   Score _____

5   believes drugs should be used to reduce pain
4   believes drugs should be used to relieve tension
3   uses drugs to relieve depression
2   uses drugs to feel elated
1   uses drugs to enhance sexual sensations

   Score _____

5   is well educated about the effects of drugs
4   is knowledgeable about the effects of drugs
3   knows something about the effects of drugs
2   knows little about the effects of drugs
1   is ignorant about the effects of drugs

   Score _____

5   does not take any drug without fully knowing its effects
4   may experiment with drug taking under a doctor's supervision
3   may experiment with drug taking if advised by a close friend
2   may take a psychoactive drug to see what it is like
1   might try LSD if it were available

   Score _____

5   educates others about the effect on health of psychoactive drugs
4   is aware of the health consequences of psychoactive drugs
3   believes that only illegal drugs have serious health consequences
2   believes that cocaine and marijuana are not addicting
1   believes that cocaine and marijuana have no effect on health

   Score _____

   Total score _____

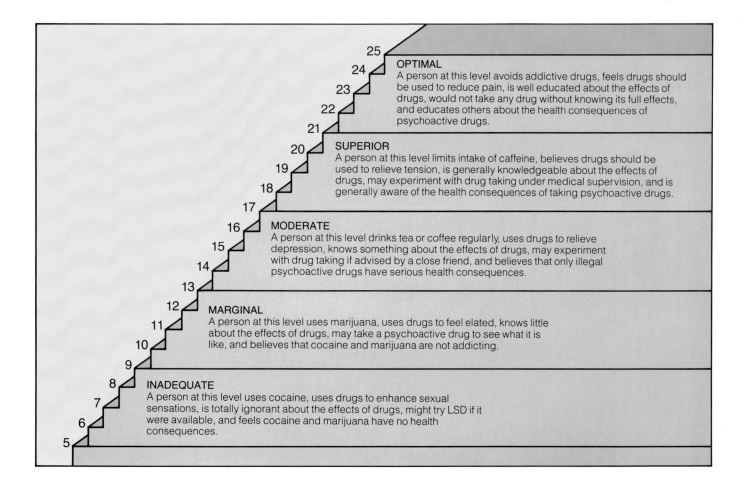

25
24
23
22
21
OPTIMAL
A person at this level avoids addictive drugs, feels drugs should be used to reduce pain, is well educated about the effects of drugs, would not take any drug without knowing its full effects, and educates others about the health consequences of psychoactive drugs.

20
19
18
17
SUPERIOR
A person at this level limits intake of caffeine, believes drugs should be used to relieve tension, is generally knowledgeable about the effects of drugs, may experiment with drug taking under medical supervision, and is generally aware of the health consequences of taking psychoactive drugs.

16
15
14
13
MODERATE
A person at this level drinks tea or coffee regularly, uses drugs to relieve depression, knows something about the effects of drugs, may experiment with drug taking if advised by a close friend, and believes that only illegal psychoactive drugs have serious health consequences.

12
11
10
9
MARGINAL
A person at this level uses marijuana, uses drugs to feel elated, knows little about the effects of drugs, may take a psychoactive drug to see what it is like, and believes that cocaine and marijuana are not addicting.

8
7
6
5
INADEQUATE
A person at this level uses cocaine, uses drugs to enhance sexual sensations, is totally ignorant about the effects of drugs, might try LSD if it were available, and feels cocaine and marijuana have no health consequences.

Take Action

Your answers to Probing Your Emotions at the beginning of this chapter and your placement level on the Psychoactive Drug Behavior Scale will, we hope, encourage you to begin a process of self-exploration and self-discovery that you will continue. Reflect on the entire chapter's content and ask yourself how each point relates to your own life. Then take action:

1. Find out what facilities are available in your community to handle drug addiction. If none is available, what facilities are needed? Locate the public health agency that is responsible for your area and communicate these needs to them.

2. Survey three older students and three younger students about their attitudes toward legalizing marijuana. Are there any differences? If so, what would account for these differences?

3. Visit a drug addiction treatment facility and interview the administrator about admission, treatment, and release procedures. Does this kind of firsthand observation affect your attitude about psychoactive drugs?

Before leaving this chapter, review the questions that open the chapter. Have your feelings or values changed? Are you now better equipped to handle the complex and very human problems associated with the use of psychoactive drugs?

Part Four

Physical Fitness

Chapter Eleven

Nutrition

Probing Your Emotions

1. How do you decide what foods you like to eat? Do you have any doubt that taste is learned? Offer a cup of black coffee to almost any child, and the child will gag and say it tastes "yucky." Yet many adults consume gallons of coffee a week. How do you explain how people learn to love coffee?

2. Consider for a moment how much eating pleasure comes not from food itself but from associated situations and emotions: interactions with other people, the ritual of dining, the environment, and so on. Does this fact help to explain why there is such passionate concern yet so little knowledge about nutritional issues?

3. Do you take vitamin pills? If so, how do you feel about taking them? If not, how do you feel about other people's taking them?

4. Do you believe there is any reason why anyone living in the United States, "the richest country in the world," should have to be nutritionally deprived? Why do you suppose that malnutrition exists in the United States?

Chapter Contents

NUTRITION AND NUTRIENTS
Nutritional needs
How the body uses nutrients
Some functions of some essential nutrients

ADEQUATE, BALANCED DIETS
How much of each essential nutrient do
    you need?
Food as a source of nutrients

CHOOSING A DAILY DIET

VITAMIN AND NUTRIENT
SUPPLEMENTATION

HUNGER AND DISEASE
Deficiency disease
Global hunger

THE FUTURE OF NUTRITION RESEARCH

Boxes

How to tell the truth about nutrition
How to keep the natural goodness in food
Additives: friend or foe?
How to cut down on sugar
Where's the nutrition?
Junk-food fans in the health-food ranks
A sheepish trend: U.S. eating patterns
    become animalistic
The vitamin C controversy

Nutrition
The process of assimilating food and using it for growth and replacement of tissue.

Caloric value
The energy value of food. A calorie is the amount of energy, in the form of heat, required to raise the temperature of 1 kilogram of water 1 degree Celsius (centigrade).

Essential nutrients
Basic substances that the body needs for building and maintaining tissue. The body cannot synthesize adequate amounts of essential nutrients from other materials, so it must get them from food or in some other form.

11 Improved nutrition of the American people during this century has probably contributed more than any other single factor to better health and an increased life span. Good nutrition is essential for optimal health, and it is important to understand how our well-being is affected by what we eat.

Some parents find it difficult to believe that their children can survive without constant coaxing: "Eat your spinach"; "finish your milk"; "don't eat that candy." Few of us escape childhood without at least a vague feeling that whatever tastes good must be bad for us and that whatever is good for us must taste terrible. Then as adults we are buried under an avalanche of nutrition advice from newspapers, magazines, books, and television. Some of the advice is reliable, much is harmless nonsense, and some is downright lethal. Many of us are left so confused about what makes up a nutritionally sound diet that we continue to eat what we like but feel guilty that we may not be eating properly.

At least some of these conflicts are unnecessary, because it is clear that nearly everyone in the United States can have a nourishing diet without having to eat food they do not like or entirely giving up food they do like. This does not mean that what people eat does not matter; it means that we have available to us many different ways to fulfill our nutritional needs.

Although nutrition is a young science, we already know most of the basic facts about the nutrients needed for an adequate, balanced diet and what foods will supply those needs. However, there is much that we still do not know, especially about how various foods and long-term eating patterns may affect different individuals depending on their environment and their genetic constitution. Because data are incomplete in these areas, equally competent nutritionists may differ in their conclusions and dietary recommendations.

Most of us, unfortunately, do not have the resources to sort out the reliable and proven from the less well established or even from the plausible-sounding but spurious claims of faddists and hucksters. (See "How to Tell the Truth About Nutrition," page 255.) A number of the basic facts of nutrition are presented in this chapter. Although some of the interrelationships between foods and nutrients are complex, the guidelines for selecting a nutritious diet are few and simple.

Nutrition and Nutrients

Some of the basic concepts in *nutrition* have existed since at least the fifth century B.C., the time of Hippocrates. Hippocrates postulated that foods contain a life-giving substance, in differing amounts for various foods, that is extracted by the body during digestion. A second important idea—that people need a variety of food in their diets—was given support by several eighteenth-century researchers. One of them was James Lind, a surgeon in the British navy, who showed in a paper published in 1759 that fresh fruits and vegetables contain a substance (now known as vitamin C) that prevents scurvy. The biggest step toward a science of nutrition, however, was an eighteenth-century discovery by the French chemist Lavoisier. He determined that the body's use of a given amount of food required approximately the same amount of oxygen and produced about the same amount of heat as simply burning that amount of food. His experiments made clear that the "life-giving substance" Hippocrates referred to was the *caloric,* or energy, *value* of a food.

Little by little, the body's specific nutritional needs came to be recognized—first protein, then minerals, and, early in this century, vitamins. After about 1912, nutritional knowledge advanced rapidly for perhaps 50 years. At first a diet was considered adequate if it included fats and carbohydrates, as potential energy sources; protein, for tissue structure; an ill-defined assortment of minerals, to build bone; and a vague substance called "vitamine." Today we know that a diet adequate for promoting normal growth and development, supporting reproduction, and preventing deficiency symptoms consists of about 50 different well-defined chemicals.

Putting it in the simplest possible terms, we can say that the digestive processes of the body extract certain substances—called nutrients—from the food we eat. The metabolic processes of the body convert the nutrients into new tissue and into energy for the body to grow, to sustain and rebuild itself, and to perform work.

Nutritional Needs   *Essential nutrients* are the basic substances that the body needs for building and maintaining tissue. They are substances that the body itself

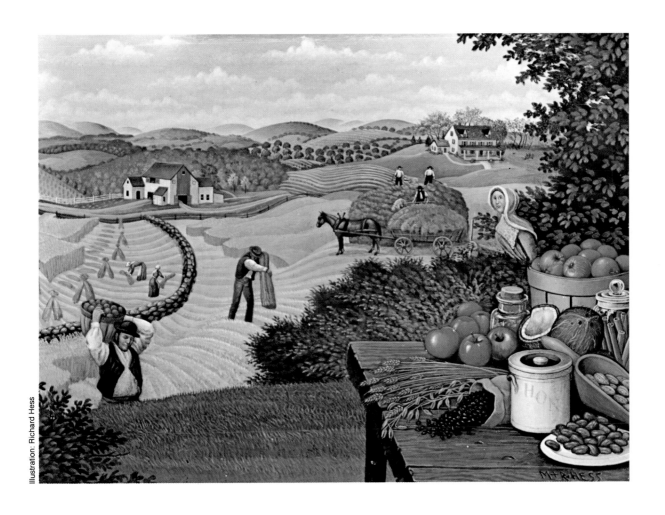

Synthesis
The combining of separate substances to form a new, complex product.

Metabolism
The physical and chemical processes by which the body uses foods, that is, converts nutrients into energy and creates new molecules for tissue.

Fats
A class of energy foods composed of carbon, hydrogen, and oxygen in specific proportions. Fats have a higher energy value than carbohydrates.

Carbohydrates
A class of energy foods containing carbon, hydrogen, and oxygen. Carbohydrates, including sugars and starches, are a primary source of fuel for the body.

Vitamins
Any of various relatively complex organic substances essential in small amounts for the effective functioning of metabolic processes.

Minerals
Inorganic substances that are needed in cellular metabolism and as structural components.

Toxic
Poisonous.

---

cannot *synthesize;* it must get them from food itself or in some other form.

The body stores some nutrients. These remain available for long periods. It *metabolizes* others rapidly, and these must be resupplied often. The body needs relatively large amounts of some nutrients, particularly the energy-supplying *fats* and *carbohydrates.* Of others, such as some *vitamins* or *minerals,* it needs only small amounts.

Some nutrients can be consumed in great quantities without apparent harmful effect; others may be *toxic* in amounts only somewhat greater than what is necessary to prevent deficiency symptoms.

Some nutritional needs are highly specific; that is, only one substance can satisfy the needs. Others can be satisfied by any of a variety of similar substances.

How the Body Uses Nutrients   All living organisms—from one-celled bacteria to multicellular human beings—need energy to create and maintain tissue structure. They obtain it in different ways. Some plants, for example, use light energy from the sun to convert the chemical elements they get from air, water, and earth into all the complex chemicals they need. Some of these chemicals are used directly and at once as tissue-building material; others are stored for use as energy sources when no light is available. Other plants that use sunlight for energy are not able to synthesize all the chemicals they need. They require certain organic substances synthesized only by other organisms.

Animals, including humans, are not able to use the sun's energy directly. They also are not able to synthesize all their tissue structures from the elements. They must depend on what they eat to supply the organic and inorganic compounds, or nutrients, necessary for both energy and structural material. The body needs, in varying amounts and proportions, about 50 such compounds, from which it extracts energy and synthesizes a variety of other compounds.

Generally speaking, the chemical arrangement of human body tissues is different from that of the plant and animal tissues we use as food substances. The body must break down those substances into simpler substances; these can then supply energy or be rearranged

into specifically human materials. In animals, the breakdown process is called *digestion.* It takes place in the alimentary tract, which consists of the mouth, pharynx, esophagus, stomach, and intestine. Techniques of food preparation, such as fermentation and cooking, affect the breakdown process in varying ways. For example, cooking is necessary to make some of the nutrients in potatoes available, but for many other vegetables it is not. Cooking may make some foods easier to digest, or it may destroy nutrients. It all depends on what is being cooked, how it is being cooked, and for how long. (See "How to Keep the Natural Goodness in Food," page 256.)

Each nutrient functions in the body in many different ways. Although the first signs of a nutrient deficiency may appear only in a single organ or system, the deficiency is actually affecting the entire body. When one of the essential nutrients is not available, body tissues are broken down to satisfy the need. This permits the body to survive for a time but at some cost to itself.

Some Functions of Some Essential Nutrients   The primary end products of fat and carbohydrate metabolism are carbon dioxide and water. The chemical transformations involved in this metabolism provide most of the energy we need. Fats and carbohydrates do more than supply fuel, however. Some portion of each fat or carbohydrate unit is transformed for use in all tissues. The weakness and fatigue experienced by people who have long-term calorie-deficient diets is caused by a general deficiency of important tissue materials, not simply by too few calories.

Digestion of *protein* in the stomach and intestine produces altogether about 22 *amino acids.* The amino acids are then absorbed from the intestine into the bloodstream and carried to the liver and elsewhere for synthesis of the extremely complex and specialized structural and functional proteins of all the tissues in the body. These proteins are the chemical basis of life, and a protein deficiency in the diet causes not just a failure to grow, but a disruption of the entire metabolic system.

The body uses iron mainly in the synthesis of hemoglobin, the pigment in red blood cells that transports oxygen. In addition, however, nearly every cell of the body uses iron-containing *enzymes* in carrying out

Digestion
Processes of breaking down foods in the gastrointestinal tract into compounds that the body can use for energy, growth, and repair.

Proteins
A class of foods that supplies nitrogen, sulfur, and other elements. Proteins are complex organic compounds made from 22 amino acids, 10 of which are essential nutrients. The body breaks down proteins and uses the amino acids to build the structural and functional components of tissue; proteins may also contribute in a minor way to fulfilling energy needs.

Amino acids
Organic compounds; the structural units from which proteins are built.

Enzymes
Proteins in cells that aid chemical reactions.

Anemia
A deficiency in the oxygen-carrying material in the blood.

Pellagra
A disease associated with a diet deficient in niacin and protein.

---

its metabolic processes. Thus, although the obvious result of iron deficiency is *anemia*—shortage of hemoglobin in the blood—many other tissues are also affected and less able to function efficiently.

Niacin (one of the B vitamins) is an important part of the many enzyme systems that are necessary for the metabolism of proteins, carbohydrates, and fats. A deficiency of niacin can cause a form of malnutrition called *pellagra*. Symptoms of pellagra are chronic diarrhea, dermatitis, and disturbances of the nervous system.

All body processes—not just some—require many different nutrients and may be affected by the lack of even one essential nutrient. The synthesis of red blood cells, for example, requires not only iron but also copper, cobalt, protein, numerous vitamins, and energy nutrients. If any of these nutrients is missing from the diet, anemia can result. Every essential nutrient is required for good health—and in the right amount. See Tables 11–1 and 11–2.

Adequate, Balanced Diets

In the past, nutritional scientists tried to establish how much of each nutrient people should have in their diets to prevent deficiency. These amounts, thought to be the same for everyone, were called "minimum daily requirements." Although certain guidelines can be useful, we now know that there is no such thing as a specific standard minimum daily requirement. No two people have precisely the same nutritional requirements, and what they do need depends on a number of factors, including their size, their sex, the amount of physical activity in their lives, and the climate they live in. People in different stages of life—childhood, adulthood, pregnancy, old age—have different needs. Genetic makeup can make a difference too. One person will thrive with an extremely small amount of a nutrient while a few others might need amounts so large as to be poisonous to some people.

Nutrients can also affect each other. Too much or too little phosphorus in the diet increases the calcium requirement, for example. An excess of one B vitamin can create a deficiency of another if the intake of the latter is marginal. Carbohydrates are necessary if fats are to be completely metabolized. Bacteria in the intestine may either produce or consume essential nutrients, and variations in bacteria can change the body's requirements, especially for vitamins.

(text continues on p. 256)

Table 11-1   Essential Nutrients

Water

Major Sources of Energy

Carbohydrates, fats.

Essential Amino Acids

Phenylalanine, tyrosine, isoleucine, leucine, methionine, cystine, valine, tryptophan, threonine.

Possibly Essential Amino Acids

Histidine, arginine.

Nonspecific Nitrogen (such as nonessential amino acids)

Alanine, glutamic acid, proline.

Protein

The essential amino acids and nonspecific nitrogen form the protein requirement.

Major Minerals (Elements)

Calcium, chlorine, iron, magnesium, phosphorus, potassium, sodium, sulfur.

Trace Minerals (Elements)

Chromium, cobalt, copper, fluorine, iodine, zinc, manganese, molybdenum, nickel, selenium, vanadium, silicon.

Fat-Soluble Vitamins

Retinol (vitamin A), calciferol (vitamin D_2), α-tocopherol (vitamin E), methylnaphthoquinine (vitamin K).

Essential Fatty Acids

Linoleic acid, linolenic acid, arachidonic acid.

Water-Soluble Vitamins

Thiamine (vitamin B_1), riboflavin (vitamin B_2), pyridoxin (vitamin B_6), cobalamin (vitamin B_{12}), niacin, pantothenic acid, folacin, biotin, choline, ascorbic acid (vitamin C).

Table 11-2   Functions and Sources of Essential Nutrients

Nutrient	Function	Problems associated with deficiency	Source
Calories	Supply energy for growth and development and normal body functioning.	Inadequate caloric intake in children is evidenced by lack of growth and energy and loss of weight.	All foods. Starchy, sweet, and fat foods are concentrated sources.
Protein	Essential for normal growth and development.	A severe or prolonged deficiency in children results in retarded growth and may retard mental development. In adults, deficiency symptoms (weight loss, lassitude, and decreased resistance to disease) are less specific.	Foods of animal origin, namely, meat, fish, poultry, and milk products. Cereals and beans are also an important source of protein.
Vitamin A	Essential for the formation of cells, particularly in the skin, and for normal vision; aids in maintaining resistance to infections.	Deficiency signs: Night blindness, and skin changes characterized by dry, rough skin. Prolonged vitamin A deficiency can lead to permanent blindness.	Whole milk and whole-milk products; dark-green, leafy, and yellow vegetables; liver.
Vitamin D	Necessary for the absorption of calcium and the normal development of bones.	Lack of vitamin D causes rickets in children.	Vitamin D–fortified milk. Vitamin D is formed in the skin upon exposure to sunlight.
Vitamin C	Important for normal tooth and bone formation and wound healing. Plays a role in normal resistance to infection.	Deficiency results in soft, spongy gums, prolonged wound healing, and, in the advanced deficiency state, the classic disease scurvy.	Citrus fruits, tomatoes, and certain vegetables such as cabbage and potatoes.
Thiamin	Essential for growth, normal function of the nervous system, and normal metabolism.	Deficiency results in retarded growth, edema, and changes in the nervous system. Advanced deficiency can result in beriberi.	Liver, eggs, whole grain or enriched cereals and cereal products, and lean meat.
Riboflavin	Essential for utilization of protein and is also involved in other metabolic processes.	Deficiency can result in skin changes such as angular lesions, tongue changes, and poor growth.	Dairy products are the major source, but meats and green leafy vegetables are other sources.
Niacin	Essential for normal digestion and utilization of food.	The classic deficiency state is pellagra, characterized by diarrhea, dermatitis, dementia, and death.	Liver, meats, whole grain, and enriched cereals and cereal products.
Calcium	Necessary for formation of bones and teeth. Also plays a role in normal blood clotting and normal functioning of nerve tissue.	Deficiency in children may be associated with rickets; in adults, calcium may be lost from the bones.	Milk and milk products, fortified cereal products, and certain leafy vegetables.
Iron	Necessary for the formation of hemoglobin, a component of red blood cells.	Iron deficiency symptoms include weakness and fatigability. Advanced deficiency leads to anemia.	Liver, green leafy vegetables, dried fruits, enriched cereals and cereal products, molasses, and raisins.
Iodine	Essential for normal function of the thyroid gland.	Deficiency results in an enlargement of the thyroid gland, which is known as goiter.	Iodized salt is probably the most widely used source. Seafood, water, and plants from certain areas contribute substantial amounts.

Source: *Ten-State Nutrition Survey 1968–70*, vol. 1, U.S. Department of Health, Education, and Welfare, p.4.

How to Tell the Truth About Nutrition

The air is blue!   It's filled with words about nutrition flying at us from all sides! Words that are knowledge, words that are near-knowledge, and words that are downright doubtful. Pity us all, trying to tell the truth from the fiction. After these many years I have some thoughts about how to recognize A FACT.

Personal experience is not it
"I cured my hangnails by eating green cheese!" Very interesting. It may be a fact that the hangnails did clear up. The nonfact is that the green cheese was responsible. This does not prove that green cheese was *not* involved, either. It simply proves nothing. That's why personal experiences are at the low end of the totem pole for credibility. But sometimes a shrewd personal observation FOLLOWED BY CARE-FUL RESEARCH does indeed lead to real facts.

Clinical experience is not it
"My doctor cured my warts with garlic!" Doctors may seem successful with nutritional treatment, often combined with drugs and other therapy. Clinical experiences of doctors are important indications of areas which deserve follow-up in careful research. But until this research is done, forget it. Here are possibilities. Not facts.

Newspaper reports are not it
Clinical studies or experiments reported in newspapers are exciting! The newspaper may even sell better if the reports are sensational! But wait. Think. Be skeptical. Often such reports are premature conclusions of preliminary studies. Alas, too often such research cannot be duplicated in another laboratory!

Population studies are not it
Researchers see different disease rates in different countries, and tie them statistically to eating habits. This points the way to promising areas for research. But until the research clarifies and confirms such relationships, we've got possibilities again. Not facts!

Money, money everywhere, and hardly a cent for nutrition
Well, that's not quite true. But it's vital to know who pays. Did the sugar industry pay for research on the safety of artificial sweeteners? Are such sweeteners competing with sugar on the market? That research needs repeating in another laboratory NOT funded by the sugar industry.

Controlled studies are it, sometimes   In a controlled study, part of the subjects receive a nutritional factor while others do not. All other factors are kept exactly the same! Even so, a well-controlled study may be possible only in limited aspects of the nutritional problems. In humans, with our complex emotional responses, great care must be taken that the researchers them-selves do not influence the results. Double-blind studies are necessary, in which neither the subject nor the researcher giving the pill knows who gets the vitamin C!

Duplication in another lab . . . Eureka!   Sometimes after painstaking, carefully designed studies done by conscientious people, their results cannot be duplicated in other laboratories. Why? Perhaps some inadvertent bias had crept in. Perhaps the subject is more complex than originally thought. When research is duplicated, a giant step towards establishing fact has been taken.

But we've got plenty of areas of non-fact   Nutritional studies of humans are hard to do, require great skill, scientific acumen, piles of nonsuspect money, and the most cautious interpretation. From us, the public, a little patience is required.

Helen Black
The Berkeley Co-op Food Book

How to Keep the Natural Goodness in Food

■ To preserve water-soluble vitamins, avoid prolonged soaking of fresh vegetables. Don't wash rice before cooking; you'll wash B vitamins down the drain.

■ Prepare salads just before serving. Also delay cutting up and cooking vegetables until the last minute to reduce the loss of vitamin C. (The most nutritious way to eat fruits and vegetables is raw.)

■ Boil vegetables until just tender in a minimum amount of water, using a pot with a tight-fitting lid to prevent vitamin loss. Do not thaw or wash frozen vegetables before cooking.

■ Pressure cooking is the least damaging to vitamins. Steaming is second best, boiling less desirable. Frying leads to some vitamin loss, but a more serious disadvantage is that it adds fat and significantly increases the ratio of calories to nutrients.

■ Broiling, frying, and roasting retain more B vitamins in meats than do braising and stewing. But in braised meats and stews, you can recapture lost vitamins by consuming the broth. Meats cooked rare retain more heat-sensitive thiamin than well-done meats.

■ Potatoes boiled or baked whole in the skin retain nearly all their vitamins. In general, the smaller the pieces into which you cut vegetables before cooking, the greater the vitamin loss.

■ Foods that are cooked ahead and later reheated can lose significant amounts of vitamins, especially C. This is not of major significance, however, as long as you have other sources of vitamin C in your diet.

■ Cooking in copper pots can destroy vitamins C and E and folacin, unless the pots are well-lined. Pots made of iron, brass, or monel (a nickel alloy) also destroy some of the vitamin C. But glass, stainless steel, aluminum, and enamel cookware do not affect nutrients.

■ Use the cooking water from vegetables and the drippings from meats (after skimming off the fat) in soups and gravy. That way you recapture many of the lost vitamins. You can also use the vitamin-rich liquid from canned fruits to prepare gelatin desserts or fruit-flavored beverages.

Jane E. Brody

Jane Brody's Nutrition Book

To complicate a complicated matter still further, nutrients often act *synergistically;* that is, one nutrient can only be used by the body if certain other nutrients are also present. Thus, for example, if we have a vitamin D deficiency, we will not be able to use all the calcium we consume.

How Much of Each Essential Nutrient Do You Need?

Many national governments have developed dietary standards for use as guides in planning or evaluating nutrition programs and designing diets. Such guidelines were first introduced in Japan shortly after World War II, and Japanese adults are now from two to four inches taller than their parents.

In the United States the Food and Nutrition Board of the National Research Council, National Academy of Sciences, publishes guidelines, known as recommended dietary allowances. *Recommended daily allowances (RDA)* are suggested amounts of some essential nutrients that should be included each day in a diet "designed for the maintenance of good nutrition of practically all healthy people in the USA." This means that if you are obtaining the recommended amounts of these nutrients from a typically varied American diet you are very likely receiving adequate amounts of all essential nutrients. It does not mean that a person receiving less than the RDA is necessarily receiving an inadequate diet or is malnour-

ished. Because of hereditary or environmental factors, these recommendations may not be appropriate for some individuals. The Nutrition Board continually reviews scientific evidence and research findings and incorporates them into recommendations that are revised about every five years.

Food as a Source of Nutrients

We could satisfy our nutritional requirements with a formula made up entirely of pure chemicals. We could take pills instead of eating food. *Synthetic diets* are valuable in treating certain medical conditions, but most of us get our nutrients from the foods we eat and drink. Generally, we know that a varied diet including both animal and vegetable foods is likely to include every important nutrient, but the knowledge we have of the specific composition of foods by nutrient is rather limited.

Compilations of the available information are known as food composition tables. They may, like the well-known calorie counters, deal with a limited number of nutritional factors in relatively few foods or they may be encyclopedic, giving data for numerous essential nutrients in a great variety of foods. However, any food table has limitations, not only because some foods and nutrients have not yet been analyzed, but also because the food one eats may have different nutrient values than that tested. For example, we all know that some

Synergy
Cooperative action increasing an effect beyond the sum of independent actions.

Recommended daily allowances (RDA)
Standard specifications of nutrient intake designed for maintenance of good nutrition; determined by the Food and Nutrition Board of the National Research Council.

Synthetic diet
A diet consisting entirely of well-defined chemicals and usually ingested as a liquid formula.

---

hamburger is more fatty than other hamburger and thus will have more calories per serving. Vegetables may be of differing genetic strains or may have been grown under differing conditions or harvested at different times. Any of these variables can affect nutrient values significantly.

Complex prepared foods present an additional problem. Refining and preparation often remove vitamins and minerals. On the other hand, the processor, by means of fortifications and supplementation, may add even more vitamins and minerals than were originally present in the basic food components. Reliable information about nutrient content must be based on analyses of the specific products. Increasingly, food producers and distributors with a concern for the consumer's right to know are providing information about the content of key nutrients on their labels. Nutrient-content labeling of all packaged foods may become mandatory in the near future, although such information is presently only legally required when the packager makes nutritional claims for the product.

Even if a food is known to contain a nutrient, there is no guarantee that we can get the nutrient simply by eating the food. Some nutrients occur in forms that people cannot use completely. Others are available only if they are processed in some way or not processed at all. Carotene in carrots, from which the body makes vitamin A, is a case in point. If you eat a carrot raw, some of the carotene will not be available to you. If you put the carrot through a juicer, the carrot cells are crushed, and the carotene is released. Carotene also becomes available if the carrot is cooked, but it is destroyed if the carrot is overcooked.

Other characteristics of foods—besides the nutrients they possess—determine how useful foods are. These characteristics, such as bulk, toughness, structure, and the presence of natural toxins, affect our ability to use the nutrients foods contain. They also have various other influences on health. For example, roughage such as vegetable fiber helps to clean the teeth and may even help prevent certain diseases.

In spite of the imperfections we have noted, food tables can be useful, although perhaps not to the average person. Trained dietitians and nutritionists can make excellent use of them to devise varied and nutritious diets to meet almost any set of conditions: low cost, vegetarian, soft, highly concentrated, low residue, or devoid of specific nutrients. The tables can also be used to plan special diets for people who are sick.

Our understanding of the function of food is gradually being expanded. Recent evidence has shown that food is more than simply a source of material to be processed. Somehow it regulates metabolism and body functions as well. This is what makes it possible for the body to make effective use of a large variety of foodstuffs and adapt to different eating patterns. We do not understand precisely how the regulatory mechanisms work, but it is clear that for the best possible nutrition we shall have to take into account the *source* and *balance* of essential nutrients, not just the quantity.

Choosing a Daily Diet

Very few people choose the food they eat on the basis of nutrient content and recommended dietary allowances. Most base their decisions on habit, what tastes good, what they feel like eating, and what packaging and advertising make "sound good." Food often means more than just the satisfaction of hunger. People eat for pleasure or out of anxiety or boredom or for any of a multitude of reasons. Familiarity, cost, status, taste, convenience, religious or cultural beliefs, associations with other times (especially childhood), advertising, and education all affect choice of foods. Food choice is an expression of personality and culture.

With the variety of foods available in the United States, it is possible for most of us to eat a nutritious diet without radically altering our present food choices. Selecting a diet that furnishes all essential nutrients does not require us to become accountants balancing nutrient content of foods eaten against recommended dietary allowances. All that is required is that we remember and apply one simple principle: Eat as large a variety of foods as possible! No one food is a super food. Neither milk or liver nor wheat germ nor yogurt can supply all nutritional needs. No single food must be *completely* avoided unless that specific food "disagrees" with one or is forbidden as part of a therapeutic diet. Even *(text continues on p. 263)*

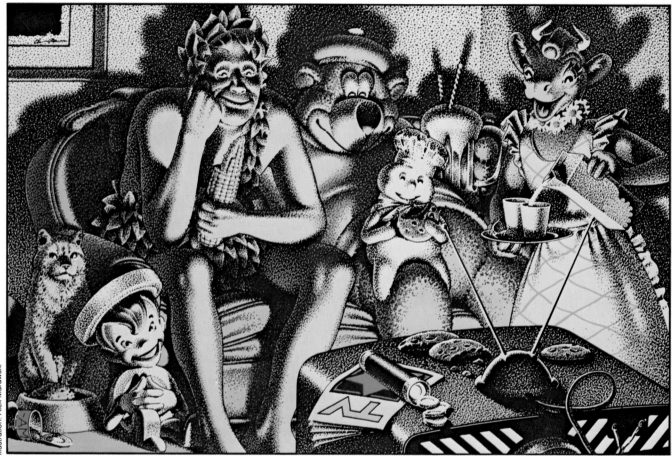

Additives: Friend or Foe?

If we are what we eat, then Americans are a processed and preserved nation of people. Consider this typical breakfast menu: packaged cereal with milk, orange juice, and decaffeinated coffee. It's likely that the cereal has added sugar, salt, and a chemical to preserve freshness; the milk has been fortified with vitamins A and D, and the orange juice could contain food coloring. Your coffee may have been decaffeinated with methylene chloride, a decaffeinating chemical.

The concern many Americans have about food additives is justified when you consider that the average American consumes over four pounds of additives each year. Over 3,000 chemicals are used in our foods, and the numbers continue to increase. Such an abundant use of additives in our food supply raises important concerns: (1) Are they necessary and beneficial, and (2) are they safe and adequately tested?

What Are Additives?

An additive is a substance that has been intentionally added to foods for any number of reasons—to improve nutritional value, to ensure freshness, or make food look and taste better. Adding an emulsifier to peanut butter keeps the oil from becoming a separate top layer, and a pink coloring agent added to peach ice cream could make it more aesthetically pleasing. When additives are used in large amounts, they may perform more as an ingredient than an additive. Sugar, salt, corn syrup and baking soda are prime examples of additives that work as ingredients.

Background   Additives have always played an important role in our food supply. Thousands of years before refrigeration, meat and fish were preserved by salt and other spices. With the advent of the industrial revolution and the ensuing mass migration from farm to city, additives made it possible to store foods for long periods of time and distribute food thoughout the country over long distances. The demand for fast, pre-packaged foods continues to increase as more women are entering the work force and spending less time preparing food in the home.

The first Food and Drug Act passed in 1906 gave our government the power to prohibit the selling of poisonous, toxic foods. This law remained the status quo until 1958 when the Food Additives Amendment and later the Color Additives Amendment (1960) shifted the burden of responsibility from the government onto the food manufacturer. It now became the manufacturer's responsibility to prove an additive was *safe;* the government no longer needed to prove it was *unsafe.*

The GRAS List   While these laws mandated that food manufacturers expose food additives to the rigors of the scientific method, two major additive lists became exempt from the testing requirement—those additives used for a long time and "generally regarded as safe" (called the GRAS list), and additives considered to be "prior sanctioned substances" (substances approved before 1958).

The GRAS list was formulated after "experts" gave their stamp of approval to almost 700 untested food additives. The list has grown since its inception, and if a manufacturer deems an additive safe, he may still use it. Only if Food and Drug Administration (FDA) tests show the additive to be unsafe will it be removed from the list—salt, sugar and many vitamins and minerals are just a few. Yet the GRAS list also contained many well-known additives that have since been removed because they are no longer "generally regarded as safe," such as saccharin, cyclamates and nitrates.

What Is Safe?

The Delaney clause (1958) clearly defines what a safe food additive is:

". . . no additive shall be deemed to be safe if it is found to induce cancer when ingested by man or animal . . ."

Interest in the safety of food additives accelerated in the 1960s when aminotriazole, a pesticide found in cranberry juice, proved to be "unsafe." Shortly afterwards, the cancer-inducing properties of cyclamates became front-page news, and in the early 70s, tests on a widely used food coloring, red dye No. 2, indicated still another compound that could be carcinogenic. Nitrites and saccharin are other well-known additives recently removed from the GRAS list because of their potential to cause cancer.

Although the bureaucratic wheels are slow to turn, in 1971 the FDA began a systematic safety review of major GRAS ingredients. Independent scientists who conduct tests on GRAS substances give the FDA safety information while categorizing many of the additives. Some categories include: "safe," "unsafe," "more information needed," or "restrictions on current usage" (as with salt). These results help determine if an additive will continue to be used.

(continued on next page)

Additives: Friend or Foe? (continued)

A Perspective

Although food additives are more strictly regulated today than at any previous time, some experts feel they are not regulated strictly enough. "I think we have a false sense of security from tests performed on additives" says Dr. Michael Jacobson, Executive Director of the Washington, D.C.–based Center for Science in the Public Interest. "When the tests are described, it sounds like the chemicals are extremely well tested, but in fact the results are not taken very seriously when there's a problem." Another challenge facing the consumer is how to avoid an undesirable additive when only a handful of the more than 3,000 additives are listed on labels. Still another issue remains: Even if a substance is tested and ordained "safe," what impact could it have on our health when it interacts with other addi-

tives and drugs over a period of years? "This is a difficult subject to deal with," says Dr. Jacobson. "For instance, there are ten million alcoholics in this country whose bodies are devastated by alcohol, and no additive used in alcoholic beverages has ever been tested in the presence of alcohol."

What to Do

As consumers, we can exercise our choice in the supermarket by reading labels and making our views known to shop managers or manufacturers. If you continue to select cookies made with saccharin because you are diabetic or interested in weight loss, you may decide not to purchase ice cream with artificial flavoring. It's all a matter of trade-offs. Other additive-minimizing tactics: do not add unnecessary additives to your foods such as

MSG, salt, or sugar; and wash fruit and vegetables to avoid pesticides.

Most food additives are safe and serve a useful purpose for many of us. We cannot completely avoid additives, but we can cut down on our intake. A majority of food additives are used in processed "convenience" foods such as sugar-laden breakfast cereals, sodas, luncheon meats and candies. Far healthier, nutrient-packed food choices would include foods as close as possible to their natural state: fresh fruits and vegetables, whole grains, legumes and unprocessed nuts and seeds. By avoiding convenience foods, intake of chemical additives will automatically be reduced. Antioxidants, benzoic acid, BHA, BHT, calcium propionate—or an apple; the choice is ours.

Deborah Kesten
Healthline

How to Cut Down on Sugar

The following tips can help you reduce your consumption of "empty" or unneeded sugar calories.

■ Don't buy sweet snacks or candy "to have in the house." Substitute popcorn, raw vegetables, or fruit for snacks.
■ Get in the habit of serving fresh fruit for desserts. If you must rely on canned or frozen fruit, choose those packed in water instead of sweet syrup. Dried fruits—raisins, dates, figs, apricots—have a high concentration of sugar (because most of their water has been removed) and are sticky, making them less desirable for your weight and teeth.

■ Instead of buying cakes, pies, or cookies, make your own. Try reducing sugar in the recipe by a third or more. Make dessert breads that contain little sugar and are loaded with nourishing ingredients like whole-wheat flour, oatmeal, nuts, raisins and perhaps a fruit or vegetable like cranberries or carrots.
■ Don't use sweets to reward children.
■ Eliminate soft drinks from your diet. Try seltzer or mineral water instead.
■ If you put sugar in your coffee or tea, gradually reduce the amount you use.
■ Read the labels on all processed foods and consider avoiding any that list sugar among the top ingre-

dients. (Ingredients are listed in order of the quantity used.) Don't be fooled, however, by manufacturers who list sugar, corn syrup, honey, and other sweeteners separately—all are sugar.
■ Try new combinations and preparations to create sweet flavors without sugar. For example, use sweet spices and herbs, such as cardamon, coriander, basil, nutmeg, ginger, or mace. Put grapefruits, bananas, onions, or tomatoes under the broiler, or let the water cook out of a pan of carrots to caramelize the natural sugars. A little sprinkle of shredded coconut makes fresh fruit taste sweeter.

Jane E. Brody
Jane Brody's Nutrition Book

Where's the Nutrition?

If junk food is food that contributes nothing but calories to the diet, fast foods aren't junk. Nutritionally, fast food is not very different from the typical American diet. The general criticisms of fast food are those often heard of the American diet: too much protein, fat, calories, sodium; not enough complex carbohydrates and fiber.

For example, take the cheeseburger-shake-fries combination that's often ordered as a fast-food meal. By our analysis, averaging samples from seven chains, here's how that meal compares with the dietary goals established by the Senate Select Committee on Nutrition and Human Needs. The table shows proportions of a day's calorie intake supplied by various nutrients:

Calories from	Fast-Food Meal	Dietary Goal
Protein	14%	12%
Fat	43	30
Complex carbohydrates	23	43
Simple sugars	20	15

That meal would supply 70 to 90 percent of the daily protein requirement for most people, whereas a person eating three meals a day needs only a third of his or her protein from one meal. Extra protein eaten in a day just means extra calories for the body to use—or to store.

And fast food offers no shortage of calories. The average meal of burger, shake, and fries would supply about 1150 calories. That's

(continued on next page)

How the fast foods compare

Item	Price	Serving Size[2]	Calories	Sodium
Cheeseburgers[1]				
Arby's	$1.45	5½ oz.	492	576 mg.
Burger King Whopper	1.83	9	663	1081
Hardee's Big Deluxe	1.49	8¼	557	900
Jack in the Box Jumbo Jack[3]	1.49	7¾	544	839
McDonald's Big Mac	1.67	7	587	888
Roy Rogers 1/4-lb.	1.48	6	416	597
Wendy's Single	1.55	7¼	547	886
Fries (small)				
Arby's	.55	2¼	195	31
Burger King	.59	1¾	158	56
Hardee's	.50	2¼	202	48
Jack in the Box	.59	2¼	217	117
Kentucky Fried Chicken	.65	3½	221	92
Long John Silver's	.58	3½	282	59
McDonald's	.62	3	268	45
Roy Rogers	.56	3	230	161
Wendy's	.72	3½	317	110
Chocolate shakes				
Arby's	.79	11	365	295
Burger King	.79	9¾	367	251
Hardee's	.70	8½	273	262
Jack in the Box	.80	11¼	324	118
McDonald's	.79	10¼	377	287
Roy Rogers	.78	13¼	518	219
Wendy's	.77	8½	367	281

Item	Price	Serving Size[2]	Calories	Sodium
Fish[1]				
Burger King Whaler	$1.34	6½oz.	502	466 mg.
Hardee's Big Fish	1.19	6¼	515	702
Long John Silver's Fish Sandwich	2.29[4]	7¼	560	1118
McDonald's Filet-O-Fish	1.20	5	373	519
Chicken[1]				
Jack in the Box Chicken Supreme	1.99	7¾	572	1272
Kentucky Fried Chicken Fillet Sandwich	1.89	5½	399	1012
Kentucky Fried Chicken Original Recipe 2-Piece Dinner	1.72	7¼	720	1445
McDonald's McNuggets	1.63	3¾	284	444
Roy Rogers Fillet Sandwich	1.65	6	526	1054
Wendy's Fillet Sandwich	1.87	6	441	699
Roast-beef sandwiches[1]				
Arby's	1.79	5½	416	887
Hardee's	1.29	4¾	294	776
Roy Rogers	1.87	5¼	298	665
Miscellaneous entrées[1]				
Hardee's Chili Dog	.75	4¾	329	879
Hardee's Ham & Cheese	1.49	4½	326	897
Jack in the Box Taco	.85	2½	174	376
Jack in the Box Super Taco	.99	4¼	311	662
Roy Rogers Ham/Swiss	1.82	6	416	1392
Taco Bell Taco	.73	2¾	194	213
Taco Bell Taco Light	1.29	4¾	375	417
Wendy's Chili (small)	1.17	10½	310	1086

[1]Burgers and sandwiches include sauce and extras, where available.
[2]Rounded to nearest ¼ oz.
[3]Jumbo Jack doesn't include cheese.
[4]Price includes fries and cole slaw.

Where's the Nutrition? (continued)

about 40 percent of the number needed to maintain the weight of a 165-pound man, 60 percent of that needed by a 128-pound woman. For someone on a diet, 1150 calories is virtually an entire day's allowance. The main reason for all those calories? Fat.

About half of a cheeseburger's calories come from fat, because of the fat found in beef, cheese, and mayonnaise-type sauces. Chicken and fish normally have a low fat content and relatively few calories, but not when they are breaded and fried. For the most part, the chicken and fish items we tested were as fatty and as caloric as the burgers. Frying has the same effect on potatoes—they get almost none of their calories from fat when raw, but about half of them from fat when french fried.

Fat contributed a slightly smaller percentage of calories in the average roast beef or ham-and-cheese sandwiches. But tacos, which look as if they are a good

part lettuce, get more than half their calories from fat, presumably from the meat, the cheese, and the fried tortilla.

Shakes get most of their 350 or so calories from sugars. An exception was Wendy's Frosty, which had less sugar and more fat than the others, but about the same number of calories.

Now that salads are available at many fast-food outlets, it's possible to choose a fairly well-balanced, even low-calorie meal. A salad adds the complex carbohydrates and fiber that are missing from most fast foods, and if you go easy on the dressing, a salad has very little fat or sugar. A salad, a diet soda, and a plain hamburger, without cheese or oily sauce, can make a meal that's fairly low in calories.

A salad, especially if you choose carrots, tomatoes, and dark green vegetables, can provide some of the vitamins—A, C, E, and folic acid– missing from ordinary fast-food fare. Shakes supply calcium (as does

milk, of course). Beef-containing items are usually rich in B vitamins such as thiamin, niacin, riboflavin, and B-12, and are fairly good sources of the minerals iron and zinc. Entrées containing chicken and fish generally supply those nutrients, too, though to a lesser extent.

A salad might be one of the few things people who have to restrict their sodium intake could choose at the typical fast-food outlet. As the table shows, many of the items we tested contained more than 500 milligrams of sodium, some more than 1000.

Generally, fries had less sodium than any other food, even shakes. The potatoes may taste salty, but saltiness is not necessarily a good measure of sodium content. Many food additives other than salt contain sodium, some of which probably account for the sodium content of the shakes.

Consumer Reports

so-called junk foods, potato chips, candy bars, and popcorn have some nutritional value and can be eaten in moderation as part of a varied diet.

The U.S. Department of Agriculture has developed a simplified guide to selecting a diet that supplies balanced, adequate amounts of all essential nutrients. This is based on the use of the four basic food groups as illustrated in Table 11–3.

Table 11–3 shows only one of the many ways of combining a variety of foods to form an adequate diet. Although most plant proteins are deficient in one or more essential amino acids, even vegetarians can easily obtain a nutritious diet by eating dairy products and eggs. Pure vegetarians (vegans) can do the same by eating meals including a wide variety of foods. For example, if legumes (peas, beans, and lentils) and cereals are eaten together, the proteins complement each other. The

maligned "fast foods" can be part of a nutritious diet if they are supplemented with fresh fruits and vegetables such as green salad or cole slaw. It is not essential that each meal be nutritionally complete as long as the other meals in the day add the desirable variety.

By and large, the problem with our food selection is not that we do not get adequate amounts of the essential nutrients. The problem is that we eat far more than is necessary to relieve hunger. Part of the reason for this is the skill of the food industry in combining seductive advertising and packaging with attractive, highly palatable products. Foods are often made more appetizing by excessive use of fats, refined sugar, and salt, not to mention flavorings and colorings. Thus, not only are we taking in more calories than we need, but also, in the opinion of many health experts, we are eating far too much fat, refined sugar, and salt. Historically, the affluent

Table 11-3   Four Basic Food Groups

Food Group	Amount Suggested and Foods Included	Nutrients Provided
Milk or milk products	Children: 3 or more glasses; smaller glasses for children under nine Teenagers: 4 or more glasses (low-fat) Adults: 2 or more glasses (low-fat)	Protein, fat, carbohydrate Minerals: calcium, phosphorus, magnesium
	1 cup milk = 1 cup yogurt = 1⅓ oz processed cheddar cheese = 1½ cups cottage cheese = 2 cups ice cream	Vitamins: riboflavin, pyridoxine, D and A (if fortified)
Meat	2 or more servings (1 serving = 2 to 3 oz cooked lean meat) Meat, poultry, fish, legumes	Protein, fat Minerals: iron, magnesium, phosphorus, zinc Vitamins: B vitamins (cobalamin, folic acid, niacin, pyridoxine, thiamin)
Fruits and vegetables	4 or more servings (1 serving = ½ cup raw or cooked)	Carbohydrate Minerals: calcium and iron (some greens)
	All fruits and vegetables (include one citrus fruit for vitamin C and one dark green or yellow vegetable for carotene)	Vitamins: A (as carotene), B vitamins (folic acid, thiamin), C, E, K
Breads[a] and cereals[a]	4 or more servings (1 serving = 1 slice fortified or whole grain bread = 1 oz fortified or whole grain dry cereal = 1 corn tortilla = ½–¾ cup cooked fortified or whole grain cereal, rice, grits, macaroni, etc.)	Carbohydrate, protein Minerals: iron, magnesium, phosphorus, zinc Vitamins: B vitamins (niacin, pyridoxine, thiamin), E

Source: University of California at San Francisco Hospitals, *Diet Manual.*
[a]Bran, whole grain breads and cereals, and, to a lesser degree, raw and dried fruits and raw vegetables will increase the amount of unabsorbable fiber in the diet.

Junk-Food Fans in the Health-Food Ranks

In this age of granola bars, there are still a lot of closet Twinkie eaters out there. . . .

"Nobody likes to admit he likes junk food," says Harry Balzer, a vice president of NPD Group, a Port Washington, N.Y.–based market research concern. Asking a sweet eater if he eats a lot of candy "is like asking an alcoholic if he drinks much," Mr. Balzer says.

NPD has developed a new study designed to get at the truth of what people eat. As part of its study, NPD distributed the usual questionnaires to the members of 1,000 households, asking them questions about their attitudes on nutrition and food. In addition, the concern asked each household to record in a diary every snack or meal consumed during a two-week period in each of the two years the survey spans. . . .

As expected, each group frequently eats:		More surprisingly, each group frequently eats:
Fresh fruit, rice, natural cereal, bran bread, wheat germ, yogurt, granola bars	**Naturalists**	French toast with syrup, chocolate chips, homemade cake, pretzels, peanut butter and jelly sandwiches
Wine, mixed drinks, beer, butter, rye/pumpernickel bread, bagels	**Sophisticates**	Prepackaged cake, cream cheese, olives (probably in drinks), doughnuts, frozen dinners
Skim milk, diet margarine, salads, fresh fruit, sugar substitutes	**Dieters**	Coffee, zucchini, squash

NPD found that its subjects divide roughly into five groups: meat and potato eaters; families with kids, whose cupboards are stocked with soda pop and sweetened cereal; dieters; natural-food eaters; and sophisticates, those moneyed urban types whose diets feature alcohol, Swiss cheese, rye and pumpernickel. The study focused mainly on the last three groups because food companies are mostly interested in them. . . .

Betsy Morris
Wall Street Journal

in most cultures have eaten more than they needed, and today in the United States most of us are nutritionally affluent; despite our concern about rising food costs, we have to spend a far smaller fraction of our earnings for food than do people in any other country.

The paperback book shelves are replete with books describing not restraint and moderation but easy ways and gimmicks to avoid the consequences of overindulgence: "calories don't count diet," macrobiotic diets, grapefruit diets, beer drinker's and candy eater's diets, high fat diets, low fat diets, and so on and on. Although one or another book with sound nutritional advice may find its way to these book shelves, the most reliable and, incidentally, most economical sources of good nutrition advice are publications of your health department or the U.S. Department of Agriculture's extension service.

Vitamin and Nutrient Supplementation

As each new vitamin or other essential nutrient has been identified and become available, there have been those who have recommended its excessive intake to achieve beneficial effects. The underlying reasoning in some instances was simply, "if a little is good, more is better." In other situations a nutrient, usually a vitamin, taken in large doses was supposed to cure or prevent specific diseases—vitamin A for arthritis and acne, vitamin B_1 for neuralgia and muscle aches, vitamin C for arthritis and the common cold, vitamin E for heart disease and sexual impotency, and so on. None of these claims has been supported by scientifically acceptable evidence. Although massive doses of nutritional supplements are not always harmful—except that they may delay individuals from obtaining the necessary competent medical attention—numerous cases of toxicity requiring hospitalization have been reported. In a sound dietary regimen there is no need for high-potency (more than the recommended dietary allowance) nutrient supplements. At these dosages vitamins are drugs and should be used only in special circumstances upon advice of a physician. Another type of nutritional quackery is represented by use of the term *vitamin* to designate substances that have no demonstrable nutritional value in humans or higher animals. These include vitamin B_{15}, or pangamic acid, and vitamin B_{17}, or laetrile.

Recent surveys of food consumption in the United

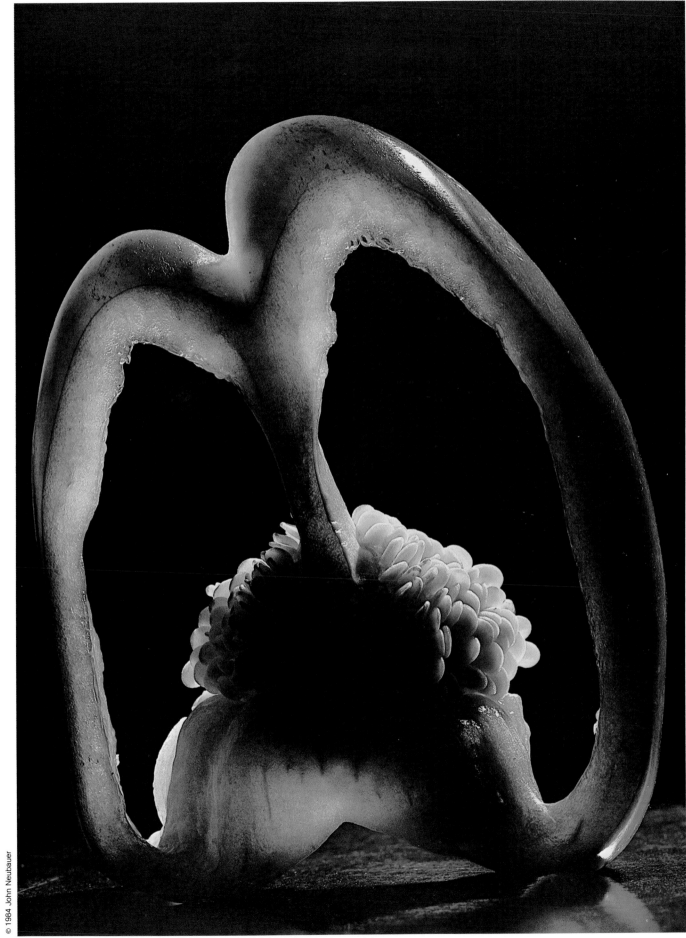

A Sheepish Trend: U.S. Eating Patterns Become Animalistic

Sandra Fried, who could afford to buy what most people would call a real lunch, is standing in the concourse of the World Trade Center eating granola-covered Tofutti, an ice-cream-like concoction made of soybeans.

Miss Fried isn't dieting, however. She's grazing.

"I don't like to eat heavily during the day," says Miss Fried, a marketer at Dean Witter Reynolds Inc., the brokerage firm. "I find that if you eat a little bit, just enough to sustain you, you have more energy to get through the day. If you eat a lot, you feel sluggish."

At the end of the day, she eats dinner, but not always a traditional one. "Sometimes I'll just have tuna fish or a salad," she says. "I'm not very into food preparation."

Intermittent Munching

For more younger working people like Sandra Fried, meals mean a munch here and munch there, rather like cattle or sheep. Hence, the food industry's name for them: grazers.

Not coincidentally, grazers are largely members of the first generation to grow up on fast foods. They eat on impulse rather than three times a day. Although they are more apt to choose foods with a healthful image, some of their choices are in fact little different nutritionally from the hamburgers and french fries of their childhood.

Leo Shapiro, a Chicago consultant who may have been the first to describe the grazing society, says the pattern has become even more common since he wrote about it in 1978 with Dwight Bohmbach. "It used to be that the family ate when the food was ready," Mr. Shapiro

says. "Now you have people eating when they're ready."

Demographic factors in the grazing phenomenon include more single people, smaller households and varying family schedules. But Anthony Adams, the director of marketing research at Campbell Soup Co., says, "I am a strong believer that the one main trend here that the other little trends are spinning off of is female careerism."

Avoiding Cooking

Michael Dundas, a clerk for Commodity Exchange Inc. in New York, says he and his wife don't cook during the week. "There's no time to cook. You're starving. You can't wait two hours to cook a chicken or a roast." Instead they eat pizza, fast food or hot sandwiches.

Many new products succeed because they respond to the desire for high-quality and out-of-the-ordinary food that can be available quickly: frozen hors d'oeuvres that can be prepared in minutes in the microwave ovens that are now in almost 30 percent of American homes and a host of finger foods that have popped up in restaurants and take-out shops.

Purveyors of these products have learned that the grazers are fickle animals. They constantly change direction in their search for the ultimate grazing ground. Because many grazers come from two-income households with plenty of cash but not much time, however, pleasing them is important to many fast-food chains, restaurants and convenience stores.

"Grazers don't make a commitment. They wander," says Anne Powell, of General Mills' restaurant group. "People grab a bite and have a beverage at one place, and

then they go to the movies or a play. Then they may go to another restaurant or even back to the first one."

General Mills believes these people will be drawn to the new oyster bars at its Red Lobster restaurants, which in addition to seafood will serve the two dishes that have emerged as specialties in the grazer's pasture: potato skins and nachos, which are cheese-covered corn chips. Both creations seem somehow to allow the practitioner to feel morally superior to the guy chomping down on a steak; they are also warm and gooey, providing more emotional sustenance than bean sprouts and carrots.

Grazers who pick here and there often are pursuing thinness, abiding by a corollary to the theorem that calories consumed while standing don't count. Grazers may eat three meals, but usually not *real* meals: They are seldom eaten at home, they don't conform to any definitions, and they are hardly ever cooked from what used to be called scratch.

"Two thirds of families eat their main meals together six or more nights a week," says Stephen Sellery of Performance Marketing Inc. "That means a third do not."

That third, however, isn't confined to choosing this restaurant or that restaurant. Increasingly these people can get anything they desire anywhere they go—at convenience stores, supermarkets or take-out operations—eliminating the time-consuming need to simultaneously feed and sit still.

Although the word *grazing* seems to be popular lately in the food industry, *nonmeal meal* is a contender, too. Jane Wallace, the editor of *Restaurants & Institutions,* dates the first use of "grazing" to the introduction of salad bars, when "the person who was eating out began participating in the selection of his own food."

Spontaneous Combinations

In a recent paper presented at an industry conference, an executive of Uncle Ben's Inc., the rice people, described grazing this way: "Each individual in the household goes through the kitchen at mealtime and grazes through the refrigerator and the cabinets, pulling together various foods to make a meal. They'll use whatever's on hand, spontaneous combinations, unusual combinations, but they want good food, not junk food. . . . "

Granted, lots of people never stand on street corners eating croissants, popcorn, pizza, chocolate-chip cookies or yogurt. But sales of such food have flourished lately. Wendy's International Inc. introduced baked potatoes with toppings in November and already sells 600,000 a day, making it the company's most successful new item

ever. "It's a versatile product that people can eat as a meal or a side item," says Brad Quicksall of Wendy's. The chain offered the potato mainly because consumers think it's good for them. "Nutrition is something we think is here to stay," Mr. Quicksall says, "and we don't think it has peaked yet."

Calorie Consciousness

Indeed, a common grazer goal is to get the greatest enjoyment and variety for the fewest calories, and if it's healthful, so much better.

To provide the variety and flexibility that grazers seek, restaurants are adding more appetizers to their menus. Houlihan's, a chain owned by Gilbert/Robinson Inc., has 30% more appetizers than it did two years ago. Increasingly, couples order two large appetizers, a bottle of wine and two desserts, and split everything.

"That's something that wasn't happening five years ago," says Frederick R. Hipp, executive vice president. "I think it's a real opportunity

for restaurants." To provide even more choice, Houlihan's will soon offer an additional menu with low-calorie dishes.

Now that grazers are adults who can ruin their appetites at whim, science is coming around to their side. Snacking doesn't have the bad reputation among nutritionists it once did. "There really isn't any consensus on whether it's better to eat six little meals a day or three big ones, as far as weight control is concerned," says Karen Morgan, a University of Missouri professor who studies snacking.

Grazing may produce new, as yet unimaginable products that are healthful and yet may be eaten on the run. Mr. Adams suggests that Campbell could develop a soup product in the form of a bar, perhaps by putting vegetables in a yogurt base.

"If breakfast can be a bar," he asks, "Why not soup? The only question is the carrier."

Trish Hall
Wall Street Journal

States have shown that as our lives become more sedentary we are eating less and less. Even with a varied diet it is difficult to obtain the recommended dietary allowances of all vitamins and minerals on, say, 1,600 calories a day. Since the RDA has a large built-in safety factor, this does not mean that you are not getting the amounts of these nutrients you need. However, if you are on a low-calorie diet that lacks variety, it would be appropriate to use a multivitamin-mineral supplement that provides the recommended dietary allowance. Avoid megavitamins and "high potency" and "stress" preparations. More is not better in this case.

Hunger and Disease

Starvation and deficiency disease have been a part of human life for a long time. They are still widespread in

many parts of the world, and the situation is likely to grow worse in the next few years as the number of people in the world increases beyond the capacity of any nation to feed them. Even in the United States both hunger and deficiency disease exist, despite our capacity to feed people well.

Deficiency Disease   The United States has an abundant food supply. It has a food distribution system so developed that all kinds of foods are available in all parts of the country throughout the year. Various organizations are engaged in long-term and extensive educational efforts in nutrition. Government welfare programs provide either food stamps or surplus foods. Even so, the United States has a malnutrition problem.

The term *malnutrition* commonly refers to conditions, symptoms, and diseases resulting from a deficiency of one or (usually) more essential nutrients. The condition

The Vitamin C Controversy

Vitamin C (ascorbic acid) plays a major role in maintaining the health and integrity of our bodies. Along with helping to heal wounds, burns, and broken bones, it also works to strengthen blood vessel walls [and] increase resistance to infection, and [it] helps to produce collagen, the substance that holds tissues together. Without it, we can become sick and die.

History

While ascorbic acid was first isolated in the lab in 1927, it was not until 1932 that its value as a vitamin was recognized. With little fanfare, research scientists explored vitamin C's role in health through the 1940s, 50s and 60s. Vitamin C entered the limelight in 1970 when two-time Nobel laureate Linus Pauling published his book, *Vitamin C and the Common Cold,* endorsing vitamin C as the long-awaited answer for the common cold.

Inspired by a colleague, Dr. Irwin Stone, and other vitamin C studies, Pauling began ingesting huge amounts of vitamin C to ward off viruses and colds—and, in his case, it appeared to work. "My wife and I began the regimen recommended by Stone," Pauling writes in his book. "We noticed an increased feeling of well-being, and especially a striking decrease in the number of colds we caught and in their severity."

For the most part, members of the orthodox medical community bristle at Pauling's suppositions. Anecdotal stories unsubstantiated by the rigors and scrutiny of the scientific method can be easy to criticize— until the evidence changes.

Rationale

Most species synthesize their own vitamin C, although man, monkeys, the guinea pig, and the bulbul (a Persian songbird) depend on external food sources for ascorbic acid. Inadequate vitamin C intake results in scurvy, with the ensuing complications of loose teeth, weakened bones, wounds that won't heal, and anemia. To insure adequate intake, the Recommended Daily Allowance (RDA) of vitamin C for a person 15 years and older is 60 milligrams a day.

Pauling and his colleagues theorize that due to a genetic accident, the human species lost its ability to synthesize vitamin C about 25 million years ago, about the time we started obtaining the vitamin from plants. Although we no longer make our own vitamin C, Pauling explains that the amount of vitamin C produced by a mouse, cat or dog, or even a house fly is proportional to body weight. Therefore, he argues, humans also need vitamin C intake proportional to their body weight. Dr. Sheldon Margen, Professor of Public Health at the University of California, Berkeley, disagrees. To say that "because it has allegedly been demonstrated that rats synthesize the equivalent of 10,000 milligrams of vitamin C each day, that our species must also consume an equivalent amount is a spurious leap in logic."

While scientific recommendations cannot be based on theoretical arguments, a growing body of medical literature is substantiating some of Pauling's claims, while other studies continue to explore vitamin C's potential health benefits. Some of the results are conclusive while others indicate the need for additional research.

Cancer

In a controversial study by Pauling and his colleague, Scottish surgeon Dr. Ewan Cameron, ten grams of vitamin C a day were given to patients with advanced cancer. Although the patients who received vitamin C megadoses lived four times longer than patients not given the vitamin, the study was criticized because a comparable group of cancer patients were not selected to receive a placebo (an inert substance identical to the material being tested). Researchers at the Mayo Clinic did not replicate Pauling's results. However, Dr. Pauling defends his study, claiming that patients who participated in the Mayo Clinic study already had impaired autoimmune systems due to chemotherapy. As a result, claims Pauling, vitamin megadoses could not work effectively.

Since there is a growing consensus that vitamin C may be biochemically suited to prevent or perhaps control the cancer process, researchers are continuing to explore ascorbic acid's cancer-inhibiting potential. "Vitamin C intake has been implicated as a protective factor against lung, colon, skin, and stomach cancers. It seems to ward off cervical cancer as well," according to a recent report in *Science News*. In addition, the National Research Council has concluded: "The limited evidence suggests that vitamin C can inhibit the formation of some carcinogens. . . . The results of several case-control studies . . . suggest that the consumption of vitamin C containing foods is associated with a lower risk of certain cancers." At this point, vitamin C research is not extensive, and further research is indicated.

The Common Cold

Vitamin C is perhaps best known for its reputation to combat colds and control infectious diseases. It does this, suggests Pauling, by activating the immune system. While numerous studies have failed to substantiate these claims, Pauling explains this is because most studies administer insufficient amounts of vitamin C for it to work effectively. For example, when a Japanese physician treated hepatitis

by increasing the ascorbic acid dosage from one and a half grams to two, it did have a protective influence. As yet, scientific studies do not show the vitamin to be effective in preventing colds, although it does appear to lessen the severity of colds, and, according to health writer Jane Brody, may control the onset of such diseases as influenza, hepatitis, and mononucleosis.

A Word of Caution

Vitamin C can be beneficial for a multitude of disorders. It may lower the risk of cancer, reduce polyps, and reduce bronchial spasms in asthmatics. Although it is considered nontoxic, large doses may activate certain health problems in

vulnerable people. For instance, vitamin C could destroy red blood cells, cause kidney stone formation, and interfere with the metabolism of certain nutrients (e.g., iron and vitamin A). And when large doses are abruptly stopped, vitamin C deficiency, or scurvy, could result.

While vitamin C is essential for our bodies to function well and large doses are indicated in certain circumstances, conclusive information on its risks and benefits is not yet available. Additionally, well-planned studies are needed to determine the proper role of vitamin C in health and medicine.

Deborah Kesten
Healthline

can often be cured simply by adequate diets. Pellagra is a classic and extreme example of deficiency malnutrition. As noted earlier, in advanced cases it is characterized by inflammation of the mouth and tongue, diarrhea, dermatitis, and severe mental impairment. Other such diseases are beriberi, scurvy, kwashiorkor, marasmus, and rickets.

Extreme deficiency disease is rare in this country but is occasionally found among certain groups—the elderly, infants, and isolated groups living in extreme poverty. Old people living alone often subsist on extremely monotonous and nonnutritious diets such as tea and toast, cereal, or baked beans and coffee. Until a few years ago deficiency disease in children had declined until it was limited to children of the illiterate poor; now it, too, is becoming more widespread, frequently because the parents of these children follow "fad" diets involving extreme restrictions. A significant number of people in the United States, especially among the economically deprived, although not actually malnourished, are eating diets that place them at risk for deficiencies.

Another kind of malnutrition, not too little food but too much of the wrong kinds, is also associated with disease. Coronary heart disease, diabetes, hypertension, obesity, and dental caries have all increased as diets have become more and more imbalanced in the direc-

tion of too many calories and too much animal fat, sugar, and salt.

An imbalance among nutrients seems to be the primary diet problem, at least in the United States. In view of the great amount and variety of foods available in this country, there is no reason for anyone to be poorly nourished, much less the great numbers who are. We know enough about what causes nutrition problems; solving them is not so easy.

Global Hunger We in the United States may have trouble deciding whether to have butter or margerine on our bread. Others, perhaps half the world's population, have no such problem. The reason is simple. There is not even any bread.

Deficiency malnutrition is a problem worldwide, especially among the poor. Many people in the poorer, less-developed countries do not have enough to eat, and what they do have often lacks vital nutrients such as proteins, minerals, and vitamins. Symptoms of deficiency vary from country to country and between rural and urban populations, depending on which nutrient is most scarce. The groups most directly affected are children from six months to five years old and pregnant or nursing women. Growth and development defects are often seen in people who survive beyond childhood.

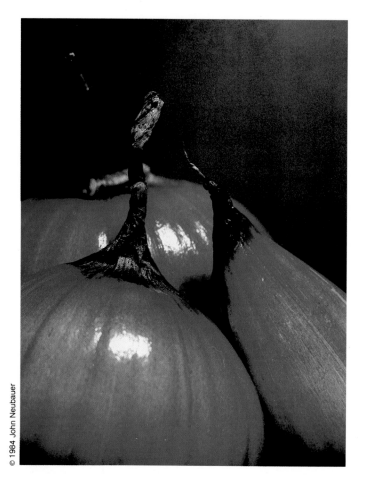

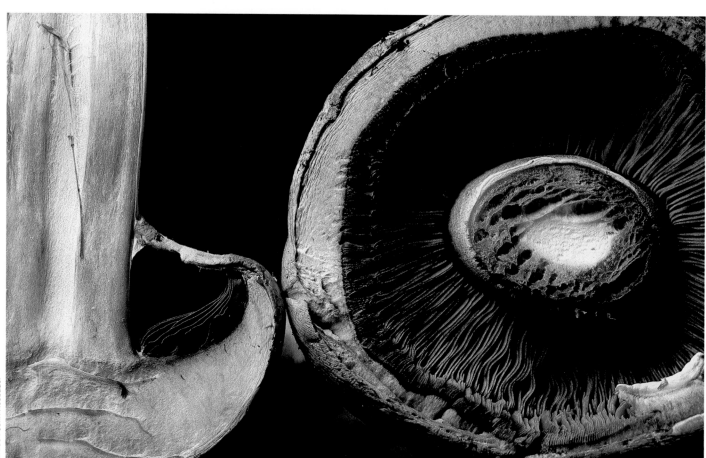

At the root of hunger and deficiency malnutrition, wherever it exists, is poverty. Contributing causes that vary in importance from place to place include severe weather conditions, poor soil, poor agricultural practices, poor distribution of goods and services, overpopulation, changing social structures, economic and cultural traditions, and governmental unconcern or mishandling. There is never a single cause or solution, and some well-meaning but poorly thought-out attempts to ease malnutrition problems have only made them worse.

Introduction of strains of high-yielding cereal grains and improved farming practices—the so-called Green Revolution—did substantially increase grain production during the 1960s, raising hopes that the global hunger problem might be solved. But changing the land use from such plants as peas, beans, and lentils, all good protein sources, to high-yield grains has in some countries made the protein deficiency problem worse. Improved farming methods have been a mixed blessing, too. The wholesale use of strains of new cereal grain seeds to produce high yields may exhaust the soil unless large quantities of chemical fertilizer are available, making any gains in production relatively short term. Then, too, chlorinated hydrocarbon insecticides (also a part of high-yield grain production) flushed into the sea by streams and rivers are threatening the world's fish supply. There is the ever-present threat of drought, lately more often a reality than not. Further failure of "wonder" crops because of drought will again widen the gap between food production and need. Difficulties of water management in underdeveloped drought-plagued nations are enormous and cannot be solved overnight, no matter how many people are starving.

There is no reason to believe that the problem of global nutrition will be solved before millions more have suffered and died, either directly or indirectly as a result of malnutrition. No nation can do it alone; even the resources of the rich, developed nations are being taxed by the continued increases in world population. Present approaches are almost totally inadequate. If we are to make any headway at all, the national, corporate, and personal self-interest that is now the rule must give over to a world view in which the needs of all people are considered, not just the needs of a few.

The Future of Nutrition Research

In the developed countries there have been some successes in preventing deficiencies, but the successes only make the failures more evident. Nutritional planners have largely been unable to solve the many complex problems of making the right nutrients available to everyone. They also have not been able to define the nutritional patterns that will contribute most to long, healthy life.

What are the lifelong effects of diet? Much research in nutrition is now directed toward answering this question and others. For example, what are the effects of what we eat as infants and children on our health as adults? Do we benefit by eating more than we need of a nutrient, especially a vitamin or mineral? Do different dietary patterns or foods have different long-term effects on health, even though each meets our nutritional needs? Will we have to choose between, say, a diet that favors growth and youthful vitality and one that favors an old age free of disease? Are some foods damaging to health over the long term?

We do not have complete answers to any of these questions, but long-term experiments with animals and intensive studies of people with different eating habits are beginning to suggest possibilities. Definite answers for human nutrition in general, however, may require observations for several generations.

Nutrition Behavior Scale

Read the following statements carefully. Choose the one in each section that best describes you at this moment and record its score at the right. (For instance, "rarely drinks milk" has a score of 1.) When you have identified five statements, total your score and find your position on the scale.

5 drinks low-fat milk
4 prefers low-fat milk
3 occasionally drinks low-fat milk
2 occasionally drinks milk
1 rarely drinks milk

Score_____

5 eats fruit twice a day
4 eats fruit once a day
3 eats fruit three to four times a week
2 eats fruit once a week
1 rarely eats fruit

Score_____

5 eats vegetables twice a day
4 eats vegetables once a day
3 eats vegetables three to four times a week
2 eats vegetables once a week
1 rarely eats vegetables

Score_____

5 avoids fast foods
4 rarely eats fast foods
3 eats fast foods three to four times a week
2 eats fast foods five to six times a week
1 relies heavily on fast foods

Score_____

5 avoids sugar
4 avoids candy
3 eats candy three to four times a week
2 eats candy daily
1 eats candy and cake daily

Score_____

Total score_____

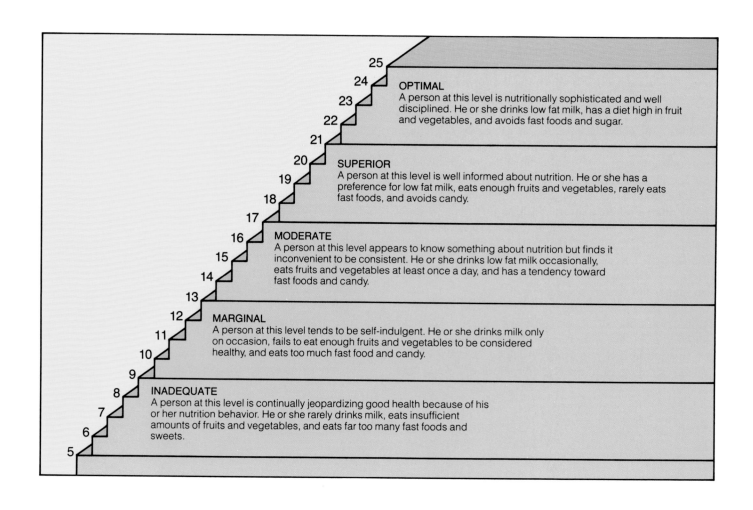

25
24
23
22
21
OPTIMAL
A person at this level is nutritionally sophisticated and well disciplined. He or she drinks low fat milk, has a diet high in fruit and vegetables, and avoids fast foods and sugar.

20
19
18
17
SUPERIOR
A person at this level is well informed about nutrition. He or she has a preference for low fat milk, eats enough fruits and vegetables, rarely eats fast foods, and avoids candy.

16
15
14
13
MODERATE
A person at this level appears to know something about nutrition but finds it inconvenient to be consistent. He or she drinks low fat milk occasionally, eats fruits and vegetables at least once a day, and has a tendency toward fast foods and candy.

12
11
10
9
MARGINAL
A person at this level tends to be self-indulgent. He or she drinks milk only on occasion, fails to eat enough fruits and vegetables to be considered healthy, and eats too much fast food and candy.

8
7
6
5
INADEQUATE
A person at this level is continually jeopardizing good health because of his or her nutrition behavior. He or she rarely drinks milk, eats insufficient amounts of fruits and vegetables, and eats far too many fast foods and sweets.

Take Action

Your answers to Probing Your Emotions at the beginning of this chapter and your placement level on the Nutrition Behavior Scale will, we hope, encourage you to begin a process of self-exploration and self-discovery that you will continue. Reflect on the entire chapter's content and ask yourself how each point relates to your own life. Then take action:

1. In your Take Action notebook keep track of everything you eat and drink for five days. Then divide a page of the notebook into two parts. On the left side of the page list the foods and drink you had that are the most nutritious; on the right side of the page list the foods and drink that are the least nutritious. Are there any surprises?

2. You have been assigned by your company to plan a menu for a group of important customers invited for dinner on Sunday. You have discovered two important facts about this group. They are nutritionally sophisticated. They are all vegetarians. Plan a menu and show it to a close friend, asking for his or her candid opinion.

3. The next time you shop for more than eight food items, read the label on each item and make a list of the top three contents. What element or substance occurs most frequently?

4. Read the following Behavior Change Strategy, and take the appropriate action.

Behavior Change Strategy

Nutrition

It is not at all unusual to hear people announcing the fact that they are trying to eat more "natural foods" or telling their friends that they are going to a particular restaurant because it serves "healthful food." At one time the content of our food was considered important primarily in terms of its calorie content. Even the term *diet* has come to mean a weight-loss program instead of its more complete definition: the food we eat. But there is a growing trend in our society toward a concern about the preparation, preservation, and derivation of our food. References to "natural" and "health" foods have become so commonplace that today these terms are used almost indiscriminately.

Establishing Baseline Levels   If
you want to alter your diet, some of the major health behavior change strategies we have already examined can help you. For example, you can keep track of your target behavior or set of behaviors by means of a diary (see Chapter 1). Let's say that you want to do two things to your diet:

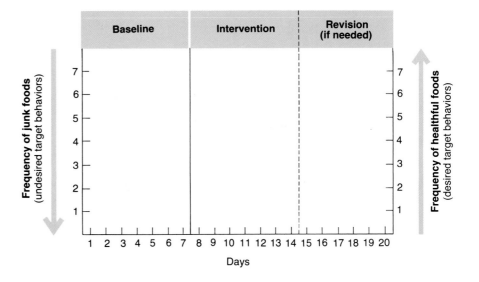

(1) you want to cut out all junk food while walking between classes or while on errands in town, and (2) you want to eat more fresh fruits and raw vegetables.

Begin by keeping track of your junk food consumption. In a diary jot down the time of day and what occurred before and after the eating event. On a chart such as the one shown here, keep track of the number of eating events. Because you also want to add more fruits and vegetables to your diet, you will want to keep notes on the kinds of foods you have been eating at meals. You can include this information on the same chart that you are already using (only on the right-hand vertical axis) or you can simply keep two graphs.

Intervention   Once you have established your "baseline" levels, begin to make some changes in those routines that seem to precede your eating of junk food. For example, you might find that you have been eating food from a vending machine that you walk by every day after class. If this is the case, try another route that allows you to avoid the machine. You might also find that you usually are hungry at one particular time of day and that you rarely have lunch or a healthful snack with you. If this is the case, try to keep a healthful snack on hand so that you will not be caught off guard and then be pushed toward eating junk food (which always seems to be available). You can use the same sort of strategy to increase the number of fruits and vegetables in your diet: specifically, you will need to shop for these food items *in advance* and prepare them *ahead of time* so that they are readily available.

Revision (If Needed)   You may discover that your initial plan works perfectly or that it works well for three weeks but then loses its effectiveness. You will have to watch out for programs that become stale and lose their strength, and, of course, you will want to revise an ineffective program entirely once you have given it a real try. The critical data from your diary can help you to decide how to revise your program. Plotting the data on a prominently displayed chart can encourage your progress.

Social Eating Events   Avoiding an attractive (seductive) candy vending machine may be a lot easier than cutting back on late-night pizza binges; the former involves only you while the latter involves you and your friends. It is harder to make adjustments in social eating patterns, but there are some strategies that you can try. First, tell your friends that you would prefer to try something new to eat instead of pizza (popcorn, etc.). Being assertive in such matters can be very helpful; you may discover some allies who share your views about the type of food you want to eat. Second, try to cut down somewhat on these group activities without eliminating them entirely. Of course, you can try to change or limit the kinds of food you eat at these times, but it is generally very difficult to refrain from joining in once you are actually in the social situation.

Systematic Changes in Other Habits   Many people take up sports activities or begin to increase their routine activity levels (walks after meals, etc.) at the same time that they try to adjust their diet. While it is not a good idea to try to make too many significant changes at one time, you may want to personally experiment with other changes while you make adjustments in what you are eating.

Chapter Twelve

Overweight

Probing Your Emotions

1. Quickly now, how do you feel about overweight people? If you are overweight, do you feel the same way about yourself? If you are thin, are you careful about your eating and exercise? Does your mood affect what you eat and how much you exercise? Does vigorous exercise change your mood?

2. Your teenage brother is shy and has trouble finding acceptance among his friends. In the last five years he has become overweight, and you have a suspicion that he has chosen to become this way as a defense against social risk taking. He seems to be blaming his solitary life on his obesity, getting some anxiety relief because something more incriminating or more personal is not the cause. Is this a coping mechanism? Is it a healthful coping mechanism? To a teenager like your brother, which do you suppose has greater value: the medical consequences of obesity or the social consequences?

3. Your best friend goes on an eating binge whenever she is under stress. To keep from gaining weight, she then makes herself vomit. You have tried to dissuade her from doing this, but she says she feels fine and is maintaining her weight. What do you feel your responsibility is in this situation? Don't answer this objectively; allow yourself to take into account your feelings for your friend. What positive action could you or should you take?

Chapter Contents

WHAT SHOULD YOU WEIGH?

WHAT IS OBESITY?

WHAT CAUSES OBESITY?

Genetic factors
Developmental factors
Metabolic factors
Physical factors
Social and emotional factors

HOW CAN WEIGHT BE CONTROLLED?
Dieting
Exercise
Medical and psychological approaches

Boxes

Anorexia nervosa and bulimia
25 tips from the Diet Center
Evaluating a fad diet
Play plans for exercise and weight loss
Eating for health

Overweight
A condition in which a person weighs more than is normal for people of the same height and sex.

Overfat
A condition in which a person has more body fat than is normal for people of the same height and sex.

Obesity
A physical condition characterized by excessive accumulations of fat in the body. Usually the term refers to weight 20 percent in excess of average.

12 Although "slim is in" in our culture, it is nevertheless clear that the American population is slowly gaining more and more weight, particularly with age. Indeed, some evidence shows that Americans are among the heaviest people in the world, gaining an average of one or two pounds a year after the age of 20. (See Figure 12–1.) Thus from 30 to 50 million Americans are *overweight*. Furthermore, the problem is not so much being overweight as being *overfat*. One can, of course, be overmuscled, but most overweight people have an excess of body fat. Obesity in particular and overweight in general are linked to a large number of health problems, including high blood pressure, high blood fats (hyperlipidemia), diabetes, heart diseases of various kinds, strokes, diseases of the blood vessels, kidney and lung problems, complications during pregnancy, and serious risks for any kind of surgery, especially surgery requiring anesthesia. Some experts consider the social and personal costs of being overweight as great as the medical hazards. Studies show that people are consistently rated as less likeable because of being overweight.

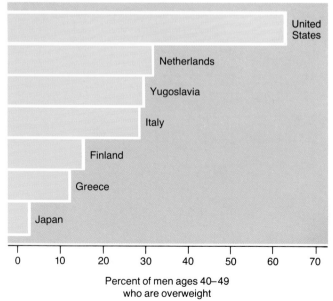

Figure 12–1 Comparison of degree of overweight in males aged 40–49 in population samples of seven countries.

Source: Redrawn from Ancel Keys, *Coronary Heart Disease in Seven Countries*, American Heart Association Monograph No. 29, fig. 56, p. 19.

What Should You Weigh?

Most weight tables list the average for Americans in terms of body build, age, and sex. However, since Americans are on the average overweight, such tables can be misleading. Ideal weight should take into consideration such things as muscle size, body structure, and tendency to retain water. Ideal weight must consider not only total weight but also the body's proportion of fat to lean tissue (such as muscle and bone). Again, the issue is the amount of "overfat"—body fat in excess of an appropriate proportion for a reasonable body weight. Generally, for females about 20 to 24 percent of body weight is composed of fat tissue, while for men, it is in the 12 to 15 percent range. Of course, athletes commonly have a much lower percentage of body fat, sometimes as low as 4 to 6 percent.

Check Table 12–1 to see approximately how much you should weigh. A range from minimum to maximum ideal weight is offered (in parentheses) for each case. Thus, for a woman who is 5 feet 6 inches tall in shoes and has a medium frame, the ideal weight is 128 pounds, with a range of 120 to 135 pounds. (If in doubt about your body frame, use the medium category.) One way to estimate overweight is to find the upper end of the range, such as 135 pounds for the woman in our example, and add 10 pounds. If you weigh more than 10 pounds above the upper limit, then you probably could stand to lose some weight. How much you should lose depends on several things. Unless you are obviously overweight—well beyond the ten extra pounds for your ideal upper limit—how much you should lose depends on how you feel and what you think about your weight and whether you are happy with how you look.

What Is Obesity?

Obesity is a physical condition characterized by excessive body weight. Usually a person is considered obese if his or her body weight exceeds 20 percent of the weight given in height-weight tables. For example, if the 5-foot 6-inch woman discussed earlier weighed more than 155 to 160 pounds, she would be considered obese. In extreme cases the condition of obesity is ob-

Table 12-1   Ideal Weight (Pounds) in Light Clothes* (and Range)

	Men				Women		
Height**	Small frame	Medium frame	Large frame	Height**	Small frame	Medium frame	Large frame
4'10''	—	—	—	4'10''	95	102	112
4'11''	—	—	—		(92–98)	(96–107)	(104–119)
5'0''	—	—	—	4'11''	98	104	114
5'1''	—	—	—		(94–101)	(98–110)	(106–122)
5'2''	116	124	134	5'0''	101	107	117
	(112–120)	(118–129)	(126–141)		(96–104)	(101–113)	(109–125)
5'3''	119	127	137	5'1''	103	110	120
	(115–123)	(121–133)	(129–144)		(99–107)	(104–116)	(112–128)
5'4''	122	130	140	5'2''	106	113	123
	(118–126)	(124–136)	(132–148)		(102–110)	(107–119)	(115–131)
5'5''	125	133	144	5'3''	109	116	126
	(121–129)	(127–139)	(135–152)		(105–113)	(110–122)	(118–134)
5'6''	129	137	147	5'4''	112	120	130
	(124–133)	(130–143)	(138–156)		(108–116)	(113–126)	(121–138)
5'7''	133	141	152	5'5''	115	123	134
	(128–137)	(134–147)	(142–161)		(111–119)	(116–130)	(125–142)
5'8''	137	145	157	5'6''	119	128	138
	(132–141)	(138–152)	(147–166)		(114–123)	(120–135)	(129–146)
5'9''	141	149	161	5'7''	123	132	142
	(136–145)	(142–156)	(151–170)		(118–127)	(124–139)	(133–150)
5'10''	145	153	165	5'8''	127	136	146
	(140–150)	(146–160)	(155–174)		(122–131)	(128–143)	(137–154)
5'11''	149	158	169	5'9''	131	140	150
	(144–154)	(150–165)	(159–179)		(126–135)	(132–147)	(141–158)
6'0''	153	162	174	5'10''	135	144	154
	(148–158)	(154–170)	(164–184)		(130–140)	(136–151)	(145–163)
6'1''	157	167	179	5'11''	139	148	159
	(152–162)	(158–175)	(168–189)		(134–144)	(140–155)	(149–168)
6'2''	162	171	184	6'0''	143	152	163
	(156–167)	(162–180)	(173–194)		(138–148)	(144–159)	(153–173)
6'3''	166	176	189	6'1''	—	—	—
	(160–171)	(167–185)	(189–199)	6'2''	—	—	—
6'4''	170	181	193	6'3''	—	—	—
	(164–175)	(172–190)	(182–204)	6'4''	—	—	—

Note: The numbers in parentheses are reproduced with permission from the Metropolitan Life Insurance Company's Desirable Weight Table.

*For adults aged 18 and above.

**Height in shoes—assume one-inch heel for men and two-inch heel for women.

Source: Peter Wood, *The California Diet and Exercise Program,* Mountain View, Calif., Anderson World Books, 1983. Reprinted by permission of Anderson World Books, Inc.

Skinfold calipers
An instrument used to measure thickness
of skinfolds in various parts of the body;
excellent means of assessing obesity.

Triceps
A muscle that runs along the back of the
upper arm.

Calorie
A unit of food energy.

vious, but in many cases, it is somewhat unclear. Several measures exist to determine if a person is obese. The obvious one is absolute body weight, that is, the number of pounds a person weighs. However, this measure fails to consider the person's height, body frame, and amount of body fat. A better method is to compute percent overweight on the basis of recommended weights for body frame and sex on standard height-weight tables. (We did this with one 5-foot 6-inch woman.) However, this method does not consider percent body fat.

An even better method is skinfold-thickness measurement. The thickness of the adipose, or fat, tissue just under the skin, called subcutaneous fat, is assessed by measuring folds of skin with constant-tension *skinfold calipers*. Certain areas of the body are particularly useful in measuring for fat, such as the area just above the hip and the skin layer on the triceps muscle of the upper arm. The triceps measurement is a particularly reliable indicator of the density of the fat that is just under the skin (altogether, about 50 percent of body fat is subcutaneous). You can perform this test yourself. Pinch a fold of your skin just behind your triceps with your thumb and index finger. Then measure the distance between your thumb and finger. A person who has a skinfold thickness of a little more than one inch is often considered to be obese.

Technically, the most precise way of determining the percentage of body fat to total body weight is to assess how much water the body displaces when submerged in a tank. Since fat tissue has a different density from muscle and bone tissue, a precise measure of body fat is possible by comparing a person's weight under water with that person's weight outside of water. The skinfold-caliper pinch test is in reasonably close agreement with the underwater test.

What Causes Obesity?

Most people believe that excessive body weight is simply caused by eating too much. Unfortunately, this is not entirely true. A number of factors influence body weight, only one of which is the amount and type of food eaten. The other major factor in determining obesity, which is often referred to as the energy equation issue, seems to be how much energy one expends in the course of daily activities, that is, how many *calories* are taken in and how many calories are used up. In a general sense, to increase weight one must take in more calories, and to lose weight one must use up more calories than are consumed.

In 1900 Americans consumed *more* calories than they did in 1975, and yet Americans are considerably more overweight nowadays than they were at the turn of the century. It would therefore appear that we are consuming fewer calories and yet weighing more. This decrease in calorie consumption appears to be continuing, as has been shown by national food surveys carried out in the United States in 1965 and again in 1978. During this 13-year period, the intake of calories dropped significantly for all age groups and for both sexes. Yet people are not losing weight; rather they are gaining. Why? The answer to this question is offered by Dr. Mark Hegsted of the Human Nutrition Center of the U.S. Department of Agriculture. He noted that we are indeed as big and as fat as ever and that obesity appears to be increasing in this country, so the only interpretation possible at this time is that Americans are becoming less physically active and more sedentary in their life-style.

A study recently completed by Dr. Peter Wood and his colleagues at Stanford University helps us to understand the major contributing factors to obesity, at least for most people in this country. Eighty-one middle-aged men, who were physically sedentary, volunteered for a year-long study in which 48 were assigned randomly to an exercise program of jogging regularly three times a week; the other group served as a control, and its members were asked to maintain their usual sedentary habits and routines. Those in neither group were encouraged to change their diet. Careful records were kept of the number of miles run each week by those in the jogging group, along with changes in their body fat (measured by the underwater procedure) and the amount of food they typically consumed. The study found that the men who had done the most jogging had lost the most body fat, a finding that could be expected. Further, those who did the most jogging also showed

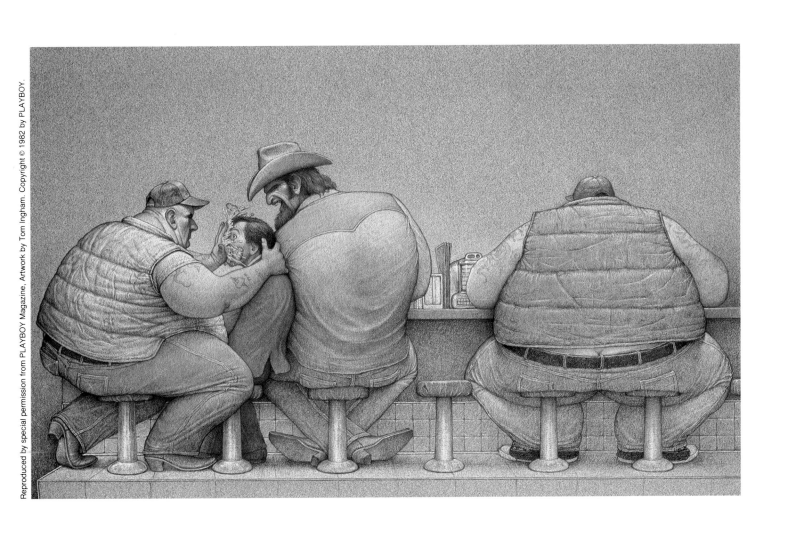

Hypothalamus
A part of the brain that helps to control
activities such as eating by stimulating the
release of many different hormones.

the largest increase in calorie consumption—again not particularly surprising. In addition, the men who were jogging and *lost* the most body fat also *increased* their food intake the most; they were eating much more but weighing much less within the one-year period.

Studies of obesity have shown that the body does seek to maintain and stabilize body weight. Volunteers, all of normal weight, ate an 8,000-calorie-a-day diet, resulting in weight gain. However, in spite of eating enormous quantities of food, the average volunteer showed only a 25 percent increase in weight; the body weights of all subjects peaked below 220 pounds. When released from this diet and allowed to choose their own food, all subjects returned to their previous weights without effort. Animal studies also show this stability in regulation of body weight. Even obese animals two or

Illustration by John Martin

three times as heavy as their nonobese counterparts did not fluctuate more than nonobese animals once they reached their maximum weight. It appears, then, that weight *is* being regulated, and the issues concerning obesity have to do in part with a better understanding of that regulation.

In trying to understand the various causes of obesity, we need to look at a number of possibilities, including genetic, developmental, metabolic, social-emotional, and physical-activity factors.

Genetic Factors   Obesity can be produced in animals through selective breeding. Since this is so, we must assume a hereditary influence in human obesity. (Unfortunately, many studies with human subjects confuse the genetic and environmental influences.) Researchers are currently studying the hereditary transmission of body types, of which there are three: lean and slightly muscular (the slender ectomorph); athletic, characterized by powerful musculature (the mesomorph); and chubby, characterized by a prominent abdomen and other soft parts of the body (the endomorph). Evidence suggests that such body types can be inherited.

Studies have noted a great variability in body weights among humans but a remarkable consistency of body weight for individual persons over time. Such findings suggest that each person may have his or her own ideal biological weight—often referred to as "set point"—and that some may have a set point that is far above what is considered to be normal or average in a particular culture. This set point acts much like a thermostat that regulates the temperature around an ideal that is set, such as 68° Fahrenheit. It has been known for many years that laboratory animals will adjust food intake and physical activity to compensate for either starvation or forced feeding. The same kind of regulation through the set point may occur in humans. Animal studies in which different sections of the *hypothalamus* have been surgically altered have shown that the set point may operate within this part of the brain, which controls emotions as well as eating and other crucial bodily functions. Depending upon what portion of the hypothalamus was surgically altered, the animals either increased or decreased body weight and then maintained that new

Resting metabolic rate (RMR)
The rate at which a person uses energy,
as measured in calories, while at rest: for
example, while sitting quietly or sleeping.

weight, as if a new set point had been established. The significance of set point theory in understanding obesity has to do with the possibility—and it is just a possibility—that some individuals may literally be fighting their own biology in the sense that they are trying to alter what the body itself ceaselessly attempts to defend, namely a certain weight level. Whether this is an "unfair" contest for the obese person trying to lose weight is a very significant question. Clearly some obese people must work much harder than others to lose weight and keep it off.

Developmental Factors   Obesity in childhood is a major problem that is becoming more prevalent. Approximately 25 percent of all children are overweight, and parents who hope an obese child will "grow out of it" are waiting for something that is highly unlikely to happen. Indeed, most obese children become obese adolescents, and most obese adolescents become obese adults. It has been estimated, for example, that if an obese eighth grader does not reduce body weight to a reasonably normal level by the end of adolescence, the odds against his or her doing so later in life are 28 to 1.

The persistence of obesity in childhood may be explained by studies showing that body weight is a function of the size and number of fat cells. Weight gain can take place in two ways: by increasing the number of fat cells, which commonly occurs in childhood, or by enlarging the size of existing cells, typically what goes on with adults.

The size and number of fat cells may influence how the hypothalamus sends signals to other organs in terms of stimulating the desire to eat and in controlling how much food is consumed. Some researchers have speculated that people who have lost weight but who have a larger number of fat cells tend to overeat in reaction to the body's tendency to refill those fat cells. One impressive study divided obese women into three categories: (1) those whose obesity was linked to having too many fat cells, (2) those with enlarged fat cells, and (3) those with both conditions. Regardless of the approach used to lose weight and regardless of the length of time used to lose weight, all of the women stopped losing weight when their fat cells reached normal size. Furthermore, the number of fat cells did not decrease. Thus women

with a large number of fat cells tended to remain obese while those whose obesity was linked more to enlarged fat cells did lose weight. Continuing studies in this area may help us understand why some individuals successfully lose and maintain weight at normal or ideal levels while others continually struggle unsuccessfully to reduce body fat and total weight. We must be careful at this point not to get prematurely discouraged about the problems of reducing body fat and losing weight. There may be combinations of weight-loss methods that will work for those with a larger number of fat cells.

Metabolic Factors   While obesity is very rarely caused by abnormal metabolic problems, such as disturbances of the thyroid that result in a lowered resting basal metabolism level or Cushing's syndrome (a disorder of the adrenal cortex), recent evidence suggests that basal metabolism plays a major role in maintaining excessive body weight.

Basal metabolism or the *resting metabolic rate (RMR)* is the rate at which the body uses energy measured as calories essential at rest (for example, sitting quietly). Normally, one pound of weight is gained or lost in relationship to 3,500 calories, although this can vary widely among individuals. This *resting* rate of calorie use ranges from about 1 to 1.5 calories per minute. (By contrast a person running vigorously may use 20 or more calories per minute.) If RMR is increased from 1 to 1.2 calories per minute, then the result over one day is an increase of almost 300 calories expended ($0.2 \times 60 \times 24 = 288$). Such an increase is equivalent to walking or running about three miles. A person making such an increase from 1 to 1.2 calories per minute RMR would lose 30 pounds of fat in one year! Of course the reverse is also true.

What is not well understood and may be at the heart of why dieting by itself consistently fails to produce permanent weight loss is what happens when the number of calories is reduced. As the body takes in fewer calories, it also adjusts its RMR to a lower level. The converse is also true: the higher the caloric intake, the higher the RMR. A number of studies have found that as a person reduces caloric intake and starts to lose weight, a 15 to 30 percent reduction in RMR takes place.

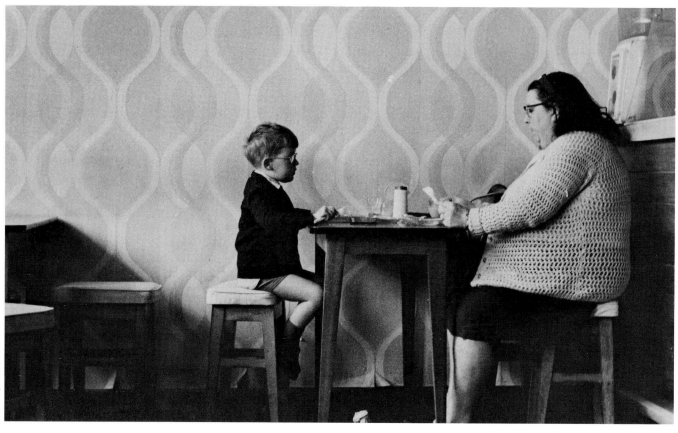

This change in RMR can occur as quickly as 48 hours after either a reduction in body weight or a reduction in caloric intake. Obviously, restricting caloric intake and not altering other factors, such as vigorous play and exercise activities, can sabotage efforts at weight loss.

Recall our earlier discussion of set point theory and how the body struggles to maintain and stabilize body weight. There is some evidence that rigorous physical activity can help offset this reduction in RMR and the body's tendency to stabilize weight. Indeed, the crucial role of vigorous physical activity has been poorly acknowledged as a major factor in the causes and cure of obesity, particularly the problem of being overfat.

Physical Factors   In terms of obesity, there are many advantages of physical activity, including (a) increasing caloric expenditures, (b) counteracting ill effects of obesity, (c) suppressing appetite, (d) increasing basal metabolism, and (e) minimizing loss of lean body tissue. It is important to note that losing weight through dieting alone, particularly through "starvation" diets of 300 to 600 calories, results in a loss of 75 percent fat tissue and 25 percent lean tissue, particularly muscle tissue. However, research indicates that when weight loss is accomplished through a combination of dieting and physical activity, the loss of lean body tissue decreases to about 5 percent.

Exercise has commonly been ignored as a major factor in obesity because it requires so many calories of physical activity to lose one pound. For example, in Scandinavia the traditional 49-mile cross-country ski race, which lasts about 10 hours, uses the energy equal to about two pounds of fat tissue. Another way of looking at the relationship of exercise to expending calories is to ask how many minutes of activity are required to use up 100 calories (keep in mind that a medium-sized piece of apple pie is about 350 calories). When running or jogging on the flat, it can take about 10 minutes to burn 100 calories. The same applies to sawing wood, playing racquetball, and swimming. Aerobic dancing requires 15 minutes of activity to burn 100 calories, as does roller skating and playing soccer; and playing volleyball, cleaning windows, washing the car, or raking leaves requires 20 minutes. Such figures are discouraging to a person who is considering physical activity as a means of losing weight. Yet a crucial fact is commonly overlooked. Exercise works slowly yet continuously in influencing body weight. Statistics show that the typical American gains from one to two pounds a year between the ages of 20 and 50. In total this amounts to about 45 extra pounds by the age of 50. An average weight gain of one and a half pounds equals 5,250 calories spread over 365 days. On a daily basis this equals a mere 14.4 calories per day. Thus, just a slight yet consistent and steady increase in physical activity over the months and years can literally make the difference between maintaining normal weight and becoming seriously overweight.

Social and Emotional Factors   Eating, like most basic human activities, tends to become a focal point, not only of whatever is happening to an individual psychologically, but also of interpersonal relationships and cultural values. If we know, for example, that a person's daily breakfast consists of two cups of instant coffee and three cigarettes taken standing up, we know a little about that person's inner life or at least that person's inner life at the moment. Other examples come readily to mind. The intimate dinner has a special significance for lovers; so does the "working lunch" for business associates or political leaders. Food is often invested with religious significance, as in the Jewish seder, or with family feeling, as in the traditional American Thanksgiving dinner.

Social and emotional meanings are also attached to the results of various patterns of eating. Thus, being obese can have a sexual significance for the individual, but the nature of that sexual significance might depend on both personal and cultural factors. It might be important to know, for example, whether the obese individual grew up in a society that considers obesity sexually attractive or in one that considers it sexually repulsive. Many social and emotional factors may be involved in obesity.

Failure to Perceive Internal Cues   Every human being is born with a tremendous capacity for self-regulation. If you need rest, you become sleepy and, as soon as

Anorexia Nervosa and Bulimia

Recent years have seen an alarming increase in the number of cases of anorexia nervosa and bulimia. These disorders, unlike obesity, are classified as psychiatric disorders. Diet is an important factor in but not the direct cause of these disorders. Psychological factors probably play the prime role, but no single psychological theory is widely supported at present. Although these disorders have certain similarities and are often confused, each has its own symptoms and treatment.

Anorexia Nervosa

Anorexia nervosa, a diet-related disorder caused by emotional problems, is characterized by loss of appetite and severe weight loss. Though it mainly affects teenage girls, older women and occasionally men may also suffer from it. People with this disorder feel fat even when they are underweight or emaciated.

Vitamin and mineral deficiencies may appear, and menstruation usually stops. If untreated, the condition may become fatal as the victims literally starve themselves to death while continuing to assert that their food intake is excessive. Treatment for anorexia involves medical procedures along with psychological therapy. Slowly increasing one's food intake is required. For those too weak to eat, feeding is done intravenously or by tube. In many cases anorexics can be restored to good physical health, particularly if treatment is begun before the condition becomes a chronic life pattern.

Bulimia

Less well known but apparently more widespread than anorexia nervosa is the disorder bulimia. Most bulimics are college students or career women in their 20s and 30s. People with this disorder

usually maintain their normal appetite, weight, and biological functions. Instead of turning *away* from food in times of stress, as anorexics do, bulimia sufferers turn *to* food. After overeating, bulimics purge themselves of calories by means of self-induced vomiting, laxatives, diuretics, or extended periods of fasting. Recent studies at the University of Chicago have indicated that over 25 percent of entering freshmen use some degree of self-induced vomiting to lose weight. In severe cases bulimics develop distended abdomens that eventually resemble those of pregnant women.

Success in treating both anorexia and bulimia has been achieved with behavior therapy. This involves a program of environmental control in which eating behavior is shaped and reinforced by very specific rewards and punishments.

---

you give in to the feeling, fall asleep. When you have had enough rest, you wake up. When you need food, you feel hunger pangs in your stomach, and the natural response is to look for something to eat. The sleepy feeling and the hunger pangs are examples of *internal cues*—sensations in your body that demand a specific response. This system of internal cues remains with you throughout life. But learned behavior patterns can modify your capacity *to be aware of* the cues. This, in fact, commonly happens in industrial societies. For example, when a child's sexual feelings are in conflict with a cultural taboo, the child learns first to pretend not to have the feelings and then to block his or her awareness of those feelings. This process of learning not to feel internal cues often goes hand in hand with learning to pay attention to *external cues*. External cues tend to reflect social demands, but once you have "internalized" them, they *seem* to be coming from inside. The internal cue "Eat something now!" is crowded out of consciousness by the external cue "It isn't lunchtime yet." The internal cue "Stop eating!" is overridden by the external cue "Clean your plate."

To study the relationship between obesity and perception of internal cues, psychologist Richard Nisbett conducted the following experiment: Each subject was given an early afternoon appointment for what he was told was an experiment to measure physiological factors. He was also instructed to eat nothing after 9 that morning. After 30 minutes of a bogus experiment, the subject was led into another room "to fill out some questionnaires." The room was empty except for a table, a chair, and a refrigerator. On the table were a bottle of soda and either one or three roast beef sandwiches wrapped in white paper. The subject was told that since he had skipped lunch he could help himself to the food on the table and that if he wanted more there were more sandwiches in the refrigerator. The experimenter then left.

The subjects had previously been classified in three groups—overweight, underweight, and normal weight. Overweight subjects confronted with three sandwiches generally ate more than other subjects; overweight subjects confronted with one sandwich ate less than normal subjects. In fact, they ate as little as the underweight subjects. One of the questions on the

Internal cues
Sensations from inside the body that
provide information.

External cues
Sensations from outside the body that
provide information.

Prevalence
The number of instances of a condition in
a specified population at a given time.

---

questionnaire was "Are you a 'clean your plate' type or are you likely to leave something?" A large percentage of the overweight subjects considered themselves plate cleaners, and their behavior confirmed it. They were less likely than other subjects to leave anything uneaten and also less likely to go to the refrigerator for more. In other words, the external cue "Clean your plate" was stronger than any internal cue that might have indicated "I'm still hungry" or "I'm full."

Emotional factors have often been cited as causes of obesity. Certainly, in times of stress, losing weight is difficult for some people. It does not necessarily follow, however, that obese people are more neurotic than normal-weight people.

Socioeconomic Status   The *prevalence* of obesity in lower-class women is 6 times that in upper-class women (37 percent, compared to 2 percent). Among men, the ratio is 2 to 1 (32 percent, lower-class to 16 percent, upper-class).

Socioeconomic factors besides those of class are involved in obesity. For example, people who are downwardly mobile tend to have a greater prevalence of obesity (22 percent) than those who remain in their parents' social class (18 percent). In contrast, those who are upwardly mobile have a relatively low rate of obesity (12 percent). Another social factor in obesity is the number of generations of one's family that have lived in the United States. Among first-generation Americans, 24 percent are obese, as compared to 5 percent of fourth-generation Americans, independent of socio-economic status.

Religion   The greatest prevalence of obesity is found among Jews, then Roman Catholics, and then Prot-estants. Among the Protestant group the greatest prev-alence is among Baptists, followed by Methodists, Lutherans, and Episcopalians.

Age   By age 50 obesity increases to three times the prevalence at age 20 and then declines, presumably because of the deaths of obese men from cardiovascular problems. More women are obese than men, and the obesity prevalence for the female population persists beyond age 50.

How Can Weight Be Controlled?

Most people think that going on a diet is the best way to lose weight—the newer the diet, the greater the fat loss. Yet such thinking is scientifically unfounded. Dieting alone is a very poor long-term solution to taking off fat and keeping it off. Diets that offer simple solutions to the complex problems of being overweight may actually be bad for you—especially by not supplying the full range of nutrients you need and, even more importantly, by possibly setting you up for long-term failure.

You do need to consider what you eat and how much you eat, but you also need to realize that the weight loss game involves many players and requires a variety of game strategies. As we have seen, the causes of being overfat involve a variety of factors. Although they may sound very complex, some strategies for losing body fat and keeping it lost turn out to be straightforward and successful when people are patient yet persistent in their efforts.

Few obese people have succeeded in controlling their weight. Many lose weight and then gain it back. Most do not even enter treatment. Of those who do, a majority stop. According to studies done in 1959, only 25 percent of those entering treatment lost as much as 20 pounds, and only 5 percent lost as much as 50 pounds. Results of routine medical treatment for obesity showed that only 12 percent lost as much as 29 pounds.

In 1980, those results were updated. Essentially the same discouraging picture prevails for the long term, but results for short-term weight loss have dramatically im-proved. Using behavioral methods—such as monitoring and recording calories *and* physical activity, establishing short-term goals about how much to eat and exercise each day, and providing self-rewards for progress—commonly leads to losses of one to two pounds per week or an average of about 12 pounds for most 8- to 12-session weight-loss programs. Further, most of the discouraging long-term results are due to people's trying to reduce body fat only by dieting. When controlled eat-ing (but not crash or rash diets) is combined with reg-ular physical activities, the results are much more encouraging.

Dehydration
A condition in which a person has less than a normal amount of body water.

Dieting   Most low-calorie diets cause a rapid loss of body water at first. The weight loss shows up on scales, and many beginning dieters think that they are losing body fat. It soon becomes obvious to all but the most blindly optimistic dieters that they cannot keep on losing weight so quickly. If they somehow manage to persist, they will suffer serious *dehydration*. Rapid weight loss stemming from loss of body water is usually followed by an equally rapid weight gain.

In general, only the calorie content of food influences weight, although people on a high-protein diet probably do lose weight slightly faster than those on a diet that includes a number of different calorie sources. Eating the right foods is important. Nonfat dairy products and low-calorie complex carbohydrates high in water and fiber are best. Foods high in fats are loaded with calories and tend to add to weight problems, especially for inactive people. Three balanced meals a day are important, especially breakfast. Skipping breakfast to save time and calories is a good example of a poor strategy in the weight-loss game. Snacks planned ahead of time also help reduce eating high-calorie fast food substitutes. By following these suggestions *and* by increasing physical activity, obese people can achieve and maintain a healthy weight.

The goal in treating obesity is twofold. The individual's first aim should be to reestablish normal weight; the second should be to maintain that weight for the rest of his or her life. Speed is not what counts, yet most popular diets promise just that, even though it is physiologically impossible. Consider a diet that promises a 220-pound man that he will lose 22 pounds in 10 days. Even if he eats nothing, his calorie deficit will only be 3,500 calories a day, or 35,000 calories in 10 days. At the rate of 1 pound of fat lost per 3,500-calorie deficit, he will lose only about 9 pounds in those 10 days. And remember, this loss is what would occur if he ate absolutely *nothing*. Also remember that almost 3 of those pounds will not be lost fat but lost muscle and lean body tissue. (That is why starvation-type diets are very dangerous.) If he did indeed lose 22 pounds, much of it would be body water, which would replenish itself once he started eating normally again.

Exercise   Some people who might be able to benefit from exercise as an alternative to dieting (or combined with it) may be passing it up because they unquestioningly accept certain popular beliefs about exercise. For example, some people falsely believe that exercise has little effect on weight. This fact would be strange if it were true, since one of the main jobs that calories do is provide energy for use in physical activity. The claim is made that people must exercise a tremendous amount to lose a small amount of weight. It is true, for example, that to lose one pound, one must walk 35 miles, but it is misleading to assume that you have to trudge each and every one of those miles in a single day. Walking one mile every day for two years will expend 73,000 calories, the equivalent of 18.2 pounds of body fat.

Probably the most widely accepted mistaken idea about exercise is that any weight loss the exercise achieves is offset by an increase in appetite (and in calorie consumption). Studies with experimental animals show that this idea has no basis in fact. When normally sedentary animals were required to perform a *moderate* amount of exercise regularly, their consumption of food *decreased* and so did their weight. Only *strenuous* regular exercise causes people to eat more, and in such instances this increase is appropriate to the increased energy expenditure. The additional food intake does not result in a weight gain; it often does not even make up weight that is lost because of expenditure.

Exercising once in a while is no more effective than dieting once in a while (see Chapter 13.). A good exercise program for weight loss does not produce spectacular results overnight, but if the program is followed faithfully over a long period of time, the total amount of weight lost will be reasonably large. Anyone beginning an exercise program should start exercising slowly and increase demands over time. The weight lost through exercise is primarily body fat (over 90 percent). Regular exercise produces a trimmer and healthier looking body and will not deplete lean muscle tissue. Including more exercise is easy if approached gradually. For example, increase daily activities by walking up stairs instead of

(*text continues on p. 290*)

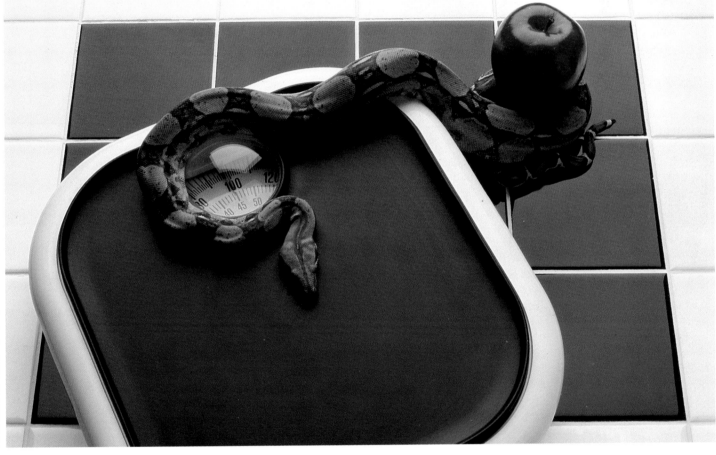

Photo: Michel Pilon; art director: Georges V. Haroutiun; client: Comac Publications

25 Tips from the Diet Center

By now, everyone knows about the Diet Center, but just in case . . . it is the world's largest weight-loss organization, with 1,758 offices across the country and a commonsense approach to diet that works so well, members lose a million pounds a month. Diet Center counselors gave us this batch of tried-and-true suggestions, practically guaranteed to keep you slim.

1. When you feel the urge to overeat, head for the nearest mirror and take a good, long look at yourself. (Do you still crave those extra calories?)

2. Parties needn't sabotage a diet: Call your hostess in advance and ask if you may bring one of your special (low-cal) dishes, beautifully prepared, to share with the guests.

3. If boredom is your downfall—if you tend to eat because there's nothing else to do—realize it's not food you want, but something to fill the void. Write letters, clean a closet, take a walk—anything to keep your mind and body occupied.

4. Midafternoon is the toughest time for many dieters. Be prepared for the four o'clock slump with an appropriate snack, such as any one of these items, each less than 100 calories: small baked potato; sliver of angelfood cake; twenty-eight chocolate chips; "Danish" made with thin-sliced bread topped with 1 tablespoon cottage cheese, 1 teaspoon sugar, cinnamon; popcorn flavored with Parmesan cheese; mug of hot chicken bouillon. (Keep snacks handy in a desk drawer if you work.)

5. Avoid the temptation to finish what the kids leave on their plates by having them, or your spouse, remove the plates and then wrap or dispose of leftovers as soon as the children have gotten up from the table.

6. Start thinking of food as fuel for your body's engine and eating as simply a way to keep your motor humming.

7. Make a "dream-come-true" bulletin board and hang it in a prominent place. Pin up pictures of how you want to look, slinky clothes you'd love to wear, things you'd like to do when you're thinner.

8. Be firm with people who "love you" with food. If your mother makes lasagna each time you visit, explain that losing weight is your top priority and she can *really* show she cares by broiling a piece of chicken for you.

9. Don't be discouraged if you're not losing pounds as fast as you think you should. When you hit a plateau, get out the tape measure and check for inch loss. Often the tape will show what the scales do not.

10. Read labels carefully when you shop for food. Bear in mind that any ingredient ending in "-ose" (dextrose, sucrose, fructose, maltose, for example) is a sugar.

11. Avoid wearing clothes you can hide in. Big, shapeless dresses and skirts with elastic waistbands disguise excess poundage, but offer little incentive to lose. Neatly fitted clothes with zippers, buttons and belts keep you and others aware of your progress.

12. Use modified "aversion conditioning" techniques to help you deal with temptation: When faced with a plate of cookies, french fries, anything you love, try to visualize the food soaking wet, covered with sand or ashes, stale or moldy.

13. Eat elegantly, even though you're counting calories. Smaller portions seem much more satisfying when arranged artfully, dressed up with colorful garnishes, served on best china and glassware.

14. Keep the fridge stocked with appropriate food so you'll never be caught with nothing but no-nos to eat. Boil a dozen eggs, cook up lots of fish and chicken breasts at once, cut up and store huge quantities of salad vegetables, etc.

15. When stress threatens to wear down your willpower, get away from the source of the tension if possible. Most important, ask yourself, "How would overeating help me in this situation?"

16. Shopping for a party? Don't store chips, cookies or other goodies where they might tempt you. Keep them out of sight and out of mind until the big day . . . locked in the trunk of your car if need be.

17. Get started on an exercise routine to burn off additional calories and tone muscles. Program your workout into the same time slot daily; don't allow anything but an emergency to interfere.

18. Shop for a really sensational dress or suit in the size that you want to be. Use the store's layaway plan and pay something on the outfit each time you lose five pounds. By the time you finally reach your weight goal, your new clothes will be paid for and ready to wear.

19. Plan meals carefully so that there will be little if any food left over for snacking later. (When entertaining, send leftovers home with guests.)

20. Hang a calendar near the bathroom scale and record your weight weekly. Take a moment or two at weigh-in time to give yourself a pep talk and plan your day's diet.

(continued on next page)

25 Tips from the Diet Center (continued)

21. Eat an apple or munch on a carrot or celery sticks if preparing the evening meal makes you ravenous. Something to nibble on while fixing dinner helps you break the destructive taste-as-you-cook habit.

22. Cooperate with a dieting friend if you're both having trouble finding the time to shop and prepare special low-cal meals. One week, you shop for the two of you; she cooks. The next week, she shops; you cook.

23. Carry a "fat" picture of yourself in your wallet. (The more unflattering the photo, the better.) Take a peek at it whenever you feel your resolve beginning to waver.

24. If you need extra help getting from Friday P.M. to Monday A.M. without bingeing, map out a weekend diet strategy, listing in detail exactly what you will eat and when. Prepare food ahead and follow your plan exactly. It's when you *don't* have a plan that problems arise.

25. Get out of the mind-set that uses food as a reward. Make a list of nonfood treats for when you need a psychic lift—a new lipstick, a paperback book, a long-distance call to your best friend, a movie. And of course, promise yourself something extra special when you reach your long-term goal.

Ladies' Home Journal

Evaluating a Fad Diet

We cannot possibly examine all the diets and reducing aids that promise quick, easy results, but there are several criteria we can use to evaluate a weight-reduction program:

1. *Does it have any real advantages over existing or conventional diets?* Most fad diets have a gimmick, such as eating grapefruit or using liquid-protein supplements. Do these gimmicks work, or are they only a means of attracting attention to the diet?

2. *Is the diet easy to follow?* Fasting, for instance, produces a weight loss, but it requires a great deal of willpower. Most people cannot keep it up for very long.

3. *Does the diet provide any long-term modification of eating habits that will allow the weight loss to be maintained after the diet is over?* Many diets, such as liquid-protein diets and fasting, and diet aids, such as drugs, can produce a weight loss. However, because eating behavior is not changed, the person usually regains the weight.

4. *Does the diet present any hazard to health?* Very restrictive diets may lead to malnutrition; others, such as liquid-protein diets, have caused injury and even death.

5. *How much does it cost?* Often the dieter is enticed into buying expensive equipment or overpriced "special" foods. Seldom are these items of any value.

6. *Does the diet promise quick results in return for little effort on the part on the dieter?* This is one of the hallmarks of a fad diet. Many of these claims simply are not true. Rapid weight losses observed on some diets, such as the low-carbohydrate diet, are because of loss of water.

7. *Are there any inconsistencies with established knowledge?* Examples include the assertion that carbohydrates rather than excess kilocalories are fattening and that grapefruit possesses some magical weight-reducing property.

William L. Scheider
Nutrition: Basic Concepts and Applications

Thyroid
A gland in the neck that controls the rate of body metabolism.

Diuretic
An agent that promotes the excretion of urine.

Gastrointestinal tract
Tissues of the stomach and intestines

using elevators, walking or cycling to school or work, or parking far enough away from destination to allow yourself to walk some distance. The benefits of weight loss via planned activities are very positive because the body's metabolism increases to offset the reduction in calorie intake from eating less. Thus the weight loss from physical play and exercise is gradual yet much more likely to be permanent. Sustaining a well-balanced routine of physical activities, especially play activities that one enjoys, is just as important as a well-balanced diet. For losing fat, some now believe that it is far more important, since the physically active body will tolerate a less than ideal diet as compared to a sedentary body.

Medical and Psychological Approaches A variety of medical and psychological methods are used in weight control. Treatment with drugs involves the use of phenylpropandamine (PPA), similar to amphetamines, to suppress appetite. In combination with a diet and under medical supervision, they have *very limited usefulness*. Further, they have a very serious potential for abuse that far outweighs their effectiveness. No scientific data support the use of drugs such as PPA and others that suppress the appetite. And their side effects may include insomnia, marked irritability, dry mouth, and addiction.

Administration of thyroid hormone is sometimes recommended for controlling obesity. For obese people whose *thyroid* is functioning normally, this treatment is useless. It is true that a genuine thyroid deficiency may cause weight gain, but such a deficiency can usually be easily diagnosed with appropriate blood tests, and it rarely causes obesity.

Some drugs act on the kidneys to promote loss of water from the body. These drugs, called *diuretics*, are also often advocated for the treatment of obesity. However, because of the threat of severe dehydration, uncontrolled use of diuretics is potentially dangerous. Besides, obesity is not simply a *weight* problem. The problem is a superabundance of body fat, and diuretics have no effect on body fat.

"Starch blockers," tablets containing the protein phaseolamin extracted from kidney beans, are another recent "solution" to weight loss. The normal enzymic digestion of starches (carbohydrates) is interfered with in the small intestine, thus preventing its absorption into the body. No scientific evidence exists that weight loss occurs or is maintained by means of starch blockers; furthermore, they may cause cramps, nausea, and diarrhea.

Total starvation as a method for losing weight first became popular in the early 1960s. Originally, people were starved (or starved themselves) for periods lasting from ten days to 2 weeks. Some people repeated the starvation episodes periodically. Then it became fashionable to starve obese people for longer periods of time. Many obese patients were once starved for periods of up to six months or a year or more, during which time they often lost more than 100 pounds. This type of treatment is no longer widely favored. In the first place, total starvation leads to substantial loss of body constituents other than fat—notably, protein. Second, the treatment may be dangerous. For it to be safe the treatment must be carried out in a hospital under strict supervision, an expense that many people cannot meet. Finally, potential dangers can become actual, and people have suffered significant complications as a result of total starvation. These include acute attacks of gout, severe anemia, sudden drops in blood pressure, and in a few cases severe metabolic disturbances. Starvation regimes do little to retrain eating habits and encourage regular physical activities, and most people who have lost weight under starvation conditions have rapidly gained it back following their return home, where they resumed their poor eating and exercise habits.

Another extreme treatment for controlling obesity is surgery—the bypassing of a major portion of the *gastrointestinal tract*. The bypass prevents food from being absorbed into the body. This form of treatment also may lead to serious complications, notably chronic diarrhea and kidney stones. It should be regarded only as an experimental and extreme form of therapy, appropriate for very few people.

Group treatment of obesity is available through self-help organizations such as TOPS (Take Off Pounds Sensibly) and commercial organizations such as Weight Watchers, which has a membership of several million. Many obese people are apparently more inclined to use the services of Weight Watchers than to seek medical or self-help group assistance. The effectiveness of

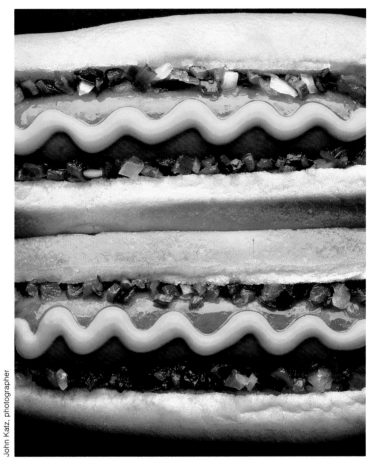

John Katz, photographer

Play Plans for Exercise and Weight Loss

Peter Wood has developed a variety of ways in which people can reduce weight and avoid unpleasant dieting. One strategy concerns using so many calories each day in play activities—doing things that are fun and interesting. If a person gets into the habit of expending a few more calories each day, then in time he or she can lose many pounds. Here are three plans, each designed to use up a different number of calories. Plan A is a minimum plan, while Plans E and J are more vigorous.

Play Plan A
(25 calories per day)

Choose *one* playful act *each day* from the accompanying list, These are *extra* play calories to *add* to your usual routine.

Walk a quarter mile (3 blocks)

Cycle a mile, slowly

Swim for 3 minutes

Dance (aerobic) for 5 minutes

Clean windows for 6 minutes

Rake leaves for 6 minutes

Scrub floor for 6 minutes

Feel free to try different activities on different days.

Playful Hints . . .

■ Get off to a good start—don't overdo!
■ Find a playful friend!
■ Don't forget—keep your play record.
■ Yes—it's easy to start with, but there's lots more fun to come!

Play Plan E
(150 calories per day)

Choose *one* activity every day:

Walk at moderate speed for 30 minutes

Cycle for 25 minutes

Swim for 15 minutes

Dance (aerobic) for 25 minutes

Dance (disco) for 30 minutes

Play volleyball for 30 minutes

Play table tennis for 30 minutes

Clean windows to music for 30 minutes

Scrub floors to music for 30 minutes

Playful Hints . . .

■ Do you have a companion to play with? Whom do you know who would like to lose weight with you?
■ Make some of your play useful: clean windows or scrub floors to music! The exercise is burning fat.
■ Think "play" whenever you have to go somewhere: Can you walk over, not ride? Is the bike handy? Why not walk to and from the restaurant? Go on, even jog a little on the way!
■ If you don't drive, you won't have a parking problem (or a parking ticket).

Play Plan J
(500 calories per day)

Choose one activity each day:

Walk five miles in 75 to 90 minutes

Run for 45 minutes

Cycle for 60 minutes

Play racquetball for 60 minutes

Dance (aerobic) for 60 minutes

Play soccer for 60 minutes

Roller skate for 65 minutes

Mow the lawn for 60 minutes

Saw wood for 50 minutes

This high level of fitness should be approached slowly. It involves playing vigorously for about an hour a day, or 4 percent of our 24-hour day. The player is very fit, eats a lot, and has banished weight problems!

Playful Hints . . .

■ Major league stuff!
■ Remember, drink more water than you feel you need when it's hot.
■ To avoid injuries, do your stretching exercises and vary your plan.
■ You are now twenty times more playful than you were at month 1.
■ You have played away 4½ pounds of fat this month!
■ This level of play will keep you slim and fit forever!

Peter Wood
The California Diet and Exercise Program

Behavior modification
Psychological techniques that make use of
learning principles to modify unwanted
behaviors.

Weight Watchers, however, is difficult to evaluate, since controlled studies are not available.

Psychotherapy can also be a treatment for obesity. Half the people seeing doctors for obesity treatment report emotional disturbances, including anxiety and depression, associated with fasting or restricted-calorie diets. Although psychotherapy may help some people lessen the stresses they feel and indirectly result in modest weight loss, there is no evidence that exploring the historical causes of overeating can reduce overeating or weight.

The real breakthrough in treating obesity was reported in 1967 when Richard Stuart described a successful obesity treatment using *behavior modification*. Eighty percent of his subjects lost more than 20 pounds and many lost 30 to 40 pounds over the year. Many other studies have demonstrated successful use of behavior modification to treat mild-to-moderate obesity.

Since Stuart's initial results, other behavioral treatments have been tried, but few have matched his impressive results. Typically, treatment programs last only three months (about 10 to 12 sessions), with an average weight loss of about 11 or 12 pounds, or 1 or 2 pounds per week. Such losses are often maintained for the first year but regaining weight after that is common.

The reasons that many behavioral programs have not produced large sustained weight losses seem clear. Substantial and sustained weight loss requires an ongoing, frequent, "intensive" treatment program (the Stuart study involved frequent contacts over the entire year). The temptation to fall back on old habits of eating and inactivity is tremendous. If people know that they will weigh-in weekly and that their food and physical activity diaries will be checked and discussed, they are more likely to adhere to their eating and activity plans. Frequent contacts also provide much needed encouragement and social support, both for progress and for inevitable plateaus in losing weight. Some positive side effects of behavioral programs are noteworthy when compared to other approaches: (a) few emotional symptoms tend to arise during behavioral treatments, (b) the drop-out rates from behavioral treatments are very low, and (c) people's overall psychological functioning tends to increase.

Behavioral treatments vary widely but often focus on the elimination of behavior associated with poor eating and physical activity habits. Such programs instruct people in specific methods of changing maladaptive eating habits. Most of these programs include the monitoring (writing down) of food intake and weight; the setting of reasonable weight-loss goals (usually from 1 to 1½ pounds per week); rewards for success in changing habits; nutritional counseling; social rewards (achieved by teaching family and friends to praise, not criticize); cognitive strategies for directing appropriate behavior and countering self-defeating thoughts; and stimulus-control procedures that reduce the presence and availability of calorie-rich foods.

A new and promising aid for weight loss is a microcomputer to be carried by the overweight person. After establishing daily calorie and physical activity goals, the person records his or her intake and physical activities into the computer four times a day. Each time, the computer displays the number of calories thus far consumed for the day compared to the total calorie goal planned for the day. ("You have used 417 calories. That's 42 percent of your goal.") Feedback on the amount of physical activity is provided in a similar fashion. The computer also offers various instructions as well as different kinds of encouragement ("Great! You're doing just fine."). Compared to subjects who used some standard behavioral methods, such as self-monitoring, those who used the computer lost twice as much weight over a two-month period. Although long-term results are not yet available, this approach holds great promise as a tool for people who are trying to be consistent in their plans to reduce caloric intake and increase physical activities. Conceivably, software programs could be developed to provide a variety of strategies for losing weight, thus allowing people to select those programs best suited to them.

Eating for Health

Overweight, anorexia nervosa, and bulimia are not the only diet-related health concerns of Americans. And being thin does not necessarily imply healthiness. Many people appear to be of normal weight yet have diets high in fat, salt, and sugar. Young people may feel especially immune to the ravages of weight gain and chronic illness that affect many Americans. The encouraging fact is that most chronic diseases, such as heart disease, high blood pressure, and some cancers, are clearly preventable. The discouraging news is that young people are already developing some of the characteristics of chronic disease, such as elevated blood pressure and plaque growth in their coronary arteries. The choices people make about diet, as well as exercise, stress, drug and alcohol use, and cigarette smoking, greatly influence their level of health now and in the future. Altering one's diet and participating in ongoing physical play activities is one way of reducing the overall risk of developing certain diseases later in life.

Despite theories about the irreversibility of the numbers of fat cells and other biological factors, most people clearly can avoid being overfat. Research has shown that diet-related diseases such as heart disease and some types of cancer can be prevented in part by adopting guidelines that minimize high fat, sugar, and salt intake and that emphasize high-fiber, complex (unrefined) carbohydrate foods. Diets that are high in fat and low in fiber have been increasingly implicated in both diseases. Fats, especially saturated animal fats (high in cholesterol), contribute to heart disease by raising cholesterol in the bloodstream, which in turn is involved in gradually blocking arteries in the heart with plaque. As plaque formations increase, hardening or closing of the coronary arteries, or atherosclerosis, occurs. A fully blocked coronary artery leads to restricted blood flow within the heart, leading to part of the heart muscle's actually dying from insufficient nourishment. If blood flow to the brain is blocked, a stroke occurs. Bowel and stomach cancer, hypertension, diabetes, and other diseases are also related to diet, but less is known about the specific relationships. Nevertheless, in 1984 the American Cancer Society announced for the first time that the evidence linking obesity and diet to various cancers was compelling. A 12-year study found a marked increase of cancers of the uterus, gallbladder, kidney, stomach, colon, and breast in obese people. In general, among people who were 40 percent or more overweight, women had a 55 percent greater risk for cancer and men had a 33 percent greater risk.

Although risk factors such as gender, genetic makeup, and family history cannot be changed, people can alter their diet, as well as their smoking, drug use, stress, and exercise.

Guidelines for a Healthy, Moderately Low-Calorie Diet

- Reduce consumption of high-fat foods by using low-fat or nonfat dairy products and avoiding butter, processed cheese, and red meats.
- Increase use of carbohydrates, such as fresh fruits, vegetables, grains (rice, oats, corn, noodles), and legumes (beans, peas). These are high in nutrients and fiber.
- Reduce consumption of red meats, organ meats, and eggs for protein. Fish and poultry are healthier sources of protein. Vegetable and grain combinations such as beans and rice, peas and noodles, peanuts and whole wheat bread also supply complete protein.
- Reduce consumption of highly processed fast foods, which are typically high in calories, fats, salt, and sugar.
- Help the body process foods effectively by developing and maintaining a vigorous plan of physical play activity.

Weight Control Behavior Scale

Read the following statements carefully. Choose the one in each section that best describes you at this moment and record its score at the right. (For example, "slender" has a score of 5.) When you have identified five statements, total your score and find your position on the scale.

5 slender
4 close to ideal weight
3 slightly above ideal weight
2 overweight
1 obese

Score _____

5 maintains regular eating schedule
4 eats three times a day
3 has irregular eating habits
2 usually snacks between meals
1 eats frequently during the day

Score _____

5 eats a balanced diet
4 emphasizes vegetables in diet
3 prefers meat and potatoes
2 eats high-fat foods
1 enjoys desserts with every meal

Score _____

5 vigorously active
4 relatively active
3 moderately active
2 minimally active
1 inactive

Score _____

5 believes weight is mostly affected by diet and exercise
4 believes weight is mostly affected by diet
3 believes exercise weight loss is offset by increased appetite
2 believes weight is mostly affected by genetics
1 believes weight is least affected by diet

Score _____

Total score _____

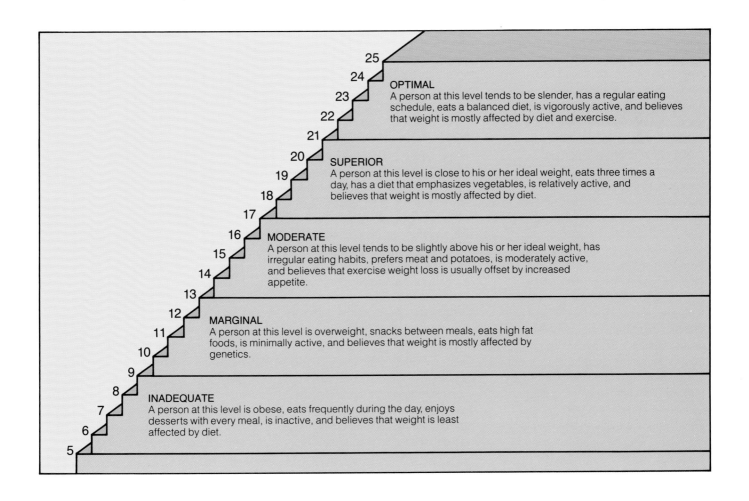

OPTIMAL
A person at this level tends to be slender, has a regular eating schedule, eats a balanced diet, is vigorously active, and believes that weight is mostly affected by diet and exercise.

SUPERIOR
A person at this level is close to his or her ideal weight, eats three times a day, has a diet that emphasizes vegetables, is relatively active, and believes that weight is mostly affected by diet.

MODERATE
A person at this level tends to be slightly above his or her ideal weight, has irregular eating habits, prefers meat and potatoes, is moderately active, and believes that exercise weight loss is usually offset by increased appetite.

MARGINAL
A person at this level is overweight, snacks between meals, eats high fat foods, is minimally active, and believes that weight is mostly affected by genetics.

INADEQUATE
A person at this level is obese, eats frequently during the day, enjoys desserts with every meal, is inactive, and believes that weight is least affected by diet.

Take Action

Your answers to Probing Your Emotions at the beginning of this chapter and your placement level on the Weight Control Behavior Scale will, we hope, encourage you to begin a process of self-exploration and self-discovery that you will continue. Reflect on the entire chapter's content and ask yourself how each point relates to your own life. Then take action:

1. Read at least three currently popular diet plans. (Your library probably has copies of several diet programs.) Evaluate each plan in terms of the seven criteria give in "Evaluating a Fad Diet," page 289. Which plan appears to be the best? Why? Would you consider going on any of the three diets? Would you recommend any of them to an overweight friend?

2. In your Take Action notebook keep track of your eating behavior for four or five days. Note the time, setting, amount of food, your mood, and what activities preceded your eating. What are the relationships between your eating and any of these elements? For instance, do you eat more food or certain kinds of foods when you are happy as opposed to upset?

3. List the positive behaviors that help you control your weight. Consider how you can strengthen these behaviors. Don't forget to congratulate yourself for these positive aspects of your life. Now, list the behaviors that tend to block your maintaining optimal weight. Consider each of these behaviors and decide which ones you can change to improve your health and life-style.

4. Read the following Behavior Change Strategy, and take the appropriate action.

Behavior Change Strategy

Weight Control

Most people first become acquainted with behavioral methods or behavior modification in relation to weight-control programs. Dr. Albert Stunkard, a respected authority in this field, has estimated that each week approximately 400,000 people are exposed to behavioral methods as a part of commercial weight-loss programs.

In part, this phenomenal activity can be attributed to the awareness and pervasive character of weight gain in our culture. Behavioral measures provide a distinct departure from the usual approach of counting calories, going on fad diets, and searching for instant results. Rather than promising overnight success (a promise that rarely can be fulfilled in lasting fashion), behavioral weight-control programs encourage slow but steady reduction at a rate of about 2 pounds per week. Such programs usually emphasize the "energy balance" concept that serves to explain the relationship between calories taken in via eating and drinking and calories burned off through physical activity. The energy balance concept represents the two central goals of any weight-control program: (1) to reduce the quantity and the high-caloric quality of food consumed and (2) to increase activities that use up excess calories. The strategies included to accomplish these goals follow the self-management format described in more detail in Chapter 1 of this book. Dietary/nutritional counseling is often included in many of these weight-control programs. However, this section will focus only on behavioral strategies.

Self-Monitoring   Keeping a chart or diary of body weight is a basic behavioral strategy. In addition to weight, a variety of additional data can be (and often is) collected. For example, one weight-control guide, *Take It Off and Keep It Off* (1977), provides instruction and blank diary pages that ask for the quantity, type, and caloric content of food consumed, as well as where the eating occurred, who was present at the time, and a description of hunger and other feelings associated with the eating episode. Moreover, the authors, Katz and Jeffrey, provide a 1,000-calorie food plan and weekly diet along with an exchange diet diary. Finally, they include a physical activity record that asks for the type and duration of activity, the estimated calories expended via that exercise, the place in which the exercise occurred, who, if anyone, was present, and the associated feelings.

Thus, there is an impressive number of ways to approach record keeping in any behavioral weight-loss program. However, it is important to keep in mind that some people find recording in such a computerlike fashion to be burdensome, a fact that does not facilitate adherence or follow-through. Self-monitoring should be linked to the specific strategies that are being used to manage weight; they should not become an end in themselves.

Stimulus Control   Eating and even internal feelings about being hungry are linked to routine situations. One way to lose weight is to try to limit the number of situations (times and places) in which food is permitted. Reestablishing—and narrowing—stimulus control over eating plays a major role in behavioral programs. Other stimulus controls involve placing high-calorie foods out of sight in the refrigerator or on shelves and prominently displaying low-calorie foods, reducing the size and appearance of food on the plate, eating more slowly, and avoiding the temptation of eating something just so it won't be thrown out.

Relaxation Methods   Eating that is linked to feelings—so-called "emotional eating"—can be a major contributor to overweight. The emotions can include tension, anxiety, boredom, depression, and anger. Although there are specific strategies for coping with these feelings, a more general approach used in most weight-control programs is to include instruction and practice in deep muscular relaxation as a coping skill.

Thoughts and Self-Statements
Many weight-control programs emphasize the role of thoughts and self-statements in sticking to a personal program or contract. For some, it is helpful to keep a diary of self-statements that pertain to losing weight. The following illustrates what such a diary might look like.

Time	Thoughts
7:30	"I'd really like a doughnut, but I'm not going to blow my day."
8:15	"It's not fair; I'm really trying and I haven't lost anything."
9:10	"Wish I had a doughnut or something; I'm hungry."
10:00	"It's not fair; it's snack time and all I get is water."
11:30	"Nothing tastes as good when I know there's no dessert."
12:10	"Look at them; they stuff themselves with sweets and stay skinny."
1:15	"Maybe I could have just a couple of cookies after school. I've earned them."
2:30	"Look at them—running off to their afternoon snacks. It's not fair."
3:15	"I don't care if I'm fat; I'll never lose anyway. It's not worth it."
4:30	"I might as well eat and enjoy it. I'll never be thin, no matter what I do."
5:45	"You pig. Now you feel stuffed and you've ruined your day."
7:30	"What a failure I am. I don't deserve to be thin."
9:00	"I'll never learn, will I? It's no use."
10:30	"I feel hopeless. I've tried everything and I always blow it."

Source: M. J. and K. Mahoney, *Permanent Weight Control: A Total Solution to the Dieter's Dilemma.* New York: Norton, 1976, p. 65.

Self-Contracts and Rewards   Contracts can also play a major role in a weight-control program. These include determining a schedule for completing major behavioral tasks, as well as weight-loss goals, and identifying the consequences of these activities.

Often the overweight individual sets aside a certain sum of money, which is managed by a "banker" who is carefully selected to help. If goals are not achieved, a portion of the money is forfeited. Because some people are not terribly bothered if they lose money to a "good cause," innovative program designers have found that the money should be sent to a previously agreed-upon "most hated" group or organization. In this way, the loss of the money becomes more unpleasant since it is not only lost but also directly helps a group that is distasteful to the person trying to lose weight. When the dieter completes certain tasks and goals on schedule, he or she is given a portion of the money to spend in a prearranged way, say, to buy an article of clothing one size too small (another incentive to lose weight).

Summary   Losing weight is quite different from many of the other target behaviors described in this book because it represents the *effective management* of a behavior rather than its total elimination. (We have to eat to survive, but we certainly do not have to smoke to survive.) For this reason, weight control presents a continuing challenge for many individuals. Programs that work for a period of time often lose effectiveness, so revised plans must be developed. The problem-solving character of effective weight management is critical. The interested reader is encouraged to review Chapter 1.

Chapter Thirteen

Exercise

Probing Your Emotions

1. How do you really feel about exercise? If you have postponed starting a regular exercise program or have had difficulty keeping at it, what are three of your excuses? How valid do you feel these excuses are?

2. You have been going to a health club for about three months. A friend asks you why you go. What do you tell your friend? If your friend joked about your enthusiasm, how would you feel?

3. How many of your friends who exercise regularly do so because of the health benefits they will enjoy in 30 years? Don't people exercise or participate in a sport because it makes them feel good rather than just because their bodies are benefiting? Many people have difficulty doing something that is "good for them" but that entails some perceived sacrifice (ask any dieter). Keeping this in mind, consider your own exercise regimen: Are you able to get out there at least three times a week? If not, what is *really* stopping you? If so, how would you go about getting a friend to join you?

Chapter Contents

WHAT IS PHYSICAL FITNESS?

WHY GET INTO SHAPE?
Emotional advantages
Physical advantages

HOW TO GET INTO SHAPE:
THE PLANNING STAGE
Choosing the appropriate activities
Buying equipment

IMPLEMENTING YOUR PROGRAM
Warm-up
Types of exercise
Cardiorespiratory endurance, or
    aerobic, exercises
Other forms of exercise
Developing skill in physical activities
Diet and fluid intake

WHAT IS ENOUGH? HOW
TO MAINTAIN FITNESS
The training effect: stress vs. distress
How to know that you are in shape
How to maintain fitness

INJURIES

Boxes

Running to Olympus
Commercial health clubs
Physiological benefits of warm-up
The five principles of a safe
    and effective exercise program
Steroids
That "extra effort" can hold you back

Physical fitness
The extent to which the body can respond
to the demands of physical effort.

13 Until a few years ago the only people who seemed to exercise in public were athletes and health nuts. Although many people watched their favorite sports event in person or on television, they rarely thought about participating in any regular physical activity themselves.

In just a short time we have gone from a nation of spectators to a nation of participants. Exercise is "in." Nowadays, if you don't backpack, run marathons, play tennis, or lift weights, people think there must be something wrong with you. Social forecasters Yankelovich, Skelly, and White have predicted that the national fitness craze will continue to escalate throughout the 1980s before it levels off. Clearly, more and more people believe that regular exercise is good for them and can be an enjoyable way to spend their leisure time.

Unfortunately, this craze has created problems for many of these new exercise enthusiasts. Some start in a wave of eagerness only to quit a few months later because of boring programs. Others are struck down by any number of overuse injuries that plague the "weekend warrior." Athletic injuries have become the scourge of many novice exercisers. In sports like tennis and jogging, over 50 percent of the participants can expect to experience injuries serious enough to interrupt their training. This, in turn, often leads to frustration and discouragement.

Most of these difficulties stem from a basic lack of understanding of the nature of exercise and training. Many people participate in inappropriate activities or do too much too soon. Approached correctly, exercise and sports can contribute to health and well-being and provide a continuing source of pleasure. With a little knowledge and planning, you can formulate a program that is good for you, that is fun, and that requires little time.

What Is Physical Fitness?

Physical fitness is the ability to adapt to the demands and stresses of physical effort. The term encompasses a wide variety of factors, such as cardiorespiratory endurance, muscular strength and power, flexibility,

body composition, speed, agility, neuromuscular coordination, and specific skill. Although there may be some overlap, each of these factors is independent of the others and each requires specific types of exercise for optimal development.

The human body has the ability to adapt to physical stress and actually improve its function. Likewise, in the absence of stress, its function deteriorates. For the most part, physical capacity tends to reflect the amount and intensity of physical activity.

The ability of the body to adapt to its level of physical activity has a profound effect on its biological well-being. If a person is chronically inactive, then his or her body reflects the inactivity: the heart and lungs have a lower capacity; the muscles, bones, and joints are weaker; and the metabolic capacity is impaired. Research studies indicate that the unfit person runs a higher risk of a myriad of health hazards such as heart disease, obesity, high blood pressure, backache, undernutrition, and a lower ability to cope with the effects of emotional stress. Likewise, if a person is chronically active, physiological function improves and the individual tends to become healthier.

Why Get into Shape?

People have a variety of reasons for exercising and participating in sports. For some, it is an attempt to stay a step ahead of the grim reaper. For others, it is an integral part of an active and exciting life-style.

Emotional Advantages Although exercise and sports enhance health and well-being, most committed participants also point out the emotional benefits of involvement. The joys of a well-hit cross-court backhand, the euphoria of a run alone in the park, or the rush of a downhill schuss through deep powder provide pleasures that transcend possible health benefits. Physical activity is an opportunity for harmonious interaction or invigorating competition with others. It provides an arena in which we strive to win or to become better than we are.

Physically fit individuals have plenty of energy. They

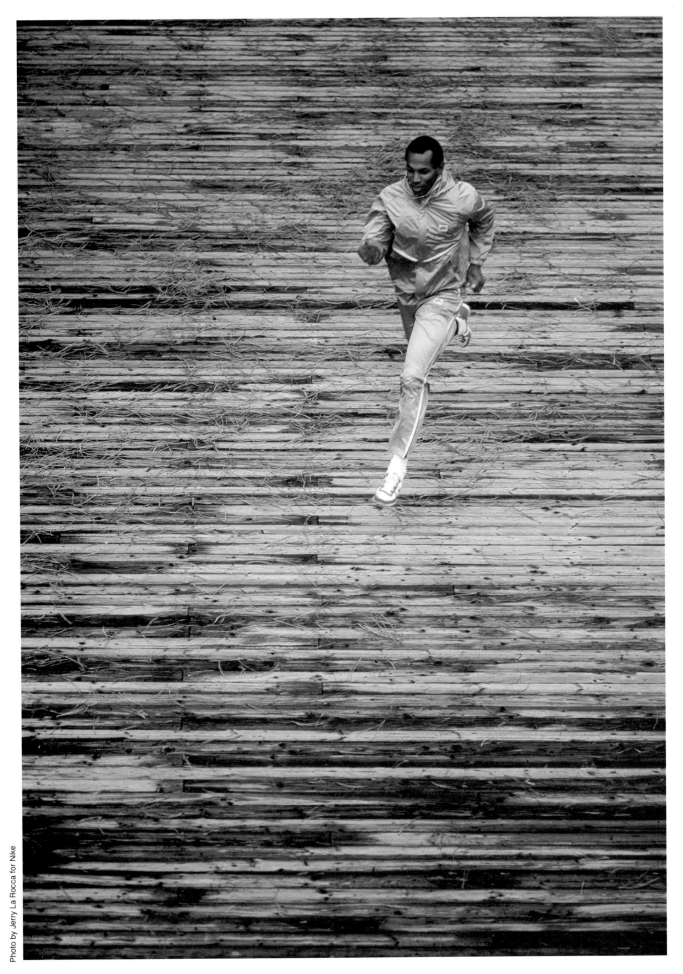

Running to Olympus

It is night, and I am running along the edge of a city park. Ahead of me is an exercise, a rite that is special, even though it has none of the trappings of ceremony.

I am not wearing shimmery polyester-blend trunks. I wear shapeless hiking shorts. I am not wearing $57 top-of-the-line-five-star-rated jogging shoes. I wear a comfortable pair of well-used Adidas found in the trash at a local high-school track. I am not wearing scientifically correct socks and head-band designed to wick up perspiration. I wear old gym socks, and a red kerchief is tied around my forehead. I do not have stereo head-phones, stopwatch and record pad—or pep pills hidden in my shoe. No, I am not your typical "magazine-cover" runner.

I am running at night because it is the best time. It is cool and quiet, the smog has settled, and no critics can view me and my un-fashionable running garb.

I run in the city, but even in these populated sprawls there are pockets of wilderness where wildlife thrives. Coyotes dart away into the darkness as I pass by. Poet birds sing. The sweet smell of sage per-fumes the moonless night.

As I meet the upcoming curve, my memory is jogged. I recall that the Hillside Strangler left one of his victims here. I feel my pocket and comfortably reassure myself that my pocket knife, designed for cutting twine and oranges, is still secure in its place.

I continue along the road, where only the whishes of the automatic sprinklers break the silence. Around the curve, headlights in the distance cause a flash of paranoia. Beads of sweat, smelling of fear, appear. The car grows closer and the headlights blind me as I instinctively run for-ward. The light is nearly upon me . . . and then it passes and disap-pears. The sound fades gradually, and so does the paranoia.

I stare into the distance on this long stretch. All the muscles are screaming, and I am keenly aware that the body machine is working well, attuned to the freedom of movement. I pass through a nominal level of pain and acknowl-edge it. Then my sensitivity focuses on the correctness of my move-ments. The even pace of the inhala-tions and exhalations . . . the knife-edge of my foot straight ahead . . . the hands relaxed . . . the toes kicking forward . . . the hips swing-ing with each stride.

As the body follows the brain's program, the mind travels a sepa-rate path. The quiet dark allows me to think deeply and inwardly. The feet drop to the pavement, one after the other, regularly, continous-ly. The mind soars as the body whizzes along.

My vision rises as I look into the heart of pain—not my immediate physical pain, but the pain of human-ity. We are born, we struggle, we fight, we love, we learn, we grow old, we die. Life is like a flash of light—at least as seen through the runner's vision at this moment of attunement. With each muscle's flex and each inhalation, I can feel the whole world, its hopes, aspirations, dreams, sorrows, disasters. I cannot feel these things when I view the 7 o'clock news while announcers chuckle and entertain.

The moving body is fully alert, fully alive, and so is the mind. The physical and mental and spiritual are all one, and now the introspec-tion moves from general to specific. I see my own life as if superim-posed on a screen in the middle distance, and I see the pain I've inflicted on others. Funny, I think of the "small" things: a glib word spoken crudely that caused crying, a rude insult that mars a friendship, acts of disobedience, a lie here, a theft there, an unloving act for no reason. I relive each of these things and cold tears splash on my cheeks. Now that I have felt the pain that I caused others to feel, I can resolve to change my ways.

The tears dry. I feel refreshed and joyous as I continue the steady pace. Suddenly a shock of cold water splatters my face and shatters my introspection. It is a misdirected jet from a broken lawn sprinkler—a baptism, a benediction.

No, I don't have bright stripes on my shorts, nor have I read The Complete Book of Running. But I have successfully accomplished an ancient rite. The body and soul are stretched, refreshed.

Tonight as the body sleeps, I shall put on my winged shoes and run to Greece.

Christopher Nyerges
Los Angeles Times

Catecholamines
Hormones secreted by the adrenal glands, especially during stress.

Enkephalin
A substance secreted in the brain and thought to produce the "runner's high" or euphoric feeling many people experience during exercise.

Degenerative diseases
Diseases that cause progressive destruction of tissues.

Cardiorespiratory endurance
The extent to which the heart and lungs can respond to physical exercise.

Aerobics
Exercise that emphasizes increased use of oxygen.

---

are productive and ready for whatever opportunities and activities present themselves. Their life-styles are interesting and varied. Sedentary people, on the other hand, miss many pleasures that life has to offer; they have less freedom. Often they don't have the stamina to enjoy many of the options open to them. A walk in the mountains, a game of volleyball, a dream vacation in Europe, or a game of Frisbee on the beach can be exhausting or impossible. Even the activities of daily life can sap the energy of inactive people.

Exercise also seems to help people cope with the effects of stress and improve their emotional health. In fact, many psychiatrists and psychologists recommend exercise as therapy for their patients. Biologically, the fit person secretes less of the "fight or flight" hormones, the *catacholamines*, in response to stressful situations. These hormones can be very destructive to the body when they are chronically secreted in the overstressed individual.

Researchers have recently identified a substance secreted in the brain called *enkephalin*. Enkephalin is thought to produce the euphoria or "high" that many people experience during exercise. It therefore appears that there is a physiological basis for what many exercise advocates previously attributed to metaphysics.

Physical Advantages Advances in public health and medicine have resulted in the eradication of many of the diseases that plagued human beings for centuries. Now we are faced with an array of perplexing *degenerative diseases* that largely demand changes in personal life-style rather than reliance on traditional medical crisis intervention. Diseases and disabilities such as heart disease, stroke, obesity, diabetes, hypertension, and backache can all be affected to a large degree by life-style factors such as diet, smoking, and exercise. More and more evidence points to the extreme importance of regular physical activity in reducing the risk of these health problems.

Convenience and reduced effort have been the aims of many of our technological advances. Driving the automobile is more convenient than walking; the gasoline mower is easier to use than the push lawn mower; and the escalator has replaced the stairs. More and more jobs require people to sit at a desk all day.

Clearly, we have to go out of our way to be physically active.

This sedentary life-style has led many to develop sedentary bodies that are ripe for a number of degenerative diseases. Over the last 30 years, researchers have been successful in establishing relationships between low levels of physical activity and the increased risk of heart disease. Usually these studies show that people in active occupations have fewer heart problems than those in sedentary positions. Still other studies show that the level of physical fitness is a critical factor in lowering the risk of heart disease. Exercise is important because it improves the body's function and reduces the severity of other factors that increase the risk of heart disease. These factors include obesity, blood sugar, hypertension, blood fats, and blood uric acid.

Benefits of Endurance Exercise Endurance exercise, also known as *cardiorespiratory endurance* exercise or *aerobics*, is most important for health. As Dr. Kenneth Cooper, developer of the system of aerobics, has said, "You can live without big muscles or a nice figure, but you can't live without a healthy heart." Table 13–1 describes some of the ways regular endurance exercise can reduce the risk or severity of heart disease. Exercise helps the body become a more efficient machine that is better able to cope with challenges from the environment. Three major adaptations seem to occur: an improvement in the body's oxygen transport capacity, more efficient body chemistry, and increased awareness of healthful living habits.

Perhaps the most important benefit of endurance exercise is the improved ability of the heart, lungs, and circulatory system to transport oxygen to the body's tissues. The heart pumps more blood per beat, the heart rate slows, red blood cells increase, tissue blood supply improves, and blood pressure decreases. The trained cardiorespiratory system doesn't have to work as hard at rest and at low levels of exercise because of its higher capacity. The trained heart can more easily withstand the stresses and strains of daily life and meet occasional emergencies that make extraordinary demands on the body's cardiorespiratory resources.

The human body survives by converting chemical or food energy into mechanical or work energy. This

Lipids
Fatty substances, such as cholesterol and triglycerides, in the blood.

Cholesterol
A fatty compound in the blood that is also found in deposits in the walls of arteries.

Triglyceride
A fatty compound that circulates in the blood; may have a role in atherosclerosis.

Plaque
A deposit on the inner wall of blood vessels. Blood can coagulate around a plaque and form a clot.

Lipoproteins
Chemicals in the blood that are made up of proteins and fat.

Preventive medicine
A branch of medicine that focuses on preventing disease rather than treating it.

Table 13-1   Endurance Exercise and Coronary Heart Disease

Endurance exercise tends to increase

1. efficiency of the heart
2. size of blood vessels
3. blood supply to the heart
4. efficiency of distribution of blood to the tissues
5. return of blood to the heart
6. enzymes in the tissues that help supply energy
7. efficiency of blood coagulation factors
8. high-density lipoprotein cholesterol
9. blood volume and number of red blood cells
10. efficiency of the thyroid gland
11. growth of hormone production, which increases the use of fats
12. tolerance to stress
13. prudent living habits
14. the joy of living

Endurance exercise tends to decrease

1. blood levels of triglycerides, total cholesterol, and low-density lipoprotein cholesterol
2. glucose intolerance
3. obesity and body fat
4. platelet stickiness (overadhesiveness in this type of blood cell has been implicated in the development of coronary artery disease)
5. arterial blood pressure
6. heart rate
7. vulnerability to dysrhythmias of electrical conduction in the heart
8. overreaction by ''stress'' hormones
9. strain associated with psychic stress

Source: Adapted from S. M. Fox, J. P. Naughton, and W. L. Haskell, ''Physical Activity and the Prevention of Coronary Heart Disease, *Annals of Clinical Research* 3 (1971): 404–432.

process involves an intricate network of hormones, fuels, and enzymes that keep the body alive. The physically fit body adapts to facilitate these chemical reactions. There is an improved ability to generate useful energy, to use fats, and to regulate hormone control systems.

Blood *lipids*, or blood fats, such as *cholesterol* and *triglycerides*, have been implicated in the development of *plaques* that can form on the inner lining of the coronary arteries. Cholesterol is carried in the blood by substances called *lipoproteins*, which exist in different sizes. Excess low-density lipoprotein (LDL) cholesterol is deposited on the walls of the coronary arteries, while high-density lipoprotein (HDL) picks up excess cholesterol in the bloodstream and carries it back to the liver

for excretion from the body. Therefore, we can speak of "good cholesterol," HDL, and "bad cholesterol," LDL. Endurance exercise increases the amount of HDL and reduces the amount of LDL. Some researchers have said that the relative amounts of HDL and LDL may be the most important factor involved in the development of coronary heart disease. (See Figure 13-1.) Endurance exercise has been shown to have a markedly positive effect on the lipid profile.

Endurance exercise also aids body chemistry in the regulation of energy balance. We need food to supply vitamins and minerals as well as energy. However, a diet high in the proper nutrients is relatively high in calories. Regular exercise enables a person to eat enough calories for an optimal diet without getting fat. On the other hand, research studies indicate that without exercise it is extremely difficult to consume a nutritious diet and maintain an ideal body weight. Sedentary people may gain weight on an optimally nutritious diet because they are taking in more calories than they are burning up.

In addition to allowing a person to eat well, physical activity tends to promote prudent living habits—a phenomenon known as the "halo effect." People seem to become more aware of their bodies when they exercise, so they tend to live a more healthful life-style. They can feel it if they smoke, are overweight, or don't get enough sleep. The halo effect should not be underestimated. Regular endurance exercise is a critical factor in *preventive medicine* because it improves other health factors in addition to exerting its own beneficial effect.

Age	No exercise	Slight exercise	Moderate exercise	Heavy exercise
45–49	1.06	0.56	0.38	0.23
60–64	4.90	2.32	1.19	0.92
75–79	16.05	6.55	3.46	1.96

Figure 13-1   Death by degree of exertion (per 100 men): Studies of heart attack victims show that people who exercise regularly are less prone to heart attack.

Electrocardiogram
A record of the electrical activity of the heart.

Benefits of Muscular Strength and Flexibility Exercises
In addition to cardiorespiratory endurance, other types of fitness exercises are important for health. Muscular strength and muscular endurance, joint flexibility, and posture are also critical to well-being. Backache affects nearly 85 percent of the population. In most cases this can be directly traced to weak abdominal and spinal muscles, poor flexibility in the spine, hips, and legs, and chronically poor posture. If people spent even five minutes a day working on these fitness factors, the amount of back trouble would be drastically reduced.

A basic principle of human movement states that if you don't use it, you'll lose it. Joint stiffness in the shoulders, neck, knees, and ankles can often be attributed to disuse; this is particularly true in older adults. Such stiffness can be reduced by regularly moving the joints through their normal range of motion.

Aside from the health benefits of strength and flexibility, these fitness characteristics are vitally important for maximum enjoyment of most sports. Strong, flexible people can move forcefully and easily with little risk of injury. Strength allows them to hit a golfball farther, water-ski more vigorously, and jump higher. Flexibility allows them to get their arm farther back for a tennis serve, move better on the dance floor, and move more efficiently in the swimming pool. Strength and flexibility are vital parts of any physical activity program.

How to Get into Shape: The Planning Stage

Exercise can be a positive factor in your life rather than a chore. Your individual program should promote good health and be fun at the same time. A little planning and reflection will go a long way in helping you achieve those goals.

It is always a good idea to have a physical examination before you start your exercise program. Exercise actually can be dangerous for some people. Others may have a medical condition that requires a modified program. Additionally, because the body experiences profound changes in capacity and function as a result of exercise, initial baseline measurements will be helpful in assessing the effects of exercise on your health.

If you are over 35 years of age or have an increased risk of heart disease because of heavy smoking, high blood pressure, or obesity, be sure to have an exercise *electrocardiogram* before beginning a program. This will help ensure that your program is a benefit to your health instead of a potential hazard.

Choosing the Appropriate Activities Although good health is an important reason to exercise, it is a poor motivator for consistent adherence to an exercise program. If you don't enjoy your program, you won't continue it for very long. It is easy to say, "If I miss this workout, it's not going to kill me." Unfortunately, that missed workout can stretch into several months. However, if you select a physical activity that you like and look forward to, you will be much more faithful to it.

Personality should have a great deal to do with your choices. If you like competitive sports and dread the idea of running around a track, you might choose activities like racquetball, basketball, and squash. Here you can get a good workout and still satisfy the competitive need. Likewise, if you are the solitary type, you might consider a sport like cross-country skiing or road running where you can go off by yourself. If you don't have a favorite sport or exercise, expose yourself to some new activities. Take a class, join a health club, go on a sports vacation. You *can* find an activity that's both enjoyable and good for you.

Try to choose activities that contribute to your general health and well-being. Improved physiological function is a major benefit of exercise. However, some activities don't do very much in this regard. Endurance exercises such as walking, jogging, swimming, and cycling produce a cardiovascular training effect, while bowling, golf, and weight lifting do not. Although a variety of activities is desirable in a well-rounded program, cardiorespiratory endurance exercises should play a central role in your routine.

Be realistic. Consider the constraints that some sports present. Factors such as accessibility, expense, and time can make many activities impossible. For example, if you live in Florida, snow skiing isn't something you're likely to do on a regular basis. Some sports, like tennis, require a lot of time to achieve a reasonable skill level; you may be better off walking to get a good workout. Similarly, if you don't have four-hour blocks of time available, you will have difficulty squeezing in eighteen holes of golf. Look at your own situation and develop a reasonable plan.

Variety is also important to an enjoyable exercise program. If you are interested in a particular sport, supplement it with conditioning activities. For example, if you are a tennis player, support your playing with strength, flexibility, and endurance exercises. Participate in new activities and try to improve in old ones. The more variety, the less boredom.

Buying Equipment When you are sure of your activities, buy the best equipment you can afford. Good equipment will enhance your enjoyment and decrease your risk of injury. Along with the recent growth in physical activity has come a wave of new equipment and clothing. Some of it is truly revolutionary: running shoes are designed according to the biomechanics of the foot; skis allow you to go faster with better control; tennis rackets make it easier to hit the ball over the net; new materials make sports clothing more comfortable and fashionable.

Unfortunately, some of these new products are either overpriced or of poor quality. A flashy but overweight tennis racket can produce an elbow injury, while a shoe that can't absorb shock can cause leg pains. Before you

invest in a new piece of equipment, investigate it. Is it worth the money? Does it produce the results it is supposed to? Ask the experts (coaches, physical educators, and sports instructors) for their opinion. Better yet, educate yourself. Every sport, from running to volleyball, has magazines devoted to every aspect of it. A little effort will be well rewarded.

Footwear is perhaps the most important item of equipment for almost any sport. Buy shoes that are appropriate for the activity. Don't jog in shoes designed for tennis or basketball and vice versa. Make sure the shoes fit; it doesn't make any difference that the shoe has a five-star rating if your feet hurt. (The characteristics of an ideal running shoe are shown in Figure 13–2.)

Implementing Your Program

When engineers build a bridge, they take into consideration the strength of the material and the stresses it is likely to encounter. They have a precise idea of the results of their efforts because the structure is subject to the laws of physics and chemistry. Likewise, the body's adaptations to the stresses of exercise are subject to the laws of science. You can predict the outcome of your fitness program if you follow some simple principles and work within your physical capacity.

Warm-Up Warming up before exercising enhances performance and decreases the chances of injury. Muscles work better when their temperature is slightly above resting level. Warm-up helps the body's physiology gradually progress from rest to exercise. Blood needs to be redirected to active muscles, and this takes time. The heart needs time to adapt to the increased demands of exercise. Warm-up helps spread synovial fluid throughout joints, which helps protect articular surfaces.

Warm-up should include stretching and low-intensity movements similar to those involved in the follow-up sport. Stretching exercises are performed for major muscle groups and joints of the body such as the calves, quadriceps, hamstrings, hips, back, neck, and shoulders. Low-intensity movements include hitting forehands and

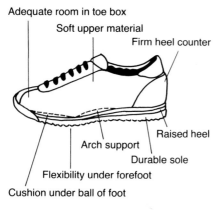

Adequate room in toe box
Soft upper material
Firm heel counter
Raised heel
Durable sole
Arch support
Flexibility under forefoot
Cushion under ball of foot

Figure 13-2 What to look for in a running shoe.

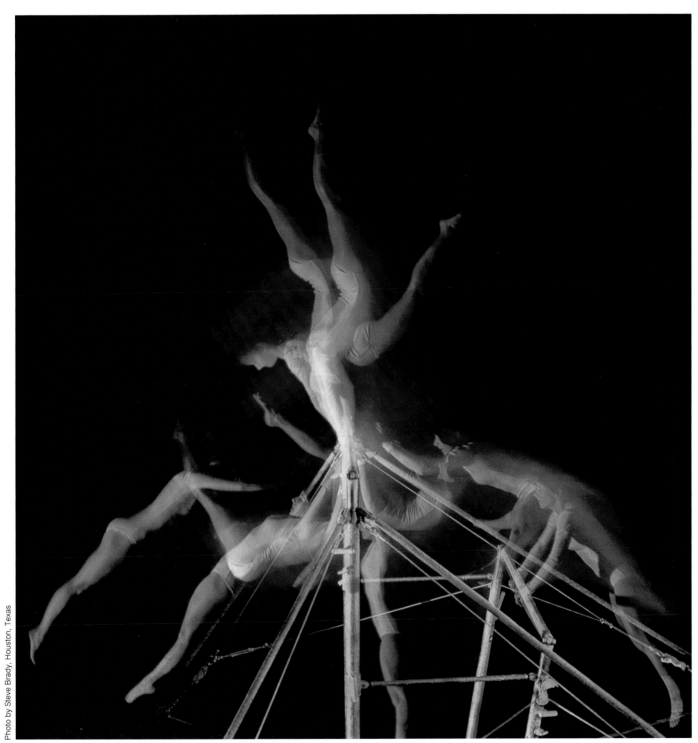

Commercial Health Clubs

. . . There are exceptions to all generalizations: some health clubs do an outstanding job and others are frauds or near-frauds. The range can be found among national chains as well as among one-person operations. It is extremely difficult to make blanket statements, but *Consumers Guide®* can at least set down some guidelines.

High-Pressure Selling   When you enter a health club, you can expect a tour followed by a high-pressure sales pitch. Be ready for it. Instructors and managers are well-schooled in making an effective representation. They want your business.

   Consumers Guide® sees nothing wrong with the health club mana-ger's making a strong case empha-sizing the value of exercise. But that's it. Under no circumstances should you feel badgered, embar-rassed, belittled, threatened, detained, or mocked. If you feel any exces-sive amount of pressure, leave or at least ask for more time. If you are told this is a once-in-a-lifetime deal or that the rates go up tomorrow, etc., forget it. It's a high-pressure outfit interested in the dollar figure, not yours.

The Contract   Read the contract carefully. If you want more time, take it. If you feel you should read it at home or want to discuss it with other members of your family or anyone else, do so. If the health club won't permit you to take the contract home, steer clear of that organization. Make sure the contract commits you to no more than two years; one year is preferable. All contracts should provide for a minimum three-day cooling-off period; look for a "use of facility" clause permitting you to use the club during those three days.

Key Considerations   During the tour, explanation of facilities, and closing, you should be aware of the following:

1.   Is there a discussion of your in-dividual problems? This should take place prior to signing the contract. Is there a discussion of your physi-cal limitations, risk factors, and the possibility of stress tests? Do they recommend that you talk to your doctor before you embark on an exercise program?
2.   Is the person conducting the tour an instructor, a manager, or what? Does he or she seem to be well trained and not just well built? Ask if he or she is a physical education or physical therapy graduate with additional training in fitness. If not, does the club have an in-service training program emphasizing cardiovascular fitness? Do you sense that the person has a genuine interest in you? Is he or she able to explain how the machines operate, their value and limitations?
3.   Does the spa manager or instruc-tor emphasize cardiovascular fit-ness, or is the focus on muscle strength and muscle endurance? If the emphasis is on muscle strength and endurance, you can eliminate that club. Be careful—even the offi-cial statement of the Association of Physical Fitness Centers notes that "the modern health spa . . . offers programs of physical fitness incorpo-rating concepts of progressive resis-tance exercise for both sexes. . . ." Progressive resistance exercise is the development of muscle endur-ance and strength. Remember, the primary focus should be on car-diovascular fitness.
4.   Visit the club *at a time of day when you plan to use it.* This is crucial. Every club has a peak-usage time. Waiting in line to run on the treadmill, ride a bicycle, or lift weights can be a serious incon-venience. Consider time and use of facilities as important factors.
5.   Before signing anything, talk to several of the people who are exer-cising (or who have just finished, if you don't want to interrupt their work). If the manager doesn't permit you to do this, cross the club off your list. Ask what they think of the program, what the emphasis is, and whether personal attention is given. Try to find out what the dropout rate is. European Health Spas claim that nearly three-fourths of their new members are referrals from other members. If the three-fourths figure is correct—and there is no way to check on it—it would indicate that this chain must be doing something right.
6.   Find out how long the club has been in your area. The longer the better, and if under the same management, that's another plus. Approach a new club with caution—especially "pre-opening" sales. There have been cases where con artists have held pre-opening sales for clubs that never opened.
7.   Find out if the club belongs to the Association of Physical Fitness Centers. This trade association for full-service health spas is dedicated to upgrading the industry. The Asso-ciation has established a code of ethics that covers programs, facilities, employees, and consumers' rights.
8.   The spa needs you more than you need the spa. Don't forget that. . . . A club is an extra. It can provide you with some social con-tacts, motivation, and a special place to exercise—if you need these things.

Charles T. Kuntzleman
Rating the Exercises

Physiological Benefits of Warm-Up

Most athletes incorporate some form of preliminary physical activity or warm-up procedure into their training routines, especially if they anticipate a strenuous workout. When questioned, athletes usually reply that they warm up to avoid stiff muscles. Few actually understand that the increase in body temperature produced by warming up may benefit their overall physical performance. Warming up seems to be particularly important for a peak effort in short-duration activities such as sprinting, weight lifting, and high jumping.

The effects of temperature are probably more important in warming up than the acceleration of the respiratory and cardiovascular systems and increases in hormone levels. In addition, increasing the temperature of the specific muscles that will be used in vigorous exercise appears to be the most advantageous method of warm-up for optimal physical performance.

Favorable Effects of Warm-Up

The favorable effects that may be derived from warming up are summarized [below].

The breakdown of oxyhemoglobin for the delivery of oxygen to the working muscle is increased.

The release of oxygen from myoglobin is increased.

The activation energy for vital cellular metabolic chemical reactions is lowered.

Muscle viscosity is reduced, producing an improvement in mechanical efficiency.

Nervous impulses travel more rapidly, and the sensitivity of nerve receptors is augmented.

Blood flow to the muscle is increased.

The number of injuries related to muscles, tendons, ligaments, and other connective tissues may be reduced.

The cardiovascular response to sudden, strenuous exercise is improved.

Frank G. Shellock
The Physician and Sportsmedicine

---

backhands before a tennis match, skiing down an easy run before tackling a more difficult one, and running a 12-minute mile before progressing to a usual 8-minute one.

Types of Exercise We spoke earlier about the desirability of selecting a variety of physical activities that you enjoy. Let's turn now to the various types of exercise and see how they enhance general health and different kinds of activity.

To develop a factor of fitness such as cardiorespiratory endurance, strength, power, speed, flexibility, or skill, you must work on specific exercises to develop those fitness characteristics. Lifting weights will not develop the heart and lungs, and running contributes little to strength and power.

Cardiorespiratory Endurance, or Aerobic, Exercises
As the name implies, cardiorespiratory endurance, or aerobic, exercises develop the heart and lungs. These exercises use large muscle groups continuously for a prolonged period of time. The best exercises for developing cardiorespiratory endurance are running-jogging, walking-hiking, swimming, bicycling, rowing, cross-country skiing, and rope skipping. Games such

as racquetball, tennis, basketball, and soccer are also good *if* the skill level and intensity of the game are sufficient to provide a vigorous workout.

Cardiorespiratory endurance exercise should play the prominent part in any physical activity program. The American College of Sports Medicine has made recommendations based on scientific research for the quantity and quality of training required for developing and maintaining cardiorespiratory fitness and body composition in healthy adults (see Table 13–2).

Frequency of Training The optimal workout schedule for endurance training is three to five days per week. Beginners should start with three and work up to five days. Training more than five days a week often leads to injury in the recreational athlete. Training less than three days a week provides little health benefit and subjects you to the risk of injury because the body never gets a chance to fully adapt to regular exercise training.

Intensity of Training The most misunderstood aspect of conditioning, even among experienced athletes, is training intensity. Problems are caused by doing too little or too much. Many recreational swimmers, for example,

Training effect
An increase in maximum oxygen consumption as the result of an exercise program.

Pulse rate
The number of pulse beats per minute.

Maximum oxygen consumption (MOC)
The maximum amount of oxygen the body can burn during strenuous exercise.

Maximum pulse rate
The fastest rate at which the heart will beat.

Target pulse rate
A heart rate above the resting rate but less than the maximum rate.

Table 13-2   The Recommended Quantity and Quality of Exercise for Developing and Maintaining Fitness in Healthy Adults

Mode of activity

Aerobic or endurance exercises, such as running-jogging, walking-hiking, swimming, skating, bicycling, rowing, cross-country skiing, rope skipping, and various game activities.

Frequency of training

3 to 5 days per week

Intensity of training

60 percent of capability range plus resting pulse rate, or 50 percent to 85 percent of maximum oxygen uptake

Duration of training

15 to 60 minutes of continuous aerobic activity. Duration is dependent on the intensity of the activity.

Source: American College of Sports Medicine, *Sports Medicine Bulletin* 13 (1978): 1-4.

get very little benefit from their exercise because they don't work hard enough—their activity is closer to bathing than swimming. On the other hand, working too hard will invariably result in injury.

Intensity is the crucial factor in attaining a *training effect*. Although several methods for calculating this effect have been devised, one of the easiest to apply

Table 13-3   Maximum Pulse Rates

Age	Age-Predicted Maximum Pulse Rates
20–24	200
25–29	200
30–34	194
35–39	188
40–44	182
45–49	176
50–54	171
55–59	165
60–64	159
65 +	153

Source: Derived from Metropolitan Life charts.

involves *pulse rate*. In order for exercise to have a training effect, the pulse rate must be elevated. A training effect is an increase in *maximum oxygen consumption* (*MOC*) as a result of an exercise program. The training effect occurs, however, at a pulse rate slower than the maximum. The *maximum pulse rate* is the fastest rate possible before exhaustion sets in.

To determine the rate at which you should exercise—your *target pulse rate*—first find out what your pulse rate is after ten minutes of complete rest. Then subtract your resting pulse rate from your maximum pulse rate. The most reliable way of calculating this maximum rate is by means of a treadmill test, which is administered in physicians' offices, hospitals, and sports medicine laboratories. Maximum pulse rate can also be estimated by subtracting your age from 220, or it can be taken from Table 13–3. Although these last two methods are usually fairly accurate, they can be grossly inadequate for some people.

The difference between your resting and maximum pulse rates is your capability range. For example:

Maximum pulse rate	200
Resting pulse rate	– 70
Capability range	130 beats

The training effect occurs when the pulse rate is elevated above the resting pulse rate by an amount that is 60 percent of the capability range. In the above example, 60 percent of the capability range is 78 beats. Adding 78 to the resting pulse rate of 70 gives a rate of 148 beats, the target rate at which the training will occur.

Measure your pulse rate either at the wrist or at one of the carotid arteries, located on each side of the Adam's apple, but be sure to take all measurements during one exercise period from the same place. Begin counting immediately after you have finished exercising. The pulse rate usually drops rapidly following exercise, so the most accurate procedure is to count beats for 15 seconds and then multiply the number by 4.

To build fitness, the pulse must be maintained at the training-effect, or target, rate for several minutes. You can speed up your pulse to 150 just by charging up stairs, but you will not be increasing your fitness. (See the following section.)

The Five Principles of a Safe and Effective Exercise Program

I. Range	Muscle and Joint Flexibility	Cardiorespiratory Capacity	Muscle/Bone Balance and Strength
II. Intensity	Execute a full range of possible motions for each of your major joints and muscles.	Engage in continuous activity at your age-adjusted target heart rate.	Selectively exert each of your major muscles.
III. Duration	15 to 30 seconds per movement (9–12 minutes total).	Build from 10 minutes or less to at least ½ hour.	8 to 12 repetitions per muscle (30–45 minutes total).
IV. Frequency	Not less than once a day.	Daily if possible, and not less than every other day.	Every other day, or not less than twice a week.
V. Progression	Extend your range of motion as your flexibility increases.	Gradually intensify your activity while maintaining your target heart rate.	Increase resistance as your strength develops.

A fully effective exercise program activates three distinct physical potentials.

Tom and Dianne Murphy
Personal Fitness Workbook

The more fit you become, the harder you will have to work to continue to improve. By monitoring your pulse rate, you will always know if you are working hard enough to improve or if you are overdoing it. For most people, a fitness program involves attaining an acceptable level of fitness and then maintaining that level. There is no need to keep working indefinitely to improve; this only increases the chance of injury.

Duration of Training   The length of time you should spend on a workout depends on its intensity. If you are walking, swimming slowly, or playing a stop-and-start game like tennis, you should participate for 45 minutes to an hour. High-intensity exercises such as running can be practiced for a shorter period of time. The recreational athlete should start off with less vigorous activities and only gradually increase the intensity. For most people, continous endurance exercise should last from 15 minutes to an hour.

Other Forms of Exercise   Exercises that will develop muscular strength and muscular endurance should also be included in any program designed for promotion of health. Your ability to maintain correct posture and to move efficiently depends in part on adequate muscle fitness. Good muscle tone is also important for appearance. After all, if you are physically fit, you want to look physically fit.

Muscular strength and endurance can be developed in many ways, from weight training to calisthenics. Common exercises such as sit-ups, push-ups, pull-ups, and wall-sitting (leaning against a wall in a seated position and supporting yourself with your leg muscles) satisfy the strength needs of most people if they practice a few exercises for the major muscle groups three to five days a week.

Resistive exercise, such as using weights or exercise machines, is required to develop a significant amount of strength. In general, one must train at least twice a week for an hour to experience significant results. Using heavy resistance with few repetitions (one to ten) builds strength and muscle size, while employing more repetitions improves muscular strength—endurance (the ability to exert force over a longer period of time). Strength training improves performance in most sports and has become a prominent part of the training program of many types of athletes.

Flexibility is perhaps the most neglected part of fitness even though it is extremely important. Flexibility is lost when the joints are not moved through their normal

Steroids

We all have steroids circulating in our bloodstreams all the time. Most of them are hormones—chemicals that regulate a variety of bodily processes. Some of these steroid hormones are made in the ovary or testicle, and they are responsible for maintaining specifically male or female traits. Other kinds of steroid hormones are produced in the outer portion, or cortex, of the adrenal glands, which are located above the kidneys. These adrenal steroids do many things, but roughly speaking they can be grouped into two classes. One type is mainly responsible for stimulating sodium retention by the kidney and thus, indirectly,

helps to control the volume of body fluids. The main day-to-day function of the other type is regulating energy supplies to cells throughout the body. These hormones also help us mount a response to stress. In addition to the various hormones, one of the vitamins we rely on, vitamin D, is a modified form of a steroid; it acts as a hormone to help regulate the absorption and distribution of calcium. . . .

The *male steroids* (or androgens) include testosterone and chemically similar substances; this is the type of steroid used by some athletes in the belief that they can build up extra muscle tissue. Good medical

practice does not support such a use of androgens. They have, at most, only a slight effect on muscle tissue in otherwise normal individuals and may predispose to tendon rupture or other disturbances, especially if used in growing bodies. In certain unusual kinds of anemia, androgens can be very helpful, and they have some other limited uses in medicine. There is no good evidence that male hormones reduce or reverse the effects of aging in men.

Harvard Medical School Health Letter

---

range of motion. Some exercises, such as running, actually decrease flexibility because they require only a partial range of motion. It is therefore important to do exercises that maintain mobility in the major joints. At least once a day, do some stretching or mobility exercises for the hamstrings, hips, lower spine, neck, and shoulders. If you get into the habit of doing these exercises regularly, you can prevent many of the aches and pains in muscles and joints that plague most of the population.

Developing Skill in Physical Activities   The ability to learn a skill and the rate at which it is learned are specific and therefore unrelated to other activities. In other words, if you want to learn a particular skill, you have to practice that skill and not something else.

Many people do not exercise or dislike exercise because they feel silly or self-conscious. They feel ridiculous hitting tennis balls over the fence instead of over the net; they are embarrassed by running a 15-minute mile or trying to touch their toes and barely getting past their kneecaps. Such people do not give themselves a chance. They try an activity once or twice and then give it up in despair. If they would take the time and effort to acquire some competence, they would begin to enjoy physical activity.

The first step in learning a skill is to get help. If you want to acquire competence in tennis, golf, or sailing, it is best to take lessons. Most sports require a mastery

of certain basic skills, so instruction from a qualified teacher can save you hours of frustration, and it can increase your enjoyment of the sport. Take a class, sign up for lessons at the recreation department, or get private instruction.

Skill is also important in conditioning activities such as jogging, swimming, and cycling. You should know your capacity and be able to gauge the intensity of exercise that will result in improvement without injury. Some help with technique from a coach or fellow participant will often help you to move and train more efficiently.

Diet and Fluid Intake   The relationship between diet and exercise is widely misunderstood. Many athletes and other physically active people waste millions of dollars on vitamins, minerals, and protein supplements. For most of these people, a nutritionally balanced diet (see Chapter 12) contains all the energy and nutrients needed to sustain an exercise program.

Long-distance runners as well as other endurance athletes benefit from diets that are higher than average in carbohydrates because carbohydrates increase the amount of *glycogen* in the muscles and liver. Glycogen is vitally important for sustaining physical activity over long periods of time. When this substance is low, the athlete feels sluggish, weak, and tired.

The body depends on water to maintain an optimal internal environment. Water is important for many

Glycogen
A carbohydrate stored in the liver and
some muscles and released when
needed.

chemical reactions and for maintaining the correct body temperature. Because sweating reduces the water level, it is important to drink fluids during exercise sessions. As a rule of thumb, if you are involved in heavy exercise, you should try to drink about a half pint of water for every 15 minutes of exercise. Increase this amount if it is hot outside.

Water, preferably cold water, is the best fluid replacement. It is cheaper and more effective than any other drink. Many of the commercially available fluid replacements are too high in sugar.

The best way to detect water loss after exercise is by weighing yourself in the nude (sweaty clothes can weigh a lot). An average endurance workout burns up about 200 calories, while a pound of fat contains about 3500 calories. The majority of weight loss after physical activity obviously is due to water loss. Relying on thirst alone, it can take 24 hours or more to replace this water loss. Ideally, you should restore your body fluids before exercising vigorously again.

What Is Enough?
How to Maintain Fitness

Your ultimate level of fitness depends upon your goals, the intensity of your program, and your natural ability. It is important to recognize when your fitness is adequate.

The Training Effect: Stress vs. Distress   When the body is subjected to a physical stress that it can tolerate, it adapts and improves its function. However, if the stress is intolerable, the body breaks down and becomes distressed or injured. This is the cornerstone of exercise training.

You won't improve unless you push yourself. For example, to improve your flexibility, you have to attempt to push the joints past their normal ranges of motion. Improved fitness is an adaption to overload; if there is no stress, there is no improvement. You have to overload your body consistently over a long period of time.

Overdoing it is just as bad as not exercising hard enough, however. No one can become fit overnight. It takes time for the body to adapt to increasingly higher

levels of stress. The process of training involves a countless number of stresses and adaptations. If you feel sore and tired the day after exercising, then you have worked too hard. Injury will slow you down just as much as a missed workout.

Consistency is the key to fitness improvement and freedom from injury. A training diary can help you apply the stresses of exercise more scientifically. A training diary is a record of your workouts. All you need are a pencil and notebook to write down the details of your program. In this way you will be able to evaluate your progress and plan your exercise intelligently.

How to Know That You Are in Shape   You are in shape when your body has reached your desired degree of adaptation. A 4-minute miler may be out of shape if he is running a mile in 4 minutes and 20 seconds, while the average person may be in adequate shape if he or she can run 2 miles in 18 minutes.

The best way to assess your fitness is in a modern sports medicine laboratory. Such laboratories are widely available and can be found in university physical education departments or medical centers. Here you will receive an accurate profile of your capacity to exercise. Typically, your endurance will be measured on a treadmill or bicycle, your body fat will be estimated, and your strength and flexibility will be tested. This evaluation will reveal whether you are in shape and provide you with an exercise program that's appropriate for your level of fitness.

Testing your own fitness is more difficult because fitness abilities such as endurance, strength, coordination, and agility are specific to an activity or task. It is meaningless to compare the number of pull-ups or push-ups you can do with the strength requirements of tennis, skiing, or jogging.

To obtain a rough estimate of your cardiorespiratory fitness, check your speed in the 1.5-mile run/walk. Keep in mind, however, that for activities such as swimming and cycling, this test may be totally inadequate. Nevertheless, it can provide an estimate of whether your fitness is consistent with good health. Table 13–4 provides standards for both men and women (see page 316).

(*text continues on p. 316*)

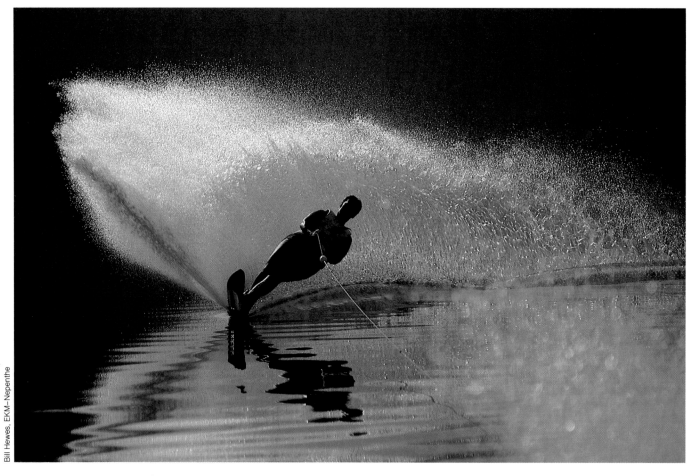

That "Extra Effort" Can Hold You Back

Whether you want to run fast or think fast, over-effort diminishes your prospects. The way to perform at your best is to learn to ease off all extra tensions by switching off all untimely reactions.

Take, for example, thinking and doing. We try to think while we're doing, which impairs the doing, and we try to do while we're thinking, which prevents us from thinking clearly.

In our ambition to succeed, we're driven to do everything at once. This isn't the way the body/mind functions. You can't abruptly "stop and think," as is so often counseled. Stopping is an active process. What you can do is stop, pause, and then think. There needs to be an interval between doing and thinking and thinking and doing.

While you perform, you mustn't think about the technique of your performance. While you think through the details involved in performing, you mustn't perform. You can do both at once, of course, but you won't do either well. To think or perform at your best, you must keep the functions separate.

When you try too hard at anything, you produce extraneous effort; you quiver and become tense; your motions are inefficient. When you play too hard, you make a business of recreation, which deprives you of its expressive, restorative benefits. Working too hard and playing too hard are roads to self-destruction. Consider the word: re-creation. That's its function.

To work hard and play hard should mean working productively and playing ecstatically. Peak experiences result when all elements fit harmoniously together and you become as one with your game or task. That state arrives spontaneously. It's almost never achieved

through extreme effort—because such striving sets up bodily forces that disorganize and burden the essentials needed for the event.

In neuromuscular terms, a gentle forcefulness is produced by just the right number of muscle fibers coming into play at just the right time in just the right organization to move the levers and joints of the body through the precise motion needed to accomplish the objective. Extra effort upsets this balance. Result: A poor performance.

The basic purpose of neuromuscular training is to refine movement to such an extent that only those motions directed toward the final action are in play. Extraneous efforts by muscle fibers that drain the organism of its energy and cause general confusion within the neuromuscular system are eliminated.

Suppose you're playing darts. If you were to throw the dart as you might throw a stone in anger—clenching, winding up, and heaving with all your might—your chances of hitting the bull's-eye with any consistency would be worlds less than if you were to take the dart gently in your thumb and forefinger and send it on its way with a relaxed and gentle motion. By refining the muscle systems in control of the dart and eliminating the extraneous ones, you have minimized your effort but maximized your prospects.

There was a period some years back when I took every opportunity I could to interview athletes who had either just broken a world's record or bettered their own record in an event to a remarkable degree. "What happened?" I asked each of them. "Tell me about that performance from beginning to end." By the time I had interviewed a dozen

athletes, I could predict almost exactly what each of them would say. The scenario went like this:

> I didn't feel well that day. I was nauseated and felt weak. As a matter of fact, it crossed my mind to ask the coach to scratch me from the event. But before I knew it, my event was called. I hardly remember starting. All I knew for sure was that I was in motion. I don't remember any particular moment during the event. It all seemed so easy. At the finish, the way the crowd was cheering told me I'd done well, but I had the feeling that if I'd only tried a little harder I could have done much better.

It was almost spooky. Here were different athletes in different events in different parts of the country, none of them communicating with any of the others, yet all of them giving me the same basic story. They were all astonished that they had broken their records on that particular day; not one of them felt he had been really putting out his best.

In the years since then, every time I've been near an athlete who had vastly improved his performance, I've asked him to comment on these stories I'd been told by other performers under similar circumstances. The inevitable reply: "I wouldn't change a word."

These athletes are telling us something about maximum performance that every one of us can apply in our daily lives. If you're exhausting yourself trying to achieve, that's about all you'll do. The lesson is as valid in the office as on the field; the executive who strains at his work is no more effective than the baseball player who tries to hit a home run with every swing of his bat. Nile Kinnick knew this. He was a legendary football player and scholar at Iowa in the late 1930s, a Heisman

(continued on next page)

That "Extra Effort" Can Hold You Back (continued)

trophy winner and a Phi Beta Kappa. When he died in a Navy training exercise at the start of World War II, a diary was found among his effects. "It is a sad mistake to try to be head man in everything you attempt," he had written. "The axiom, 'If it is worth doing at all, it is worth doing well,' has its limitations. Stay on the ball most of the time, but learn to coast between moments of all-out effort."

Kinnick was years ahead of his time in his understanding of maximum performance. Most ath-letes of his day associated great performances with pain, struggle, and exhaustion. Today's enlightened athletes aren't like that. They don't spend their energy on needless histrionics. When their race is called, they shake out their hands and feet to get loose, kick their knees up and down, run a few easy spurts, and try a few starts. . . .

The record books tell us which is the sounder approach. The times and distances of today's supercool athletes are far better than those of athletes in an earlier day who gave everything to win. Certainly, the excitement of a winning basket or touchdown or a record-breaking time is just as intense today as it has ever been. But the execution is done with much more grace and ease.

Exhaustion is no longer the mark of top-class performance. It shouldn't be the mark of yours.

Lawrence Morehouse and Leonard Gross
Maximum Performance

How to Maintain Fitness Fitness can be maintained only by exercising on a regular basis at a consistent intensity. Three days per week seems to be the minimum number of days to maintain most types of fitness. You must work at the intensity that brought you to your desired fitness level. If you don't, your body will become less fit because less is expected of it. In general, if you exercise at the same intensity over a long period, your fitness will level out and can be maintained easily.

Psychologically, people seem to be able to do this only if they have a goal. The goal can be anything from fitting into a dress bought last year to skiing down a new slope.

The important thing to remember is that you can have goals without striving to improve your fitness.

Varying a program is another good way to maintain interest. For example, you might consider competitive sports (swimming, running, racquetball, volleyball, golf, and so on) at the recreational level. Exposing yourself to new experiences can add zest to any program.

Injuries

Injuries can occur even to the most careful physically active person. Although annoying, they usually are neither serious nor permanent. However, if an injury isn't cared for properly it can escalate into a chronic problem, sometimes serious enough to cause permanent curtailment of the activity.

Proper first aid is extremely important for rapid rehabilitation from athletic injuries. Soft-tissue injuries (injuries to muscles and joints) should be treated with ice compresses and the affected part of the body elevated to minimize swelling. A doctor should be consulted for head and eye injuries, possible ligament injuries, broken bones, and internally related disorders such as chest pain, fainting, and intolerance to heat.

Before returning to full exercise participation, the injured person should meet the following criteria: (1) full range of motion in the joints, (2) normal strength and balance among muscles, (3) normal coordinated patterns of movement, with no injury compensation movements, such as limping, and (4) little or no pain.

Table 13-4   Standards for the 1.5-Mile Run/Walk (Min:Sec)

	High	**Good**	**Fair**	**Poor**
Males				
20–29	9:45	12:00	13:00	15:00
30–39	10:00	12:15	13:30	16:00
40–49	10:30	12:30	14:00	16:30
50–59	11:00	13:30	15:00	18:30
60 +	11:15	14:30	16:30	19:00
Females				
20–29	11:00	13:15	14:15	16:15
30–39	11:15	13:30	14:45	17:15
40–49	11:45	13:45	15:15	17:45
50–59	12:15	14:45	16:15	19:45
60 +	12:30	15:45	17:45	20:15

Note: This test should not be attempted without at least six weeks of conditioning. Check with your doctor if you are over 35.

Fitness Behavior Scale

Read the following statements carefully. Choose the one in each section that best describes you at this moment and record its score at the right. (For example, "firm, toned body" has a score of 4.) When you have identified five statements, total your score and find your position on the scale.

5 maintains a regular exercise program
4 often engages in physical activity
3 occasionally exercises
2 rarely exercises
1 is sedentary

Score _____

5 trim, highly toned body
4 firm, toned body
3 firm, poorly toned body
2 slack body
1 flabby body

Score _____

5 vigorous
4 energetic
3 active
2 excessive sleep pattern
1 awakes tired

Score _____

5 feels exhilarated after vigorous exercise
4 recovers rapidly after vigorous exercise
3 is tired after vigorous exercise
2 overweight
1 sluggish

Score _____

5 excellent stamina
4 good stamina
3 limited endurance
2 easily tired
1 easily exhausted

Score _____

Total score _____

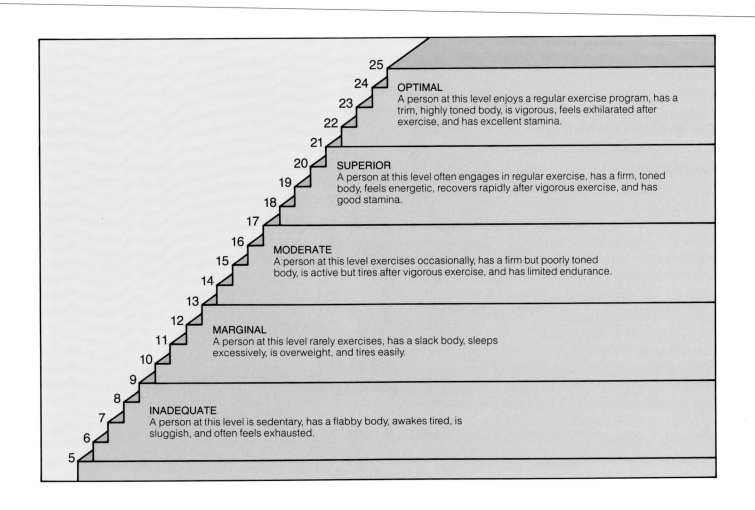

25
24
23
22
21 **OPTIMAL**
A person at this level enjoys a regular exercise program, has a trim, highly toned body, is vigorous, feels exhilarated after exercise, and has excellent stamina.

20
19
18
17 **SUPERIOR**
A person at this level often engages in regular exercise, has a firm, toned body, feels energetic, recovers rapidly after vigorous exercise, and has good stamina.

16
15
14
13 **MODERATE**
A person at this level exercises occasionally, has a firm but poorly toned body, is active but tires after vigorous exercise, and has limited endurance.

12
11
10
9 **MARGINAL**
A person at this level rarely exercises, has a slack body, sleeps excessively, is overweight, and tires easily.

8
7
6
5 **INADEQUATE**
A person at this level is sedentary, has a flabby body, awakes tired, is sluggish, and often feels exhausted.

Take Action

Your answers to Probing Your Emotions at the beginning of this chapter and your placement level on the Fitness Behavior Scale will, we hope, encourage you to begin a process of self-exploration and self-discovery that you will continue. Reflect on the entire chapter's content and ask yourself how each point relates to your own life. Then take action:

1. On the left side of a page in your Take Action notebook list the positive behaviors that help you avoid a sedentary life-style and keep you fit. How can you strengthen these behaviors? On the right side of the page list the behaviors that block a physically active life-style. Consider which ones would be easiest to change and start to change them.

2. Track and monitor your physical activity during the next two weeks by doing the following: Indicate in your Take Action notebook the activity and the time, date, and duration of the

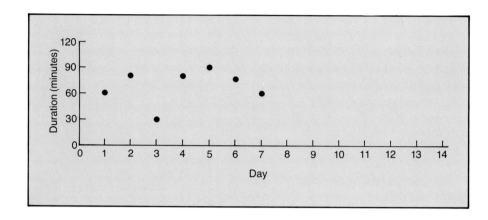

activity. After you have accumulated this information, draw a graph that looks like the one above, adding your own appropriate dots. At the end of the two weeks, connect the dots with a solid line. This line is called a trend line. Is your trend line generally up, down, or horizontal?

3. Look in your closet and take out the shoes you use for your most

frequent physical activity. Consider whether they are appropriate for the activity. Find an expert (coach, physical educator, or sports instructor) and ask his or her opinion.

4. Read the following Behavior Change Strategy, and take the appropriate action.

Behavior Change Strategy

Exercise

Perhaps more than any other topic area in health promotion, exercise has caught the spirit of the 1980s. Books on running and other forms of exercise appear almost daily. Exercise spas and special sports centers have become a major business enterprise in many parts of the country. With all of this frenetic development and the apparent ground swell of popular interest, it may come as a bit of a surprise that there has been relatively little behavioral research to provide tested guidelines for following personal exercise programs. The research that has been published has focused, instead, upon the physiological changes and benefits associated with training. Moreover, most of this

limited research has reflected the training experiences of special groups of subjects like athletes, armed forces personnel, students in physical education classes, and people recovering from seriously debilitating health events like heart attacks.

What, then, can be recommended to individuals who do not have the external incentives or intrinsic motivation of these special groups? The best recommendations are drawn from the literature on behavior self-management approaches to exercise enhancement.

Diary (Self-Monitoring) As with the other behavior change strategies suggested throughout this book, the best first step involves collecting

detailed information, in this case about beginning or "baseline" activity levels. There are a number of ways to go about measuring your personal exercise activity. For example, you can measure the number of times per week (*frequency*) you participate in a certain type of exercise. You can also measure the *duration* of your activity (for example, how much time you spend walking or swimming laps). By combining frequency and duration, you begin to assess the *intensity* of your usual exercise. This approach is satisfactory if you are trying to increase only one or possibly two types of exercise, but it grows more complicated if you want to increase your general level of activity, including a range of different types of behavior, such as walking, running, climbing stairs, swimming, and lifting weights.

Dr. Kenneth Cooper has devised an aerobic point system to handle specifically the complexity that comes with increasing different types of physical activity. *Aerobic* refers to the amount of oxygen the body can process per unit of time, and it reflects upon the conditioning of the lungs, heart, and vascular system. In essence, Cooper has assessed the relative fitness benefits from different activities in terms of aerobic impact—the amount of oxygen the activity requires at different levels of training. By awarding points to various forms of activity, Cooper's system allows for a varied "menu" of activities while linking practice to physiologic indices of fitness. Cooper has also made use of a standardized fitness self-test that permits classification into fitness levels. More specifically, in a special running exam, the participant merely measures the distance he or she can cover in 12 minutes. Based on that distance, it is possible to determine his or her level of fitness (excellent, very poor, or somewhere in between). With a gradually increasing range of activities and the associated aerobic points accumulated per week, this system builds upon self-monitoring to encourage significant personal changes in exercise habits.

Cooper offers four key guidelines: progress slowly, warm up properly before exercising, exercise within your personal tolerance, and cool down slowly following exercise.

Stimulus Control There are a number of ways to change your personal environment that will encourage you to follow through with an exercise program. For example, you might put your jogging shoes in an obvious place where you cannot miss them (in the hallway or by the bedroom door). This compels you to think about jogging. Although *thinking about* jogging is not the same thing as jogging (thoughts do not merit aerobic points), it is part of the

Aerobic Points

Activity	Distance or Time	Min/Sec	Points
Walking/Running	1 mile	19:59–14:30	1
		14:29–12:00	2
		11:59–10:00	3
		9:59–8:00	4
		7:59–6:31	5
		6:30–5:45	6
		under 5:45	7
Cycling	2 miles	12:00 or longer	0
		11:59–8:00	1
		7:59–6:00	2
		under 6:00	3
Swimming	200 yards	6:40 or longer	0
		6:39–5:00	1
		4:59–3:20	1.5
		under 3:20	2.5
Handball	10 minutes		1.5

Source: Adapted from K. H. Cooper, *The New Aerobics* (New York: Bantam, 1970).

chain of events that leads to that behavioral goal. This use of stimulus control is similar to the way in which we use alarm clocks to help us awaken at the desired hour of the morning—setting up the environment to assist us at a later time.

Another example of stimulus control is posting your diary of practice on the bedroom door or some other highly visible place. This will serve as a *reminder* and provide you with additional incentive to increase your activity. You can even set up special study areas, or "dedicated activity zones," to make other work more efficient so that you have enough time in your daily schedule to participate in physical activities.

Cognition (Self-Statements)
Thoughts can play a critical role in a personal exercise program. Rationalizations can discourage your efforts. ("The more I play tennis, the more uncoordinated I become." Or, "I'm just making a fool out of myself!") Thoughts don't need to be so personal, however, to undermine your enthusiasm. ("It's too cold outside to

run right now." Or, "I just don't want to take too many showers in one day—I'll just wait until tomorrow to do x, y, and z.") As in all behavioral programs, it is wise to begin by keeping a list and identifying such thought patterns and *then* to directly attack negative thoughts in order to reduce their frequency.

Self-Contracts and Reward Systems Personal contracts can provide an important and added incentive to your exercise program. A typical contract specifies in detail the target behaviors of concern: the kinds of exercise activities you want to increase and by how much. It identifies the day and time of practice and usually includes your signature. Of course, there are benefits that come directly from improving your personal fitness level—in terms of both psychological and physical improvements—but these benefits are often delayed. A reward system can provide more immediate positive consequences and can even be related to your target behavior (for example, paying yourself a certain amount of money for each day you follow your program and with the money you "earn" buying new jogging shoes or a subscription to a jogging/running magazine).

Exercising with other people often offers the incentives of both structure and companionship. However, this happens only if the other person or members of the group maintain a thorough and regular exercise schedule. In any case, you must be prepared to exercise independently should the group break apart or become less conscientious.

Available research suggests that many—perhaps most—people who initiate a program of increased physical exercise fail to stick with their plan for very long. They "relapse" and often try again later. These findings reveal that it isn't as easy to maintain regular activity as books and personal testimonials would have us believe. The problem-solving approach described more fully in Chapter 1 of this book combined with the specific strategies outlined in this section can improve your chances of becoming more physically fit.

Part Five

Consumer Health Issues

Chapter Fourteen

The Consumer and Medicine, Fads, and Quackery

Probing Your Emotions

1. Your friend has lung cancer. Her doctor has told her that chances of recovery are small, and he recommends treatment involving radiation, chemotherapy, and surgery. Your friend begins treatment but is horrified and depressed by the side effects. In her despair she considers abandoning the treatment in favor of a program of animal cell injections and large doses of vitamins administered by a clinic you feel is suspect. What do you tell your friend? How do you feel about her desperate search for alternative therapy? What would you do in a similar situation?

2. How much sympathy do you have for people who follow the principles of a new fad diet only to be disappointed in the results a few weeks later? Are you occasionally tempted by what such diets promise—despite what you know about caloric balances?

3. Do you feel that a spokesperson's authority is heightened if his or her ideas appear in print? Should you question the accuracy of everything you read (including *this* book)?

4. Have you ever purchased food or a drug, cosmetic, or medical device that turned out to be unsatisfactory—perhaps mislabeled, unsanitary, even potentially dangerous? If so, did you feel—ripped off, helpless, furious? Did you let your emotions interfere with your doing something about the product? What could you have done? What *did* you do?

Chapter Contents

THE SCIENTIFIC TRADITION

THE PAST AS PROLOGUE

ORTHODOX MEDICINE
Allopathy
Osteopathy
Choosing medical advisers

ALTERNATIVE APPROACHES
TO MEDICINE
Acupuncture
Chiropractic
Faith healing
Homeopathy
Naturopathy
Holistic medicine

QUACKERY TODAY
Laetrile
Other unproven methods
Diet and food faddism

DECISION MAKING

CONSUMER PROTECTION
The Food and Drug Administration
The Federal Trade Commission
The U.S. Postal Service
Other consumer protection
    agencies and organizations

GOVERNMENT ATTEMPTS TO
REDUCE HEALTH CARE COSTS
Professional Standards Review
    Organizations (PSROs)
Health Maintenance Organizations (HMOs)
Health Systems Agencies (HSAs)
Diagnosis-Related Groups (DRGs)

Boxes

Recognized specialties and subspecialties
    of allopathy and osteopathy
How to cut health care costs
Taking responsibility

Hypothesis
A tentative assumption made to test its
logical consequences.

14 In our society a peculiar dilemma faces us if we are ailing. Unless a problem is extremely clear-cut, like a broken arm that needs to be set, we may find ourselves adrift in a sea of choices. Our symptoms may be mild or ambiguous. Should we forget them, or take two aspirin, or see a doctor? A doctor may find nothing wrong. Or two doctors may make conflicting diagnoses. Should we see a specialist? How can we decide what kind of specialist to see? Would that new miracle capsule advertised on TV help? The manufacturer wouldn't be allowed to make those extravagant claims if the claims weren't true, would it? On the other hand, if we listen to the "small print," there does seem to be some hedging ("*may relieve minor symptoms*"). Maybe it would be better to see a chiropractor or an osteopath. Or go to bed earlier. Or take up running. Or cut out sugar. Or meditate. Or see a therapist or a clergyman, or just talk to a friend. Maybe acupuncture would help. To the best of the sufferer's knowledge, there may be no choice he or she can make with any real assurance that it will bring relief. Even the best efforts of conventional Western medicine cannot always provide that assurance. It should come as no surprise, therefore, that in this bewildering situation people often buy worthless health products or useless health services.

During 1983 Americans spent $322.4 billion on health and health products as compared to $39 billion in 1965. Although much of this increase is the result of inflation, we can clearly see the upward spiral of health care costs in terms of the gross national product. The portion of the GNP devoted to health care rose from 5.9 percent in 1965 to 10 percent in 1982.

Roughly three-quarters of the nonsurgical care provided by physicians (both general and specialist) is supportive, not curative. Supportive techniques are those used for the sophisticated management of diseases such as cancer and heart disease. These techniques have been vastly improved by the development of new technology— very expensive new technology. Yet our own behavior is largely responsible for many diseases, including stroke, heart attack, certain forms of cancer, atherosclerosis, cirrhosis of the liver, and emphysema. Our total bill for health costs could be cut substantially if the people of the United States would change just one behavior pattern—stop smoking!

When traditional medicine offers no hope, a patient or his or her family may be ready to try anything. In the fall of 1980 many people were shocked to hear that Steve McQueen, a popular, rugged movie actor, was reportedly dying of a rare and virulent form of lung cancer, mesothelioma. Most doctors considered this condition incurable. Conflicting reports started surfacing from Tijuana, Mexico, where McQueen had gone to undergo unorthodox therapy that consisted of Laetrile, intramuscular injections of animal cells, vitamins, coffee enemas, and rubdowns with castor oil.

The first newsbreak following rumors of McQueen's illness came from the director of a clinic south of Tijuana. He stated that the cancer had been checked and the patient was making satisfactory progress to full recovery. A personal friend of McQueen countered by saying that McQueen was like an old man—barely able to move— and the friend feared for McQueen's life.

Finally, in November news was flashed around the world that the 50-year-old actor had suffered a fatal heart attack following surgery to remove massive tumors. The director of the clinic stated that he opposed the surgery because he felt that McQueen's body had been making progress against the cancer. The surgeon who performed the operation stated that McQueen had massive tumors that should have been removed when they were discovered. Without the surgery, McQueen's days were limited as he had difficulty breathing without special equipment. The surgeon concluded that it is reasonable to assume that the cancer had caused the death—when we die, we all die because our heart stops beating.

A former wife of Steve McQueen lashed out at the people at the clinic where the unconventional treatment was prescribed, calling them "charlatans and exploiters." No one knows why McQueen went to Mexico for his final days, but two American doctors who work in Juarez said that American doctors had told him to just go home and die. Mexico at least offered him some hope.

The Scientific Tradition

Wherever medical research is pursued, it is likely to have certain elements: observation, trial and error, and the forming and testing of *hypotheses*. The Western scientif-

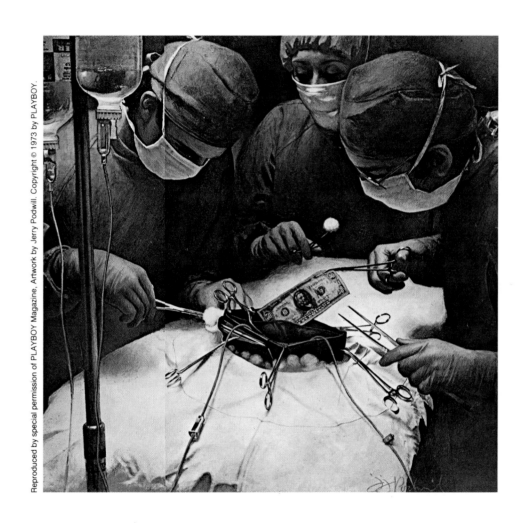

Placebo effect
The effect achieved when a patient takes a harmless concoction but thinks it is an active drug.

Fad
A craze or fashion that passes with time.

Quackery
The fraudulent practice of medicine or the healing arts.

Empirical approach
Based on observation.

Demonic theory
The theory that disease is caused by demons who enter the body.

Humoral theory
The theory that disease is caused by an imbalance of four fluids–blood, phlegm, yellow bile, and black bile–in the body.

Pathogenic model
The theory that disease is caused by invading organisms.

---

ic tradition prides itself, rightfully, on its rigorous testing of hypotheses. The insistence on persuasive and verifiable answers to the question "How do you know?" greatly reduces the number of ineffective remedies that enter medical practice and continue in use. Nevertheless, it would be a mistake to assume that traditional medicine has all the answers or that everything outside the tradition is mere superstition.

The medical establishment is not immune to changing fashions, and (in rare cases) yesterday's standard practice may be tomorrow's quackery—or vice versa.

The search for healing methods that work is complicated by several basic but often overlooked facts about human sickness and health:

1. The human body is extremely capable of healing itself, with or without medical treatment.
2. Human health is influenced by a large number of interacting factors, such as activity levels, diet, environmental stresses, and the like.
3. Psychological factors contribute to, or can cause, physical ailments.
4. Belief and imagination can have a profound effect on a person's health, as demonstrated by the so-called *placebo effect* (the tendency of some people to recover from an illness when given placebos, or sugar pills, that they think are drugs).

Sick people are likely to get well in the normal course of things, even without treatment. They are also likely to attribute their recovery to any treatment they might have taken. The recovery is seen as proof of the treatment's effectiveness, and the result may be a convert to the latest fad or a testimonial for a (usually) harmless but ineffective quack remedy.

We shall apply the label *fad* to any brief wave of popularity for a healing method. A typical example would be almost any of the succession of weight-loss diets that have swept the country in recent years. We assume here that most fads are promoted by people with a sincere belief in their effectiveness.

We shall define *quackery* as the fraudulent misrepresentation of ability and experience in diagnosing or treating disease or as the misrepresentation of the effects of the treatment offered.

The Past as Prologue

Little is known about the very earliest beginnings of medical science in any of the world's major cultures. Nevertheless, we can make some educated guesses on the basis of the information we do have.

Many primitive cultures believed that illness was caused by demons who had gained entry into the body. Common treatment was to drive out the evil spirits through exhortations by a medicine man or witchdoctor. In some cultures holes were drilled in the skull to allow the demons to escape. Though the human body is surprisingly capable of healing itself—sometimes in spite of medical treatment—we should also remember that belief, imagination, and faith are important to the healing process. The medicine man and witchdoctor were also the religious leaders of their day.

Studies indicate that in some primitive cultures an *empirical approach* may have existed along with magic and superstition. "Primitive" research was sometimes based on observation and experience, and "primitive" remedies sometimes work.

Medical science evolved from the *demonic theory* to the *humoral theory*, which held that the body contained four humors, or fluids; a balance in these fluids supposedly resulted in health; an imbalance, in disease. From the time of Hippocrates (about 400 B.C.) to the mid-1800s, bloodletting was the accepted treatment for the so-called fluid imbalance.

Quackery thrives on confusion, and the mid-nineteenth century was a period of maximum confusion among both the lay public and professionals. During the period from 1830 to 1850 phenomenal advances were made in medicine. Doctors abandoned the accepted doctrine of hundreds of years—that bleeding the patient was a cure for all diseases. Debates continued over the origin of disease. And—perhaps most importantly—doctors admitted that they could cure few diseases. Quacks were claiming to cure all ills.

The modern theory of disease that forms the basis of Western medical science was developed over a period of centuries. This theory, which is based on the *pathogenic* (germ) *model*, holds that disease is caused by invading organisms. Research guided by this model even-

Antibiotics
Drugs based on substances originally produced by living organisms and used to kill microorganisms.

Allopathy
A system of medical practice based on producing a condition that is incompatible with the disease.

Osteopathy
A system of medical practice similar to allopathy; sometimes mistakenly associated primarily with manipulative therapy.

Manipulative therapy
Manual adjustment of the spine to relieve ailments.

---

tually led to the use of *antibiotics*. From Fracastoro, who in the year 1530 suggested that the disease he called syphilis was caused by a microorganism, to the confirming work of Pasteur and Koch in the late 1800s and early 1900s, the pathogenic model has been scientifically tested and expanded to include orthodox approaches to modern medicine and the treatment of disease.

Orthodox Medicine

Today there are two philosophies in the approach to orthodox medicine, allopathy and osteopathy. Although these approaches are quite similar in terms of scientific investigations leading to the present practice of medicine, there are slight differences between them.

Allopathy   The term *allopathy* is frequently applied to the method of treatment practiced by the holders of the degree of doctor of medicine (M.D.).

To obtain the M.D. degree requires four years of training at a medical school accredited by a joint committee (Committee on Medical Education) of the American Medical Association and the Association of American Medical Colleges. The first two years cover the basic sciences, and the last two years are devoted to work in a variety of hospital and clinic settings. In addition, most states require a one-year hospital internship following medical school. While standards for admission into medical school vary somewhat from state to state, three to four years of premedical college work are generally required, and most entering students have baccalaureate or higher degrees. Before a physician is allowed to practice, he or she must be licensed by a board of medical examiners. This occurs only after the individual successfully completes state or national board examinations.

The rapid expansion of technology in modern medical knowledge is forcing most medical school graduates into specialty education. A physician who elects to specialize faces an additional two to five years of graduate study and residency under specialists in his or her field of choice. See "Recognized Specialties and Subspecialties of Allopathy and Osteopathy," page 328.

Osteopathy   Osteopathic medicine was formally organized by Andrew T. Still when he established the American School of Osteopathy at Kirksville, Missouri, in 1892. Still, who had little formal education, was the son of a traveling Methodist preacher and doctor. He served his apprenticeship with his father and attended medical lectures in Kansas City. Following the Civil War he became disillusioned with the humoral system of medicine and formulated a new concept of healing based on a theory of structural disturbance. His basic idea was that the living body is a vital machine that will produce the necessary remedies to protect itself against disease as long as it is in correct mechanical adjustment.

Modern osteopaths are quick to point out that osteopathic manipulation was never synonymous with *osteopathy*. Still did not set out to establish a therapy that was to represent all of medical knowledge. Rather, his study and contemplation led him to conclude that an individual should be treated as a unit; a person cannot become sick in one area of his or her body without having the other areas affected. Osteopaths contend that osteopathy is not a fad competing with conventional medicine but a reform movement started *within* the medical practice in midwestern America.

The first doctors of osteopathy graduated in 1894, and within three years a national organization was formed. In 1901 this became the American Osteopathic Association. Almost immediately battle lines were formed, and the conflict between the American Medical Association and the newly formed American Osteopathic Association spread to organized medicine at state levels. The early leaders of osteopathy did not perceive the movement as antimedicine but as a movement for a new orientation within medicine.

Much of the conflict resulted from confusion about whether *manipulative therapy* was indeed the keystone of osteopathy and from the apparent relationship between it and chiropractic philosophy. This still causes confusion in the minds of the general public. There is no philosophical, scientific, or technological agreement between osteopathy and chiropractic.

Today the conflict between traditional medicine and osteopathy has been, for the most part, resolved. Osteopathic physicians have unlimited practice rights in all 50

Recognized Specialties and Subspecialties of Allopathy and Osteopathy

Administrative medicine: Operation and management of organizations and institutions such as health departments, hospitals, clinics, and health-care plans

Allergy: A subspecialty of internal medicine

Anesthesiology: Administration of drugs to prevent pain or to induce unconsciousness during surgical operations or diagnostic procedures

Aviation medicine: A subspecialty of preventive medicine that deals with problems of aviation and space flight

Cardiology: A subspecialty of internal medicine that deals with the heart and blood vessels

Child psychiatry: A subspecialty of psychiatry that deals with nervous and emotional problems of children

Dermatology: Diagnosis and treatment of skin diseases

Family practice: General medical services for patients and their families

Forensic pathology: A subspecialty of pathology that deals with medicine and the law

Gastroenterology: A subspecialty of internal medicine that is concerned with disorders of the digestive tract

General surgery: Surgery of parts of the body that are not in the domain of specific surgical specialties (some overlapping areas)

Internal medicine: Diagnosis and nonsurgical treatment of internal organs of the body of adults

Neurological surgery (neurosurgery): Diagnosis and surgical treatment of diseases of the brain, spinal cord, and nerves

Neurology: Diagnosis and nonsurgical treatment of diseases of the brain, spinal cord, and nerves

Nuclear medicine: Use of radioactive substances for diagnosis and treatment

Obstetrics and gynecology (ob/gyn) Care of pregnant women and treatment of disorders of the female reproductive system

Occupational medicine: A subspecialty of preventive medicine that is concerned with the special physical and psychological risks in industry

Opthalmology: Medical and surgical care of the eyes, including the prescription of glasses

Orthopedic surgery (orthopedics): Care of diseases of the muscles and diseases, fractures, and deformities of the bones and joints

Otolaryngology (ent): Care of diseases of the ears, nose, and throat

Pathology: Examination and diagnosis of organs, tissues, body fluids, and excrement

Pediatric allergy: A subspecialty of pediatrics

Pediatric cardiology: A subspecialty of pediatrics that is concerned with diseases of the heart

Pediatrics: Care of children from birth through adolescence

Physical medicine and rehabilitation (physiatrics): Treatment of convalescent and physically handicapped patients

Plastic surgery: Surgery to correct or repair deformed or mutilated parts of the body or to improve facial or body features

Preventive medicine: Prevention of disease through immunization, good health practice, and concern with environmental factors

Proctology: Diagnosis and treatment of disorders of the lower digestive tract (colon and rectum)

Psychiatry: Treatment of mental and emotional problems

Public health: A subspecialty of preventive medicine that is concerned with promoting the general health of the community

Pulmonary disease: A subspecialty of internal medicine that is concerned with diseases of the lungs

Radiology: Use of radiation for the diagnosis and treatment of disease

Thoracic surgery: Surgical treatment of the lungs, heart, and large blood vessels within the chest cavity

Urology: Treatment of male sex organs and urinary tract and treatment of female urinary tract

---

states. The training of traditional medical doctors and osteopaths is nearly identical. California has classified most of its osteopathic physicians as medical doctors, and all former California osteopathic schools now grant the M.D. degree to their graduates. Specialty requirements are the same as for M.D.s.

Choosing Medical Advisers "You can never get a doctor when you need one!" is a complaint frequently heard in many communities. However, this is most often the case for those who wait for an emergency before they attempt to contact a physician. In seeking medical care, people must decide what their needs are. The most

Acupuncture
Using needles to puncture the body in order to relieve pain or cure disease.

Loci
Specific places; plural of *locus*.

Chiropractic
A system of healing that emphasizes the manipulation of the spinal column.

---

frequently recommended plan is for a family to select a family practice physician to deal with the family's medical problems and to rely on his or her program of referral to qualified specialists when their services are required. On the other hand, a young family may choose to turn to specialists to provide their general medical care. It may be desirable to select several specialists—for example, a pediatrician for the children and an internal medicine specialist for the adults.

College students should investigate services that are available through the student health center. Services may be provided free of charge or for a nominal fee. The college health center can serve a vital role in the health care of students because its personnel are familiar with the problems of students; if additional medical care is needed, the health center can serve as the referral agency to obtain necessary specialized treatment and care.

For more specific information on selecting medical advisers, see "How to Choose a Doctor," page 367. Many of these suggestions can also serve as a guide in choosing a dentist.

Alternative Approaches to Medicine

The term *alternative approaches* is used to signify that the following philosophies are unorthodox in that they have never been based upon acceptable scientific evidence—the rigorous testing of hypotheses. It would be impossible to discuss all of the alternative approaches, so discussion will center on a few of the better known philosophies.

Acupuncture   According to the definition of Chinese traditional medicine, *acupuncture* is the treatment of disease—not just the alleviation of pain—by inserting very fine needles into the body at specific points called *loci*. The practice of acupuncture dates back to 2500 B.C. and is described in the oldest book of Chinese medicine.

According to this philosophy, human beings are subject to universal laws. The forces behind life and death are in the form of Ch'i (vital energy). The general flow of Ch'i through the body is controlled by the interplay of two opposing forces, the yin and the yang.

Yin represents negative: night, cold, dark, female, and the interior of the body. Yang is the opposite: positive, day, hot, light, male, and the exterior of the body.

In human beings, health results from the balance of yin and yang. All diseases, the philosophy says, are due to an imbalance of these forces. An acupuncture practitioner first locates the energy imbalance and then seeks to restore the balance by inserting needles into one or more loci and by leaving the needles in place for a designated period of time. The equilibrium of yin and yang is then expected to be restored and the disease cured.

Considerable interest in acupuncture surfaced in 1971 after the doors of China were once again opened to Western visitors. From extensive research, however, it appears reasonably clear that acupuncture does not cure organic disease, and its anesthesia benefits seem to be limited. The AMA views acupuncture as an experimental medical procedure that should be performed only in a research setting by a licensed physician or under a physician's supervision.

Chiropractic   The *chiropractic* movement was born on September 18, 1895, when Daniel D. Palmer of Davenport, Iowa, allegedly performed a spinal adjustment that restored a man's hearing. Harvey Lillard was the janitor of the building in which Palmer's office for the practice of magnetic healing was located. While examining Lillard, Palmer, a former grocer with no formal education, located a painful vertebra that appeared to be out of place. Lillard said this was where he had hurt his back 17 years earlier when he had lost his hearing. Palmer applied a sharp thrust that repositioned the bone, and a short time later Lillard claimed that he could hear better than ever.

Anyone attempting to study chiropractic is immediately confronted with the problem of definition. There is no consensus among chiropractors as to what constitutes chiropractics. The definitions range from a "scientific method of healing based on a theory that most human ailments or diseases are the results of the displacement

How to Cut Health Care Costs

When the average health consumer approaches the system, he is faced with a bewildering array of providers and a very complex set of decisions regarding treatment. Most commonly, the family physician is asked to guide him through the system. But an informed consumer can himself make the decisions that give him the highest quality service at the lowest possible costs by carefully implementing the following:

1. Have a family physician. This will reduce costs and time when illness does strike. A trusted family physician is still the best source of medical information available to the average consumer.

2. Never use an emergency room when a physician's office visit will suffice. Emergency room costs average more than $50 per visit in most areas. The quality of emergency room care can be inconsistent and sporadic because of different professionals' being on duty at the time of each visit. Emergency rooms are equipped and staffed for traumatic emergency care. A patient with a routine, nonemergency problem is not likely to receive the best care and would be much better off in his doctor's office.

3. Only licensed medical personnel should be used for health care services. Most state licensing laws are very good. Any individual offering health services who is not properly licensed should be reported to the state health licensing agency. Be

wary of claims of "guaranteed" quick and easy cures.

4. If at all possible live in an area where you have access to a major medical center. For very serious, uncommon, or complicated illnesses and injury, you should have access to a major teaching facility. Often *indigent services* will be available to those who live within the political boundaries of the entity that supports the hospital. If there is a possibility that you would not be able to pay a very large hospital bill, and you live within a county that supports a large teaching facility, you could probably be admitted and a large portion of your bill adjusted. If, however, you live in another county and could not pay the bill, there is a chance you would not be allowed admittance at all. If you are ever unable to pay a large hospital bill, go to the hospital controller's office and find what the hospital policy is on indigent care. Often larger teaching hospitals have legal requirements from their funding agency to accept indigent patients.

5. Match the illness with the hospital. As stated above, if you have an uncommon illness, you may be better off in a major teaching facility. If you are, however, less seriously ill, you will receive better and cheaper service in one of the many fine community hospitals available.

6. Understand your treatment. Understand the nature of your illness, what treatment you are

receiving, and why you are receiving it. Knowledge of your illness may help with your recovery and thereby help cut costs.

7. Like it or not, the health care institutions of this country have a wide range of quality, from poor to adequate to the very best. For most major illnesses, there are one or two institutions that have a higher success rate than other hospitals in the country for treatment of certain diseases. Finances permitting, a patient who is seriously ill should consider seeking the best possible care available.

8. Consider joining a health maintenance organization (HMO). In a health maintenance organization, a subscriber pays an annual premium, and all of his family's health care needs are taken care of during the year. The HMO's have a real motivation to prevent expensive treatment, so they theoretically place more emphasis on preventive services. The physicians are generally paid on a salary basis, regardless of services performed. There are more than 170 HMO's in 36 states, with a total enrollment in excess of 6 million.

9. Consider outpatient surgery for minor procedures. Outpatient surgery reduces the cost of the inpatient stay.

J. Stephen Lindsey
Life & Health

of the vertebrae of the spinal column" to "a science based on the premise that good health depends upon a normal functioning nervous system"; and there are two major professional organizations that disagree with each other. The common way of differentiating between chiropractic factions is the straight/mixer dichotomy: the "straights" adhere to a strict definition, limiting the scope of practice

to manual manipulation of the spine. The "mixers" advocate, in addition to spinal adjustments, the use of heat, light, water, electricity, vitamins, colonic irrigation, and other physical and mechanical adjuncts.

The goal of some chiropractors is to be considered as primary health care providers for Medicare and future national health care plans, and in this they have been

Faith healing
Belief that religious faith or faith in the
healer can result in a cure.

Homeopathy
The use of medication that would produce
in healthy people symptoms of the disease
to be treated.

---

highly successful. They enjoy limited benefits (they may
not prescribe drugs or perform surgery) in all states and
have the recognition of the U.S. Commissioner of
Education for a provisional accrediting Council on
Chiropractic Education.

A primary concern of many, and this includes some
chiropractors, is that the present political efforts of
chiropractors to be included among providers of primary
care through physical examinations would have disastrous results. In essence they and many other concerned individuals are saying that chiropractors do not
have the training, knowledge, or experience to recognize, identify, or differentiate human pathology or disease processes that must precede any treatment.

Faith Healing   History is replete with widespread examples of belief in *faith healing*. From the early demon
model to the miracles of Jesus to the healing shrine of
Lourdes in France, people have reported miraculous,
spontanous episodes. Whether today's believer follows
the teachings of Mary Baker Eddy, Katheryn Kuhlman,
or Oral Roberts, the basic tenet is that religious faith or
faith in the healer can result in a cure through divine
intervention.

Mary Baker Eddy, founder of the Church of Christ,
Scientist (Christian Science) in 1879, believed that she
was a recipient of a cure through "truth in Christ." The
philosophy of Christian Science holds that people are
spiritual ideas and therefore cannot be sick. Poor health
or illness is equated with faulty beliefs, and prayer heals
by replacing bad thoughts with good ones.

Today there are approximately 4,000 Christian
Science practitioners (healers) in the United States.
Christian Science is legal in all states, and some
insurance companies cover practitioner fees. The fees
are deductible as a medical expense for federal tax
purposes.

For many years Katheryn Kuhlman, who claimed to
be an instrument of the Holy Spirit, was known as the
"queen" of faith healers in the United States. Although
she maintained that she believed in the medical profession and had a number of physicians who would certify
her cures, none could be found who would state that
anyone with organic disease had ever been cured by
Kuhlman. More recently a well-known evangelical

preacher and healer, Oral Roberts, has tried to blend
prayer and scientific medicine and to that end has
built a medical center at Oral Roberts University.

Homeopathy   *Homeopathy* was one of the most
notable of the many nineteenth-century fads. Its founder,
Samuel Hahnemann, received his medical degree in
Germany in 1779. While practicing in Leipzig, he studied
the action of quinine. Pondering a statement that
quinine, widely used to treat fevers, would also produce
a fever of several days' duration, he concluded that a
disease could only be cured by a remedy with a tendency
to produce a similar disease. The concept "likes are
cured by likes" became the basic tenet of Hahnemann's
new medical system.

Forming his doctrine were two additional beliefs—
that medicines increase in potency with their dilution
and that a large number of diseases are due to a
condition that he called *psora* (an itch or some kind of
skin disease). Hahnemann lectured and wrote numerous
articles and gained many converts to his new system.
Although he also had many opponents, the movement
spread—from Germany to France, England, and the
United States.

Dissension soon appeared in the homeopathic
schools between the pure Hahnemannians, who had
discarded the lance and scalpel, and those who adopted
some principles while rejecting others. The conflict, along
with a growing realization that the basic principles were
false, caused the ranks to diminish. Another phase of
the movement hastened its end. The United States and
England were flooded with homeopathic books on
"domestic practice" for family use. Many of these books
were sold with a case of medicine containing remedies
so diluted (one to one-millionth) that they could not
harm a baby and were, of course, absolutely useless.
This was true quackery, and it led to the discrediting of
the movement.

Medical historians are quick to point out that
homeopathy appeared at an opportune time. The practice of orthodox medicine had made rapid advances
during the early nineteenth century, but many physicians
would not accept the new techniques and still clung to
the old concepts. Hahnemann and his followers
crusaded against the principles of the Greek humoral

Naturopathy
A system of healing that is based on the belief that disease is caused by the violation of nature's laws. Treatment is generally limited to natural substances and forces.

Holistic
Emphasizing the organic relationship between the parts and the whole. In medicine the term often signifies treatment of the patient, not just the disease.

Remission
A significant decrease of symptoms.

Regression
A reduction of symptoms in a disease process.

Laetrile
A drug derived from apricot kernels and used for cancer therapy; of no proven value.

model—emetics, purgatives, and frequent bleeding. Most important, they proved that the body had natural healing powers. Also, the philosophical debates spurred on by efforts to prove, or disprove, various theories led to many scientific advances in anatomy, physiology, and chemistry, helping to place the study of medicine on a sound scientific footing.

Homeopathy is experiencing a revival. Although it is more popular internationally than in the United States, U.S. homeopathic organizations report growing membership lists.

Naturopathy   The philosophy underlying *naturopathy* is that the basic cause of disease is the violation of nature's laws in thinking, breathing, eating, drinking, working, and resting, as well as in social, moral, and sexual conduct.

Treatment consists of "natural food" diets, vitamins, herbs, tissue minerals, sea salts, manipulation, massage, exercise, colonic enemas, and the use of such natural forces as rest, heat, air, sunlight, and electricity. Drugs (except those that are components of body tissue) and surgery are not allowed.

Naturopaths are licensed in only seven states and in the District of Columbia. Some naturopaths claim to practice "classical homeopathy" in addition to their basic philosophy—a trend that does not please homeopaths.

Holistic Medicine   At this point it might be helpful to briefly discuss the term *holistic* (or *wholistic*) in conjuction with alternative approaches. A great deal of confusion appears to surround the term. Generally speaking, holistic means emphasizing the organic relationship between the parts of something and the whole.

Many people see the holistic movement as an important development in the health field. Others state that the concept of holistic medicine has been the underlying force of all medicine. They point out the statement attributed to Sir William Osler, a Canadian-born physician (1849–1919): "The good physician treats the disease; the great physician treats the patient who has the disease."

It would be prudent for the health consumer to examine the practitioner who espouses the holistic trend and what he or she means by the term. Is it legitimate or is it a guise under which unorthodox practitioners attempt to fool the unwary?

Quackery Today

The snake oil salesman with his medicine show operating from the back of a covered wagon has faded into history, but medical quackery is still with us. The snake oil salesman's successors are much more sophisticated in appearance and appeal. They speak knowledgeably about a wide variety of topics and use correct medical language. Their walls are covered with diplomas, some legitimate, others from notorious degree mills. Some quackery is so sophisticated that it has been supported by research studies and huge advertising budgets for product promotion. The modern quack knows the psychology of consumers, how much they know about their own level of health, and what their fears and superstitions are.

Quacks *always* represent themselves as successful in treating ailments not yet understood by medical science. Arthritis and cancer are good examples. Both have other characteristics that help to support the quack's testimonial claims. They are subject to *remission* and *regression*. Some cancer patients have remissions, and arthritis may suddenly flare up and then subside, leaving the sufferers free of pain for weeks or months. If treatment is attempted just before a remission, the patient may be seduced by the *post hoc, ergo propter hoc* (after this, therefore because of this) fallacy.

Laetrile   The Steve McQueen story, one in a long series of Laetrile tragedies, focuses attention on a continuing controversy—do we have the right to choose our own treatment and, quite possibly, our own path to death? The proponents of Laetrile say yes!

Laetrile, which is short for LAE-vomandelo-niTRILE-beta-glucuronic acid, also known as amygdalin and vitamin B_{17}, is derived from apricot kernels. Laetrile was discovered in 1920 by accident in an attempt to improve the taste of bootleg whiskey. It was allegedly purified as an anticancer drug in 1952 by a San Francisco biochemist, Ernest Krebs, Jr., and has been a subject of controversy ever since. The theory and claims behind

Amygdalin
A substance found in the bitter almond; formerly incorrectly thought to be the same thing as Laetrile.

Adipose tissue
Connective tissue that stores fat.

Laetrile have been changed repeatedly. The original claim was that Laetrile sought out cancer cells and then released hydrocyanic acid to kill them. Later it was claimed that cancer is caused by a deficiency of vitamin B_{17} and Laetrile *is* vitamin B_{17}; therefore, Laetrile can prevent, control, or cure cancer.

An interesting twist to the Laetrile story came in a 1981 announcement that the drug Laetrile has actually not existed until recently. Dr. David Rubin and colleagues at the Israeli Medical Research Foundation claim that for the past two decades the drug that has been called Laetrile is *not* the same thing as *amygdalin* (a natural substance that is chemically related).

The Laetrile that has been synthesized, they claim, is derived from a patent that was originally developed by Krebs as he expanded the work of his late physician father. The younger Krebs developed a formula to concentrate on a fact known since the early 1940s—that most cancers contain high levels of an enzyme, beta-glucuronidase. A substance developed from this formula should be able to attack cancer cells without injuring normal cells. Krebs, however, was never able to make the substance he described in his patent. So he substituted amygdalin and the controversy was on. It would truly be unfortunate if the confusion caused by Krebs's substitution has masked a brilliant discovery for so many years.

Other Unproven Methods Since the passage of the Food, Drug, and Cosmetic Act of 1938, at least one major cancer fraud seems to have surfaced in every decade. In the 1940s it was William F. Koch, who did business as the Christian Medical Research League; in the 1950s it was Harry Hoxsey's clinic in Dallas, Texas; in the 1960s it was Krebiozen; and in the 1970s it was Laetrile.

The reason for the continued onslaught of quackery is quite simply money. Quackery is big business in the United States today, with Americans reportedly spending millions of dollars annually on worthless products and services.

It would be impossible to mention all of the questionable practices existing today, but here are a few more examples.

Cellulite is a name that quick weight-loss or spot reducing proponents have given to the dimply, waffled-looking fat that is found predominantly on the thighs and buttocks. Advertisements for products to reduce or remove "cellulite" appear regularly in newspapers, magazines, and books. Yet scientific needle biopsies have shown that no difference exists between fat that has the characteristic appearance of so-called cellulite and other types. Genetics determines how our extra *adipose tissue* will look.

A recent entry into the arthritis quackery field, where blatant quackery exists, is the green-lipped mussel remedy. This "natural" treatment is an extract from the green-lipped mussel, a shellfish found only in the waters of New Zealand. The mussel extract, sold in capsule form under a variety of names (Seatone, Freedon, Aquatone) in health food and drug stores, is claimed to aid in mobility and pain reduction. Books and pamphlets state that it has been shown effective as an arthritis remedy even though it is being touted as a "secret" remedy and is *not* being released for testing by qualified experts.

The Arthritis Foundation states that over 31 million Americans suffer from arthritis and spend $950 million each year on unproven remedies such as copper bracelets, "immunized" milk, and now green-lipped mussel extract. If you have any doubt about any new treatment, contact the Arthritis Foundation at 3400 Peachtree Road, N.E., Suite 1101, Department P, Atlanta, GA 30326.

Diet and Food Faddism Nowhere is the consumer beset with more confusion than in deciding what to eat (see Chapter 11). Nutrition is still a young science so riddled with controversy that one can with very little effort quote respected experts to support either side of almost any of its many issues. Since food products are sold for profit, there are also vested interests on both sides of most of those issues. Inevitably, this situation has spawned a succession of fads, especially in the form of weight-reduction diets. Most of these diets promise dramatic weight loss in a short time. Since sustained weight loss is a slow process (the weight was not gained overnight either), the really effective methods—reducing caloric intake from food below the level expended in activity or increasing the caloric expenditure in activity above the intake from food—are less appealing to many than fad diets.

Fad diets are often promoted extensively in the mass media. Another factor promoting diet and food faddism is the rapid proliferation of unqualified nutrition consultants. The California Council Against Health Fraud noted that in 1980 the number of "degree mills" offering mail order diplomas in nutrition counseling was rapidly increasing. According to the CCAHF, one California degree mill has 3,700 enrollees. Graduates advertise themselves as "nutritional consultants" with academic credentials when they are nothing more than salespeople armed with nutritional misinformation preying on an unsuspecting public.

Nutritional supplements come closer to the classic picture of a health fad. Even nutritionists who are alarmed at the consumption of refined and processed foods generally consider such supplements unnecessary except in special cases. Nor is any evidence available that vitamins extracted from foods ("natural vitamins") are any more effective than vitamins produced in the laboratory, since the chemical composition is the same in both cases.

Decision Making

What the quack is marketing is hope. The push to legalize Laetrile sparked debates about the right of a terminally ill patient to have some hope, even if it is based on a worthless drug. But 70 years of experience in the fight against ineffective cancer treatments show some important trends. First and foremost, no matter how harmless their ingredients, all such products are death traps for those whose cancers are curable by effective methods. The lesson learned long ago is quite simple: The only way to protect the public from medical fraud is to keep dubious products and schemes out of the marketplace. So-called freedom of choice, in this area, is actually freedom to swindle the sick. The operational code of the quack is to make healthy people think that they are sick, while telling sick people that he or she will make them healthy.

With the increasing incidence of sophisticated quackery and the possibility of widespread growth of quack or fraudulent schemes if a freedom-of-choice law is passed, consumers need decision-making guidelines. The many published lists of tips on how to spot a quack all seem to include these seven factors:

1. *Secrecy.* The machine or product has been developed by a special formula. Purchasers of the Drown radiotherapeutic device had to promise to have their machines repaired only at the Drown offices. The actual circuit was so simple that a junior high school science student would have recognized its simplicity.

2. *Cure.* While orthodox medicine uses the term *cure* guardedly, the quack sometimes guarantees a cure for many or all diseases.

3. *Spurious degrees.* The quack's offices are covered with degrees that the unsuspecting victim believes are legitimate indications of special skills in medicine.

4. *Scare tactics.* The quack speaks of horrible medical consequences if treatment is delayed for as much as an hour. Be wary of signing any contracts for a specified number of treatments. Such contracts are a sure sign of quackery. Any time speed is emphasized, the patient should become immediately suspicious.

5. *Testimonials.* "Case histories" depicting a long line of successes appear as advertisements, as planted stories in newspapers, or on television talk shows. Talk show hosts like to interview quacks because they tend to "liven" things up. This gives the quack instant exposure to millions of people. There is little incentive for giving equal time to scientists to refute the quack's claims because the scientist must be more cautious in his or her statements and is therefore a less entertaining figure.

6. *Medical conspiracy.* Quacks are quick to claim that they are being persecuted by the medical community because their cures will cut into the incomes doctors make "by keeping people sick." They are also quick to state publicly that they are willing to make their substances, machines, or other products available for testing, but the material is rarely delivered.

7. *Law suits.* Many quacks are legally belligerent and travel with an entourage of lawyers. Whenever someone challenges the quack's claims, he or she threatens to sue.

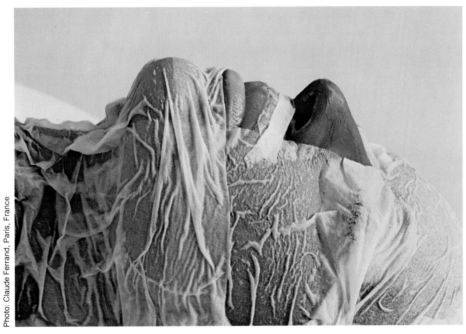

Taking Responsibility

We all need to accept the responsibility for our health. We cannot squander the good health that we are born with and then expect to buy back this precious commodity at some later date. Conclusions drawn from a study by Lester Breslow and others at the UCLA School of Public Health indicate that by following seven simple rules

a man can extend his life by eleven years on the average and a woman by seven. Here are the seven rules:

1. Do not smoke cigarettes.
2. Get some regular exercise.
3. Use alcohol moderately or not at all.
4. Get seven to eight hours of sleep nightly.
5. Maintain proper weight.

6. Eat breakfast.
7. Do not eat between meals.

If and when you decide that medical care is necessary, seek orthodox treatment first. A delay in obtaining competent care, especially in the case of cancer, can produce disastrous results.

Consumer Protection

The individual consumer usually does not have the time or resources to check the truthfulness of every service or claim for a health product. Fortunately, many federal, state, and local agencies do have those resources and use them in a continuing effort to protect consumers from fraudulent claims and dangerous products.

In many communities complete lists of federal, state, and local consumer protection agencies are available, with phone numbers and addresses. We shall limit our discussion here mostly to the three largest federal agencies: the Food and Drug Administration (FDA), the Federal Trade Commission (FTC), and the U.S. Postal Service. The FDA, a branch of the Department of Health and Human Services, is concerned primarily with the ingredients and labeling of products that move in interstate commerce. The FTC is concerned with all cases of deceptive advertising, and the Postal Service has primary jurisdiction where mail fraud may be involved.

The Food and Drug Administration   The FDA's authority is limited to laws passed by Congress and assigned to the agency for enforcement. Its principal responsibility is enforcement to ensure wholesome foods, safe and effective drugs and medical devices, harmless cosmetics, and truthful labeling of such products.

What do you do if you run into a food, drug, cosmetic, or medical device that you feel is unsanitary, mislabeled, or potentially harmful? You can complain to the FDA! Complaints can lead to recalls and even to improved products.

Before registering your complaint, first check to see that you have used the product for its intended purpose and have properly followed instructions. Check to see if the product was outdated. Save any unused portion for FDA review.

To call the FDA office nearest you, look in the phone book under U.S. Government, Food and Drug Administration. Or you can write to Product Complaints, FDA Office of Consumer Affairs, HFE-88/P, 5600 Fishers Lane, Rockville, MD 20857.

To understand how the FDA does its job and why the government can never completely protect the consumer, it is necessary to examine what "safety" means. What may be safe for one person is not necessarily safe for another. Nothing can ever be completely safe. Any product, if used incorrectly, has a potential for harm.

The FDA's approach can be simply stated: To be considered safe, a product must have more benefits than risks, and any risk must be justified. It is the FDA's job to set the conditions under which a product's benefits must be shown to outweigh any possible risks. If such conditions cannot be set, then the FDA must seek to prohibit sale of that product.

The *benefit-risk ratio* applies to every product regulated by the FDA. For example, in reviewing the scientific studies conducted for a new drug, the FDA determines whether the proved benefits from the drug when used as specified on the approved label are sufficiently greater than the potential risks. Only if the benefits outweigh the risks will the FDA approve the drug for marketing.

The same judgment applies when the FDA reviews data for a food or color *additive* or for any other product.

In applying this safety concept, the FDA has a number of alternatives, depending on the type of product and the degree of regulation authorized by Congress. The FDA can prevent the sale of some products, such as unproved new drugs and harmful food additives. It can require products to be redesigned, reformulated, relabeled, or packaged in a safer way. It can take action against false or misleading labeling. The FDA can order removal of products from the marketplace whenever new scientific data reveal risks that are not acceptable.

Benefit-risk-ratio
The relative amounts of benefits and risks of a product or procedure.

Additives
Chemicals added to or found in food that are not normal constituents. Some, such as preservatives, coloring agents, and sweeteners, are deliberately added; others, such as insecticides and antibiotics, often appear as incidental additives.

Adulterate
To make impure or inferior by adding improper ingredients.

Extradition
The legal surrender of an alleged criminal to a jurisdiction of another state, country, or government for trial.

Finally, the FDA can go to court to seize illegal products; to obtain injunctions against violators; or to prosecute the manufacturer, packer, or shipper of *adulterated* or mislabeled products.

Since seizures are court procedures, they take time and do not always result in the most efficient consumer protection. Recall of a defective or hazardous product has become the quickest and most practical way to get an unsafe or unacceptable product off the market.

Many people have the impression that the FDA conducts such recalls. Actually, a recall is conducted by the company that made or distributed the product. The agency may request a company to recall a product, and the FDA monitors the recall to make sure it is accomplished. But in most instances firms decide to recall the product without a request.

The Federal Trade Commission The FTC tries to protect the consumer against untruthful or fraudulent advertising. Although the commission has specific responsibilities for law enforcement, its fundamental purpose is to guide rather than prosecute. The commission's job, as assigned to it by Congress, is to step into the marketplace when necessary to keep consumers from being cheated.

But the FTC is in trouble. For over 50 years FTC performance had been generally slow and ineffective. In 1970 the FTC was reborn. Young, activist attorneys were brought in who, in turn, brought a sense of mission to the agency. In 1974, armed with a new trade regulation rule, the agency was able to set standards to prohibit certain practices in an entire industry whenever there was a general pattern of industrywide consumer abuse. After five years of intensive work, two trade regulation rules had been enacted and 16 more FTC actions were ready. Suddenly Congress stepped in and stalled the actions.

The growing "get-government-off-our-backs" movement plus extensive business lobbying had succeeded in blocking a three-year funding for the FTC in 1977. Following one-year continuing resolutions in 1978 and 1979, Congress finally approved the Federal Trade Commission Improvements Act of 1980, which appropriated funding for another three-year period.

An important limitation placed on the FTC from its inception is that it cannot bring any action directed toward the settlement of private controversies, and it cannot act merely in the interest of a private party. Any action the FTC brings must involve the public interest. But this should not stop you from complaining about false or deceptive practices, because your single complaint added to many others becomes the public interest. As in the case of the FDA, check your telephone directory or write to the Bureau of Consumer Protection, Federal Trade Commission, Rm. 256, 6th St. and Pennsylvania Ave., N.W., Washington, DC 20580.

Obviously the FTC would be overwhelmed by its task if it did not receive considerable help from three principal sources: (1) the majority of people in business, who voluntarily comply with the law themselves and through organized effort encourage others to do so; (2) advertising media and advertising agencies, which generally maintain high ethical standards; and (3) private and civic organizations, which identify and expose deceptive practices.

But in light of the recent attempts to handcuff the FTC, consumers should pay close attention to Congress and its dealings with regulatory agencies.

The U.S. Postal Service The U.S. Postal Service, through its Postal Inspection Service, operates to prevent the mails from being used to defraud the public. It reports that Americans, mostly those in low-income brackets, are being bilked of $500 million a year through mail fraud.

The Postal Inspection Service is the oldest of all federal investigative agencies. It is staffed by about 1,100 inspectors (of a total of 700,000 postal employees). The postmaster general, through the inspection service, is responsible for enforcing the postal laws. The prevalence of medical fraud and quackery during the middle of the nineteenth century, as well as the related legal problems of *extradition*, prompted the enactment of the first mail fraud statutes in 1872. These statutes were the first federal effort to protect the public from quacks and swindlers. Before that time a swindler could set up shop in one place and victimize individuals throughout the rest of the country with relative safety. Now it is prohibited to use the mails to obtain money or property by means of false or fraudulent representations, pretenses, or promises. Conviction on charges of postal fraud brings felony penalties of up to five years imprisonment and/or a $1,000 fine for each mailing made in attempting to continue a fraud. The Postal Service can also refuse to deliver mail to a promoter, forcing the shutdown of his or her mail-order operation.

Other Consumer Protection Agencies and Organizations   Many other agencies operate to protect the consumer. At the national level the Department of Health and Human Services houses, besides the FDA, the Office of Consumer Affairs, the Public Health Service, the National Institute of Health, and the Health Services Administration. Each of these agencies offers extensive consumer services. The Consumer Product Safety Commission works directly to protect the consumer against unreasonable risks that are associated with products. Several private organizations also work for consumer protection. The National Better Business Bureau promotes voluntary self-regulation of business in their advertising and sales representations. Consumers Union is a nonprofit organization that publishes *Consumer Reports,* a magazine that reports evaluative research conducted through laboratory and use tests on many products. The American Medical Association, American Cancer Society, American Heart Association, and others provide free educational materials and services to anyone who requests such information.

At the state and local levels we find many branch offices of the large national organizations. Most states and counties have medical associations. State offices for the large voluntary health agencies are found in large metropolitan areas. It is at this level that the individual can usually request and get prompt action in cases of fraud or quackery.

Government Attempts to Reduce Health Care Costs

On page 330 you read about what you, the health consumer, can do to cut the cost of your own health care. Here we examine what the federal government is doing in an effort to combat rising costs of health care in the United States. Public health experts agree that the

principal cause of spiraling health care costs, even more than general inflation, increased insurance coverage, and new expensive technology, is the fee-for-service system that dominates American health care. This system rewards the physician for providing more and more costly services. Hospitals are paid a markup over costs. More costs mean more revenue.

The federal government has long been concerned with the issue of rising health care costs, which becomes a political football in every presidential campaign. A number of federal plans that have been implemented and show some promise of success sound much like alphabet soup: PSROs, HMOs, HSAs, and DRGs.

Professional Standards Review Organizations (PSROs)   In 1972 Congress directed what was then known as the Department of Health, Education, and Welfare to create professional standards review organizations. PSROs are charged with organizing physicians to review hospital use under Medicare and Medicaid programs.

This peer review system has been evaluated by several studies, but the results are inconclusive. There seems to be a consensus, however, that the PSRO is only marginally successful as a cost control mechanism. Given the high cost of operating a PSRO, the current benefits are questionable. The potential of the program looks promising only with congressional financial assistance, good management, and a willingness on the part of practicing physicians to accept change.

Health Maintenance Organizations (HMOs)   In 1973, after many years of debate and over the serious objections of the American Medical Association, Congress passed the Health Maintenance Organization Act. This act overturned state laws that prevented prepaid group medical plans. It requires employers who offer health insurance benefits and have 25 or more employees to include an HMO option if an HMO exists in the area. Generally, the client (health consumer) prepays a fixed fee, and the HMO agrees to provide comprehensive health care services. The HMO concept is designed to emphasize maintenance of the positive health picture as opposed to the negative sickness care emphasized in the predominant fee-for-service arrangement.

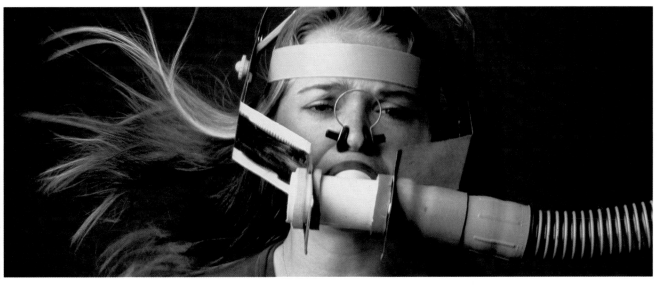

Chuck Kuhn, photographer; William Cain, Inc., agency; Blue Ribbon Sports/NIKE, client

Although HMOs have 10 to 40 percent lower costs than the conventional fee-for-service system, the reasons for such lower costs are unclear. Undoubtedly, a lack of financial incentives for physicians to admit patients to hospitals plays a significant part. Still, the growth rate of HMOs has not met the expectations of its promoters. Apparently consumers are reluctant to change from a traditional health insurance program that has met their needs. Nevertheless, the situation is slowly changing. There is an increasing public demand for a system, such as HMOs, that has built-in incentives for economy and consumer satisfaction.

Health Systems Agencies (HSAs)   The National Health Planning and Resources Development Act was signed into law in 1975. It mandates a system whereby states and the newly created health systems agencies establish a mechanism (certificate of need) to approve new hospital construction or substantial remodeling, as well as the purchase of expensive "new technology" equipment. As in the case of the PSROs, studies about the benefits of the HSAs' certificate-of-need procedure are inconclusive. HSAs are made up of consumer representatives, provider representatives, and a staff of professional planners. A possible reason for the inconclusive performance of the HSAs is that health planning is a political process that involves bargaining, negotiating, and favor trading. Consumer and provider representatives are rarely united. It does appear that in some areas, however, the HSA movement has been successful in curtailing capital investment and a large increase in the number of hospital beds. HSAs have also been successful in bringing the issue of health care costs to the community's attention.

Diagnosis-Related Groups (DRGs)   In 1982 Congress authorized Medicare payments to be based on what Medicare thinks specific treatments should cost. The Tax Equity and Fiscal Responsibility Act (TEFRA) mandates that hospitals must accept Medicare payments based on the figures of diagnosis-related groups rather than the traditional method of reimbursement for total costs. Hospitals receive a fixed fee for designated services. (There are 467 Medicare treatment categories.)

New Jersey was chosen as a test state for diagnosis-related payments. For four years all payers, including Medicare, used the DRGs. This program has led health insurers to begin to adopt the same system in other states. As a result, hospitals are attempting to adopt cost-tracing methods. These procedures based on the New Jersey experience have had a major impact on slowing the spiraling costs of health care.

Consumer Behavior Scale

Read the following statements carefully. Choose the one in each section that best describes you at this moment and record its score at the right. (For instance, "relies on chiropractors for medical advice" has a score of 3.) When you have identified five statements, total your score and find your position on the scale.

5   has family doctor (M.D. or D.O.)
4   prefers M.D. or D.O. for medical problems
3   relies on chiropractors for medical advice
2   uses unorthodox medical care, such as acupuncture
1   prefers faith healers to orthodox medicine

Score _____

5   is well informed about prescription and over-the-counter drugs
4   seeks expert advice before buying medicines
3   reads label before taking medicine
2   takes medicine without reading label
1   likes whatever cure-all fad comes along

Score _____

5   looks for solid evidence before making a health decision
4   looks for some evidence before acting
3   relies on TV programs for health information
2   likes to be viewed as having the latest health products
1   relies on unqualified others for health decisions

Score _____

5   selects comprehensive health insurance after careful review
4   selects health insurance on the recommendations of friends
3   selects health insurance for no particular reason
2   is unsure if covered by health insurance and what it covers
1   is not covered by health insurance

Score _____

5   believes diet with variety and balance is healthful
4   believes diet should emphasize fruits and vegetables
3   believes vitamin supplements are necessary
2   believes all white bread is unhealthful
1   believes the most healthful foods are in health food stores

Score _____

Total _____

25
24
23
22
21
OPTIMAL
A person at this level has a family doctor (M.D. or D.O.), is well informed about prescription and over-the-counter drugs, looks for solid evidence before making a health decision, including health insurance, and believes that a diet that has variety and balance is healthful.

20
19
18
17
SUPERIOR
A person at this level prefers an M.D. or D.O. for medical problems, seeks expert advice before buying medicines, looks for some evidence before making a health decision, buys health insurance on the recommendations of friends, and believes a healthful diet should emphasize fruits and vegetables.

16
15
14
13
MODERATE
A person at this level relies on chiropractors for medical advice, reads label before taking medicine, selects a health insurance plan without a particular reason, relies on TV programs for health information, and believes vitamin supplements are necessary for good health.

12
11
10
9
MARGINAL
A person at this level uses unorthodox medical care such as acupuncture, takes medicine without reading the label, likes to be viewed as having the latest health products, is unsure whether he or she is covered by health insurance, and believes that white bread is unhealthy.

8
7
6
5
INADEQUATE
A person at this level prefers faith healers to orthodox medicine, likes whatever cure-all comes along, relies on others for health decisions, has no health insurance plan, believes that the most healthful foods are in health food stores.

Take Action

Your answers to Probing Your Emotions at the beginning of this chapter and your placement level on the Consumer Behavior Scale will, we hope, encourage you to begin a process of self-exploration and self-discovery that you will continue. Reflect on the entire chapter's content and ask yourself how each point relates to your own life. Then take action:

1. Take detailed notes on or make a tape recording of several radio or TV commercials for health care products. On the basis of your reading of this chapter develop a set of criteria or rules to evaluate the commercials.

2. Do some research and find out what health insurance programs are available for college students. Which ones would you most recommend?

Which ones would you least recommend? Why?

3. Go to the student health center and briefly evaluate the quality and kinds of services it offers. Consider such things as waiting time, health literature available, referral services, and so forth. Give a copy of your evaluation to the manager or appropriate official.

Before leaving this chapter, review the questions that open the chapter. Have your feelings or values changed? Are you now better equipped to handle the complex and very human problems associated with consumer health issues?

Chapter Fifteen

Prescription and Over-the-Counter Drugs

Probing Your Emotions

1. When you visit the doctor, do you expect to receive a prescription for some kind of medication? If no drugs are prescribed, do you feel "cheated"?

2. When you have a headache, do you immediately reach for an aspirin tablet? When you have a common cold, do you immediately take a cold remedy? Do you consider *not* taking medication for these ailments? If you don't take medication, how do you treat these problems?

3. Do you know what *generic* drugs are? Do you request generic drugs when you have a prescription filled or when you purchase over-the-counter drugs, or do you prefer to use brand-name drugs? Why do you feel more comfortable taking one rather than the other? Why do you suppose so many people continue to purchase brand-name drugs when generic drugs are less expensive?

4. What prescription or over-the-counter drugs do you use regularly? (Remember: Aspirin, birth control pills, and the medication you take to keep yourself awake to study for exams are all drugs.) Do you feel you are a responsible drug user? If not, why do you feel you use the drugs you do?

Chapter Contents

PRIMITIVE DRUGS AND MODERN DRUGS

PATENT MEDICINES IN AMERICA

GOVERNMENT REGULATION OF THE DRUG INDUSTRY

HOW NEW PRESCRIPTION DRUGS ARE TESTED

THE MARKETING OF OVER-THE-COUNTER DRUGS

DANGERS OF SELF-MEDICATION
Drug interactions
Vitamin overdoses and imbalances
Drugs can deplete vitamins from the body

HOW TO SELF-MEDICATE SAFELY
Drug safety precautions
Drugs recommended for informed self-medication

EMERGENCY TREATMENT FOR POISONING OR DRUG OVERDOSE

POSSIBLE FUTURE SAFEGUARDS

Boxes

The placebo—an ethical problem
Using over-the-counter drugs
Drugs and alcohol
Aspirin use

Primitive
A word sometimes used to describe earlier, less "civilized" times; refers to cultures that are not technologically
advanced.

Infusion
The liquid produced by soaking a substance in water and extracting its soluble
parts; also the injection of a fluid into a
vein.

Poultice
A hot, soft mush prepared by wetting pow-
ders. Poultices are placed or spread on a
sore or inflamed part of the body to
soothe it.

Tonic
Something that restores or refreshes.

Patent medicines
Drugs that can be sold legally without a
doctor's prescription.

---

15 People almost everywhere believe that certain medicines have the power to heal and
cure and to promote well-being. In a primitive society
a medicine man may use magic, as well as drugs (some
of which work), in treating the physical, emotional, and
spiritual problems of his clients. Technological societies,
on the other hand, supposedly reject magic, although the
word sometimes appears in advertising copy.

When a medicine is believed to be effective but that
belief has not been proved, the belief can be called a
theory. Western science started to advance when people
began continually testing theories by experiment and
observation—in other words, empirically.

Belief confirmed by empirical evidence is called
knowledge; belief contradicted by empirical evidence is
called superstition. In our society we judge knowledge
to be more valid than superstition, but in both technological societies and primitive ones, beliefs in the power of
certain medicines cover a wide range and may or may
not be justified. We have some wonder drugs that work,
and so do they. They have some magical cures that do
not work, and so do we. Western societies may have
more medicines that work better simply because we
have an immense experimental technology. The medicine man, in comparison, has only limited equipment
and a few possibilities for trial-and-error testing.

Primitive Drugs
and Modern Drugs

Most drugs used in *primitive* medicine come from
plants. These are prepared as teas, *infusions,* or *poultices*
and swallowed, inserted, applied, inhaled, or administered in every possible way. Many of these drugs were
developed empirically; that is, they were tried and they
worked. Others do not work but are still used because
a belief or theory says they *should* work.

Many primitive medicines have survived the introduction of modern science, although for varying reasons.
Quinine, for example, was discovered actually to have
the medical properties assigned to it in primitive medicine. Belladonna was originally used to enlarge the
pupils of the eyes because people thought that large

pupils were attractive. It is now used (in modified form)
to enlarge the pupils so the eye can be examined with
an opthalmoscope. Other primitive medicines are no
longer used—the mandrake root, for example. This root
was used as a *tonic* ("stomachic," as it was called) almost
to the middle of the twentieth century—because it
resembled a human shape.

During the nineteenth century, medicines were developed by experiment with and observation of human
subjects. If the drug cured the disease, it was used
thereafter to treat that disease. Laboratory evaluation and
animal tests were not part of the method.

Patent Medicines
in America

In the United States, the sale and development of *patent
medicines* have roots in early colonial times, when
patent medicines were imported from England and
France in great quantities. Balsam of Life, one of these
early medicines, was promoted in the United States by
an Englishman named Robert Turlington, who claimed
that it cured a long list of disorders, including sprained
fingers and "dropsy" (now more commonly called edema, accumulation of fluids in the body). Daffy's Elixir,
another patent medicine popular in the mid-1700s, sold
for a steep price (then) equal to about a dollar. American
druggists who did not want to pay the high price bought
empty bottles of the same shape as Daffy's, filled them
with their own concoctions, and sold them as Daffy's
Elixir.

The druggist was safe, at least from the law, because
the cheated consumer had no legal protection. In fact,
consumers had no protection of any kind against fraud,
misrepresentation, or dangerous or harmful products.

Imported patent medicines gradually became less
common. They were supplanted by cheaper imitations.
Domestic producers were also quite successful in convincing the public that drugs made at home were better
and purer than drugs made abroad.

Why were patent medicines so popular in the
eighteenth and nineteenth centuries? The average consumer might have felt that he or she had little choice.

The Placebo—An Ethical Problem

Significant ethical problems surround all aspects of medicine, and several of the most troublesome ones involve drugs. Consider, for instance, the widespread use of placebos in medical practice. *Placebo* is the term applied to any harmless concoction (e.g., sugar and water) given to a patient under the pretense that it is an active drug. If [the] definition is broadly construed to include things like vitamins (when no vitamin deficiency is apparent), it appears that a significant proportion of all prescriptions are placebos. One British physician who kept a careful record of his prescriptions reported that 30 percent were in the placebo category.

Why do physicians prescribe placebos? To some extent because they constitute the safest therapy for treating hypochondria. By prescribing a placebo and thus pretending to acknowledge the seriousness of the patient's condition, the physician may be preventing him from resorting to harmful self-medication or to treatment from some unqualified or unscrupulous third party. Some physicians defend their practice of prescribing placebos by arguing that it "cements the physician-patient relationship": The patient who expects to be given a prescription may feel that the physician who fails to write one hasn't really done anything for him or doesn't really care to.

Cynics might say that physicians prescribe placebos in order not to lose customers, but the practice is also widespread in charity clinics and other settings where the question of patronage loss is less relevant.

Because of the strong psychological component in many illnesses, placebos often in fact work—i.e., have a favorable effect on health. On the other hand, they can of course be downright dangerous—by being totally useless—if prescribed after inadequate diagnosis or as a substitute for concentrated efforts to deal with serious problems.

The use of placebos undoubtedly adds to the public's expenditures for drugs, but it is not clear whether there is any less expensive way of dealing with the cases for which they are typically prescribed. Some might argue that if no prescription is indicated, the physician should take the time to explain the situation carefully to the patient in order to save the patient's money. But this may not be the most cost-effective way of dealing with the case; the physician's time also costs money—if not to the patient, then to the physician. Under fee-for-service, where the patient pays for the drug separately, the physician's impulse is to write a prescription and get on to the next case without unnecessarily wasting time. Under a prepayment plan that covers the cost of prescriptions, the physician is more likely to weigh the cost of his time against the cost of a placebo.

Victor R. Fuchs
Who Shall Live?

Doctor's fees were expensive; patent medicines were cheap. Doctors wrote in Latin and acted mysteriously. Besides that, they often gave the patient no information at all about his or her ailment. The patient was simply told to take the medicine prescribed. Patent medicine makers, in contrast, gave detailed descriptions of symptoms and ailments their products would cure. Doctors were reluctant to promise cures; patent medicine makers had no hesitation about promising everything. Doctors' patients all died sooner or later; so did drinkers of patent medicines, but at least they had the promise of everlasting health.

Doctors were sometimes brutal—they cut open boils, gave patients enemas, bled them, and peeled off quantities of skin. Still, many of their patients died. Many patients felt that a medicine had to taste bad to do good. Doctors often ignored this expectation and prescribed medicines to suit ailments without regard to how they tasted. Disappointed and, perhaps, distrustful patients could turn back to patent medicines, and many of them did. These medicines at least tasted the way people felt they should—awful.

If a patient expected a medicine to make him or her feel good right away, he or she could choose from an endless assortment of patent medicines containing cocaine, opium, morphine, heroin, or alcohol—usually 40 to 80 proof.

Certainly advertising played its part in helping to push patent medicines. For example, one nineteenth-century ad managed to exploit both the suspicions and the gullibility of the consumer.

> Most doctors prescribe BAD-EM-SALZ, but some of them don't. One doctor, more honest than the rest, explained it this way: "BAD-EM-SALZ? Yes, I used to prescribe it a great deal but I stopped. Why? Simply because the patients didn't come back to me anymore. If I had kept on prescribing BAD-EM-SALZ, they would all be getting well without my assistance."

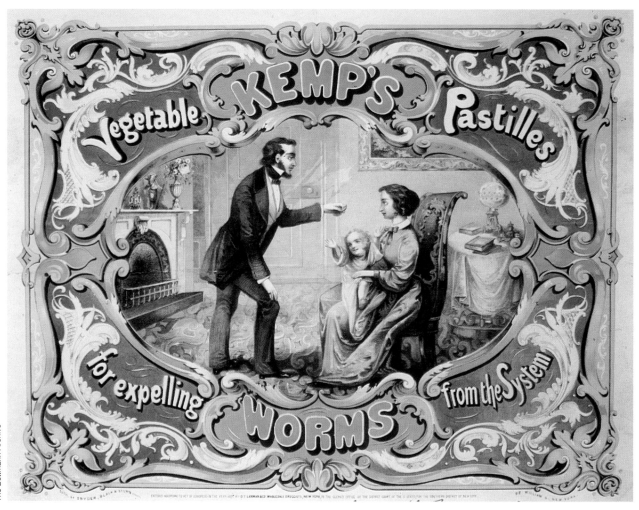

Thalidomide
A drug once used as a sleeping tablet and sedative that has been found to cause serious birth defects.

Data
Any group of facts from which deductions can be made.

Metabolize
To chemically transform food and other substances in the body into energy and wastes.

Toxic
Poisonous.

Side effect
Any effect of a drug accompanying its intended effect.

Government Regulation of the Drug Industry

The government first became interested in patent medicines because of their alcoholic content. Many remedies were being served over the bar in taverns—at low prices because they were not being taxed as liquor. The Treasury Department moved to change this situation but was forced to compromise by an association of medicine makers. The result was that medicines were subject to liquor tax only if they were sold by the glass.

The original Pure Food and Drug Act of 1906 did nothing to control the introduction of new drugs. This act forbade the adulteration and mislabeling of drugs moving in interstate commerce.

It was not until many people died as a result of using a drug called Sulfanilamide Elixir that the Food, Drug, and Cosmetic Act of 1938 was passed. This act required that companies planning to market a new drug submit an application showing the drug to be safe if used as directed on the label. It did not require any proof that the drug worked as stated.

It took tragedy to produce additional drug legislation. In the early 1960s many pregnant women (mostly in Europe) were taking a sedative called *thalidomide*. Use of this drug resulted in the birth of many seriously deformed babies. To increase protection against another such occurrence, Congress passed, in 1962, the Kefauver-Harris Amendment to the Food, Drug, and Cosmetic Act. This amendment included the following provisions:

1. All experimental drug studies must be registered.
2. Manufacturers must submit *data*, in a new drug application, supporting both safety and effectiveness.
3. Advertising of prescription products would be supervised by the Food and Drug Administration (FDA).

The amendment also extended the requirement for establishing effectiveness to drugs introduced between 1938 and 1962, but it went no further. Drugs marketed and sold, whether prescription drug or patent medicine, *before 1938* were exempted from the new provisions. The buyer must still beware.

Why should the FDA have confidence in research conducted by companies that have a financial interest in seeing their new drugs approved? Although the FDA does not want to undertake the expense of testing a new drug, it is very concerned about the public's safety. The company that develops a drug has similar concerns but for additional or different reasons. Even when a drug has been scrupulously tested, the company is still liable if the drug causes injury. Also, drug companies are extremely competitive. Newly approved drugs get immediate attention from competitors, who test them extensively in order to reduce whatever competitive advantage may exist.

How New Prescription Drugs Are Tested

Before a new prescription drug can be sold, it must undergo from five to ten or more years of development, clinical testing, and investigation, a process that can cost the manufacturer as much as $50 million.

First the physical and chemical properties of the drug are studied in a laboratory. Then the drug is tested on animals to see how it might work against disease and to study other effects: how it is *metabolized* in the body, how it affects the functions of various organs, how *toxic* it is, and what the safe levels of dosage are.

Many factors have to be considered in evaluating these tests. If the drug shows potential for treating or curing a life-threatening disease that has no other treatment, *side effects* may be ignored. For example, streptomycin is effective in treating tuberculosis, but a possible side effect is deafness. If streptomycin is the only available drug that works, the risk of deafness may be worth taking. Brochures provided with many drugs list conditions in which the drug should not be used unless a person's life is in danger. No known drug is free of side effects, so it is often necessary to weigh the risk of undesirable side effects against the benefits of using the drug.

If animal tests indicate that the benefits are worth the risk, tests with human subjects are begun. These tests are usually conducted in three phases.

1. Minimum amounts of the drug are given to healthy subjects who have had thorough physical and labora-

Metabolic pathways
The chemical changes that a substance undergoes in its passage through the body.

Over-the-counter (OTC) drugs
Drugs that can be sold legally without a doctor's prescription; also known as patent medicines.

Interaction
Action on each other; reciprocal action.

Potentiated
A process in which one drug affects another, possibly increasing the risk of harmful side effects.

Negated
A process in which one drug cancels the effect of another.

---

tory examinations for normal functioning of the liver, kidney, and other organs. These examinations are repeated during and after use of the drug to see whether there are side effects and whether the drug itself is causing them. The drug dose is slowly increased until a safe and effective range for dosage can be established. Studies are done to see how humans absorb, distribute, metabolize, and excrete the drug. Once the *metabolic pathway* is established, studies are started in animals that metabolize the drug the same way.

2. The drug is given to hospital patients who have the disease or condition the drug is intended to treat.

3. The drug is given to clinic patients who are not hospitalized. In this way the drug can be evaluated under actual everyday life conditions. Not all eventual users of the drug will be hospital patients.

After all this groundwork, the manufacturer submits a new drug application and the results of the tests to the FDA. If the FDA gives its approval, the manufacturer can sell the drug.

The Marketing of Over-the-Counter Drugs

Manufacturers of patent medicines, more commonly known as *over-the counter (OTC) drugs*, do not usually go through such a slow and costly development process. Their products are made up of certain standard ingredients. The traveling medicine show of the nineteenth century has given way to the TV commercial, but the emphasis in selling OTC drugs is the same—on the selling, not on the drug. According to figures supplied by the Federal Trade Commission, up to 26.3 percent of the gross profits on OTC drugs goes into advertising. And 75 percent of the public receives its education on OTC drugs solely from TV, radio, newspaper, and magazine advertisments. An amazing number of people naïvely believe that claims for drugs could not be printed if they were not true. They *can* be printed because federal action against advertising by drug manufacturers can take as long as 10 to 15 years. By that time, the manufacturer may well have stopped the advertising and may possibly even have quit making the product.

Actual ingredients of drugs do not change very much, although new product names constantly appear. The half million drug products made and sold in the United States use a total of only 216 active ingredients. Most of them contain, as basic ingredients, such substances as gentian (a bitter tonic), gums, resins, roots of one type or another, oils, tars, or other extracts, and, of course, alcohol.

Dangers of Self-Medication

Taking drugs can be dangerous. Most doctors are aware of the hazards and try to reduce them as much as they can. There is only so much doctors can do without the patient's help, however. Doctor and patient must communicate with each other, and the patient must tell the doctor what drugs he or she is taking. The patient may be quite ignorant of the possible effects of medicines or combinations of medicines. Especially if he or she bought the drugs in a supermarket, the patient is likely to think that they are not really drugs. After all, drugs are something one buys in a *drug*store. The fact is, any substance that changes any normal physiological process or function is a drug. Some drugs sold over the counter, whether in drugstores or in supermarkets, can interact with each other or with prescription drugs in dangerous ways. Others are dangerous, to some people, all by themselves.

Drug Interactions   The more drugs a person takes, the greater the risk of a harmful, unpredictable reaction caused by the *interaction* of two, or even all, of the ingredients. If a person is taking more than one prescription drug, or taking prescription drugs together with over-the-counter drugs, a dangerous reaction is not only possible but also probable. The risk is not limited to a few high-powered drugs. It is there with cold remedies (see Table 15–1), kidney pills, laxatives, alkalizers, or any other drug.

Potentiation   If one drug causes a second drug to be metabolized more slowly than normal, the second drug is *potentiated*. This term means that the drug remains in the system longer than it is supposed to, and additional doses taken later can build up the concentra-

Using Over-the-Counter Drugs

Federal law requires that over-the-counter drugs be accompanied by a label giving directions for proper use of the drug. Also, read the circulars that are packaged with the drugs; do not throw them away. They are considered part of the label. OTC drug labels must provide the following information:

1. Name of the product.
2. Name and address of the manufacturer, packager, or distributor.
3. Adequate directions for safe use of the drug for each of the drug's intended purposes, including any necessary cautions.
4. Names of all active ingredients and quantities of the active ingredients.

5. Net contents of the container, usually in grains, milligrams, and/or the number of capsules.

In addition to thoroughly reading the label, take a few other precautions when using OTC drugs:

1. Consult your pharmacist if you have any questions.
2. Never use an OTC drug for an extended period of time unless you are following your doctor's orders.
3. Never take several OTC drugs at the same time without consulting your doctor or pharmacist. Like prescription drugs, these drugs could react negatively in your body and cause unforeseen, harmful effects.

4. Do not combine OTC and prescription drugs.
5. Remember that most OTC drugs do not cure illnesses; generally they only relieve symptoms.
6. Many OTC drugs, including aspirin, can be harmful to pregnant and nursing women and to fetuses. Check with your physician or pharmacist about possible side effects.
7. Never give or take medication from an unlabeled bottle, or in the dark when you can't read what the label says.
8. Never force a child into taking a drug by describing it as candy.

California Department of Consumer Affairs

---

tions to dangerous levels. Also, two drugs can potentiate each other.

Negation If one drug causes a second drug to be metabolized so rapidly that it is excreted before it can do its job, the second drug is *negated*. Two drugs can also negate each other.

Let's take a look at a hypothetical case—a patient with diabetes, a disease in which the blood sugar is often too high for the body to function properly. Suppose he is taking a potent oral antidiabetic drug under close medical supervision. He wakes up one day feeling stiff and sore, decides he must be getting arthritis, and while grocery shopping, buys some pills he saw advertised on TV the night before.

After several days of pill popping (strictly according to label directions), he realizes he is feeling tired, dizzy, and somewhat nauseated. What is more, his self-diagnosed "arthritis" has not improved.

If he is lucky or smart, he calls his doctor, who orders him to her office for immediate blood tests and a checkup. Unless the doctor knows that her patient is taking the home-remedy pills, she will assume that the dosage of the antidiabetic is too high and is causing low blood sugar. This process is indeed what is happening, but not because the dosage is too high by itself. It is happening because large quantities of aspirin in the home remedy are potentiating the antidiabetic—causing it to build up in the patient's system. When blood tests

do show a low blood-sugar level, the doctor cuts down the dosage of the antidiabetic.

If the patient then stops taking the home remedy, the antidiabetic will no longer be potentiated by the aspirin in the patent medicine. His blood-sugar level will skyrocket dangerously, which may lead to diabetic acidosis, a possibly life-threatening condition. Aspirin also potentiates insulin, a drug given by injection for controlling diabetes. The same runaway blood-sugar level can be the result.

In our hypothetical case the doctor had no way of knowing that her patient was dosing himself with a pain-killer, and the patient had no way of knowing that what he was doing was dangerous. The warning on the label said only

Caution: If pain persists for more than 10 days, or redness is present, or in arthritic or rheumatic conditions affecting children under 12 years of age, consult a physician immediately.

If the diabetic patient had taken the remedy for 10 days without seeing his doctor, he could have killed himself.

If the label had warned against use by diabetics, the danger would have been reduced—*if* the patient had read the label. The Food and Drug Administration insists on label warnings, but in our case the label warning would not have been enough. And even if it had been, there is no way that the Food and Drug Administration can force the buyer to *read* the label.

Hallucinations
False perceptions that do not correspond to external reality. A person who hears voices that are not there or sees visions is having hallucinations.

Antihistamines
Drugs used to counteract the effects of histamine, a chemical the body releases in allergic reactions. Some antihistamines also have a sedative action.

Stramonium alkaloids
Atropine-like drugs derived from the jimson weed.

Phenylpropanolamine
A drug marketed for the oral treatment of nasal and sinus congestion.

Salicylamide
A pain-killing drug used to relieve mild pain in rheumatoid conditions or to reduce fever. It works much like aspirin.

Excrete
To separate from the blood or tissue and eliminate from the body.

Anticoagulants
Drugs, including aspirin, that hinder the clotting of blood.

Table 15–1 lists possible interactions for a sampling of drugs. No attempt has been made to list all drugs that might interact dangerously. A drug that is not listed in this table is not necessarily a safe drug. In fact, it is best to assume that *any* drug you can buy can be dangerous, either by itself or in interaction with other drugs.

Hallucinogenic Reactions   Another little-known danger of some over-the-counter drugs is *hallucinations*. There is no way of knowing in advance who is susceptible and to what drugs, but hallucinations are by no means uncommon. A few of the drugs most likely to cause hallucinations are Compoz, Contac, Doze-Off, Nytol, Femicin, Sominex, and Tranquil. There are many others. They contain such ingredients as *antihistamines* (pyrilamine and chlorpheniramine), belladonna or *stramonium alkaloids* (hyoscyamine, scopolamine, homatropine, atropine), *phenylpropanolamine*, and *salicylamide*.

In recent years the Federal Trade Commission has taken the stand that OTC drug manufacturers must back up their advertising claims with clinical testing and proof or change their advertising. A case in point is the so-called extra strength pain reliever. Products labeled "extra strength" are not any stronger than plain aspirin. Aspirin is aspirin, regardless of brand or claims, and is still generally the most effective drug for treating minor pain or fever. Even aspirin has its dangers, however, as noted in our hypothetical case of the diabetic. Harmful reactions to aspirin are rare, but they do occur, the most common being indigestion, nausea, vomiting, and internal bleeding. If you are taking aspirin and you see blood in your fecal matter, you should see a doctor immediately. If the bleeding lasts long enough, it can lead to iron-deficiency anemia, a condition that can be treated successfully and should not be ignored.

Vitamin Overdoses and Imbalances   Vitamins are organic compounds that occur naturally in many foods. They are a kind of nutrient the body needs only in very small amounts. Some people do have specific vitamin deficiencies, but most people should be able to get all the vitamins and minerals they need from four food groups: the milk group, the meat group, vegetables and fruits, and breads and cereals.

Excessive amounts of certain vitamins and minerals cannot be taken without either overburdening the system or creating an imbalance. For example, the body is not able to *excrete* large amounts of vitamins A and D. Because of this inability, an overdose is possible. Some of the B vitamins must be taken in certain proportions. An excess of one B vitamin can create a deficiency of another. Some minerals must also be taken in the right proportion to each other. Most notable of these are calcium and phosphorus. Excess amounts of some vitamins can cause serious problems.

Vitamin A   Overuse of vitamin A for long periods of time may result in fatigue, bone pain, dry skin, loss of body hair, weight loss, enlarged liver or spleen, anemia, and headache, among other conditions. Children of parents who have taken too much vitamin A may show symptoms of overall retarded growth.

Vitamin B Complex   Too much vitamin B complex may cause allergic disorders that, although usually not serious, can be extremely uncomfortable. It also increases the time necessary for the liver to produce prothrombin, a substance required in the clotting of blood. Taking vitamin B with *anticoagulants* may cause hemorrhaging.

Vitamin B_{12}   Great amounts of vitamin B_{12} may cause acnelike pimples. B_{12} accentuates the blood deficiency produced by pyrimethamine, a drug used in the treatment of malaria and certain serious infections.

Vitamin C   People whose systems tend to form kidney stones should avoid large doses of vitamin C, which can make their condition worse. Pregnant women or nursing mothers should take no more than the *recommended daily allowance* (100 milligrams). The metabolism of the fetus or infant will adapt to high levels of vitamin C, and scurvy may be the result when the intake drops to normal.

Vitamin D   Too much vitamin D can make the body calcium too high. It can also cause, among other conditions, mental deficiency, excess urination, abnormal thirst, nausea, vomiting, diarrhea, too much acid in the system, potassium loss, and increased blood pressure.

Table 15-1   Decongestants (Nasal and Liquid), Cough Suppressants with Antihistamines and Sympathomimetics as Main Ingredients

Any of these products

Allerest[a]	Coricidin Demilets[a]	Ornex[a]	Triaminicol
Cheracol D	Coricidin Medilets[a]	Sinutab	Trind
Coldene	Dristan[a]	Super Anahist[a]	Ursinus[a]
Contac[b]	Novahistine	Super Anahist Syrup	Vicks Formula 44
Coricidin[a]	Novahistine-DH	Triaminic	
Coricidin D[a]	Nyquil	Triaminicin[a]	

When taken with	May cause	Comments
Alcoholic beverages	Central nervous system depression; sedation.	Effects add on to those of antihistamines. Large amounts of alcohol combined with sympathomimetics may cause high blood pressure.
Anticoagulants	Decreased effects of anticoagulants.	Antihistamines may reverse anticoagulant effects by stimulating formation of enzymes that destroy the drug.
Anticoholinergics (drugs that inhibit secretions)	Excessive dryness; blurred vision; atropine-like toxicity.	Liquid decongestants and cough suppressants may have additive effects, which are especially hazardous in glaucoma.
Barbiturates	Central nervous system depression; sedation.	Barbiturates have additive effects with antihistamines; continued use may lead to lessening of the effects of either and possible barbiturate tolerance and habituation.
Doxepin	Sedation; atropine-like toxicity.	Doxepin may strengthen the effects of antihistamines because it is additive.
Monoamine oxidase inhibitors (MAOs)	Sedation; atropine-like toxicity.	MAOs may enhance the effect of antihistamines because they inhibit the enzyme that destroys the drug in the body. Severe high blood pressure is a possibility.
Narcotics	Sedation.	Antihistamines and narcotic drugs enhance each other's effects.
Reserpine	Central nervous system depression; sedation.	Antihistamines and sympathomimetics have a synergistic effect with reserpine; sympathomimetics may reverse the effect of reserpine, which is usually given to lower high blood pressure.
Sedatives	Central nervous system depression; enhanced sedation.	One of the side effects of antihistamines is sedation. Combined with a sedative drug, the effect of each is multiplied.
Steroid hormones	Decreased steroid effect.	The steroids are rapidly metabolized because of the enhanced activity and formation of enzymes stimulated by antihistamines.
Tranquilizers	Central nervous system depression; atropine-like toxicity (especially with certain kinds).	There may be additive sedative effects between antihistamines and tranquilizers; anti-high blood pressure effects of phenothiazines may be reversed by phenylephrine and/or phenylpropanolamine.
Tricyclic antidepressants	Enhanced effects of each.	Tricyclic antidepressants and antihistamines/sympathomimetics in combination may potentiate each other.

[a]These products contain salicylates as well.
[b]People who have glaucoma should not take Contac because it contains belladonna, a drug that makes glaucoma worse.

Vitamin K (synthetic) Vitamin K has caused hemolytic anemia, a kind of anemia in which red blood cells are destroyed faster than the bone marrow can replace them. Too much vitamin K can also lead to enlargement of the liver and impairment of its function. It has caused deaths in newborn babies as well as in fetuses.

Vitamins in excessive doses have been known to alter the metabolism of prescribed drugs—some necessary for the maintenance of life—such as anticoagulants, antibiotics, hypnotics, and iron salts.

The recommended daily allowances are, of course, average figures. Individuals vary greatly in their nutritional needs and also in their tolerance for large amounts of vitamins. Tolerance depends on such factors as general diet, amount of exposure to ultraviolet light, how much calcium is in the diet, and which hormones are secreted and in what quantities.

It is dangerous to take vitamin mixtures to treat self-diagnosed disorders. A person who "always feels tired" should go to the doctor. It is always a mistake to take vitamins indiscriminately. Reasons for taking them, either to supplement the diet or to correct a specific deficiency, should be clearly understood and choice of a supplement should be based on a rational approach to a specific problem.

Drugs Can Deplete Vitamins from the Body Some drugs prescribed by doctors for the treatment of various diseases may reduce the effect of certain vitamins. Does this mean that you should not take the drugs? Or does it mean you should not take the vitamins? Most drugs are taken to get well; vitamins are taken to stay well. The answer is to take both. All drugs are not incompatible with vitamins.

Certain drugs can interfere with the body's utilization of both vitamins and other nutrients. These drugs can cause a form of malnutrition by blocking the body's use of vitamins as well as other nutrients. Nutritional vitamin deficiencies are more likely to develop in people who are taking medicines and are poorly nourished, for example, alcoholics or persons who are hospitalized. (Even though hospital food is balanced nutritionally, sick people do not eat well or very much.)

One mechanism by which vitamins may be depleted from the body is the competition of two different chemicals for the same receptor site in the body. Similarly, certain drugs such as aspirin or tetracycline or alcohol may deplete the tissues of vitamin C or vitamin B. A remedy, of course, is to take larger amounts of vitamins C and B to resaturate the receptor sites.

A drug also can interfere with the body's synthesis of various other vitamins, such as vitamin K, which is necessary for proper blood-clotting mechanisms. To be utilized, vitamins must be absorbed into the circulatory system. Mineral oil, for example, can inhibit the solubility and absorption of the fat-soluble vitamins, such as vitamins A, D, E, and K. Another method by which vitamins are prevented from being absorbed is through the use of laxatives, which hasten the departure of the nutrients from the body.

Many drugs and vitamins must be converted into a usable form by a metabolic chemical reaction in the body. Prednisone, phenobarbital, and certain other drugs may hasten or block the metabolism of these drugs or vitamins so that they pass in an inert state from the body, depriving it of their benefits.

Situations that require increased vitamins are growth, fever, high metabolic rate (as caused by *hyperthyroidism,* for example), and some cancer treatments. Ingesting a *variety* of foods and supplements is important because deficiencies occur in multiples, not individually. Table 15–2 lists a number of vitamins and the drugs that can block or deplete them.

How to Self-Medicate Safely

If everyone suddenly stopped using OTC drugs and began making appointments with doctors for every cold or headache or sore throat, doctors could not possibly handle the load. Some OTC drugs *are* useful in relieving some symptoms and in treating some disorders, as we shall see. Doctors themselves may recommend OTC drugs where they can be helpful. *Self-medication,* in other words, does serve a useful purpose. If you self-medicate, you should know what you are taking and why, and you should understand how drugs work and what their dangers are.

Drug Safety Precautions   You will be much more likely to benefit from self-medication with the least possible danger if you keep these rules in mind:

1. If you go to more than one doctor, tell each of them about all the medications you are taking, including without fail those you buy without a prescription. Drugs you buy at a supermarket are "real" drugs. If they are misused, they can kill you just as dead as any other drug. If you are taking drugs, prescription or otherwise, keep a record and carry it with you all the time. Correct the record when you stop taking a drug or start taking a new one.

2. Tell your doctor or dentist about any reaction you have had to any drug.

3. Don't take any drugs at all that your doctor doesn't know you're taking. Drug interactions within your body can be harmful, and even "ordinary" drugs like laxatives and aspirin can cause extreme interactions.

4. Follow your doctor's instructions exactly, especially those regarding when and how often you should take the medicine. If he or she tells you to take a medicine an hour before a meal, do so. The food you eat can alter the effects of a drug, as can the body's chemistry. If the prescription calls for you to take one pill, take only one. Two are not better.

5. After you start taking a new medicine, call your doctor immediately if you have any unusual reactions or symptoms.

6. Don't stop taking a prescription drug unless your doctor tells you to stop. Some drugs are not entirely effective until a complete course of treatment has been followed. Don't continue taking a medicine indefinitely unless your doctor tells you to do so.

7. Don't save old prescriptions "in case you get sick again." All drugs begin to deteriorate when they are exposed to air and moisture. For example, an aspirin bottle that has been opened many times is likely to have a vinegary odor. This indicates that the aspirin is combining with water vapor and releasing acetic acid, which is what causes the stomach upset that sometimes accompanies taking aspirin. If you smell vinegar in an aspirin bottle, throw it away and buy a fresh bottle. If you buy in

bottles of 100 tablets or fewer, deterioration is less likely to occur. Some antibiotics, including tetracycline, become toxic as they deteriorate. It is safest simply to destroy unused medicines as soon as you have stopped taking them and to clean out your medicine chest at regular intervals. Flush drugs down the toilet. Many children and pets have been poisoned by drugs they found in the garbage can or the wastebasket.

8. Never give your medicine to someone else, or take someone else's medicine. When your doctor prescribes a medicine for you, he or she takes into account your age, weight, sex, other medications you are taking, and other factors.

9. When you are traveling, take along written prescriptions for any medicines your doctor has prescribed

Table 15-2   Vitamins and Minerals Blocked or Depleted by Drugs

Viamins, Minerals	Drugs
Folic acid	alcohol, diuretics, antimalarials, anticonvulsants, anticancer drugs, aspirin, oral contraceptives
Vitamin B_6	hydralazine (for hypertension), L-dopa (for Parkinsonism), oral contraceptives, aspirin, anticonvulsants
Vitamin B_{12}	potassium chloride, oral antidiabetic drugs, neomycin
Vitamin A	mineral oil (as laxative, sometimes used in no-calorie salad dressing)
Vitamin D	mineral oil, anticonvulsants
Niacin	alcohol, some antibiotics
Vitamin B_1	alcohol, diuretics
Vitamin K	many antibiotics, mineral oil, warfarin, dicumarol, aspirin
Vitamin C	oral contraceptives
Minerals: magnesium, potassium, sodium, zinc	alcohol, diuretics, oral contraceptives

Drugs and Alcohol

Recent events have highlighted the importance of physicians and health professionals giving greater attention to possible dangers of prescribing certain drugs to individuals who use alcohol. During the past several years there has been a major increase in this country in the medical and nonmedical use of drugs. A parallel increase in the use of alcohol by both men and women increases the probability that alcohol will interact with another drug, causing potentially fatal consequences. Indeed, alcohol use in combination with other drugs accounts for approximately 20 percent of the total number of accidental and suicidal deaths per year which are drug-related.

Concern over these trends prompts me to alert the medical profession to the special problems of prescribing certain drugs for patients who consume alcohol.

I wish to remind all physicians and health professionals that

■ Many commonly prescribed drugs have altered therapeutic and/or adverse medical effects when taken with alcohol. These drugs include not only sedatives, hypnotics, narcotics, antidepressants and tranquilizers, but also certain antihistamines, analgesics, anticoagulants and antiinfective agents.

■ Minor tranquilizers as well as other CNS depressants are frequently used by patients in combination with alcohol despite warnings to the contrary. This combined use may produce adverse medical consequences. Moreover, the resultant potentiation of CNS depression can impair performance of tasks requiring alertness—such as driving—increasing the likelihood of injury and even death. The combination itself can lead to death by accidental overdose or by suicide.

■ The use of marijuana and other illicit psychoactive substances is widespread, and this use often occurs in combination with alcohol, or other licit psychoactive drugs. Therefore, I urge all physicians and health professionals to

1. routinely document the history and scrutinize the pattern of alcohol consumption for individual patients to determine the possible relationship between presenting complaints and mixing drugs with alcohol;

2. be alert to the possible interaction of prescribed, over-the-counter, or illicit drugs—singly or in combination—with alcohol;

3. pay careful attention to the section in the package insert that deals with drug-alcohol interactions and consult the current medical literature and references for specific problems;

4. limit as much as is practical the quantity of drugs dispensed with any one prescription and monitor the patient with regular follow-ups for unexpected reactions to the medication;

5. consider, both in the choice of therapy and in the evaluation of the patient, the likelihood of the patient's adherence to your admonition (and that of the warning label on the prescription) against using alcohol while taking medication.

Julius B. Richmond, M.D.
Surgeon General
U.S. Public Health Service

---

for you. If your luggage is lost, or if you run out, you might be able to get more.

10. Don't drink alcoholic beverages if you are taking drugs. If you drink regularly, make sure your doctor knows about it; he or she may be able to save your life. More than one person has taken a cold capsule, an allergy pill, a sleeping pill, and a couple of drinks, and gone to sleep for good. (See "Drugs and Alcohol," above.)

11. Consider all drugs potentially dangerous. If the drug was not prescribed for you, you take it at your own risk. There is no way you can be sure that all possible dangers are spelled out in the label warning, but read the label warnings anyway. If you are still in doubt, don't take the medicine. If you take an OTC drug and the symptoms you are treating with it don't go away, see a doctor. If you want advice about an OTC drug, ask a doctor or a pharmacist, not the salesperson behind the drugstore cosmetics counter or the stock clerk in the supermarket.

12. Keep all drugs and medicines where children cannot possibly get to them. This isn't easy, but the consequences of not doing so can be tragic. Thousands of children die every year from sampling the pills in the family medicine chest.

Drugs Recommended for Informed Self-Medication

There are a few drugs that work and are safe if they are used intelligently. If you have these drugs in your medicine chest, you should not need any others unless you have a special medical problem.

1. *Aspirin.* Useful for occasional headaches and for the aches and pains caused by colds. (See "Aspirin Use," page 356.)

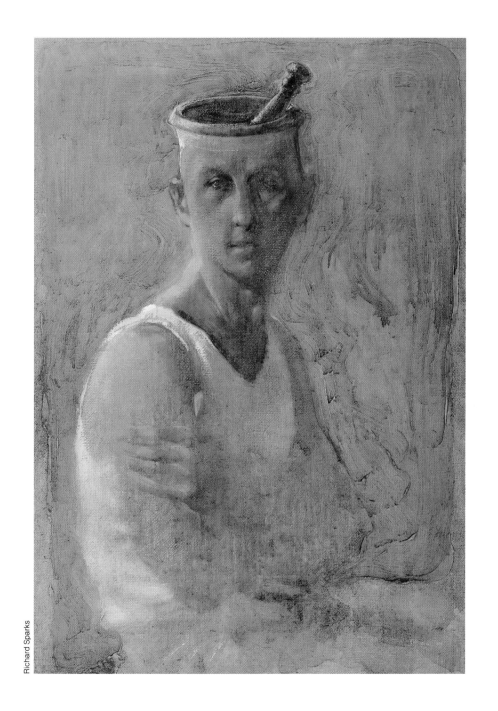

355

Aspirin Use

Aspirin's caveats are important.

- Prolonged use of aspirin for chronic conditions, such as rheumatoid arthritis, should be monitored by a physician. The FDA panel's recommendation for the label warning on aspirin and all analgesic products states: "Do not take this product for more than 10 days. If symptoms persist, or new ones occur, consult your physician."*
- Drink a full glass of water or other liquid with aspirin to minimize possible stomach irritation. If you experience mild stomach distress when you take aspirin, consider acetaminophen or a soluble form of aspirin, which can be dissolved in a glass of water before you take it.
- The FDA advisory panel recommended that the standard dosage for aspirin and acetaminophen be 325 mg or 5 grains per tablet. And if a tablet does not contain the standard dosage, it must be clearly labeled "nonstandard."
- Unless instructed to do so by your physician, do not take more than 10 to 15 grains (two or three tablets) at a time, do not take aspirin more often than every four hours, and do not take more than ten tablets in twenty-four hours. One of the earliest symptoms of chronic aspirin overdosage is ringing in the ears, sometimes accompanied by a decrease in hearing ability. These effects are reversible when the dosage is lowered.
- Some people are sensitive or allergic to aspirin (shortness of breath and wheezing, skin rash, hives). If

*The antirheumatic properties of aspirin have been purposely omitted by the panel in its consideration of safety and efficacy. The diagnoses and treatment of rheumatic diseases should be left to a physician and should not constitute any part of a label claim for aspirin.

you are among them, acetaminophen is a reasonable alternative. Since a wide variety of combination OTC products contain aspirin, be sure to read labels. The panel's recommended label warning states: "This product contains aspirin. Do not take this product if you are allergic to aspirin or if you have asthma except under the advice and supervision of a physician."

- Patients with a history of stomach ulcers or gout as well as those on oral antidiabetic medications should consult a physician before taking aspirin. The panel's recommended label warning for such patients is: "Caution: Do not take this product if you have stomach distress, ulcers, or bleeding problems except under the advice and supervision of a physician."
- Aspirin retards blood clotting in several ways. Hence patients with bleeding disorders and patients using anticoagulants such as warfarin (Athrombin-K, Coumadin, Panwarfin) should take aspirin sparingly, if at all.

There is also some evidence that pregnant women should not take aspirin during the last three months of pregnancy because of possibly affecting the blood-clotting mechanism of the newborn. Among pregnant women taking high dosages of aspirin there is some evidence of added risk of prolonged labor and an increase in the average duration of pregnancy.

- Patients due to undergo elective surgery should not take aspirin one to two weeks before they are scheduled for hospitalization because of aspirin's effect on blood clotting.
- Keep in mind that aspirin and alcohol are not a safe combination. Since each of these drugs is an irritant to the stomach lining, CU's

medical consultants warn that combining the two (e.g., treating a hangover with aspirin) may increase the risk of gastrointestinal bleeding from either drug. As for acetaminophen, it may have its potential for liver toxicity enhanced when taken by chronic alcoholics who have liver disease.

- For children's doses, consult the label. . . . Children can be given the recommended dose crushed in a little applesauce or honey if they dislike taking it straight. If children prefer to take their aspirin adult-style, be sure they drink a full glass of liquid along with it. CU's medical consultants warn against keeping flavored aspirin in the home because a child could mistake it for candy.
- Keep aspirin and other drugs out of reach of children. In 1976, the latest year for which statistics are available, twenty-five children under five years of age died after ingesting overdoses of aspirin or other salicylates. This total accounted for about 21 percent of all accidental deaths from poisoning among children in that age group. However, the number of children under the age of five years who were hospitalized for longer than one day as the result of aspirin or salicylate ingestion has decreased from 373 in 1973 to 168 in 1976 mainly as a result of the 1972 law on poison prevention packaging.
- The use of so-called timed-release aspirin preparations is not advised. As with so many of these products, absorption may be irregular and adverse reactions prolonged.

Consumers Union
The Medicine Show

Acid
Any compound that reacts with an alkali to form a salt. Acids turn blue litmus paper red.

Alkali
Any compound that reacts with an acid to form a salt. Alkalis turn red litmus paper blue.

Solvent
A substance, usually a liquid, that can dissolve other substances.

Strychnine
A poison that stimulates the central nervous system and can be lethal.

2. *Calcium carbonate.* Excellent for occasional heartburn or simple acidity or indigestion.
3. *Calamine lotion.* Useful for treating mild skin itches, poison ivy or poison oak, skin inflammations, insect bites, and the like.
4. *Milk of magnesia liquid or tablets.* Useful as a laxative, and, in smaller doses, for acid stomach.
5. *Alcohol.* To be used as an antiseptic and for rubbing. Mixed half-and-half with a cup of warm water and used as a sponge bath, alcohol works quite well to reduce high fevers.

You should also have some medical supplies on hand: both oral and rectal thermometers, adhesive bandages, adhesive tape, scissors, tweezers and a cake of soap. Note that we have not included in the list antiseptics such as iodine, merthiolate, and methaphen. Soap and water is the best antiseptic first aid. Burn ointments and cough medicines are not included, either. Ointments can do more harm than good; it is often better not to take cough medicines. Any cough that cannot be relieved by lozenges, hot drinks, or inhalating steam (carefully) should be checked by a doctor.

In some cases there are effective methods of self-diagnosis, and Table 15–3 (see page 358) provides examples of informed self-medication. It is imperative to realize, however, that these cases are limited to *simple* conditions that are readily treatable. If you have any doubt whatsoever, if all symptoms do not fit the suspected condition, do *not* attempt treatment but seek competent medical advice. Above all do not allow yourself to be influenced by media adverstising.

Emergency Treatment for Poisoning or Drug Overdose

In case of poisoning or drug overdose, the most immediate first-aid measure is to have the victim—if he or she is conscious—drink several glasses of water. The purpose is to dilute the toxic substance. Dilution slows down absorption of the toxic substance into the bloodstream, which gives time for other emergency measures. Do not try to force water down an unconscious patient. It is likely to go into the lungs.

Call a poison control center. Every city, large or small, has at least one listed in the phone directory. Write down this number now and put it near the phone. Be prepared to identify the substance, if possible, and state the amount taken. You will be given instructions for immediate first aid, and the call will also alert the hospital or medical center that the victim is on the way. When you take the victim to the hospital or medical center, take along the container from which the substance was taken.

In poisonings the two primary emergency measures to be taken are

1. Dilute the poison (with water).
2. Remove the poison. Cause vomiting with warm salt water, or mustard powder in water, *except* when the poison is caustic—as in *acids* or *alkalis*—or a *solvent,* or contains *strychnine.* Vomiting may cause solvents, acids, or alkalis to be inhaled into the lungs; in strychnine poisoning, vomiting can lead to convulsions.

The American Red Cross gives excellent information on emergency treatment of poisonings. Another source of information is the American Druggist Counterdose Chart, which is continually updated by experts. You might be able to get one from a pharmacist, or if the pharmacist does not have it, he or she can probably tell you who does. The chart can be pasted on the inside of a medicine-cabinet door.

Possible Future Safeguards

The dangers of drugs are compounded by general ignorance about their effects and by poor communication between doctor and patient. Widespread use of the personal medication record will go a long way toward reducing the dangers, especially if the doctor keeps the record updated for prescription drugs, and the patient keeps it updated for over-the-counter drugs. Further safeguards may eventually be fed into computers in such a way as to signal immediately when a drug or a combination of drugs will be dangerous to a particular patient.

Table 15-3 Examples of Informed Self-Medication

Condition	Acne	Cold Sores	Poison Oak, Poison Ivy	Hyperventilation
Symptoms:	pimples and/or blackheads; confined to face, chest, and back	ulceration or blisters confined to lips or gums; pain	redness; itching; minor swelling; blisters; oozing	feeling of inability to get enough air into the lungs; sensation of being out of breath; feeling of numbness and tingling of the hands (may extend to the feet and be noted around the mouth)
Treatment:	practice cleanliness and hygiene; reduce oiliness of skin; remove keratin plugs	relieve pain; help heal sores; prevent further or new infection	remove plant oil from skin as soon as possible, preferably within 4 to 6 hours after exposure; relieve symptoms	get carbon dioxide back into the lungs
Products Available:	Neutrogena Acne Soap (hypoallergenic) (1); Fostex Soap (2); Fostex (3); Pernox (4); Oxy-5 or Oxy-10 (benzoyl peroxide lotions) (5); Brasivol, Acnaveen Bar; Buf-Kit (6); sun lamp (7)	Orabase; Campho-Phenique; Blistex; Neosporin ointment; Bacitracin ointment; Anbesol	rubbing alcohol (ordinary); strong bar soap (Fels Naphtha, Lava, or other cake); Domeboro Powder packets or tablets; Aveeno Bath (special oatmeal); hydrocortisone cream	small paper bag
Actions:	wash at least twice daily with a good hypoallergenic soap (1) or (2) and with an abrasive soap at least once daily (6); apply a drying agent in the morning and at bedtime (3), (4), or (5)	apply Orabase as protective coating to help relieve pain inside mouth; apply Blistex or Campho-Phenique to provide relief for cold sores on the outside of the lips; apply Neosporin or Bacitracin ointment to external sores to guard against infection and give protection	apply alcohol to chemically neutralize phenolic acid base of oils; apply alkali in soap to remove and neutralize oils; apply Domeboro solution as cool compresses to soothe inflammation; apply Aveeno Bath in bath for soothing and healing; apply hydrocortisone cream to reduce inflammation	because anxiety usually causes hyperventilation, the sensation of being out of breath causes overbreathing and thus a loss of normal carbon dioxide present in the blood; breathing into and out of a paper bag restores the carbon dioxide level in the blood to normal
Dosage:	one to three times daily, according to severity	apply Anbesol for mouth pain; treat 3 to 4 times daily	thorough cleansing with strong soap and water, repeat at least once; cool Domeboro compresses 3 to 4 times a day; Aveeno Bath in cool tub water	5 to 15 minutes of rebreathing exhaled air
Note:	a sun lamp may be used to advantage following a physician's recommendation (*wear eye shields or ultraviolet goggles*); should these measures fail to control the problem, consult your physician or dermatologist	Orabase may be applied over Anbesol; Orabase may *not* be applied over Campho-Phenique or Blistex; if the external sores crust over, apply cool water to remove crust	if symptoms are present and there has definitely been no exposure to poison oak, ivy, or sumac, consult your physician immediately	
Contra-indications:	if itching, rash, or other signs of sensitivity occur, discontinue treatment immediately and consult your physician	if any of these preparations seems to cause further irritation, discontinue use immediately and see your physician	calamine lotion may help if used early, but it may spread plant oil on skin; if lesions are extensive or if home treatment is ineffective, see your physician	
Warnings:	see Contraindications	do not scratch or pick off crusts as this may lead to infection and/or bleeding; if infection develops, see your physician; any sores that persist beyond 2 to 3 weeks should be seen by a physician	if a violent, eruptive rash occurs, see your physician immediately; hypersensitivity may occur with repeated exposures; see your physician immediately	if the victim is under 15 or over 40 years of age, if there is abdominal pain, or if the victim is not normally a tense or anxious person, consult a physician immediately

Condition	Cough, Congestion	Piles (Hemorrhoids)	Impetigo	Mumps
Symptoms:	exhausting cough, spasms; dry, nonproductive cough (no mucus coughed up)	rectal pain; itching; bleeding	sores covered with soft, thick yellowish crusts (dried pus) on arms and legs	one or two days of low fever (may rise to 104°); pain behind the ear when chewing or swallowing; malaise (tiredness, fatigue); the pain worsens when sour substances are taken
Treatment:	control coughing; convert dry, nonproductive cough to a productive cough	soften stool; keep area clean; protect against further irritation	removal of crusts; healing of sores	relief of fever and/or pain, disappearance of parotid gland swelling
Products Available:	Novahistine Cough Formula; Robitussin-DM; Cheracol-D	Metamucil; milk of magnesia; Tucks (medicated moist pads); benzocaine; zinc oxide	Domeboro powder packets or tablets (to make Burow's solution); Bacitracin ointment; Neosporin ointment	aspirin tablets (325 mg); aspirin suppositories; acetaminophen tablets (325 mg) or liquid
Actions:	take cough formula to suppress cough reflex and liquefy mucus secretions to permit expectoration	take Metamucil for a more slippery bowel movement, or milk of magnesia for a more fluid, softer movement; use Tucks pads or a shower instead of toilet paper to prevent irritation; use benzocaine or zinc oxide to protect against irritation and to promote healing	use Burow's solution to soak off crusts and scabs; use Bacitracin or Neosporin ointment as antibiotic treatment; observe cleanliness	take aspirin or acetaminophen to reduce pain and fever
Dosage:	adults and children over 12: 2 teaspoons every 4 hours; children 6 to 12: 1 teaspoon every 4 hours; children 2 to 6: ½ teaspoon every 4 hours	Metamucil or milk of magnesia daily, according to directions on package until condition is healed; protective agents after bathing when area is clean and dry until no longer needed	soak crusts 2 or 3 times daily, using Burow's solution as a compress until scabs and crusts are loosened	adults or children over 12: 2 tablets every 4 hours; children 9 to 12: 1½ tablets every 4 hours; children 6 to 9: 1 tablet every 4 hours; children 4 to 6: ¾ tablet every 4 hours; children 2 to 4: ½ tablet every 4 hours
Note:	take no more than four doses in a 24-hour period; for children under 2, consult a physician	it is not recommended that preparations containing benzocaine or other ''-caine'' medications be used for more than one or two days as these compounds may sensitize, irritate, and prolong healing	if lesions do not show prompt improvement or if they seem to be spreading, see your physician without delay	take no more than five doses in a 24-hour period; with pain or difficulty in swallowing, switch to a liquid diet; for children under 2, consult a physician
Contra-indications:	for persistent or chronic cough or for cough accompanied by excessive secretions, do not take cough formula except on the advice of a physician	if hemorrhoids and bleeding persist, see your physician; if itching or pain persists, even if no hemorrhoids are present, see your physician	none known	hypersensitivity to aspirin or acetaminophen; use aspirin with caution in presence of peptic ulcer, asthma, or with anticoagulant (blood thinner) therapy
Warnings:	if cough persists for more than a week, tends to recur, or is accompanied by high fever, rash, or persistent headache, consult your physician	if relief from above treatment is not complete within one week, see your physician	do not scratch or pick off crusts as this may lead to infection and/or bleeding; if there seems to be sensitivity to the treatment, discontinue it immediately and consult your physician; do not use any preparations containing hydrocortisone to relieve itching as this may aggravate the infection	if there is pain in the testicles or abdomen or difficulty in hearing, consult a physician immediately

Prescription and OTC Drug Behavior Scale

Read the following statements carefully. Choose the one in each section that best describes you at this moment and record its score at the right. (For example, "throws out old medicines once a month" has a score of 5.) When you have identified five statements, total your score and find your position on the scale.

5   is well educated about drugs
4   is informed about drugs
3   relies on friends for drug information
2   knows little about drugs
1   is totally ignorant about drugs

Score _____

5   avoids taking medicines unless necessary
4   considers other alternatives before taking medicines
3   takes aspirin and cold medicines regularly
2   sees a doctor only to get drug prescriptions
1   buys OTC drugs almost daily

Score _____

5   takes drugs exactly as prescribed by the doctor
4   reports symptoms or side effects to doctor
3   is relaxed about complying with an exact medical regimen
2   complies with medical regimen only when convenient
1   frequently fails to comply with doctor's orders

Score _____

5   is knowledgeable about drug interactions
4   seeks expert advice when taking new medicine
3   knows that one drug may affect another
2   is unaware that one drug may affect another
1   takes several OTC drugs at the same time

Score _____

5   throws out old medicines once a month
4   occasionally throws out old medicines
3   keeps some medicines after expiration date
2   rarely throws out any old medicines
1   hoards all medicines

Score _____

Total score _____

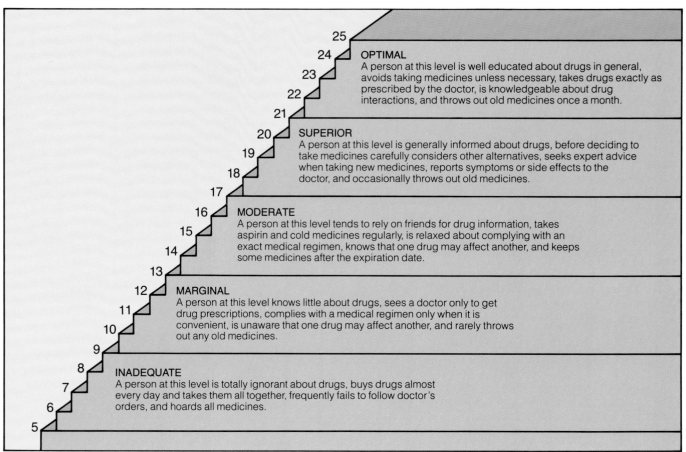

Take Action

Your answers to Probing Your Emotions at the beginning of this chapter and your placement level on the Prescription and OTC Drug Behavior Scale will, we hope, encourage you to begin a process of self-exploration and self-discovery that you will continue. Reflect on the entire chapter's content and ask yourself how each point relates to your own life. Then take action:

1. Go to your medicine cabinet. Make a list of everything in it. Divide the medicines on your list into the following three categories: unexpired prescription medicines, unexpired OTC medicines, and all expired medicines. Now throw out the expired medicines.

2. Turn to page 351. Note the products listed in Table 15–1. Do you have any of these products in your medicine cabinet? If so, make a list of the ones you may have taken together with another medicine. Note the ones that may have caused a side effect or harmful drug interaction effect.

3. Have you ever noticed the warning on aspirin containers telling you to stop taking aspirin if you experience a ringing in your ears? Have you ever noticed that some medications indicate that a particular drug has a ''half life'' of so much time? Begin today to read the labels on all medications before taking any of them. Ask your pharmacist what ''half life'' means.

4. Read the following Behavior Change Strategy, and take the appropriate action.

Behavior Change Strategy

Monitoring and Managing Medication

Medicine plays an important role in almost everyone's life—drugs sometimes alleviate symptoms of distress almost as if they were magic. The apparent potency of drugs and the relative ease with which they can be obtained over the counter or via prescription encourages the collection of large personal caches of medications.

There are at least three problems with setting up your own personal pharmacy in your medicine cabinet: (1) drugs often lose potency with the passage of time, (2) it is easy to look for one medication in the medicine cabinet only to end up taking another one that is not intended for the condition or problem you seek to relieve, and (3) it is all too convenient to use medications for the quick and easy ''magic bullet'' cure when in fact your personal distress is signaling the need for changes in your routine habits.

Action Plan   A list of steps has been developed to increase your personal awareness of and control over your use of medications. Follow the steps and ask yourself the questions.

Step 1:   Place all medications on a table for review; be sure to include pills from your purse, car, medicine cabinet, closet shelves, nightstand drawers, etc.

Step 2:   Make a detailed list of all of the prescription medications that you find, noting the name of the prescribing physician, the date, and the type of medication.

Step 3:   Throw away all of the medications that were obtained via prescription for medical problems or physical conditions that no longer exist. Remember these have been noted in your overall listing from Step 2.

Step 4:   If you discover that some prescription medications need to be renewed or refilled, promptly visit your pharmacy to obtain a new supply.

Step 5:   Answer these questions.

Q.   What do you do when you are tense?

Q.   What do you do when you can't fall asleep?

Q.   What do you do to lose weight?

Q.   What do you do when you have an upset stomach?

Q.   What do you do when you try to stay awake?

Q.   What do you do when you have a headache?

The questions listed in Step 5 of the Action Plan are often answered with references to taking medication. Yet there are alternative approaches— behavioral self-management approaches—that you can use to reduce the frequency and the severity of problems like tension or stress and insomnia or to accomplish personal goals like losing weight. Some specific nondrug plans are outlined in Chapter 1 and elsewhere in this book. The general problem-solving steps that help you identify patterns associated with problems and desired goals provide the clues to tackling behavioral tasks by using behavioral methods—not chemical solutions.

It is interesting to consider that the

body is an amazingly complicated biocomputer that sends us messages (biofeedback) in the form of physical symptoms. We can try to ignore or gloss over these messages or even seek temporary "band-aid" solutions through medicine, but we often miss "hearing" the content of the body's messages, and thus we only forestall the more important adjustments in our behaviors that will be necessary later—when damage and ill health have become continuing problems.

For example, repeated episodes of stress and sleep disturbance probably signal the need for significant life-style adjustments that if not made will result in more serious medical problems.

Sensible and Careful Medication Management

Medicine is a helpful tool that improves our ability to function and enjoy life. At the same time, this tool can be overused and abused so that it directly subtracts from function and enjoyment. Be mindful of how you use drugs to solve behavioral problems—consider using behavioral means to achieve behavioral goals.

Chapter Sixteen

Medical Diagnosis

Probing Your Emotions

1. Your appointment is for 3:00 P.M. At 4:00 P.M. you are still waiting for the doctor. You have read all the magazines within reach. A nurse calls you. You are ushered into a white examining room and told to strip. For eight minutes you shiver and read the diplomas lining the wall. The doctor finally arrives and begins the physical. He taps and listens and feels your body. Occasionally he fires a question at you. Occasionally he grunts. With the examination over, you and the doctor have a brief conversation. There is a buzz from an intercom and the doctor leaves. You have just your annual contact with the health care delivery system. Consider the details of your own last visit to your physician; concentrate on how you *felt* regarding the process. Try to focus on blocks that may have existed in your personal interaction and communication with your physician.

2. A friend tells you she has noticed a lump in her breast but is afraid to see a physician and would rather risk cancer than face its possible confirmation. How do you counsel her? Remember that a friend swayed by such powerful and apparently illogical rationalization is not going to respond to your saying, "See a doctor!"

3. You are a parent and your child is in a traffic accident and needs an emergency operation. Minutes before surgery you are asked to sign a consent form, but no one has advised you of the risks and benefits of the operation. What should you do?

4. Who is really responsible for your health?

Chapter Contents

WHEN TO GO TO THE DOCTOR
METHODS OF DIAGNOSIS
Medical history
Physical examination
Laboratory examinations
PRINCIPLES OF DIAGNOSIS
POPULATION SCREENING
SABOTAGING THE DIAGNOSTIC PROCESS
TRENDS IN MEDICAL DIAGNOSIS
PATIENT RESPONSIBILITIES AND RIGHTS

Boxes

How to choose a doctor
Guidelines for the wise use of medical X rays
Getting a second opinion
Patient's bill of rights

Symptom
A subjective change in bodily function that
indicates disease.

Checkup
A routine medical examination.

16 When a patient arrives at a doctor's office with a new complaint, neither the patient nor the doctor knows, usually, what ailment the patient needs to be treated for. The patient knows how he or she feels, but not what particular sensations or other symptoms mean. The doctor must rely on the patient for the extremely important subjective information that no tests or instruments can reveal.

Ordinarily, doctors have the task of trying to overcome communication barriers by their selection of questions and evaluation of patients' replies. Once a clear picture of a patient's complaint emerges, the doctor can use various techniques to narrow the list of possible causes.

Barriers to communication can be attacked from another direction. Most patients feel more secure and are more cooperative when doctors take the trouble to explain in some detail what they are looking for and what their conclusions are. Some explanation of the processes of the patient's disease and the treatment is also reassuring. If the patient knows something about diagnostic procedures, he or she may be able to supply the kinds of information needed at the outset. Knowing the reason for an uncomfortable, embarrassing, or painful medical procedure makes it more bearable, and a realistic idea about how the diagnostic process works helps relieve some of the anxiety patients feel when faced with the prospect of a number of tests.

When to Go to the Doctor

Apparently, the only time it is easy to decide whether to go to the doctor is when the *symptoms* are extreme. A study of students' use of a college health clinic showed, for example, that students almost always reported promptly to the clinic when they had severe disabling symptoms. When symptoms were minor, however, a student's willingness to go to the clinic depended more on his or her cultural background and level of anxiety about school performance.

People make two kinds of mistakes in deciding when to go to the doctor: (1) They either go too often because they imagine they have physical ailments; or (2) they ignore symptoms of diseases that should be treated at

once. Sometimes the only way to make a decision is subjectively. The individual's knowledge about what symptoms mean is usually severely limited. Various confusing feelings may also be involved: "Am I foolishly making a mountain out of a molehill if I go?" "Am I taking chances with my health if I don't?" Objective guidelines would be helpful.

Setting up guidelines is difficult because the severity or type of the symptom does not necessarily bear any relationship to the seriousness of the ailment. We can, however, definitely establish two guidelines.

1. Everyone should have a *checkup* or screening examination at regular intervals, whether or not any distress or symptoms are present.
2. The following symptoms indicate an immediate visit to the doctor.

Fever. One symptom that should not be ignored is fever. Fever is an objective sign of disease process, and, unless it is obviously associated with a cold and stuffy nose, it should be diagnosed and treated.

Internal bleeding. Any signs of internal bleeding, such as blood in the sputum, in vomit, or in a bowel movement, are extremely important. Bear in mind that the digestive juices of the stomach and intestine turn blood to a black color, so that blood in the stool may appear as a black tarry substance as well as in red streaks.

Abdominal pain. Persistent pain in the abdomen, especially when it is consistently in one spot and is associated with nausea and vomiting, should be reported.

Stiff neck. A stiff neck, if not associated with any physical strains or injuries, is also reason for a quick trip to the doctor.

Many diseases are without symptoms at certain points in the course of the illness. For example, the initial symptoms of syphilis disappear entirely, yet the disease continues in a potentially dangerous form if it is not treated. Hypertension, cancer, diabetes, tuberculosis, heart disease, and anemia, among other diseases, present no symptoms initially. This is why checkups at regular intervals are important.

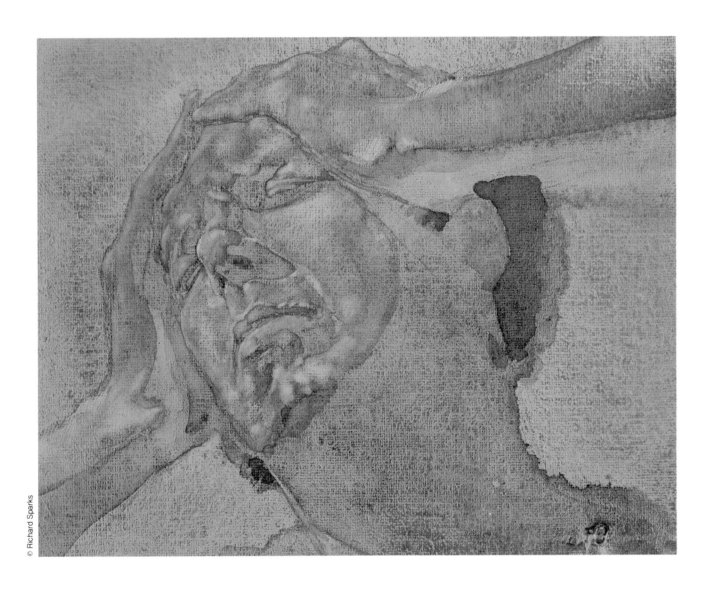

Pap smear
A preparation of cells from the cervix that are examined under the microscope to detect cancer.

Medical history
Historical account of a patient's past medical problems.

Cancer is a prime example of a serious disease that presents only minor symptoms in the beginning. The American Cancer Society lists the following danger signals of cancer:

1. Change in bowel or bladder habits
2. A sore that does not heal
3. Unusual bleeding or discharge
4. Thickening or lump in breast or elsewhere
5. Indigestion or difficulty in swallowing
6. Obvious change in wart or mole
7. Nagging cough or hoarseness

Often a cancer is felt as a lump or thickening, but since these lumps are not painful, they are often disregarded. In fact, even when people are aware that they may have cancer symptoms, they may hesitate to see a doctor in the self-defeating fear of getting bad news.

Doctors do not agree on how frequent or how complete checkups should be, but usually both men and women should have a general examination every two or three years until they are 50 and every year thereafter. Women 20 years of age and over should have pelvic and breast examinations once a year. Generally, a Pap smear should be included. A *Pap smear* is a test that detects early forms of cancer of the cervix, a kind of cancer that attacks women. Recently the American Cancer Society has said that a Pap smear can be skipped for two years if previous smears were negative two years in a row.

What is involved in a checkup varies from doctor to doctor, but certain tests, known to provide reliable information on certain conditions, are commonly part of all checkups.

Although this chapter emphasizes examinations performed by medical doctors, self-examination of the breasts or testicles at regular intervals is important too. These procedures are described on pages 419 and 421.

Methods of Diagnosis

Medical doctors have three main sources of information on which to base their diagnoses. The first is the patient's description of his or her experience. The second is the doctor's examination of the patient. The third is the results of various laboratory tests that are available to the doctor. Doctors do not usually run laboratory tests themselves. They only interpret the findings.

Medical History   The most important part of all medical diagnosis is the patient's *medical history,* including a history of symptoms and a description of his or her way of life. The amount of detail that will be included in the history depends greatly on the medical problem the patient presents, and the history may or may not be complete. A complete medical history is usually taken in a standard manner.

The first step is to record the patient's chief complaint, preferably in his or her own words. Other information about the chief complaint should include how long the patient has had it, whether it comes and goes or seems more evident at some times than others, factors that tend to make it worse or better, and a description of related complaints.

Then follows the patient's past medical history. What major illnesses has the patient had? When? Does the patient always have the same kind of problem? Answers to these questions may reveal specific vulnerabilities. For example, if the patient has had a large number of colds or has had pneumonia a number of times, the respiratory system should be given special attention. Past history may also indicate immunities to disease. A person who has had measles, for example, is not likely to get it again. Past history can also have a significant bearing on how the rest of the checkup is directed. A medical history of diabetes, rheumatic fever, tuberculosis, or abdominal operations, for example, can be important in suggesting additional questions that should be asked, in interpreting certain test findings, and in directing the course of the general evaluation (often called a workup). The patient may not be able to supply all the information needed for a complete medical history, in which case the doctor may ask for permission to request past medical records from other doctors.

The next portion of the history is the review of systems. The questioner (who may be a doctor, a nurse, a questionnaire, or even a computer terminal) asks if the patient has experienced specific symptoms associated with each of the body's physiological systems. This procedure gets at symptoms the patient forgot to mention or discarded as unimportant. The musculoskeletal, cardiovascular, respiratory, neurological, and geni-

How to Choose a Doctor

Here are some practical suggestions on finding a physician if you're new in town or you're searching for a specialist.

Don't overlook the obvious. Ask for recommendations from friends and neighbors, business associates, and anyone you know who is part of the medical community—nurses or hospital technicians, for example. They're often willing to help. The nurse who frequently recommends certain doctors to friends—based on her first-hand knowledge of their work—is not unusual.

Your family physician can help if you need a specialist or are moving to a new community. Your company doctor may have some leads, too.

Another approach is to call the secretary to the department chairman at a reputable hospital and ask for the names of staff members. "One of the best ways to choose doctors is first to choose a good hospital and then choose the appropriate doctor in its staff," writes Dr. G. Timothy Johnson in his book, *Doctor! What You Should Know About Health Care Before You Call a Physician.*

If you live in an urban area with several hospitals to choose from, be sure the one you select is accredited by the Joint Commission on Accreditation of Hospitals. This indicates that at least minimal standards of care are being met. Check with the hospital's administrative office or write to JCAH (837 North Michigan Ave., Chicago, Ill. 60611).

Ask whether the hospital is affiliated with a medical school or at least has a training program for interns and residents. So-called "teaching hospitals" usually have up-to-date physicians and the best equipment and facilities. Howard J. Robbins, vice-president of international marketing at Rohr Industries, has moved 10 times in the last eight years to job locations as diverse as France, Washington, D.C., and California. He says he always looks for a doctor associated with a major teaching institution in a new locale.

Failing that, look to nonprofit community hospitals, which are generally preferable to privately owned, proprietary hospitals or government-operated institutions.

Regardless of his or her affiliation, check the doctor's credentials. To a great extent, of course, your final choice will be based on how you mesh with the physician. But don't let compatibility outweigh qualifications. "Most people are impressed by a doctor's personality rather than his skills," says Dr. Johnson. "I'm concerned with what's between his ears."

If you are looking for a specialist, you can be reasonably sure he has had adequate training if he has been "board-certified" in his particular field. Each medical specialty has its own regulatory staff or board that supervises training and administers exams. If the doctor is "board-eligible," he or she has completed a formal training program but has not taken the exam—which is not necessarily critical.

Membership in an honorary "college" of a given specialty is another indication of advanced achievement. The initials after a doctor's name are your clue: FACS, for example, means "Fellow in the American College of Surgeons."

A doctor who teaches at a university is also usually a good bet, according to Dr. Sidney M. Wolfe, director of the Ralph Nader–sponsored Health Research Group in Washington. And the number of years he or she spent in residency is often more important than the school attended.

If you don't want to question the doctor directly, you can probably learn all you need to know by calling his or her staff. Your county or state medical society can provide some of the information as well.

Business Week

tourinary systems are the systems considered. Typically a review of the cardiovascular system would include questions about such symptoms as chest pains, shortness of breath, difficulty in breathing while lying down, and swelling in the feet. Each of these symptoms relates to disturbances in blood circulation and may be significant.

Finally, the examiner may ask about family history and social history. Some diseases are inherited or tendencies to them are inherited. Diabetes is one such disease. Others, such as viral or bacterial pneumonias, are contagious and spread within a family. Social history is information about the patient's occupation, travel experience, and living conditions. A history of travel in Africa might give a decisive hint in diagnosing a mysterious periodic fever as malaria. Exposure to asbestos in certain occupations might help in diagnosing a respiratory disease.

Why all these detailed questions? The answer is that people often are unable to supply the necessary information no matter how much they want to. Some people are alarmed by the slightest change in sensation, while others do not even notice severe pain unless they are specifically asked about it. People also tend to make their

Inspection
Detecting physical abnormalities by using the sense of sight. It includes both careful observation with the naked eye and observation using special instruments such as an ophthalmoscope (for looking into the back of the eye) or an otoscope (for looking into the ear).

Palpation
Detecting physical abnormalities by using the sense of touch. For example, systematic palpation of the breast can reveal tumorous masses.

Auscultation
Detecting physical abnormalities by using the sense of hearing, most often aided by use of a stethoscope.

Systolic blood pressure
The pressure when the heart is pumping blood and the ventricles are contracting; the higher of the two blood pressure numbers.

Diastolic blood pressure
The pressure when the heart and ventricles are relaxed; the lower of the two blood pressure numbers.

---

own guesses about what is causing their symptoms, guesses that are as often wrong as right. Questions help to establish accurate connections between symptoms. Even though the examiner may ask the questions in rapid succession, it is important for patients to listen to each one and to try to answer it accurately according to their own experience. Technology has not yet brought medical diagnosis to the point where a patient's subjective experience can be by-passed. Only the patient knows how a symptom feels.

Physical Examination　Traditionally, physical examination consists of inspection (looking), palpation (feeling), and auscultation (listening). Inspection and auscultation usually involve special tools.

Inspection　Inspection of the body begins with the unaided eye. Many diseases besides skin diseases produce changes in the skin. When the unaided eye is not sufficient to make a determination, the examiner uses special "scopes." A device called an otoscope is used to look inside the ear and see the tympanic membrane. The ophthalmoscope is a similar device for looking through the pupil into the back of the eye. Using an ophthalmoscope, the examiner can see small arteries and veins directly and study them for signs of atherosclerosis and other vascular diseases. The examiner can also assess the condition of the optic nerve. The laryngoscope and the bronchoscope can be used to look into the larynx and the bronchial tubes. The proctoscope and the sigmoidoscope permit inspection of the rectum and the sigmoid colon, the part of the colon immediately above the rectum. Many cancers that occur in middle and later life start in the sigmoid colon, and examination of this part of the body is an important part of diagnosing intestinal complaints. The cystoscope is used to look into the bladder.

Palpation　Examination by touch, or *palpation*, is done in a number of ways. The most familiar of these is counting the pulse by feeling the pulsations of the radial artery at the wrist. Arterial pulsations can be felt at many places on the surface of the body, and it is possible to tell by palpation if an artery is functioning the way it should or if it is affected by a vascular disease such as atherosclerosis. Palpation of the chest can reveal that the

heart valves are not working efficiently; it can also indicate the presence of mucus in the passages of the lungs. Tumors can often be felt beneath the skin before they can be seen. Many internal organs, including the thyroid gland and the liver, can be examined through the skin by touch. The prostate gland, a gland that contributes to the formation of ejaculatory fluid, can also be palpated. In older men, the prostate gland has a tendency to enlarge and may become a site for cancer. The examiner can detect abnormalities by a finger inserted in the rectum. Cancers of the rectum can be detected in the same way. The uterus and the Fallopian tubes can often be palpated through the wall of the vagina.

Auscultation　Auscultation is listening to the sounds of body processes, usually with the aid of a stethoscope. The standard stethoscope is constructed of a small metal cup and two ear pieces connected to the cup by hollow rubber tubing. For hearing sounds of high frequency, a thin metal disk is used instead of the cup.

One of the most important measures made by auscultation is of blood pressure. Blood pressure is checked by means of a stethoscope and an instrument called a sphygmomanometer, or more commonly, a blood pressure cuff. A sphygmomanometer consists of an air bag, or cuff, and a column of mercury marked off in millimeters. The cuff is wrapped around the upper arm and pumped full of air. The air supports the column of mercury; as air is let out of the cuff, the column of mercury falls. When the cuff is no longer tight enough to prevent the passage of blood through the artery, the examiner will hear a pulse. The height of the column of mercury when the pulse is heard is a reading of the pressure at which the heart can pump blood through the squeezed place. This pressure is called the *systolic blood pressure*. After noting the systolic blood pressure, the examiner continues to let air out of the cuff until the pulse can no longer be heard. The pressure at this point is the *diastolic blood pressure*, the pressure when the heart is in a state of relaxation. Blood pressure is given as two numbers, for example, 120/80. The first and larger number is the systolic blood pressure, and the second number is the diastolic blood pressure.

Auscultation at certain places on the chest can be used to check the functioning of each of the four heart valves.

Radiopacity
Not permitting the passage of X rays.

X rays
Slang for the films produced when X
radiation is used to make a picture.

Radioactive isotopes
Chemical elements that give off radiation.

It is possible to hear a heart murmur, establish what part of the cardiac cycle it belongs to and diagnose a corresponding valvular defect. Abnormalities in blood vessels can be established by listening to the sounds heard through a stethoscope that is placed where those vessels pass close to the surface—for example, on the head, eyelid, or abdomen.

Sounds produced by air passing in and out of the lungs can be important diagnostic clues. In illnesses such as bronchial asthma, the bronchial tubes become partly closed, so that when a patient breathes out, wheezing sounds can be heard. People who have infections such as bronchitis produce sounds somewhat like snoring. Faint crackling sounds at the bases of the lungs indicate an abnormally large amount of liquid moistening the inner surfaces of the lungs. Rubbing sounds indicate that the inner surfaces of the sac that encloses the lungs are inflamed. When normal breath sounds cannot be heard over a part of the lungs, it is a sign either that the airways to this part are blocked or that this part is filled with something that does not allow air to enter. To determine which, the examiner uses a technique called percussion. He or she presses a finger of one hand against the chest and strikes the finger sharply with a finger of the other hand. If the resultant sound is low-pitched and resonant, the underlying lung tissue is filled with air. If the sound is high-pitched and dull, the tissue is filled with a liquid or solid.

Gurgling sounds from the intestines can often be heard without a stethoscope. These sounds are normal. If there are no sounds even when a stethoscope is used, the patient may have an emergency condition such as an infection in the sac that surrounds the intestines.

Additional Tests   Inspection, palpation, and auscultation are used in various combinations to examine reflexes, to give pelvic examinations, and to test for hernias. The knee-jerk reflex is the reflex most commonly tested. It is a normal involuntary response to a blow to the tendon just below the kneecap. The blow (usually with a rubber hammer) causes nerve impulses to be sent to the spinal cord. The nerve impulses are relayed back a fraction of a second later to the quadriceps muscle, causing it to contract and the dangling leg to kick forward. The knee-jerk reflex action brings many parts of the nervous system into play, and a malfunction can indicate problems in the nervous system or in the quadriceps muscle. Stroking other tendons or muscles can elicit other reflexes.

In women the pelvic examination includes inspection and palpation. A device called a vaginal speculum is inserted in the vagina, and its two spoonlike blades are spread apart to separate the vaginal walls so that the cervix and the walls can be visually inspected. Palpation is used to examine the uterus and Fallopian tubes (oviducts). As part of the examination, loose cells for the Pap smear are collected with a cotton swab.

Male patients are tested for hernia by pressing a finger at the small opening between the scrotal sac and the abdominal sac and asking the patient to cough. Coughing increases the pressure on the abdomen, and any tendency for the contents of the abdomen to push through the opening is felt as pressure on the fingertip. The examination is conducted on both the left and right sides of the scrotum.

Laboratory Examinations   The diagnostician can take advantage of a number of testing procedures. Not all are equally useful, and they vary in cost and in the amount of discomfort or risk they involve for the patient. The general categories of tests are radiological, electrophysical, bacteriological, immunological, chemical, and microscopic. We shall describe a few of the tests in each category.

Radiological Tests   X-ray photographs are shadow pictures made when X rays are directed at the body. X rays pass through some substances more readily than others and through dense, heavy substances such as bone least readily of all. Substances that obstruct the passage of X rays in varying degrees (called the *radiopacity* of the substance) show up on the photograph as shadows of varying clarity. Parts of the body that cannot usually be seen except during surgery can be examined by means of X-ray photographs (also called simply *X rays*) and *radioactive isotopes*. The chest X ray is the most common kind of X ray (see Figure 16–1). X rays can also be taken of any other part of the body in which disease of the joints or bones is suspected.

Bones show up clearly on X rays in contrast to softer tissues. It is more difficult to discriminate among softer

Arteriogram
An X-ray picture of a vein or artery obtained by injecting a radiopaque material into the vein or artery.

CT scan
A computer-generated cross-sectional image of any part of the body produced by a specialized X-ray instrument.

Electrocardiogram (EKG or ECG)
A record of the electrical activity of the heart.

Electroencephalogram (EEG)
A record of the electrical activity of the brain.

Electromyogram (EMG)
A record of the electrical properties of skeletal muscles.

tissues such as the stomach, intestines, kidneys, and blood vessels. To highlight organs or other soft tissues, the patient swallows (or is injected with) a radiopaque material. Barium sulfate, for example, which casts a heavy shadow, is used to produce clear photographs of the walls of the gastrointestinal tract. The patient swallows the barium sulfate in a solution, and its progress through the digestive system can then be tracked by X rays. Radiopaque materials can also be injected into a vein or artery, producing an X-ray picture called an *arteriogram*. A relatively new method of making X-ray pictures called *CT scans* (from *Computerized Tomography*) is revolutionizing X-ray diagnosis. This method has two advantages over conventional techniques. It can make an image of a cross section of any part of the body, and it can visualize soft tissue without radiopaque substances or isotopes. CT scans are especially good for looking for abnormalities in the brain.

Isotopes are forms of chemical elements that give off radiation. This property makes it possible to use certain isotopes in diagnostic testing. For example, an isotope

of iodine can be used to assess the functioning of the thyroid gland. The isotope is injected intravenously, and the rate at which it appears and the places where it appears in the gland are measured by a radiation counter. The radiation counter is systematically moved over the gland, providing a picture of its "hot" and "cold" areas, hence, its functioning. Isotopes can also be used to assess the functioning of other parts of the body, including the brain, lungs, kidney, and liver. See "Guidelines for the Wise Use of Medical X Rays," page 372.

Electrophysiological Tests Electrical activity in the body occurs mainly in the heart, the nervous system, and the muscles. A graph of electrical activity in the heart is called an *electrocardiogram (EKG or ECG)*. A graph of electrical activity in the brain is called an *electroencephalogram (EEG)*. A graph of electrical activity in a skeletal muscle is called an *electromyogram (EMG)*.

For an electrocardiogram, the patient lies on his or her back, and one electrode (electrical conductor) is attached to each of the limbs. The examiner moves a fifth electrode from place to place on the chest. The result is a millisecond-by-millisecond record of electrical impulses through the heart. See Figure 16-2 (*a*). Many heart diseases produce characteristic patterns on the EKG.

For an electroencephalogram, a dozen or more electrodes are pasted at certain locations on the scalp. Recordings are made from various combinations of these electrodes. The EEG can be used to diagnose epilepsy, which shows up as a storm of spike-shaped brain waves. Brain tumors can also be detected, but they show up as a difference between brain waves on the left side and on the right side of the head. The EEG is not as easy to interpret as the EKG. Not all epileptics show an abnormal EEG, for example, and many people with abnormal EEGs are physically and mentally healthy. The EEG is not used nearly as often as the EKG, not only because it is difficult to interpret but also because heart disease is more common than diseases detectable by the EEG. See Figure 16–2 (*b*).

Electromyograms are used even less often, although they are invaluable for detecting certain types of nerve and muscle disease. For an electromyogram, pin electrodes are inserted in the muscle in such a way as to make it possible to observe the electrical discharge of individual muscle fibers. Nerve conduction studies are

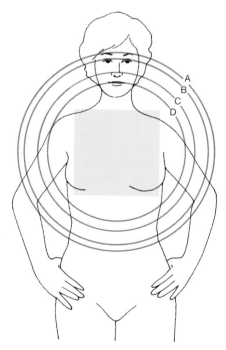

Figure 16-1   The square indicates the correct beam size for a chest X ray. Circles show excessive beam size caused by incorrect coning.

Antibiotic
An antibacterial drug that is based on substances originally produced by living organisms.

often done in conjunction with EMGs. A nerve is stimulated by a brief electrical shock, and the speed of electrical transmission up and down the nerve is measured from strategically placed electrodes.

Bacteriological Tests   Antibiotics have been used so successfully to treat bacterial infections that identification of the infecting organism might seem unnecessary. Some doctors simply prescribe an antibiotic when symptoms of an infection are present, and sometimes

this procedure is justified. Many other times, however, a specific diagnosis is necessary. Symptoms such as fever or sore throat may indicate either a bacterial or a viral infection, and antibiotics have no effect on viruses. Vaginal discharge can be caused by a fungus infection, which is aggravated rather than helped by antibiotics. (Antibiotics destroy the bacteria that normally control the spread of fungus.) Even when the infection *is* caused by bacteria, it may respond to some antibiotics but not to others, or the bacteria may be a drug-resistant strain.

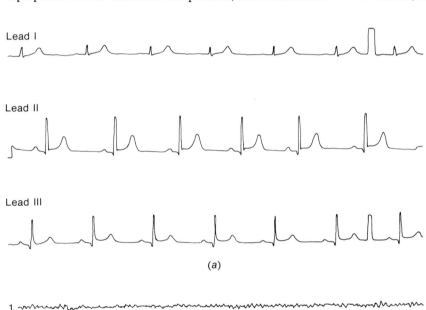

Lead I

Lead II

Lead III

(a)

1

2

3

4

5

6

|___1___|
second

(b)

Figure 16-2   An EKG tracing from a healthy young man is shown in (*a*). The electrical discharge and recharging of the cells of the heart muscle is the basis for the EKG. Each of the repetitive patterns corresponds to a single heartbeat. Different leads "look at" the electrical field of the heart from different directions and provide added information. A modern EEG tracing (*b*) includes simultaneous records from different scalp locations. Each of the lines comes from a different pair of electrodes. Alpha rhythms are especially prominent in the three lower channels.

Sample
An example or representative of something.

Specimen
A sample; in a medical context, often a urine or stool sample.

Growth medium (media, plural form)
A substance used for growing bacteria. It contains nutrients and other essential chemicals.

Culture (bacterial)
Bacteria grown artificially in a growth medium.

Antigenic substance
A chemical to which the body is sensitive.

Antibodies
Proteins in the blood that are generated in reaction to foreign proteins. Antibodies neutralize the foreign proteins, producing immunity from them.

Guidelines for the Wise Use of Medical X Rays

1. If you do not understand why X rays are being ordered, do not hesitate to ask your physician.

2. If you are concerned about the radiation you may receive from any X-ray study, your radiologist or technician ought to be able to provide you with information. They may compare the dose to that received from a chest X ray, for instance.

3. Elective (not urgent) abdominal examinations in females of childbearing age should be restricted to the first 14 days of the menstrual cycle to avoid the possibility of an early pregnancy.

4. Pregnant females should avoid all nonessential medical radiation, especially of the abdomen.

5. Young adults should avoid repetitive X-ray exposures of the gonads unless medical indications are clear.

6. Keep track of the dates and locations of previous X rays. They may be useful to you in the future and reduce the need for additional X rays.

7. No diagnostic X-ray study gives "too much" radiation *when* there are important medical reasons for it.

Harvard Medical School Health Letter

The basic method of bacteriological diagnosis is to obtain a *sample* of the bacteria from the patient and grow them under controlled conditions in a laboratory. Sterile containers are used for collecting the samples to avoid mistaking a random contaminant for one that came from the patient. If the patient has a lung infection, he or she is asked to cough up some sputum into the container. For urinary tract infections, urine is collected in as sterile a manner as possible. The area around the urethral opening is washed, and then the stream of urine is directed into a bottle, which is immediately closed. Blood samples obtained under sterile conditions are required in testing for infections that result from bacteria in the blood. Fecal matter is used to establish the cause of gastrointestinal infections.

Samples of the *specimen* to be tested are diluted and spread thinly over various *growth media* that have been prepared with a substance called agar. The media are then incubated in a warm environment. After one or two days, visible colonies of bacteria, called a *bacterial culture*, begin to appear. They show up as round spots on the agar. The color and texture of the spots indicate the species of bacteria, and their number is related to the concentration of bacteria in the original specimen. Different growth media promote the growth of different species of bacteria, so growth of an organism in one medium but not in another helps identify it. Once the species has been identified, its sensitivity to various antibiotics can be tested. One method is to spread a thin film of bacteria over the surface of a medium and then cover it with small disks containing various antibiotics. Bacteria will not grow around the disks containing effective antibiotics.

Immunological Tests   Many diagnostic tests are based on the immunity the body develops to certain foreign substances it has been exposed to. Immunological testing usually consists of skin tests and blood tests. Skin tests depend on the allergic reaction of the skin to *antigenic substances* (substances that stimulate the immune mechanism), while blood tests depend on *antibodies* (proteins formed in reaction to an antigen) that circulate in the blood.

In the skin test for tuberculosis (the most common skin test), a small amount of material derived from killed tuberculosis bacteria is injected under the surface of the skin. If the site of injection becomes swollen and hard within 48 hours, the patient is having a "positive" reaction and is allergic to the material. A person who has a positive reaction may or may not have an active tuberculosis infection, and an interview is needed before a firm diagnosis can be reached. Skin tests are also used to determine whether an adult has ever had mumps and to identify substances that make bronchial asthma worse.

The most common form of immunological blood test is the typing of blood for transfusions. Tests for blood type classify red blood cells as type A, type B, type AB, or type O and as Rh positive or negative. Blood types must match for transfusions to work. If they do not, the

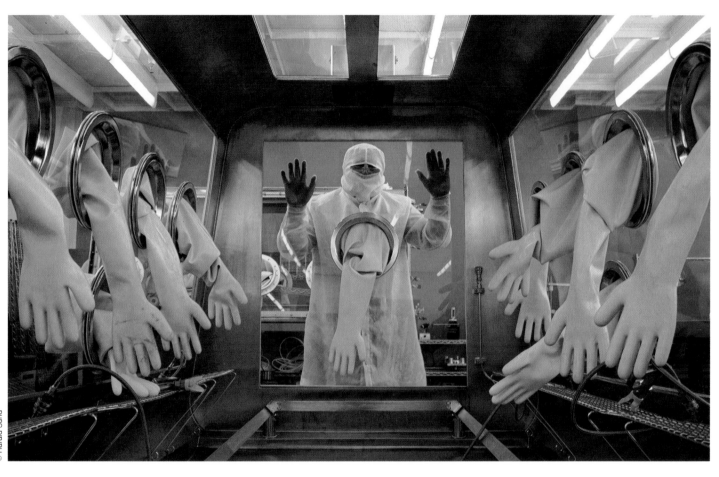

Plasma
The fluid portion of the blood.

Serum
The clear portion of a liquid separated from its solid part.

Enzymes
Chemicals that speed up the body's reactions.

immune system of the person who is receiving the blood will form antibodies against it. Blood also contains antibodies to bacteria and viruses that have infected the body in the past or are infecting it at present. Rising amounts of antibody in tests taken a few days apart are strong evidence of an active infection. Typhoid fever is one of several diseases that can be diagnosed from blood antibodies.

The various blood tests for syphilis depend on antibodies. The most specific is the TPI. TPI stands for *Treponema pallidum* immobilization; *Treponema pallidum* is the name of the bacterium that causes syphilis. Less specific blood tests are the Wassermann, the STS (serological test for syphilis), and the VDRL (Venereal Disease Research Laboratory) tests. A test is specific if it identifies antibodies found only in one disease. For example, an increased concentration of antibodies to the typhoid fever bacterium can result only from typhoid fever. Other antibody tests can give positive reactions for several diseases in addition to the one being tested for. These positive reactions are called false positives.

Chemical Tests   Analysis of the kinds and quantities of various elements and compounds in body fluids gives important diagnostic information. For example, tests for four simple ions—sodium, potassium, chloride, and carbon dioxide—are important in managing any disease that affects the amount of water in a person's body, the acid-alkali balance of the blood and tissue fluid, or the functioning of the kidneys. (Almost any serious disease affects one or more of these.) Blood is tested chemically to determine the concentrations of certain compounds in the *plasma* or a part of the plasma called *serum*. Urine is tested for glucose (a simple sugar) or protein. Normally there is no protein in the urine, and its presence there calls for further investigation. Glucose in the urine may indicate diabetes.

Some chemical tests measure processes influenced by many organs. Others are quite specific, reflecting the functioning of a single organ. An increased BUN (blood urea nitrogen) usually indicates poor kidney function. An increase in the amount of ammonia in the blood is a sign of liver failure. An increased level of serum cholesterol can indicate liver or gall bladder abnormalities as well as susceptibility to atherosclerosis. A higher

than normal concentration of uric acid in the body fluids can be indicative of gout. Calcium and phosphorus concentrations are related to the metabolic activity of the bones. Imbalances of these elements suggest possible malfunctioning of the parathyroid glands, the kidneys, and the pancreas, as well as bone disease.

Levels of hormones in the blood or urine can be important in diagnosis. The presence of abnormally large or small amounts of a hormone usually indicates a malfunction of the gland that secretes it. The test for protein-bound iodine (PBI) is one of the most common hormone tests. This test measures the amount of a thyroid hormone in the blood. Both thyroid deficiency and overactivity of the thyroid gland can cause serious problems. Pregnancy tests are based on the presence in the blood or urine of a special hormone manufactured by the placenta. The functioning of the adrenal glands can also be assessed by chemical means.

Tests for *enzymes* may also be part of the diagnostic process. Enzymes are protein molecules that act as catalysts in certain biochemical reactions. Their concentration is highest in the organ at which a particular reaction is occurring, but they may appear in the blood or urine as well. For example, amylase and lipase are ordinarily released into the small intestine, but they appear in the blood if the pancreas is diseased.

Levels of many chemicals in the body vary widely from time to time. For an accurate reading, it may be necessary to take several samples over a 24-hour period. Levels of glucose in the blood vary as much as 100 percent, depending on food intake, so the glucose tolerance test, a test used mainly for diagnosing diabetes, is done under precisely defined conditions. A patient does not eat or drink anything for a certain period of time and then is given a measured amount of glucose in a drink. A series of blood and urine samples is taken over the next few hours to measure the body's use of sugar. In other tests, special substances are given intravenously and the rate at which they are excreted is measured.

Microscopic Tests   Examination of body tissue under a microscope is a powerful method of diagnosis. Some disease processes, of which cancer is one, change tissues in specific and recognizable ways.

Cytology
The study of cells.

Biopsy
A procedure for taking a sample of tissue from a living organism.

Tonometry
The measurement of tension or pressure.

Gastric aspiration
A technique used to determine the contents of the stomach.

Lumbar puncture
A procedure for getting a sample of cerebrospinal fluid by inserting a hollow needle in the back between the vertebrae; also called a spinal tap.

Blood cells are frequently analyzed microscopically. Blood samples, taken either from a prick in the finger or from a vein, are a rich source of diagnostic information. For example, blood cells and plasma can be separated in an instrument called a centrifuge to determine the percentage of blood by volume that is made up of cells. Should anemia be indicated by a low percentage of red cells, the red cells are studied under a microscope for abnormalities of size or shape. Such abnormalities may point to the cause of the anemia. Microscopic examination is also used to determine the white count (the concentration of white blood cells), the differential (the percentage of different types of white cells), and the platelet count (microscopic blood elements necessary to prevent or stop bleeding).

Microscopic examination of the sediment from a urine specimen is a common diagnostic procedure. White cells in the sediment indicate an infection in the urinary tract. Red cells point to the possibility of kidney stones. Other microscopic elements such as bacteria and crystals provide additional information.

Lung cancer can sometimes be detected by microscopic examination of loose cells from the respiratory tract. Cells from the female reproductive tract are collected on a cotton swab and analyzed under a microscope for cancerous change, a technique called a Pap smear. The study of individual cells is called *cytology*. Techniques such as the Pap smear that depend on the recognition of aberrant cell types are known as cytological methods.

Sometimes it is necessary to do a *biopsy* to obtain a sample of cells. A biopsy is removal of a bit of tissue from the living body. Several types of biopsies involve extracting tissue with a needle. In a bone marrow biopsy, the patient is given a local anesthetic, and a needle is inserted into the marrow of one of the bones. A bit of the content of the marrow is sucked into a syringe and prepared for microscopic examination. Needle biopsies can also be done on the kidney and the liver.

Many types of biopsies require surgery. Skin lesions are biopsied easily with the patient under local anesthesia. Biopsies of suspicious lumps in the breast are usually done in an operating room with the patient under general anesthesia. The tissue is immediately examined under a microscope, and surgery may proceed, depending on the findings.

Other Tests   Some diagnostic techniques do not fall in any of the general categories we have discussed. *Tonometry* is the measurement of pressure within the eyeball. Higher than normal pressure may indicate glaucoma, a disease that can cause blindness. Visual acuity is tested by asking the person to read letters on a chart from a specified distance. Audiometric testing determines a person's ability to hear sounds at different frequencies.

Tests of the pulmonary function measure the movement of air in and out of the lungs and the exchange of oxygen and carbon dioxide across the lung membranes. In such a test, the patient wears an airtight mask or breathes through his or her mouth into a tube. A special apparatus measures the rate and depth of respiration and the concentration of gases in the expelled air and the arterial blood. A lung disease like emphysema can affect all the factors measured in a test of pulmonary function.

The contents of the stomach can be sampled by a technique called *gastric aspiration*. A flexible plastic tube about the diameter of a pencil is passed through a nostril and down the back of the throat into the esophagus and stomach. Gastric juices are extracted through the tube and checked chemically for the presence of certain substances. Hydrochloric acid, for example, which is a normal stomach secretion, is secreted at a high rate in patients who have ulcers. A low rate is associated with other diseases.

The *lumbar puncture*, or spinal tap, is a procedure in which a sample of cerebrospinal fluid is withdrawn from the spinal canal through a hollow needle. Cerebrospinal fluid bathes the surface of the brain and spinal cord; meningitis and many other diseases that affect the central nervous system can be diagnosed by examining it.

Principles of Diagnosis

Two basic principles govern the diagnostic process. The first principle of diagnosis concerns increasing and decreasing probabilities. Each symptom, physical examination finding, and laboratory test finding increases the probability that some diseases are present and decreases

Screening examination
A medical examination designed to detect
diseases before they show symptoms.

the probability that others are present. Each additional diagnostic fact should move these probabilities closer to certainty. Tests should be chosen on the basis of which ones are most likely to increase the probability of the most probable disease and decrease the probability of the second most probable disease.

The second principle is that the risk of any diagnostic procedure must be weighed against the value of the information it gives and the possibility of treating a disease, should a correct diagnosis be reached. For example, a biopsy of the brain might shed light on a neurological disease, but the procedure itself might cause brain hemorrhage, infection of the biopsy site, or other serious complications. If it is impossible to treat any of the diseases that a biopsy would reveal, biopsy is not justified. Not all diagnostic procedures are risky, but some are extremely so.

The diagnosis of treatable diseases has the highest priority. Certain symptoms of multiple sclerosis, for example, mimic those of disorders of the nervous system, such as infections. Multiple sclerosis is largely untreatable, but an infection can quite possibly be cured with the appropriate antibiotics. Clearly, more effort should be spent in making sure the infection is not present than in probing for the presence of multiple sclerosis.

These two basic principles used with specific information about a multitude of diseases guide the diagnostician in choosing the diagnostic procedures at each stage of the diagnostic process. Doctors do not carry formal tables of probabilities in their heads; rather, their experience and training give them a sense of the odds and their consequences. This sense they use mainly in an intuitive way. The diagnostic process is partly art and partly science.

Population Screening

Entire groups, or populations, are sometimes screened, or tested, for the presence of disease. Tests to be used in *screening examinations* are selected according to the principles that apply to individual diagnosis. Other criteria are used as well. The person planning a program of screening examinations must decide who in the

population to screen, what diseases to look for, and how much the program is going to cost.

Some segments of the population have a higher risk than others for certain types of disease. In general, the incidence of disease increases with age, but some diseases, such as sexually transmitted diseases (see Chapter 20), are more common in young adults. Geographic factors and socioeconomic class influence the prevalence of disease. Smokers are more susceptible to lung and heart diseases than are nonsmokers. Public health campaigns supported by the government or promoted by private organizations are usually aimed at one of the high-risk groups.

Which tests are to be used in a screening examination depends on the diseases that are to be uncovered, and these are usually the diseases most likely to occur in the group being screened. Examination of stool specimens, for example, is a highly effective method of diagnosing the kinds of diseases that occur in the underdeveloped countries. In most of the United States, use of the same method would be wasteful. Diseases likely to spread to other people, such as sexually transmitted diseases and tuberculosis, should have a high priority because treating one case can prevent others. Whether or not diseases can be treated, and when, are other important considerations in planning a screening program. It would be pointless to test a population for asymptomatic rheumatoid arthritis because that disease cannot be treated until it causes symptoms. Screening for asymptomatic hypertension, on the other hand, is important because it can be treated effectively and should be treated as early as possible.

The costs of screening examinations in time and money may determine what is practical. Individual medical procedures vary greatly in cost. The argument that one's health is one's most precious possession and that one ought to be willing to spend any amount of money to maintain it is not acceptable to most of the American public. Unfortunately, the patients who have the least money to pay for screening examinations are often those in a high-risk group.

An example of a screening program in operation is the one Kaiser-Permanente medical centers make available to members of their health plan. Technicians can administer all the tests, and doctors are needed only to interpret the results, which saves a substantial amount

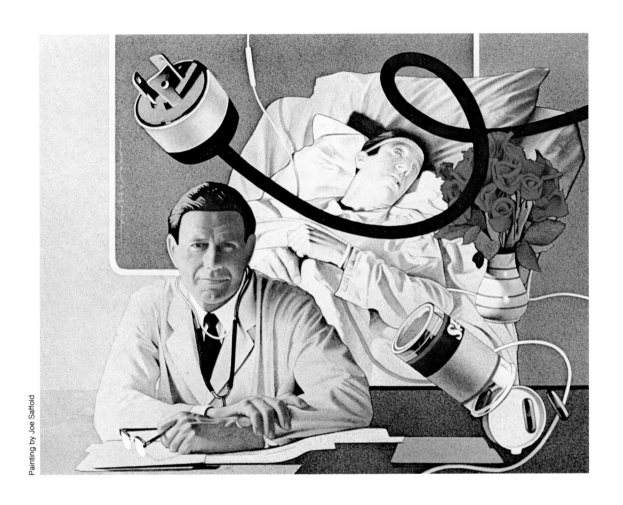

377

Hypochondriac
A person who is convinced he or she has
diseases of which there is little likelihood
or who worries about his or her body
and tends to overreport symptoms.

of money. For example, instead of listening to the heart directly, the doctor examines a phonocardiogram, an electronically produced graph of the sounds of the heart. Although a phonocardiogram provides less information than direct auscultation, it can be interpreted more quickly and conveniently. A screening battery is not a complete substitute for a physical examination. Certain important tests may be omitted, such as, in the Kaiser-Permanente battery, pelvic and rectal examinations and a Pap smear.

Some tests are ordered by physicians more than they should be for routine screening. EKGs need not be part of routine physical examinations. After one EKG has been taken as a baseline at about age 35, another should not be necessary for five or ten years if the earlier one was normal and no cardiac symptoms appear. A stress or exercise EKG is an EKG taken when a person is walking on a treadmill or pedaling a stationary bicycle. This test is expensive, and its results often ambiguous. Though it can be useful in special circumstances, it should not be given routinely. Chest X rays need be taken no more often than EKGs. Even smokers rarely benefit from frequent chest X rays because lung cancer detected first on a chest X ray is usually too widespread to cure.

Sabotaging the Diagnostic Process

People can sabotage the diagnostic process. They can do so generally in two ways. The first is illustrated by the person who is oblivious to his or her symptoms. Such people resist any suggestion that they might be vulnerable to disease. Some of them may actually have an unusually high threshold of pain; others, however, may be masking a fear that some fatal disease will be discovered. Their assumption is that, at least in health matters, ignorance is bliss.

The second kind of saboteur is the person who cannot be convinced he or she is well. Such people arrive at the doctor's office prepared to recite a long list of symptoms, and in many cases to deliver their own diagnosis. They watch their bodies closely and see the slightest deviation from previous patterns of body functioning as evidence of disease. As far as *hypochondriacs*

are concerned, the only good doctor is the doctor who finally confirms their worst fears, and many hypochondriacs spend their lives searching for just such a doctor. Hypochondriacs are not immune to sickness, however, and doctors must constantly remind themselves that one among the multitude of symptoms may be significant.

Extreme worry over physical symptoms can come from various causes. It may be a plea for attention; it may be a disguise for another worry; it may be a refusal to accept responsibility for one's own life; or it may be a way to manipulate others.

Not all worried or doubting patients are hypochondriacs. Doctors who are unsympathetic or who do not take the time to explain things to patients can cause patients to distrust them. With increased specialization and mechanization of the diagnostic process, patients may think, quite accurately, that their feelings are being disregarded. Unfortunately, the "personal touch" will probably become an increasingly distant memory as new and more complicated diagnostic procedures are introduced and as mass screening becomes widespread.

Trends in Medical Diagnosis

Diagnostic procedures are constantly being improved and revised. Chemical tests that once required transferring solutions from test tube to test tube by hand have been totally automated. Samples from many patients are given a series of analyses on an assembly line under the control of a small computer. It is now possible to run tests on smaller samples of blood or urine and to detect minute concentrations of compounds. Enzymes that formerly could only be measured together can now be separated.

Some electrocardiogram procedures are being developed to record heart activity while people are engaged in their daily routine or in standardized physical activity. The EKG can be broadcast from a tiny transmitter taped to the patient's chest or recorded on a miniature tape recorder worn on the patient's belt. These methods provide information that often does not show up when the patient is monitored for only a short time while connected by wires to a heavy machine.

Informed consent
Agreement based on full knowledge.

Computers will become increasingly important. Computers can rapidly scan physiological data in quantities that defy human analysis. Scanning of microscopic specimens and X rays for abnormal features will also be possible. Computer technology will be extremely useful in transmitting, storing, and retrieving data in the patient's permanent medical record. Even the final process, the weighing of test results and deciding on the probable diagnosis and the course of action, may eventually be done by a computer.

Rapid advances in making cross-sectional pictures of the body with CT scans also depend on computers. New methods of making CT scans with radioisotopes permit visualization of on-going chemical reactions in organs such as the brain and heart. Beams of ultrasonic sound waves are also being used to make images of organs in the body.

Patient Responsibilities and Rights

The complexity of modern medical diagnosis and health care can be bewildering to consumers. In their bewilderment they may let representatives of the medical establishment—physicians, hospital administrators, and insurance companies—make crucial decisions. In fact, some people do not like to be involved in deciding about their care or even in knowing what is wrong with them. Anxiety about sickness can result in a childlike, unquestioning faith in a doctor who is imagined to be omniscient, or all-knowing. Although this defense against anxiety is understandable, many of us are able to play an active role in the decision and treatment process.

We participate in our treatment in a responsible and critical way when we choose our doctor, make an appointment for a physical examination, examine our breasts or testicles for cancer (see pages 419 and 421), follow or disregard medical advice, or when we ask for a second opinion (see "Getting a Second Opinion," page 380).

One point at which we as patients must participate in our own treatment is when we are asked to sign permission statements for operations or other medical procedures with significant risks. In legal terms *informed*

consent is required. For informed consent to be legally valid, we must understand what we are signing. We must be informed of both the benefits and risks of procedures. For example, if a woman is to have her uterus removed (a hysterectomy), she must understand that this means she will not be able to have children and that such an operation can entail infection, inadvertent blood loss, complications from the general anesthesia such as sudden drops in blood pressure, and so forth. Informed consent cannot be given by children or senile elderly who are unable to understand. Although the right of patients to give informed consent is important for their protection, it is illusory to believe that patients can make completely independent decisions about whether to have dangerous procedures. A doctor, by virtue of his or her training and experience, is likely to have a better understanding than the patient of the relative risks and drawbacks of an operation for that patient at that time; and the patient may simply have to trust the doctor's judgment. Furthermore, a long and detailed description of all the highly unlikely but remotely possible ways the treatment could go wrong may frighten a patient unnecessarily.

The right to consent implies that we as patients also have a right to refuse. Jehovah's Witnesses or Christian Scientists may refuse certain medical procedures on religious grounds. Some people may refuse treatment because they do not trust a doctor or hospital, some out of rational or irrational fears about the treatment, and some because they are depressed and see all help as futile or even want to die. Complicated legal, moral, and ethical issues surround the concept of "dying with dignity." Many people feel that heroic attempts to prolong the life of the terminally ill are misplaced and that a person should be allowed to die at home with his or her loved ones instead of in the sterile and socially isolated environment of an intensive care unit. The difficulty of making such decisions is in being certain that a person really is near death and that no treatment will result in another period of enjoyable life. Even when a person has lost intellectual function, it is possible that he or she enjoys life in a primitive way. Often the decision to terminate life-support systems cannot be made by patients themselves because of their diminished understanding.

Getting a Second Opinion

Because the number of cases of surgery in a given geographical area increases with the number of surgeons in that area, some people have concluded that unnecessary "elective" surgery is performed more often where surgeons are plentiful. In 1977 Massachusetts passed a law requiring Medicaid recipients to get a second opinion before elective surgery. Such laws are motivated by a desire to cut down on the costs of medical care and to improve its quality. The health care consumer should consider three questions:

1. *When should I get a second opinion?* If you do not have confidence in your doctor's judgment or ability to perform the procedures he or she recommends, you should seek a second opinion. Although it is often difficult to judge a doctor's abilities, some guidelines are given on page 367. He or she should have had a good deal of experience with your health problem. Doctors who are certified as specialists and who have appointments at

teaching hospitals are the best bet if your problem is serious.

The indications for certain surgical procedures are controversial. If these procedures are recommended, a second opinion may be in order. In cases that do not involve cancer, the following operations may be unnecessary: tonsillectomy and adenoidectomy (removal of the tonsils and adenoids), hysterectomy (removal of the uterus), and cholecystectomy (removal of the gall bladder). Most operations on the nose, back, and knee and the removal of varicose veins and hemorrhoids also fall into this category.

2. *Where should I go to get a second opinion?* The doctor you consult should have as good or better qualifications than your own doctor. Getting a second opinion is not the same as changing doctors. The second doctor should not be sought as another possible surgeon, for example. Instead, he or she is only to give an opinion as a person who is disinterested in the sense

that there will be no personal financial gain in recommending surgery.

3. *What should I do with a second opinion?* If both doctors agree, the reasonable course would be to go ahead with the treatment. Surprisingly, some patients get a second opinion in the hope of rationalizing avoidance of a needed treatment, and even if the second doctor recommends it, the patient may refuse. If the doctors disagree, you are left with a difficult choice. You could get a third opinion, but that might not make matters any clearer. Essentially, when doctors disagree, you have to make your own decision based on the risks and benefits of the treatment as it has been explained to you. Follow-up studies of compulsory second opinions for participants in health care plans have concluded that most physician disagreements about whether surgery should be performed are honest differences of opinion in gray areas of medical knowledge where an expert consensus has not been reached.

In California patients' rights have been codified by the state, and a 16-point list of these rights is posted in each hospital. Besides the right to give and refuse permission for procedures and to leave a hospital against medical advice, other rights relating to decision making, confidentiality, and billing are listed. Patients have the right to know the names of the doctors who have primary care for them, and those doctors are to keep patients informed, in understandable terms, about their illnesses and their prospects for recovery. In large hospitals patients may be seen by so many doctors that they may not be able to tell who is in charge of their care. Each of these doctors may think someone else has explained the patient's illness and treatment. What patients say and what is written in their charts are to be kept confidential. Patients must give written permission for the release of medical information. Any procedures that are experimental must be labeled as such. Patients have the right to

examine and to receive an explanation of their bills, even though the bills are being paid by a third party such as an insurance company.

The responsibilities of patients are not matters of legal definition, with the exception of financial responsibility for bills. Patients can often avoid exercising their rights and maintain passive attitudes. Such patients may be regarded as "good" and easy to care for in hospitals, but they may fail to follow any treatment program after they are discharged. They may fail to take prescribed medication, to follow necessary diets, or to return for follow-up appointments. Such patients are often those who are uninformed about the reasons for their treatment, because the information was never given them or they avoided listening to it. Thus, individualized instruction in responsible self-care by medical professionals, educators, or lay self-help groups is an essential element in improving health standards.

Patient's Bill of Rights

The American Hospital Association presents a Patient's Bill of Rights with the expectation that observance of these rights will contribute to more effective patient care and greater satisfaction for the patient, his physician, and the hospital organization. Further, the Association presents these rights in the expectation that they will be supported by the hospital on behalf of its patients, as an integral part of the healing process. It is recognized that a personal relationship between the physician and the patient is essential for the provision of proper medical care. The traditional physician-patient relationship takes on a new dimension when care is rendered within an organizational structure. Legal precedent has established that the institution itself also has a responsibility to the patient. It is in recognition of these factors that these rights are affirmed.

1. The patient has the right to considerate and respectful care.

2. The patient has the right to obtain from his physician complete current information concerning his diagnosis, treatment, and prognosis in terms the patient can be reasonably expected to understand. When it is not medically advisable to give such information to the patient, the information should be made available to an appropriate person in his behalf. He has the right to know by name the physician responsible for coordinating his care.

3. The patient has the right to receive from his physician information necessary to give informed consent prior to the start of any procedure and/or treatment. Except in emergencies, such information for informed consent should include but not necessarily be limited to the specific procedure and/or treatment, the medi-

cally significant risks involved, and the probable duration of incapacitation. Where medically significant alternatives for care or treatment exist, or when the patient requests information concerning medical alternatives, the patient has the right to such information. The patient also has the right to know the name of the person responsible for the procedures and/or treatment.

4. The patient has the right to refuse treatment to the extent permitted by law, and to be informed of the medical consequences of his action.

5. The patient has the right to every consideration of his privacy concerning his own medical care program. Case discussion, consultation, examination, and treatment are confidential and should be conducted discreetly. Those not directly involved in his care must have the permission of the patient to be present.

6. The patient has the right to expect that all communications and records pertaining to his care should be treated as confidential.

7. The patient has the right to expect that within its capacity a hospital must make reasonable response to the request of a patient for services. The hospital must provide evaluation, service, and/or referral as indicated by the urgency of the case. When medically permissible a patient may be transferred to another facility only after he has received complete information and explanation concerning the needs for and alternatives to such a transfer. The institution to which the patient is to be transferred must first have accepted the patient for transfer.

8. The patient has the right to obtain information as to any relationship of his hospital to other health care and educational institutions

insofar as his care is concerned. The patient has the right to obtain information as to the existence of any professional relationships among individuals, by name, who are treating him.

9. The patient has the right to be advised if the hospital proposes to engage in or perform human experimentation affecting his care or treatment. The patient has the right to refuse to participate in such research projects.

10. The patient has the right to expect reasonable continuity of care. He has the right to know in advance what appointment times and physicians are available and where. The patient has the right to expect that the hospital will provide a mechanism whereby he is informed by his physician or a delegate of the physician of the patient's continuing health care requirements following discharge.

11. The patient has the right to examine and receive an explanation of his bill regardless of the source of payment.

12. The patient has the right to know what hospital rules and regulations apply to his conduct as a patient.

No catalogue of rights can guarantee for the patient the kind of treatment he has a right to expect. A hospital has many functions to perform, including the prevention and treatment of disease, the education of both health professionals and patients, and the conduct of clinical research. All these activities must be conducted with an overriding concern for the patient, and, above all, the recognition of his dignity as a human being. Success in achieving this recognition assures success in the defense of the rights of the patient.

American Hospital Association

Medical Diagnosis Behavior Scale

Read the following statements carefully. Choose the one in each section that best describes you at this moment and record its score at the right. (For example, "has checkups at regular intervals" has a score of 5.) When you have identified five statements, total your score and find your position on the scale.

5 has checkups at regular intervals
4 saw doctor within last two years
3 saw doctor within last four years
2 tends to ignore severe symptoms
1 avoids doctors regardless of symptoms

Score _____

5 follows medical regimens as prescribed
4 follows treatment programs with few exceptions
3 follows treatment programs according to mood
2 rarely follows prescribed treatment programs
1 ignores prescribed treatment programs

Score _____

5 fully questions doctor if any doubts exist
4 usually questions doctor if any doubts exist
3 reluctantly questions doctor if any doubts exist
2 rarely questions doctor if any doubts exist
1 avoids questioning the doctor

Score _____

5 always gets (or would get) second opinions for major medical decisions
4 usually gets second opinions for major medical decisions
3 reluctantly gets second opinions for major medical decisions
2 rarely gets second opinions for major medical decisions
1 follows one doctor's recommendation for all medical decisions

Score _____

5 refuses X rays except for a good medical reason
4 keeps track of previous X rays
3 asks doctor if X rays are necessary
2 is unconcerned about exposure to X rays
1 is frequently exposed to X rays without knowing why

Score _____

Total score _____

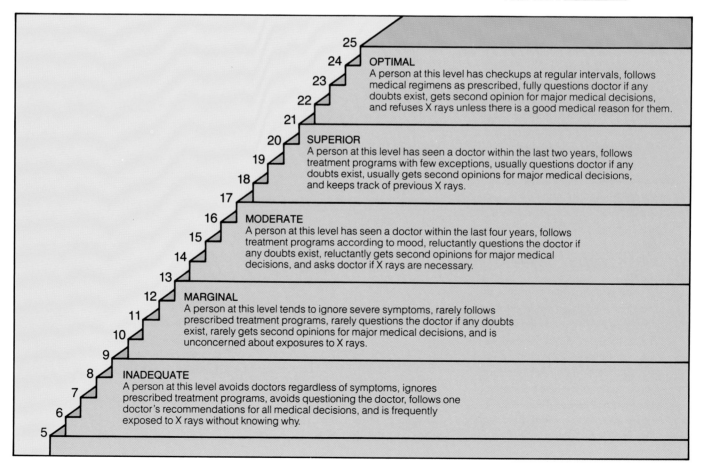

25
24 **OPTIMAL**
23 A person at this level has checkups at regular intervals, follows
22 medical regimens as prescribed, fully questions doctor if any
21 doubts exist, gets second opinion for major medical decisions, and refuses X rays unless there is a good medical reason for them.

20 **SUPERIOR**
19 A person at this level has seen a doctor within the last two years, follows
18 treatment programs with few exceptions, usually questions doctor if any
17 doubts exist, usually gets second opinions for major medical decisions, and keeps track of previous X rays.

16 **MODERATE**
15 A person at this level has seen a doctor within the last four years, follows
14 treatment programs according to mood, reluctantly questions the doctor if
13 any doubts exist, reluctantly gets second opinions for major medical decisions, and asks doctor if X rays are necessary.

12 **MARGINAL**
11 A person at this level tends to ignore severe symptoms, rarely follows
10 prescribed treatment programs, rarely questions the doctor if any doubts
9 exist, rarely gets second opinions for major medical decisions, and is unconcerned about exposures to X rays.

8 **INADEQUATE**
7 A person at this level avoids doctors regardless of symptoms, ignores
6 prescribed treatment programs, avoids questioning the doctor, follows one
5 doctor's recommendations for all medical decisions, and is frequently exposed to X rays without knowing why.

Take Action

Your answers to Probing Your Emotions at the beginning of this chapter and your placement level on the Medical Diagnosis Behavior Scale will, we hope, encourage you to begin a process of self-exploration and self-discovery that you will continue. Reflect on the entire chapter's content and ask yourself how each point relates to your own life. Then take action:

1. Turn to page 381 and read the material on patient rights. Note the items that are most relevant to your personal experiences. What, if anything, would you add or delete?

2. In your Take Action notebook keep track of the dates and locations of X rays you have had, including dental X rays. Write down all the previous X rays you can remember. If you think you have been overex-posed to radiation, communicate your concern to your doctor and ask his or her advice.

3. Make an appointment for the physical or eye examination or dental checkup that you have been putting off.

4. Read the following Behavior Change Strategy and take the appropriate action.

Behavior Change Strategy

Following Through with Suggestions: Compliance and Adherence

Many of the chapters in this book describe steps that an individual can take to accomplish health goals. Personal responsibility for change makes good sense when we look at topics like quitting smoking, losing weight, managing stress, and so on. But when people seek and receive medical care they tend to give away their personal responsibility—to resign their fate to "omniscient, modern medicine." Of course it is reasonable to heed the advice of one's physician since there is clearly a difference between recommendations received from a competent medical expert and ideas obtained from unqualified others. But following medical advice still requires the individual to manage his or her behavior. For example, in outpatient or ambulatory situations, the patient is often asked to attend meetings in regular fashion, told to take medications according to a certain schedule, asked to engage in special exercise or stretching movements, and asked to make modifications in the selection and/or preparation of foods.

Medicine has recognized the important role of self-management in health care and contains an area of research called patient adherence or compliance. The kinds of strategies that have been tested and found to be helpful include the following: (a) using reminders placed in one's personal environment (home, car, work place) that improve follow-through in taking medication and keeping scheduled appointments, (b) using diary systems and other forms of self-monitoring to keep a detailed account of a wide variety of health behaviors like diet, pill-taking, exercise practice, and so on, (c) using self-reward systems so that practice of certain self-change programs is encouraged by access to desired activities or items (emphasizing the extrinsic short-term incentives to complement the important but oftentimes too distant long-term intrinsic benefits for change), and, finally, (d) using the process of shaping, which is really a method of using self-monitoring and self-rewards to encourage small changes at first followed by larger ones (beginning with only one pill per day, for example, in the first week followed by the needed two-pill-per-day regimen in the second week).

Communication stands as one of the key requirements of improved adherence. The patient must fully understand what needs to be done, and the physician (or physician staff member) must listen to the scheduling and personal concerns about the regimen from the patient's perspective. A sharing of information contributes to a sense of shared responsibility for following through with the medical regimen. Successful medical care necessarily involves more than following doctor's orders; there has to be an accommodation of what is needed from a medical care perspective with a person's individual schedule and habits. While changes in packaging and recommendations from medicine are being made to help ease this process (for example, availability of pills that can be taken fewer times and still have the same pharmacologic benefits), the patient must recapture the sense of responsibility for self-management that characterizes so much of health and behavior.

Part Six

Current Health Concerns

Chapter Seventeen

Cardiovascular Health

Probing Your Emotions

1. There is a history of cardiovascular disease in your family. Your grandfather had a heart attack when he was 42, your father had a heart attack when he was 50, and your uncle had a stroke when he was 53. Although you are much younger, you are worried. Because you are much younger, however, you are not taking any preventive action. How do you feel about putting off the consequences of your life-style, which will inevitably affect your heart's health? At what age will you take action? Why haven't you started?

2. You are eating your favorite Sunday breakfast, steak and eggs, and your daughter says to you, "My science teacher says steak and eggs are not good for your heart." How do you respond to this, knowing that parents are important models for their children's behavior?

3. A classmate of yours suffers from persistent high blood pressure (hypertension), for which the doctor has prescribed drugs and regular exercise. However, your classmate is somewhat sedentary, doesn't believe much in taking medicine, and tends to neglect his problem. How does such apparently irrational behavior make you feel? How can you help him understand the seriousness of his disease and the necessity for taking the medication without alienating him?

Chapter Contents

THE CARDIOVASCULAR SYSTEM

MAJOR FORMS OF ADULT CARDIOVASCULAR DISEASE
Atherosclerosis
Hypertension
"Heart attack"
Stroke
Congestive heart failure

CARDIOVASCULAR DISEASE, PERSONALITY, AND LIFE-STYLE

HEART DISEASES IN CHILDREN
Congenital heart disease
Rheumatic heart disease

Boxes

Heart surgery may not be necessary
Lowered cholesterol lowers heart disease
A system for estimating your risk from
  high blood pressure
Climbing stairs is best
What you should know about heart attack
The warning signs of stroke

Cardiovascular system
The heart and blood vessels.

Cardiovascular disease
Diseases of the heart and blood vessels: hardening of the arteries, high blood pressure, and heart attacks.

Atherosclerosis
A form of arteriosclerosis in which the inner layers of artery walls are made thick and irregular by deposits of a fatty substance. The internal channel of arteries becomes narrowed, and blood supply is reduced.

Plaque
A deposit on the inner wall of the blood vessels. Blood can coagulate around a plaque and form a clot.

Coronary thrombosis
A clot in a coronary artery, often causing sudden death.

---

17 Most of us are familiar with the stereotype of the future heart attack victim: the harried, frenzied, superambitious executive. We nod and say, "He's working on a coronary." He knows the stereotype, too, and may acknowledge it with a wry grin before hurrying on to his coronary. But that stereotype is only part of the truth. The other part may be closer to home for all too many of us—the overweight and underactive person sprawled in front of the television set after too much dinner, with a cigarette in one hand and a potato chip in the other. This person is also working on a coronary. Until more of us make changes in our living habits and begin to move toward a healthier life-style, cardiovascular disease will continue to be the number one killer in America.

The Cardiovascular System

The heart is a four-chambered muscle, about the size of a man's fist, shaped roughly like a cone. Its two upper chambers are usually called the atria (plural of *atrium*) but are sometimes called auricles. Blood enters the atria from the pulmonary veins, large veins leading from the lungs. The two lower chambers, called ventricles, pump blood through the pulmonary arteries, the large arteries leading to the lungs. The wall of the heart has three layers. The interior layer, called the endocardium, is a membrane lining the chambers of the heart. The middle layer, the "muscle," is called the myocardium. The third layer, a membrane called the epicardium, covers the heart. The heart and the blood vessels (veins, arteries, and capillaries) together make up the *cardiovascular system*. See Figure 17–1.

The heart pumps blood through the blood vessels. When blood flows into the ventricles from the atria, the heart muscle contracts, squeezing blood out into the pulmonary artery and the largest artery, the aorta. Valves prevent the blood from flowing in the wrong direction.

Blood vessels are classified by size and function. Veins carry blood *to* the heart; arteries carry it *away from* the heart. The main trunk of the arterial system, the aorta, branches into smaller arteries, which in turn branch into even smaller arteries. The smallest arteries, called arterioles, branch still further into the smallest blood vessels, the capillaries.

By way of the capillaries, blood from arterioles is transferred to small veins called venules, then to larger veins, which return it to the heart. Two important blood vessels supply blood to the heart itself, directly to the myocardium. These blood vessels, branching from the aorta, are the coronary arteries.

Major Forms of Adult Cardiovascular Disease

The diseases that affect the heart and blood vessels are called collectively *cardiovascular diseases*. Chief among them are atherosclerosis, hypertension (high blood pressure), stroke, congestive heart failure, rheumatic heart disease, and congenital heart disease. Cardiovascular disease was once considered a disease of old age. This is no longer the case, since many men in their forties die from cardiovascular disease. Although often hereditary, these early deaths can also be traced to self-indulgent life-styles and common misconceptions of what "the good life" is. Many early deaths could be prevented if people changed their patterns of daily living, especially their smoking habits, exercise programs, diets, and control over such problems as hypertension and diabetes.

Atherosclerosis *Atherosclerosis* is a slow progressive disease process that begins early in life, sometimes before puberty. In this disease arteries become narrowed by deposits of cellular debris, fatty cells, calcium, and other substances. As these deposits, called *plaques*, accumulate on the walls of the arteries, the arteries lose their elasticity and are unable to expand and contract. The flow of blood through the narrowed arteries is restricted. A clot (thrombus) may form, blocking the artery and depriving the heart, brain, or other organ of the vital oxygen carried by the blood. When a coronary artery is blocked, the result is a *coronary thrombosis*, which is one kind of heart attack. When an artery leading to the brain is blocked, the result is a cerebral thrombosis, a kind of stroke.

Cholesterol
A fatty compound in the blood that is also found in deposits on the walls of arteries.

Platelets
Microscopic disk-shaped cell fragments in the blood. These disintegrate on contact with foreign objects and release chemicals that are necessary for the formation of blood clots.

Blood plasma
The fluid portion of the blood.

Antibodies
Proteins in the blood that are generated in reaction to foreign proteins. Antibodies neutralize the foreign proteins, producing immunity from them.

Several factors have been linked to the development of atherosclerosis in susceptible individuals. These include high concentration of blood lipids (fats and fatlike substances), of which *cholesterol* is one, genetic disorders, cigarette smoking, diets high in animal fats, and hypertension. The interaction of these factors is not yet fully understood.

The Growth of Arterial Plaques   One theory advanced to explain the growth of arterial plaques is called the response-to-injury theory. Apparently, the narrowing of an artery is not caused solely by the accumulation of substances forming the blockage. Studies with animals suggest that arterial blockages can begin with repeated or chronic injury to the endothelium, a thin layer of cells lining the inner surface of the artery. The injury to the inner surface allows the smooth muscle cells of the middle wall to come into contact with the blood. The muscle cells then multiply, forming a plaque.

Arterial plaques resembling but not identical to those occurring in people have been brought on in animals by injuring their arteries in several ways, among them (1) mechanically, by inserting catheters (tubes); and (2)

by increasing the amount of the blood lipids carrying cholesterol.

The direct cause of atherosclerosis may not, however, be the injury itself. It may instead be the presence of some substance in the blood that causes the smooth muscle cells to multiply.

When the endothelium is injured, *platelets* (particles in the blood that are involved in the clotting mechanism) cluster around the exposed smooth muscle cells and release chemicals into the *blood plasma*. One group of investigators has shown that one protein released by the platelets can cause smooth muscle cells to divide and that when this protein is absent the muscle cells do not divide. This research was done in tissue cultures, however, not in live animals.

Other investigators have shown (in rabbits) that when the platelets are destroyed by *antibodies,* injury to the endothelium no longer causes plaques to form. Evidence implicating platelets in the formation of plaques in people is less direct and still inconclusive. Data on humans are more difficult to obtain because experiments must not produce atherosclerosis or injure the subject in any way.

Figure 17-1   Cross section of the heart and lungs showing paths of blood flow.

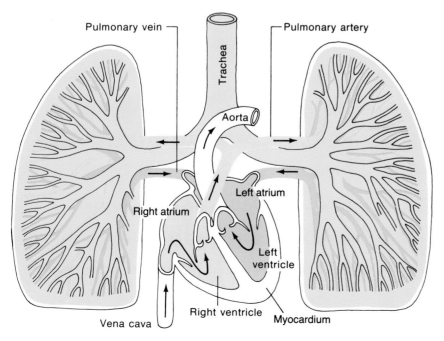

Pulmonary vein

Pulmonary artery

Trachea

Aorta

Left atrium

Right atrium

Left ventricle

Vena cava

Right ventricle   Myocardium

Hypercholesterolemia
An excess amount of cholesterol in the blood.

Low-density lipoproteins (LDLs)
Blood fats that carry cholesterol that accumulates on artery walls; may eventually block the flow of blood to the heart and brain.

High-density lipoproteins (HDLs)
Blood fats that help keep cholesterol in a watery state and thus are protective against heart diseases.

Lipoprotein
A protein and lipid connected as one chemical.

Another substance implicated in the multiplying of smooth muscle cells is the blood fat, cholesterol. One of its functions is as a building block for cell membranes. Cholesterol has been found to be a major component of plaques. People suffering from the genetically transmitted disease *hypercholesterolemia* have abnormally high concentrations of cholesterol in their blood plasma and frequently die of atherosclerosis as young adults.

Two kinds of blood fats have been identified as having opposite effects on the development of atherosclerosis: *low-density lipoprotein (LDL)* and *high-density lipoprotein (HDL)*. LDL cause arteries to thicken by accumulating on artery walls. HDL help to keep LDL in solution, or in a watery state, so that blood can pass freely through the arteries to the heart. Carefully conducted medical surveys have indicated that high concentrations of LDL in the blood plasma are a risk factor for atherosclerosis. See Figure 17–2.

Cigarette Smoking   Studies have firmly established that cigarette smoking is a risk factor for atherosclerosis. One mechanism by which smoking may increase the incidence of the disease has been suggested by Edwin Bierman of the University of Washington Medical School: Plaques that are associated with atherosclerosis contain smooth muscle cells with very high concentra-

tions of *lipoproteins*. Normally, the lipoproteins that deliver cholesterol to the cells are broken down by the cell. Bierman discovered that the breakdown process slows when the concentration of oxygen is diminished. Cigarette smoking produces carbon monoxide, which enters the blood and tends to replace oxygen, thus lowering its concentration. Thus, cigarette smoking may promote the accumulation of lipoproteins in the cells and facilitate the formation of plaques. In addition, passive smoke (smoke generated by others) has been strongly implicated in the development of atherosclerosis, as well as lung cancer. Consequently, just being around smokers for long periods of time may in itself be a risk factor for heart disease.

Diet   Does lowering the concentrations of blood lipids or cholesterol prevent or reverse plaque formation? In one controlled study with monkeys, a low cholesterol diet retarded progression of atherosclerosis. In a study of men who had already suffered one heart attack, the use of drugs that lowered blood cholesterol levels did not lessen the likelihood of a second attack. However, in a recent 10-year study of 3,800 middle-aged men with abnormally high cholesterol levels, it was conclusively demonstrated that for every 1 percent reduction in chlolesterol, there was a 2 percent drop in heart attacks.

Figure 17-2   Stages of plaque development.

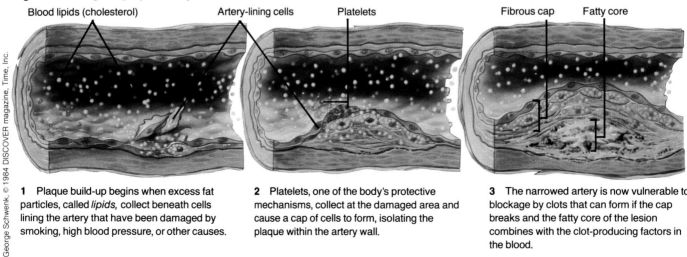

George Schwenk, © 1984 DISCOVER magazine, Time, Inc.

1   Plaque build-up begins when excess fat particles, called *lipids,* collect beneath cells lining the artery that have been damaged by smoking, high blood pressure, or other causes.

2   Platelets, one of the body's protective mechanisms, collect at the damaged area and cause a cap of cells to form, isolating the plaque within the artery wall.

3   The narrowed artery is now vulnerable to blockage by clots that can form if the cap breaks and the fatty core of the lesion combines with the clot-producing factors in the blood.

Heart Surgery May Not Be Necessary

Fifteen years ago, cardiac surgeons developed an operation that gave a new lease on life to Americans whose coronary arteries had become so clogged with fatty deposits that they could no longer supply enough blood to the heart to permit this vital muscle to function properly.

The operation, called coronary bypass surgery because it creates detours around blocked arteries, has since been performed on more than one million Americans, most of them men past the age of 50. With each year, as the surgery became more successful and surgical complications and deaths declined, the number of patients undergoing bypass surgery rose, reaching 170,000 [in 1983] at a medical cost of more than $3 billion.

Now, however, a major new study . . . has indicated that for perhaps 13 percent of these patients, surgery may not be the appropriate course of action, at least not at the time it is undertaken and perhaps not ever. The study, conducted at 15 medical centers in the United States and Canada, involved patients with mild to moderate chest pain, indicating a deficient supply of blood and oxygen to the heart muscle, and those without pain who have already suffered one heart attack and are shown on diagnostic tests to have significant blockages in one or more coronary arteries.

Although the pain of mild angina can largely be controlled by medication, such patients have long been a source of worry to their physicians, their families, and themselves. Since one or more of their coronary arteries is known to be diseased, is it only a matter of time before they suffer a serious and perhaps fatal heart attack? If so, wouldn't it be wise to forestall this event by undergoing surgery right away to bypass the blockages?

Despite the apparent logic behind the operation, evidence of lifesaving benefit has been lacking for these patients, about 60,000 of whom are identified each year. Thus far, the operation has proved to be lifesaving for only one group of heart patients: those whose left main coronary artery has a serious blockage. Even for patients with severe, incapacitating angina, for whom only bypass surgery can significantly improve the quality of their lives, it is not known whether the operation actually makes them live longer.

Still, the chest pains of angina, no matter how mild, are frightening and repeated reminders that all is not well in the coronary circulation, and more than 40 percent of patients with mild angina have opted for surgery, especially when two or more of their coronary arteries had major blockages.

But the question remained: Just how explosive was their coronary powder keg, and was it any safer to have a bypass operation, which in itself results in a heart attack or death in 7 to 10 percent of cases? The new American study, funded and coordinated by the National Heart, Lung, and Blood Institute, has shown no lifesaving value of surgery for mild angina patients over a period of at least five years.

As Dr. Eugene Passamani, project officer for the study and an institute cardiologist, pointed out, "Bypass surgery only fixes the plumbing. It does nothing to stem the progression of the underlying disease," which tends to get continually worse with time. No matter how good the surgeon, within a decade in about 40 percent of patients the newly implanted blood vessels become as clogged as the old ones they bypassed. And in half of the remaining 60 percent of surgery patients, other coronary blood vessels become seriously blocked.

Passamani said experience has shown that bypass surgery is most successful and safest the first time it is done. Thus . . . it may be best to wait to operate until it is absolutely necessary: if and when the left main artery becomes blocked or angina worsens to the point where drugs are no longer able to control the pain adequately.

"The next event after mild angina does not seem to be a heart attack or sudden death, but a worsening of the angina," Passamani said. He added that waiting until surgery was unquestionably necessary and beneficial did not increase the risks of the operation.

There may be other reasons for delaying surgery. New techniques are being introduced and studied that may be able to reopen coronary arteries without the hazards and considerable expense of a bypass operation, which costs on average between $15,000 and $25,000. Possible alternatives to surgery include stretching the narrowed arteries with a balloon, injecting a clot-dissolving enzyme directly into blocked arteries, and an experimental laser technique to ream out the vessels.

And there is the question of heading off further deterioration of the coronary vessels and perhaps even reversing some of the blockages. Studies in people as well as laboratory animals have shown, for example, that restricting dietary

(continued on next page)

Heart Surgery May Not Be Necessary (continued)

fat and cholesterol, perhaps in conjunction with taking cholesterol-lowering drugs, can cleanse out clogged arteries in the legs and may do the same in the arteries that feed the heart. Stopping smoking reduces the risk of a fatal heart attack almost immediately after cigarettes are abandoned. Properly designed exercise programs can greatly improve the ability of even a diseased coronary circulation to deliver oxygen to the heart muscle and thus increase the workload the patient's heart can withstand. And studies are now under way to determine whether learning to control noxious stress reactions will also forestall a coronary.

Jane E. Brody
Science Times

Lowered Cholesterol Lowers Heart Disease

After 3,806 middle-aged men with high cholesterol levels made 193,000 clinic visits, gave 341,000 blood samples and had 72,000 electrocardiograms, researchers are now willing to state what they've suspected all along—"the risk of coronary heart disease can be reduced by lowering blood cholesterol."

While the association between high cholesterol and heart disease has long been established, this 10-year study of the effect of a cholesterol-lowering drug is the first proof on a large scale that lowering cholesterol levels will protect against the development of heart disease. The men who lowered their cholesterol levels by 25 percent suffered only half the expected incidence of heart attacks. The effect was graded—the lower the cholesterol, the less likely a heart attack. Study director Basil M. Rifkind of the National Heart, Lung, and Blood Institute (NHLBI) in Bethesda, Md., estimated that going after cholesterol aggressively could eliminate 100,000 of the 500,000 fatal heart attacks in the United States each year.

Over 400,000 men between the ages of 35 and 59 were screened for the study, and those selected were from the group with the top 5 percent of cholesterol levels. Half were instructed to take six packets daily of cholestyramine, a cholesterol-lowering drug, while the other half took a placebo. Both groups were put on a low cholesterol diet—three eggs per week; avoidance of fatty meats; restriction of whole milk, cheese, and butter; and use of vegetable instead of animal fats.

The overall cholesterol reduction in the cholestyramine group was 13.4 percent compared to 8.5 percent in the diet-alone group. LDL-cholesterol, thought to be the harmful constituent of cholesterol, dropped 20.3 percent in the treated group and 12.6 percent in the others. With these differences, men on the drug had 19 percent fewer heart attacks and 24 percent fewer fatal heart attacks than the placebo group.

The drug is not a license to grab for the ice cream—it was used in conjunction with diet, it has a not-particularly-pleasant powdery taste, and it has to be taken six times a day. At current prices, the continual treatment necessary costs $150 per month. Side effects are apparently not serious—some of the men suffered constipation and heartburn, but they responded to treatment. Other cholesterol-lowering drugs are currently being developed, says Rifkind.

Though the results for the study population were obtained with a cholesterol-lowering drug, the take-home lesson for the general public applies to diet, the researchers say: "The trial's implications . . . could and should be extended to other age groups and women and, since cholesterol levels and coronary heart disease risk are continuous variables, to others with more modest elevations of cholesterol levels."

J. Silberner
Science News

Hypertension
Abnormally high blood pressure.

Systole
A period of contraction of the heart.

Diastole
A period of relaxation of the heart.

Sphygmomanometer
An instrument for measuring blood pressure.

Although the study used a cholesterol-lowering drug to achieve its results, the researchers concluded that their findings should apply to the general population with elevated cholesterol levels.

Hypertension The medical term for persistent or sustained high blood pressure is *hypertension*. Hypertension is in itself the primary cause of more than 60,000 deaths each year in the United States. It also contributes to one and a half million yearly heart attacks and strokes. See Figure 17–3.

Hypertension is a "silent killer," so called because it presents no symptoms. Victims thus have no way of knowing without testing that they have the disease. Recent studies have shown that more people have become aware of their hypertension and are being treated for it. Control of high blood pressure is thought to be a significant contributing factor to the recent decline in heart attacks.

Hypertension cannot be cured, but it can be treated and controlled. Lack of treatment can result in serious damage to vital organs, particularly the heart, brain, and kidneys. Blood vessels in the kidneys, for example, may rupture from constant high blood pressure, making it difficult if not impossible for them to clear waste material from the bloodstream. In the eyes, pressure on the capillaries in the retina may cause swelling and tiny hemorrhages and may eventually result in blindness. Hypertension may also cause arteries to lose their elasticity from being constantly stretched.

Blood Pressure Defined Blood pressure is the force per area exerted by blood against the walls of the arteries. This force is created by the pumping action of the heart. Every time the heart contracts, or beats (called *systole*), blood pressure increases. When the heart relaxes between beats (*diastole*), the pressure decreases. Blood pressure is highest in the arteries, which transport blood away from the heart, and lowest in the veins, which return blood to the heart.

Measuring Blood Pressure Blood pressure is measured with a stethoscope and an instrument called a *sphygmomanometer*. A sphygmomanometer consists of an airbag or cuff and a column of mercury marked off in millimeters. The cuff is wrapped around the upper arm and inflated by squeezing an attached rubber bulb. The inflated cuff depresses the brachial artery in the arm, stopping the flow of blood. Air pressure supports the column of mercury. As air is slowly released from the cuff, the column of mercury falls. When the cuff is no longer tight enough to prevent the passage of blood through the artery, the examiner will hear with the stethoscope a thudding sound as blood flow resumes. The height of the mercury when the sound is first heard is the reading of the systolic blood pressure, the pressure when the heart is contracting. After noting the systolic blood pressure, the examiner continues to release air until the sound can no longer be heard. The pressure at this point is diastolic blood pressure, the blood pressure when the heart is relaxed. Blood pressure is expressed as two numbers—for example, 120/80. The first and larger number is the systolic blood pressure, and the second number is the diastolic blood pressure.

(*text continues on p. 396*)

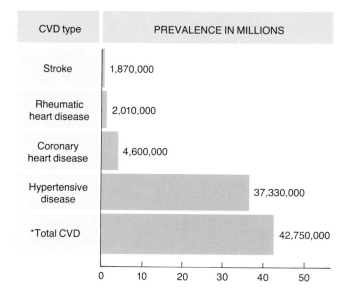

CVD type	PREVALENCE IN MILLIONS
Stroke	1,870,000
Rheumatic heart disease	2,010,000
Coronary heart disease	4,600,000
Hypertensive disease	37,330,000
*Total CVD	42,750,000

Source: American Heart Association.
*The sum of the individual estimates exceeds 42,750,000 since many persons have more than one cardiovascular disorder.

Figure 17-3 Estimated prevalence of the major cardiovascular diseases in the United States, 1981.

A System for Estimating Your Risk from High Blood Pressure

The Meaning of Risk from High Blood Pressure

High blood pressure increases the probability that damage to the cardiovascular system will occur in any given period of time. This damage often shows up as a serious event such as a heart attack or stroke. The likelihood that you will have an adverse event due to high blood pressure is called your "risk" from high blood pressure. Risk tends to increase with age as well as with blood pressure. The effect of age differs for men and women.

A useful concept to help you understand the implications of high blood pressure is that of "risk ratio." This is the ratio of your own risk to that of all persons in the United States of your same age and sex. If your risk ratio is less than 1.0, then blood pressure is less a problem for you than for the average person in your age and sex group; if your risk ratio is more than 1.0, it is more a problem.

Figuring Your Risk

Only your doctor can give you a detailed interpretation of what your high blood pressure might mean, but in the simplest sense, high blood pressure means risk. From the information provided here, you can determine approximately what that risk is.

By following the process outlined below, you will learn something more about your own risk and something more about the general implications of high blood pressure. The easiest way to get a clear reading of the various factors involved in risk is by means of a graphical analysis. Use the nomogram (a type of chart) on page 395 and work out your own risk as we go along.

Systolic and Diastolic Blood Pressure

Blood pressure is clinically defined by two numbers. For the purpose of risk assessment, we can take the average of the two numbers.

Add systolic pressure to diastolic pressure and *divide by* 2; for example:

$$140 + 90 = 230 \text{ and } 230/2 = 115.$$

Enter the average for your own blood pressure on the left-hand scale of the nomogram.

Blood pressure measures are different at different times, so the best measure will be an average of several readings. We strongly recommend that you use an average of several readings to determine your risk ratio and percentile rank.

Effect of Your Age and Sex

Both age and sex affect your blood pressure level and are factors in determining your relative risk. Blood pressure, especially systolic blood pressure, tends to increase with age, particularly in persons over age 40. The rule of thumb is that your systolic blood pressure should not exceed 100 plus your age.

Blood pressure goes up with age more rapidly in women than in men, but this does not mean that women necessarily have a greater risk. The effect of sex on risk is taken into account on the nomogram. Enter your age on the appropriate scale on the right side.

Reading the Nomogram

The bar in the middle of the nomogram defines your approximate risk from high blood pressure relative to others of the same age and sex. It also defines your risk percentile ranking in your peer group.

You can estimate your own risk by drawing a straight line with a ruler between your blood pressure on the left side of the nomogram and your age on the right side. The point at which this line crosses the risk ratio bar defines your relative risk and your ranking.

A relative risk of 1.2 means that your chance of having some adverse event related to high blood pressure is 1.2 times the average risk for someone in your peer group. A percentile ranking of 85 means that 85 percent of your peer group are below you in risk, while 15 percent are above.

We have divided the full range of risk into six broad categories. Find your risk category by noting the point at which your line intersects the arrow.

Knowing What to Do: The Meaning of Risk

Information about risk helps you to know what to do about high blood pressure. Check your category in the table below.

These criteria will refer young people to their doctors when their blood pressures do not seem to be high compared with the average blood pressure for all ages. But this is appropriate, since high blood pressure is very rare in young people.

Your doctor may or may not recommend drugs, but for young people in the higher risk categories (3, 4, and 5), some intervention such as diet changes, exercise, or relaxation will usually be indicated. Blood pressure in a higher risk range at an early age tends to lead to blood pressure in a higher range at a later age—and should not be ignored.

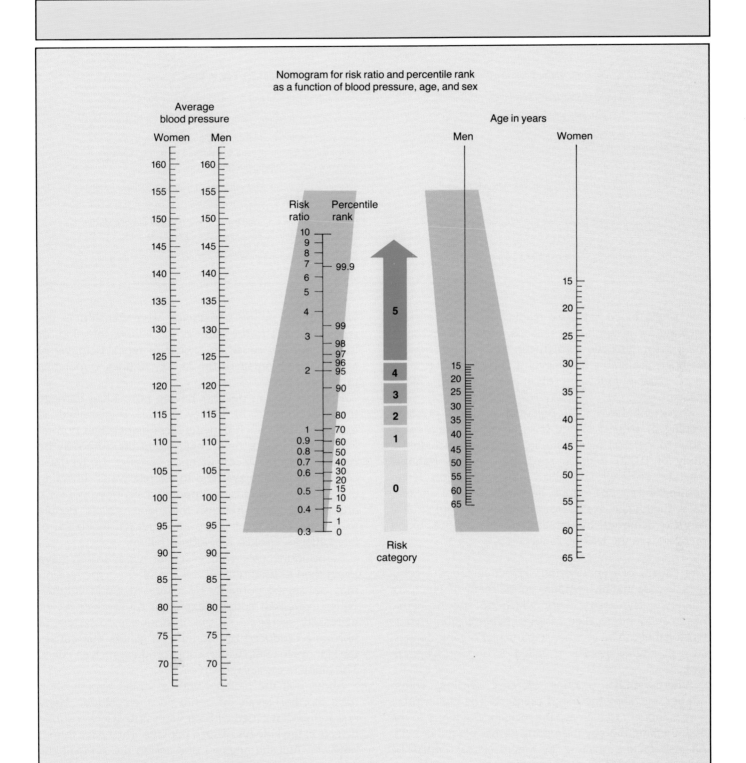

Nomogram for risk ratio and percentile rank as a
function of blood pressure, age, and sex.

(*continued on next page*)

A System for Estimating Your Risk from High Blood Pressure (continued)

Category	High Blood Pressure Risk	Actions for You to Take
0	Less than average—essentially negligible	Have blood pressure checked periodically for changes.
1	About average—not a matter of concern	Have blood pressure checked periodically for changes.
2	About 1.3 times average—should be watched closely	See your physician if blood pressure remains on the high side for any length of time or starts to drift into category 3; may not call for medical intervention.
3	About 1.6 times average—should be watched closely	See your physician; will often call for medical intervention; follow physician's recommendations.
4	About 2 times average—abnormally high	See your physician; medical intervention will almost always be called for; follow physician's recommendations.
5	About 3 times average—abnormally high	See your physician immediately; medical intervention is needed without delay.

A single blood pressure reading is not necessarily accurate for a number of reasons, including measurement error, anxiety, excitement, and so on. Several readings, preferably taken over a period of time, are a more reliable indication of a person's "real" blood pressure.

Physicians have long regarded a blood pressure reading of 160/95 as the level at which treatment is required. Several recent studies, however, including a study of 8,000 patients sponsored by the National Institutes of Health and called the Hypertension Detection and Follow-up Program, have indicated that substantial reductions in deaths from heart attacks and strokes can be achieved by treating people whose blood pressure is in the 140/90 range.

The Causes of Hypertension Hypertension is a complex disease that has various causes, many of which are unknown. Hypertension for which no specific cause has been found is called *essential hypertension*. Hypertension that can be ascribed to particular organic defects, such as kidney disease, is called *secondary hypertension*.

Atherosclerotic plaques increase friction within arteries, elevating the blood pressure. The higher pressure is thought to increase the incidence of injury to the endothelium, thereby promoting further plaque growth. All risk factors relating to atherosclerosis must be regarded as risk factors of hypertension.

The kidneys release the enzyme renin, which promotes the formation of angiotensin proteins. These in turn cause the blood vessels to constrict. The release of renin is inhibited by high pressure in the kidney arteries. If these arteries have been narrowed by atherosclerosis or by some other cause, their pressure will be low, so renin will continue to be secreted, proteins will continue to be produced, and all arteries

will continue to be constricted. Hypertension is the result. Damage to the kidneys by wound, infection, or tumor can also cause an excess of renin. Removal of the kidney or repair of the kidney arteries sometimes produces a cure.

Hypertension in patients having no evident damage to either kidneys or kidney arteries is classified as essential. Some such patients have higher than normal levels of renin. For them, high blood pressure may be caused primarily by constriction of arteries. Under these conditions the kidneys tend to excrete water, lowering blood volume, increasing blood viscosity ("syrupiness"), and placing great stress on the blood vessels. People with high renin levels have an increased incidence of heart attacks, strokes, and kidney failure.

Some individuals with essential hypertension have lower than normal renin levels. For them, hypertension may be caused primarily by increased blood volume. Either decreased sodium excretion by the kidneys or increased secretion of the hormone aldosterone (a hormone produced by the adrenal glands that causes the kidneys to retain water) could produce such an effect. The ultimate causes remain elusive.

About half the patients with essential hypertension have normal levels of renin in their blood. Many researchers have tried without success to discover subtle defects in the kidneys of such patients. They *have* found, however, that the angiotensins act on the sympathetic and central nervous systems as well as on the blood vessels, so the search for causes has broadened.

Hypertension appears to have a strong genetic component. But Harvard University researchers have found in young children an environmental influence on blood pressure as well. Whatever is responsible for essential hypertension may be acquired in childhood, but separating genetic from environmental factors has been traditionally a knotty problem in human biology. The Na-

Essential hypertension
Persistently elevated blood pressure without known or specific cause.

Secondary hypertension
High blood pressure due to disease such as kidney dysfunctioning or tumor.

Antihypertensive drugs
Drugs used to lower blood pressure.

Diuretic
An agent that promotes the excretion of urine.

tional Heart, Lung, and Blood Institute is now researching high blood pressure in children and adolescents, investigating the effects of diet, psychological factors, life-styles, genetic factors, and physical activity.

Recent experiments suggest that trace metals may be involved in the development of hypertension. Among these metals, cadmium, which is found in small quantities in many foods and beverages, is a prime suspect. When ingested, it tends to accumulate in the kidneys. Autopsies of patients who have died from hypertension have revealed a higher than normal concentration of cadmium in their kidneys. If cadmium proves to be an underlying cause of hypertension, it may be possible to reverse the disease by giving patients an agent that will help them excrete cadmium from the kidneys.

Treatment of Hypertension   Treatment of hypertension often consists of *antihypertensive drugs* and changes in diet. Recent studies have shown that regular exercise also lowers blood pressure.

One group of antihypertensive drugs is the *diuretics*, which increase fluid excretion by the kidneys. Use of diuretics is recommended for low renin patients, whose hypertension is thought to be due primarily to increased blood volume.

Another group of antihypertensive drugs blocks the action of angiotensin proteins. This treatment is appro-

priate for patients with higher than normal renin levels. Other drugs under study as possibly having an effect on hypertension are prostaglandins (hormones secreted by the prostate gland) and kinins, protein fragments that seem to cause dilation (widening) of blood vessels.

Mild hypertension can frequently be treated by changes in diet alone, such as the restriction of salt intake in salt sensitive people, caloric intake, or both. Overweight people are more susceptible to hypertension because added weight places greater demands on the cardiovascular system. Adipose (fatty) tissue, such as organ and muscle tissue, requires blood to nourish it. In overweight people the heart must pump more blood through a more extensive system of blood vessels. Restricting salt intake tends to curb fluid retention, thus reducing blood volume.

Patients with mild hypertension who fail to respond to drugs or changes in diet may be taught progressive relaxation. The patient learns to relax systematically by concentrating on muscle groups and relaxing them progressively, one by one. Such relaxation has been extremely effective with many patients. (See Chapter 2.)

"Heart Attack"   A "heart attack" is the end result of a long-term disease process. It does not just happen, although the attack itself may come without warning. (See Figure 17–4.) The most common form of heart

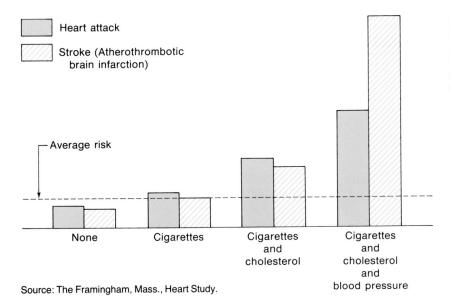

Figure 17-4   Risk of heart attack and stroke increases with the number of risk factors present. As an example, this chart uses risk factors of an abnormal blood pressure level of 180 systolic and a cholesterol level of 310 in a 45-year-old man.

☐ Heart attack

▨ Stroke (Atherothrombotic brain infarction)

Average risk

None   Cigarettes   Cigarettes and cholesterol   Cigarettes and cholesterol and blood pressure

Source: The Framingham, Mass., Heart Study.

Coronary occlusion
Partial or total obstruction of a coronary artery, as by a clot; usually resulting in myocardial infarction.

Myocardial infarction
A heart attack in which the heart muscle is damaged through lack of blood supply.

Collateral circulation
The movement of blood by a system of smaller blood vessels when a main vessel is blocked.

Angina pectoris
A condition in which the heart muscle does not receive enough blood, causing severe pain in the chest and often in the left arm and shoulder.

Stroke
An impeded blood supply to some part of the brain resulting in the destruction of brain cells (also called cerebrovascular accident).

Cerebral thrombosis
A clot in a vessel that supplies blood to the brain.

Cerebral embolism
Blockage of a blood vessel in the brain, caused by blood clots or other material carried in the blood from other parts of the body.

Cerebral hemorrhage
Bleeding in or near the brain.

Climbing Stairs Is Best

Climbing stairs is a strenuous activity that burns up more calories than jogging, swimming, or cycling for an equal amount of time. It is also an extremely effective cardiovascular exercise. But how do we get people to climb stairs when elevators and escalators are so convenient? A study conducted by the Department of Psychiatry at the University of Pennsylvania School of Medicine has shown that placing an eye-catching sign between an escalator and a stairway causes a significant increase in the number of people who use the stairs. In another study 21,000 observations were made of people going up the stairs or escalator at a shopping mall, a train station, and a bus station. The findings revealed that stair use increased from 5.3 to 13.7 percent when this sign was posted: YOUR HEART NEEDS EXERCISE— HERE'S YOUR CHANCE.

disease is coronary artery disease caused by atherosclerosis. When the coronary arteries are unable to supply oxygenated blood to the heart muscle because of a blood clot, a heart attack results. A heart attack caused by a clot is called a coronary thrombosis, a *coronary occlusion,* or a *myocardial infarction.* In myocardial infarction, part of the heart muscle (myocardium) may suffocate from lack of oxygen. If the heart attack is not fatal—that is, if enough of the muscle is undamaged to permit life to continue—the muscle begins to repair itself. It does this through a process called *collateral circulation,* in which small blood vessels open to take over the functions of the blocked artery and move more blood through the damaged area. As healing takes place, scar tissue replaces part of the injured muscle. Collateral circulation can be developed even before a heart attack takes place. Aerobic exercise (discussed in Chapter 13) increases collateral circulation and may delay or prevent heart attacks due to blocked coronary arteries.

Arteries narrowed by disease may still be open enough to deliver blood to the heart. However, at times—chiefly during emotional excitement, stress, or physical exertion—the heart requires more oxygen than narrowed arteries can accommodate. When the need for oxygen outstrips the supply, the heart's electrical system may be disrupted, also causing a heart attack. Chest pain, called *angina pectoris,* is a signal that the heart is not getting enough blood to supply the oxygen it needs. Angina pain is felt as an extreme tightness in the chest and heavy pressure behind the breastbone or in the shoulder, neck, arm, hand, or back. This pain, although not actually a heart attack, is a warning that the load on the heart must be reduced. Angina may be controlled in a number of ways (with diet and drugs), but its course is unpredictable.

Stroke   For brain cells to function as they should, they must have a continuous and ample supply of oxygen-rich blood. If brain cells are deprived of blood for more than a few minutes, they die. A *stroke,* also called a cerebrovascular accident, occurs when the blood supply to the brain is cut off. Stroke can be particularly serious because injured brain cells, unlike those of other organs, cannot regenerate themselves.

A common cause of stroke is the buildup of a blood clot in one of the cerebral arteries of the brain. This condition, called *cerebral thrombosis,* is likely to occur when the cerebral arteries become damaged by atherosclerosis. Deposits formed on the artery walls encourage the formation of clots. The risk of stroke is much higher among hypertensives than among those with normal blood pressure. If an artery to the brain is clogged from atherosclerotic deposits, the high blood pressure accelerates the disease.

Occasionally a wandering blood clot, called an embolus, is carried in the bloodstream and becomes wedged in one of the cerebral arteries. This is called a *cerebral embolism.* Another type of stroke, called cerebrovascular occlusion, occurs when a clot plugs up a cerebral artery.

Sometimes a diseased artery bursts in the brain. Blood pours into the surrrounding tissue, and cells normally nourished by the artery are deprived of blood and cannot function. This is called a *cerebral hemorrhage.* Patients

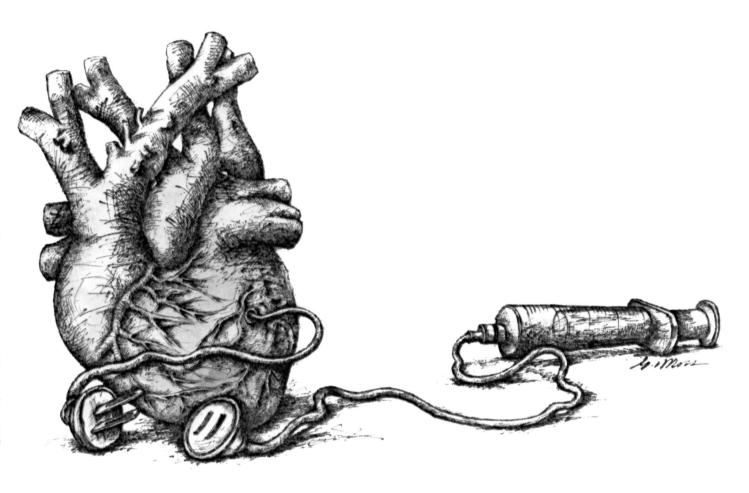

What You Should Know About Heart Attack

An estimated 4,600,000 people have coronary heart disease. An estimated 559,000 died of heart attack in 1981—350,000 before they reached the hospital. Many thousands of these might have been saved if the victims had heeded the signals.

Delay spells danger. When you suffer a heart attack, minutes—especially the first few minutes—count.

Know the Signals

The signals of heart attack are:

- Uncomfortable pressure, fullness, squeezing, or pain in the center of the chest lasting two minutes or more.
- Pain may spread to shoulders, neck, or arms.
- Severe pain, dizziness, fainting, sweating, nausea, or shortness of breath may also occur. Sharp, stabbing twinges of pain are usually not signals of a heart attack.

Emergency Action

If you are having typical chest discomfort that lasts for two minutes

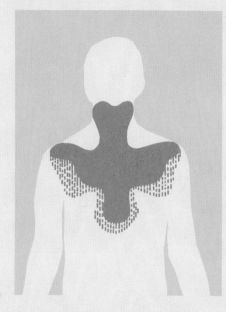

or more, call the local emergency rescue service immediately. If you can get to a hospital faster by car, have someone drive you. Find out which hospitals have 24-hour emergency cardiac care and discuss with your doctor the possible choices. Plan in advance the route that's best from where you live and work. Keep a list of emergency rescue service numbers next to your telephone and in a prominent

place in your pocket, wallet, or purse.

Be a Heart Saver

If you are with someone who is having the "signals," and if they last for two minutes or longer, act at once.

Expect a "denial." It is normal to deny the possibility of anything as serious as a heart attack—but insist on taking prompt action.

1. *Call* the emergency rescue service, or
2. *Get* to the nearest hospital emergency room that offers 24-hour emergency cardiac care, and
3. *Give* mouth-to-mouth breathing and chest compression (CPR) if it is necessary and if you are properly trained.

who suffer from both atherosclerosis and high blood pressure are more likely to suffer cerebral hemorrhage than those who have only one condition or neither.

Bleeding of an artery in the brain may also be caused by a head injury or by the bursting of an aneurysm. An *aneurysm* is a blood-filled pocket that bulges out from a weak spot in an artery wall. Aneurysms in the brain may remain stable and never break, but when they do, the result is a stroke.

An interruption of the blood supply to any area of the brain prevents the nerve cells there from functioning. Nerve cells control sensation and most of our bodily movements. Which parts of the body are affected by the stroke depends on the area of the brain affected. A stroke may impair speech, cause walking disability, or cause loss of memory. The severity of a stroke and its long-term effects depend on which brain cells have been injured, how widespread the damage is, how effectively the body can restore the blood supply, and how rapidly other areas of brain tissue can take over the work of damaged cells.

Congestive Heart Failure A number of conditions, including high blood pressure, heart attack, atherosclerosis, rheumatic fever, and birth defects, can cut down on the heart's pumping efficiency. When the heart is not able to maintain its regular pumping rate and force, fluids begin to back up and collect in the lungs and other parts of the body. When this extra, collected blood seeps through capillary walls, edema (swelling) results. Blood accumulating in the lungs causes swelling there, and this is called pulmonary edema. Pulmonary edema, in turn, causes shortness of breath. The entire process is *congestive heart failure*.

Aneurysm
A sac formed by a distension or dilation
of the artery wall.

Congestive heart failure
A condition resulting from the heart's
inability to pump out all the blood that
returns to it. Blood backs up in the veins
leading to the heart, causing an accumulation
of fluid in various parts of the body.

When people with impaired heart function stand or sit upright for long periods of time, the effect of gravity causes excess blood to accumulate in the legs. But in the prone position that people usually assume while resting, gravity no longer keeps the extra blood in the legs, and it goes into the lungs. There it interferes with breathing, which becomes extremely labored. If the heart weakens further, congestion in the lungs may be present all the time.

Congestive heart failure can be controlled. Treatment includes reducing the work load on the heart, modifying the person's intake of salt, and using drugs that help the body eliminate excess fluid. Heart stimulants taken orally, particularly digitalis, will improve the heart's efficiency.

The Warning Signs of Stroke

1. Sudden, temporary weakness or numbness of face, arm, or leg.
2. Temporary loss of speech or trouble in speaking or understanding speech.
3. Temporary dimness or loss of vision, particularly in one eye.
4. An episode of double vision.
5. Unexplained dizziness or unsteadiness.
6. Change in personality, mental ability, or the pattern of headaches.

Cardiovascular Disease, Personality, and Life-Style

"At the earliest moment at which we catch our first glimpse of Man on Earth, we find him not only on the move but already moving at an accelerated pace. This crescendo of acceleration is continuing today. In our generation it is perhaps the most difficult and dangerous of all current problems of the human race." These statements were made by historian Arnold Toynbee.

Harvard nutritionist Jean Mayer says: "We are again in the age of the great pandemics. Our plague is cardiovascular." We are social animals. We respond to the world with our hearts, our arteries, and our internal juices. Even while we lie in bed, a random thought can make our heart race and our blood pressure rise. It is hardly any wonder that many of us will eventually become disabled or die from cardiovascular disease.

The increased occurrence of cardiovascular disease has essentially been restricted to populations that are industrially and socially advanced. Perhaps the most widely publicized research linking cardiovascular disease with life-style comes from cardiologists Meyer Friedman and Ray Rosenman—*Type A Behavior and Your Heart* (1974). After extensive studies of thousands of working men, they concluded that men vulnerable to cardiovascular disease have much in common. They

tend to be people who are extremely punctual and greatly annoyed if kept waiting. They are individuals with few hobbies; they find routine jobs at home bothersome because they feel the time could be spent more profitably. They walk rapidly, eat quickly, and attempt to do several things at one time. They are impatient, often anticipating what others will say, frequently interrupting before questions or replies are fully completed. These coronary-prone individuals (whom Friedman and Rosenman call type As) seem to aspire to some vague, ill-defined achievements in their social environments. Add to this portrait a sedentary life, with little or no exercise, a tobacco-smoking habit, and one deadline after another, and you have the perfect candidate for a heart attack or stroke. In contrast, type Bs are more relaxed, and competition has no priority in their lives. They have more patience and more time for recreational activities. (See Chapter 2, pages 49-51 to find out if you are type A or B.)

In a sense some of us choose our diseases by the way we live. If we see no options, we can choose only one road. A society that is competitive, that values status and material wealth, is likely to foster only certain kinds of behaviors. Within such a society few of us can resist these important influences. If we can see that we have a choice and are able to exercise it, however, our road will have a fork. Figure 17-5 shows only the economic costs of cardiovascular disease.

Congenital heart disease
Disease present at birth due to malformation of the heart or its major blood vessels.

Blue baby
A baby with a bluish coloration of the skin due to insufficient oxygen in the blood.

Rheumatic fever
A disease, mainly of children, characterized by fever, inflammation, and pain in the joints; often causes damage to the heart muscle.

Heart Diseases in Children

Congenital Heart Disease Out of every 125 children born in the United States, one has a defect or malformation of the heart or major blood vessels. These conditions are referred to collectively as *congenital heart disease.* The development of the heart can go astray at any point, but in most cases medical scientists do not know why. German measles contracted by the mother during the first three months of pregnancy is believed to be a prime cause of abnormal fetal development. Other viral diseases may also contribute. There may be a genetic component, too, although rarely is more than one child in a family affected.

The most common congenital defects are holes in the ventricular septum, the wall dividing the lower chambers of the heart. Holes may also occur in the atrial septum, the wall between the upper chambers. With these defects, the heart produces a distinctive sound, making diagnosis relatively simple.

Other defects cannot be diagnosed without elaborate tests. One such defect is patent ductus arteriosus, a condition in which the prenatal channel between the coronary artery (the artery delivering blood to the body) and the pulmonary artery (the artery delivering blood to the lungs) fails to close as it should. Another defect,

coarctation of the aorta, is a narrowing, or constriction, of the largest artery of the body. Heart failure may result unless the constricted area is repaired by surgery. Another common defect results when the arteries delivering the blood to the body and lungs are transposed and attached to the wrong ventricles. Victims of this condition are often called *blue babies.* The red, oxygen-rich blood that should be going to the body is returned to the lungs. The blue, oxygen-poor blood going to the body fails to supply enough oxygen for essential cell functions.

Most of the common congenital defects, including that causing the blue baby condition, can now be accurately diagnosed. Important in saving lives is the early recognition that the newborn infant distressed with blue appearance, respiratory difficulty, or failure to thrive may be suffering from congenital heart disease. Surgery to correct defects is also possible. Although such operations are hazardous, they give many children the chance for a normal life that would otherwise be denied them.

Rheumatic Heart Disease Ninety percent of heart trouble in children can be attributed to *rheumatic fever,* a disease associated with the bacterium hemolytic streptococcus. The symptoms of rheumatic fever are generally vague, making diagnosis rather difficult. Among the symptoms observed in children are loss of weight or failure to gain weight; a low but persistent fever; poor appetite; repeated nosebleeds without apparent cause; jerky body movements; pain in the arms, legs, or abdomen; fatigue; and weakness. Antibiotics can usually prevent rheumatic fever. One attack of rheumatic fever will not prevent another and, in fact, often predisposes the child to later attacks. A child who has had an attack will usually have to take a daily dose of antibiotics for several years.

Rheumatic heart disease sometimes develops as a secondary response to rheumatic fever. This disease cripples the heart by scarring the muscle or damaging the heart valves. Treatment of rheumatic heart diseases often consists of surgery to restore the efficiency of damaged valves.

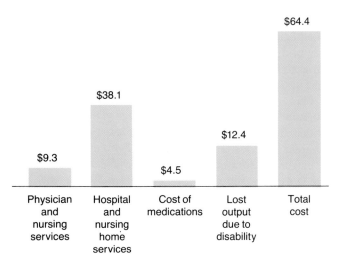

Figure 17-5 Estimated economic costs, in billions of dollars, of cardiovascular diseases by type of expenditure, United States, 1984. Source: American Heart Association.

Cardiovascular Health Behavior Scale

Read the following statements careful-ly. Choose the one in each section that best describes you at this moment and record its score at the right. (For example, "blood pressure and cholesterol level normal" has a score of 5.) When you have identified five statements, total your score and find your position on the scale.

5   blood pressure and cholesterol level normal
4   has had blood pressure and cholesterol level checked within the last year
3   does not know blood pressure or cholesterol level
2   blood pressure or cholesterol level is elevated or unknown
1   blood pressure and cholesterol level are elevated

Score _____

5   is trained in CPR
4   knows how to administer CPR
3   plans to learn CPR
2   is familiar with CPR
1   has never heard of CPR

Score _____

5   discourages others' smoking
4   has no-smoking signs in house
3   is vocal about smoking
2   is indifferent to others' smoking
1   offers cigarettes to others

Score _____

5   eats no red meats
4   eats low-cholesterol foods
3   eats few eggs
2   eats eggs daily
1   eats eggs and red meats daily

Score _____

5   knows the risk factors for car-diovascular disease
4   knows how cholesterol level and blood pressure are measured
3   knows how blood pressure is measured
2   doesn't know what causes heart disease
1   is unconcerned about heart disease

Score _____

Total score _____

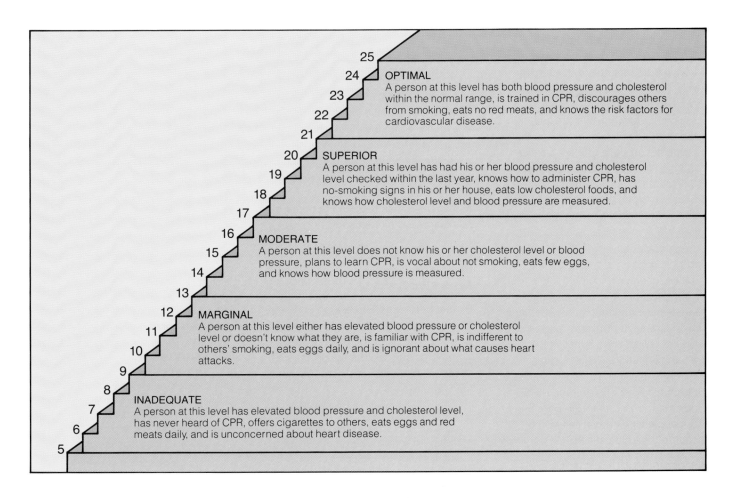

25
24   OPTIMAL
23   A person at this level has both blood pressure and cholesterol within the normal range, is trained in CPR, discourages others from smoking, eats no red meats, and knows the risk factors for cardiovascular disease.
22
21
20   SUPERIOR
19   A person at this level has had his or her blood pressure and cholesterol level checked within the last year, knows how to administer CPR, has no-smoking signs in his or her house, eats low cholesterol foods, and knows how cholesterol level and blood pressure are measured.
18
17
16   MODERATE
15   A person at this level does not know his or her cholesterol level or blood pressure, plans to learn CPR, is vocal about not smoking, eats few eggs, and knows how blood pressure is measured.
14
13
12   MARGINAL
11   A person at this level either has elevated blood pressure or cholesterol level or doesn't know what they are, is familiar with CPR, is indifferent to others' smoking, eats eggs daily, and is ignorant about what causes heart attacks.
10
9
8   INADEQUATE
7   A person at this level has elevated blood pressure and cholesterol level, has never heard of CPR, offers cigarettes to others, eats eggs and red meats daily, and is unconcerned about heart disease.
6
5

Take Action

Your answers to Probing Your Emotions at the beginning of this chapter and your placement level on the Cardiovascular Health Behavior Scale will, we hope, encourage you to begin a process of self-exploration and self-discovery that you will continue. Reflect on the entire chapter's content and ask yourself how each point relates to your own life. Then take action:

1. Blood pressure is extremely variable. Have your blood pressure measured four times on four different occasions. Average the measurements to get an accurate picture of your blood pressure level. Then turn to page 395 and use the nomogram to determine your percentile and risk ranking.
2. Call the American Red Cross and sign up for a brief course in cardio-pulmonary resuscitation (CPR).

3. Find out the route to the nearest hospital or clinic that has a coronary care unit. Educate family members and friends about the hospital and the route.
4. Read the following Behavior Change Strategy and take the appropriate action.

Behavior Change Strategy

Behavioral Management of High Blood Pressure

Because high blood pressure apparently produces few noticeable symptoms, many who suffer from it never seek or follow medical advice. In addition, high blood pressure is an ongoing, chronic problem that requires a course of treatment of long—possibly, life-long—duration. Furthermore, the recommended medical treatment often calls for the use of antihypertensive medications that frequently produce unpleasant side effects. When all of these factors are considered, it is clear that treatment may assume the role of "problem" for people who must manage their blood pressure.

A considerable and still-growing body of behavioral research has looked for ways to help people manage blood pressure. In many instances the results have not been consistent, and considerable controversy exists in making any specific behavioral recommendations. Nevertheless, current behavioral strategies seem to assume at least one of three roles: (1) they may *substitute* for drug treatment for people who cannot (or will not) tolerate drug side effects, (2) they may be used as *adjuncts* to medication in

that they may help to reduce the dosage needed to effectively manage blood pressure, or (3) they may play a *preventive* role in work with "at risk" groups such as children with elevated blood pressure readings and the relatives of patients already diagnosed as having hypertension.

Some of the strategies currently being used include the reduction of salt (sodium) intake, weight reduction, increased physical exercise, and relaxation techniques. Behavioral programs for several of these topics have already been described in detail. By far the greatest amount of research on methods of blood pressure management has been in the areas of relaxation and biofeedback.

Biofeedback and Relaxation Training

Biofeedback experiences can be used in conjunction with relaxation training or alone. The following excerpt (taken from Agras and Jacobs by Miller 1979) describes a session of biofeedback training:

> This intelligent 33-year-old [woman] had had a stroke producing brain stem damage (a complication) approximately four months before she entered the

[hospital] for rehabilitation of disabling motor deficits. There, [we] gave her training in voluntary control over her high blood pressure. A special device indirectly recorded diastolic blood pressure automatically on a beat-to-beat basis and sounded a tone that served as a reward by signalling to her that she had achieved the correct change of her blood pressure. . . . First, we rewarded her for a small decrease and then changed to reward for a small increase so that she could again succeed in producing another decrease. We also hoped that the contrast of successive reversals would help to teach her voluntary control.

At first she was able to produce changes of only 5–6 mm Hg. As she learned, we required larger changes. Then, in order to be sure that the change was not produced by any transient maneuver of skeletal muscles we required her to hold it. . . .

In spite of daily medication with 750 mg of the antihypertensive drug Aldomet (alpha-methyl-dopa) plus 100 mg of . . . Hydrodiuril, her diastolic pressure averaged 97 mm Hg during the 30 days in the hospital before training started. During this period, the pressure was variable but there was no appreciable trend. When training started, her pressure came down. . . . After her blood pressure had come down to normal, she was taken off medication. During the three days while the effects of Aldomet were wearing off, her pressure rose but then decreased to an average level of 76 mm Hg.

By means of biofeedback training, the woman described in this example apparently was able to significantly reduce her intake of medications. It is extremely important to note, however, that this occurred while she was under close medical supervision. Antihypertensive medication should not be discontinued during biofeedback or relaxation training without close medical supervision.

Is biofeedback better than relaxation training? In an incisive review of the available literature that allows for a comparison of these two popular approaches. Dr. Bernard Silver and Dr. Edward Blanchard (1978) concluded that there was "no consistent advantage for one form of treatment over the other" but that relaxation was somewhat more convenient to use and decidedly less expensive. Furthermore, they found that relaxation was probably the more fundamental approach (the "final common pathway") in the sense that it produces a more general decrease in heart rate, blood pressure, and muscle activity, which are attacked separately and narrowly by specialized biofeedback training.

Chapter Eighteen

Cancer

Probing Your Emotions

1. What is "acceptable risk" to you? Are there any habits or behaviors that you now have that may lead to cancer (living in a city with severe air pollution, having a roommate who smokes, sun bathing without a sun screen, and so on)? How do you feel about the possibility of exposing yourself to cancer through these aspects of your life-style? How certain are you of the probabilities of cancer associated with these risks? Is denial of real risk an emotional reaction or an informed decision for you?

2. You have a friend who has cancer and is in the hospital. You know that he is afraid and lonely and you want to visit him. What are your emotions? What will you say to your friend?

3. You discover that your girl friend has never given herself a breast examination. How can you help her to learn the procedure and practice it regularly? How do you feel about doing this?

4. We still have much to learn about the causes, prevention, and elimination of cancer. Perhaps you have heard someone say, "If we can send a man to the moon, why can't we find a cure for cancer?" What is your emotional reaction to this statement? What is your intellectual reaction?

Chapter Contents

HOW MANY PEOPLE DEVELOP CANCER?

WHAT CAUSES CANCER?
Ingested chemicals
Diet factors
Alcohol and drugs
Inhaled chemicals
Radiation
Viruses

DETECTION AND DIAGNOSIS

PREVENTION

Boxes

Cancer and personality
Interferon research:
   new hope for cancer control
If you won't read these 7 signals of
   cancer . . . you probably have the 8th
Breast self-examination
Breast cancer surgery:
   from radical to conservative
Testicle self-examination

Cancer
A malignant growth of cells that multiplies at an uncontrollable rate; disease caused by uncontrolled multiplication of body, lymph, or blood cells; can occur in nearly any portion of the body.

Tumor
An abnormal mass of tissue that grows more rapidly than normal.

Benign tumor
A tumor that does not spread or invade other tissue.

Malignant tumor
A tumor that invades surrounding tissues and usually is capable of producing metastases; likely to recur after attempts have been made to remove it.

Chromosome
Genetic material carried in cells that causes new cells to be like the original cell.

Primary tumor
The abnormal growth at the original site of the cancer.

Metastasize
To spread a disease or its manifestations from one part of the body to another; in cancer, the appearance of new tumors in parts of the body remote from the primary tumor.

---

18 The term *cancer* refers to disorders of cell growth. These disorders, sometimes called malignant tumors, or neoplasms, all involve unregulated, unrestrained growth of the body's cells. Normally (in adults), cells divide and grow at a rate sufficient to replace dying cells. When you cut your finger, the cells around the wound divide more rapidly to heal the wound. When the wound is healed, the rate of cell growth and division returns to normal. The process is controlled by the nucleus of the cell. If nuclei lose their ability to regulate, the cells divide at random, resulting in growth called *tumors*.

Tumors serve no known physiological purpose. Some are made up of cells similar to the surrounding cells and are enclosed in a membrane that prevents them from penetrating other tissues. Such tumors, called *benign tumors*, are dangerous only if their physical presence interferes with bodily functions. For example, a benign tumor can cause death if it blocks the blood supply to the brain.

Cancers are *malignant tumors*. They kill by invading normal tissues, eventually destroying normal cells. The nuclei of cancer cells are larger than those of normal cells. They also have a greater number of *chromosomes*. Some researchers have suggested that an increase in the number of chromosomes produced may be the first detectable sign of cancer.

Cancer cells do not stick as closely together as normal cells or as tightly to their original site, called the *primary tumor*. They break away easily, which enables them to invade nearby tissues directly or spread to other parts of the body, where they establish new colonies of cancer cells. This traveling process is called *metastasizing*, and the new tumors are called *secondary tumors*, or metastases. Traveling cancer cells can follow two courses. They can produce secondary tumors in the lymph nodes or they can invade the veins (which are less resistant to invasion than arteries) and circulate through the veins to colonize other organs. (See Figure 18-1.)

This ability of cancer cells to metastasize is what makes early cancer detection crucial. To control the cancer and prevent death, every cancerous cell must be removed. Once cancer cells enter either the lymph or the blood system, it is usually impossible to stop their

Figure 18-1 Cancer spreads in three basic ways: Malignant tumors enlarge and extend into neighboring tissue (*a*). Cancer cells break loose easily and are carried through blood vessels and lymphatic vessels to other parts of the body (*b*). Dislodged cancer cells implant themselves in neighboring organs (*c*).

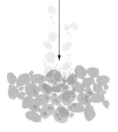

By direct extension into neighboring tissue

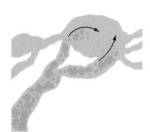

By permeation along lymphatic vessels

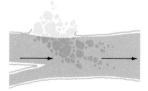

By embolism via blood vessels

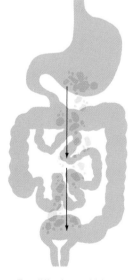

By diffusion within a body cavity

(*a*)   (*b*)   (*c*)

Secondary tumor
A metastasis; a tumor that has grown in a part of the body remote from the original site.

Carcinoma
A malignant and invasive epithelial tumor that spreads by metastasis and recurs after excision.

Sarcoma
Cancerous growth arising from bone, cartilage, or striated muscle.

Lymphoma
A tumor of the lymphatic tissues.

Leukemia
An almost uniformly fatal cancer of the blood characterized by excessive production of white blood cells, usually in increased numbers in the blood, and accompanied by often severe anemia and enlargement and hyperactivity of the spleen and lymphatic glands.

Pap smear
A preparation of cells from the cervix that is examined under the microscope to detect cancer.

---

spread to other organs of the body. Cancer cells can ravage a formerly strong and healthy body with frightening speed, depending on which part of the body they choose to invade. They may take over an artery, stopping the flow of blood to the kidneys, liver, and heart. Cancer cells growing in the pancreas or bone marrow may reduce the blood's ability to clot. If this happens, the victim may die from any ruptured blood vessel. Cancer in the lymph system weakens the body's ability to fight even the simplest fungus infection.

Malignant tumors are classified according to the types of cells that give rise to them. The most common cancers are carcinomas, sarcomas, lymphomas, and leukemia (*-oma* means "tumor"). *Carcinomas* are the most common form of cancer. They arise from epithelial cells—the cells forming the skin; glands, (breast, uterus, prostate); and membranes lining the respiratory (lungs, bronchial tubes), urinary, and gastrointestinal tracts (mouth, stomach, colon, rectum). Carcinomas metastasize primarily via the lymph vessels.

Sarcomas occur less often than carcinomas. They arise from more varied sources, such as connective fibrous tissues: muscle, bone, cartilage, and membranes covering muscles and fat. Sarcomas metastasize primarily via the blood vessels.

Lymphomas are cancers of the lymph nodes, the body's infection-fighting structures.

Leukemia is cancer of the tissues that form blood: an uncontrolled multiplication and accumulation of abnormal white cells.

How Many People Develop Cancer?

Cancer is second only to heart disease as a cause of death in the United States and is the leading cause of death among women aged 30 to 54 and among children aged 3 to 14. In 1900, 6 percent of the deaths in the United States were attributed to cancer; by 1975 cancer deaths had risen to 18 percent. More than 1,100 people a day die of cancer in this country. And at the present rate, one person in four will develop cancer in his or her lifetime.

Of the 800,000 people who were diagnosed as having cancer in 1982, about one third will be "cured"; that is,

they will be alive five years after treatment. Instead of saving a third, however, we could save half. Half the people who develop cancer could be cured if they learned what to look for and if they sought medical attention immediately.

Who gets cancer and what kind? The answers to these questions depend on sex, age, occupation, and geography, among other factors. Leukemia is the leading cause of death among children aged 3 to 14. For men the leading cancer sites are lungs, prostate, large intestine, stomach, and pancreas. The cancer death rate for black men has increased over 50 percent since 1950; for white men the increase is 20 percent. This increase is due mainly to the increasing incidence of lung cancer. (See Table 18-1, p. 410, and Figure 18-2, p. 411.)

For women the leading cancer sites are the breasts, large intestines, uterus, lungs, and ovaries (Table 18–1 and Figure 18–2). Since 1950 the overall death rate has declined 5 percent for black women and 10 percent for white women, mainly because of the increasing use of the Pap smear. The *Pap smear* is a laboratory technique that permits early recognition of cancerous cells in the reproductive tract. Unfortunately, the decreasing rate of death from cancers in the female reproductive tract is being somewhat offset by the rising rate of lung cancer (and subsequent deaths) among women. This increase, which is outrunning the increasing incidence of lung cancer among men, can be accounted for by an increase in the number of women who smoke tobacco. The number of teenage and preteenage girls who smoke tobacco is also increasing, so it is likely that the incidence of lung cancer in women will continue to rise.

Stomach cancer has become less common in the United States over the past 50 years and intestinal cancer more common. Intestinal cancer occurs much more often in the United States and Europe than in other parts of the world. Dietary habits may be partly responsible.

What Causes Cancer?

We do not know exactly what causes all the various types of cancer. A few uncommon types, including tumor of the retina, are inherited. And evidence is building to suggest that families inherit tendencies toward one type of cancer rather than another. But the

Table 18-1   Reference Chart: Leading Cancer Sites, 1984[a]

Site	Estimated New Cases 1984	Estimated Deaths 1984	Warning Signal: If You Have One, See Your Doctor	Safeguards	Comment
Breast	114,000	37,000	Lump or thickening in the breast.	Annual checkup; monthly breast self-examination.	The leading cause of cancer death in women.
Colon and rectum	126,000	58,000	Change in bowel habits; bleeding.	Annual checkup including proctoscopy, especially for those over 40.	Considered a highly curable disease when digital and proctoscopic examinations are included in routine checkups.
Lung	135,000	117,000	Persistent cough or lingering respiratory ailment.	80 percent of lung cancer would be prevented if no one smoked cigarettes.	The leading cause of cancer death among men and rising mortality among women.
Oral (including pharynx)	27,000	9,150	Sore that does not heal. Difficulty in swallowing.	Annual checkup.	Many more lives should be saved because the mouth is easily accessible to visual examination by physicians and dentists.
Skin	17,000[b]	7,100	Sore that does not heal or change in wart or mole.	Annual checkup; avoidance of overexposure to sun.	Skin cancer is readily detected by observation and diagnosed by simple biopsy.
Uterus	55,000[c]	10,000	Unusual bleeding or discharge.	Annual checkup, including pelvic examination with Pap test.	Uterine cancer mortality has declined 65 percent during the last 40 years with wider application of the Pap test. Postmenopausal women with abnormal bleeding should be checked.
Kidney and bladder	56,700	19,200	Urinary difficulty; bleeding—in which case consult doctor at once.	Annual checkup with urinalysis.	Protective measures for workers in high-risk industries are helping to eliminate one of the important causes of these cancers.
Larynx	11,000	3,700	Hoarseness—difficulty in swallowing.	Annual checkup, including laryngoscopy.	Readily curable if caught early.
Prostate	75,000	24,100	Urinary difficulty.	Annual checkup, including palpation.	Occurs mainly in men over 60; the disease can be detected by palpation and urinalysis at annual checkup.
Stomach	24,500	13,900	Indigestion.	Annual checkup.	A 40 percent decline in mortality in 25 years, for reasons unknown.
Leukemia	24,000	16,000	Leukemia is a cancer of blood-forming tissues and is characterized by the abnormal production of immature white blood cells. Acute leukemia strikes mainly children and is treated by drugs that have extended life from a few months to as much as 10 years. Chronic leukemia strikes usually after age 25 and progresses less rapidly.		
Other blood and lymph tissues	40,300	20,800	These cancers arise in the lymph system and include Hodgkin's disease and lymphosarcoma. Some patients with lymphatic cancers can lead normal lives for many years. Five-year survival rate for Hodgkin's disease increased from 25 percent to 54 percent in 20 years.		

Source: Incidence estimates are based on rates from American Cancer Society, *ACS: Cancer Facts & Figures 1984.*
       [a]All figures rounded to nearest 100.
       [b]Totals do not include nonmelanoma skin cancers (400,000 new cases).
       [c]Totals do not include cases in which the carcinoma is confined to the epithelium (over 40,000 new cases).

Carcinogen
Any substance that produces cancer.

majority of cancers appear to result from the introduction into the body of electromagnetic radiation or chemical or biological agents from the environment.

Life-style is an important element of a person's interaction with the environment. Not surprisingly, it plays a major role in the incidence of cancer among various groups of people. For example, Mormons and Seventh-Day Adventists are much less likely to develop cancers than most. Church doctrine of both groups forbids tobacco and alcohol use and recommends exercise and a nutritious diet. Seventh-Day Adventists who are vegetarians appear to have an even lower incidence of some kinds of cancer than do the meat eaters.

Agents that cause cancer are called *carcinogens*. Some carcinogens occur naturally in the environment (the ultraviolet rays of the sun, for example). Others are manufactured or synthesized substances. Some are present in the home environment—in the food we eat, the drugs we take, or the tobacco smoke we inhale.

Others are present in the work environment of certain industries. (See Table 18-2, p. 412.) Most carcinogens are physical or chemical irritants.

Ingested Chemicals   Some of the substances we eat, drink, or inhale are themselves carcinogenic. Others combine with chemicals present in the body to produce carcinogens. A great deal of money is invested in the production and marketing of these substances, and debates over their possible dangers have been long and bitter. The usual position taken by a manufacturer of a product suspected of being carcinogenic is that laboratory tests of the product were done on animals, not people, and that amounts of the substance given were much larger than a person would consume. The usual counterposition is that tests with laboratory animals have often been good predictors of results in people and that high doses are the best way we have of simulating the cumulative long-term effects of low doses.

Changes that have come about since World War II in

Figure 18-2   Cancer incidence by site and sex, and cancer deaths by site and sex. Percentages shown are estimates for 1984.

Male

INCIDENCE		DEATH
1%	Skin	2%
4%	Oral	3%
22%	Lung	35%
14%	Colon and rectum	12%
3%	Pancreas	5%
18%	Prostate	10%
9%	Urinary	5%
8%	Leukemia and lymphomas	8%
20%	All other	20%

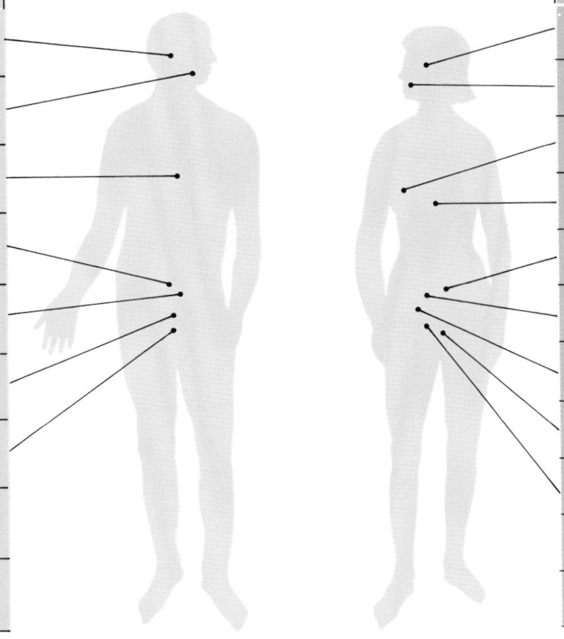

Female

INCIDENCE		DEATH
2%	Skin	1%
2%	Oral	1%
26%	Breast	18%
9%	Lung	17%
15%	Colon and rectum	15%
3%	Pancreas	5%
4%	Ovary	6%
13%	Uterus	5%
4%	Urinary	3%
7%	Leukemia and lymphomas	9%
15%	All other	20%

Preservatives
Food additives used to retard spoilage.

Additives (food)
Chemicals added to or found in food that are not normal constituents. Some, such as preservatives, coloring agents, and sweeteners, are deliberately added; others, such as insecticides and antibiotics, often appear as incidental additives.

Diethylstilbestrol (DES)
A drug used to treat menopausal symptoms but found to cause cancer in future female offspring.

Nitrosamines
Various chemical substances that can cause cancer.

methods of marketing and distributing food have greatly increased the length of time it takes food to travel from its source to the consumer. In the process, food may become stale and unappetizing or it may become spoiled and unsafe. The food industry has generally solved the spoilage problem by using *preservatives* and the staleness problem by using "cosmetic" *additives* —chemicals that disguise the look or the taste of staleness in food. Additives are, of course, used for many other reasons as well—as stabilizers, emulsifiers, fillers, or binders, for example. Some of the additives, such as salt, sugar, and saltpeter (potassium nitrate or sodium

nitrite) have been used for centuries; others, such as BHT, BHA, and MSG, are new products of the chemical industry. Dangerous chemicals may also make their way into the food supply as residues from insecticides and as traces of *diethylstilbestrol* (*DES*) or other synthetic hormones given to stimulate growth in cattle or other animals. (The United States has now banned that use of DES.)

Nitrates are a good case in point. Many food processors add sodium nitrate or sodium nitrite to ham, bacon, hot dogs, bologna, and other luncheon meats. The nitrates do two things: They preserve a pink color, which has no bearing on taste but looks more appetizing to many people, and they inhibit growth of bacteria that cause botulism, a disease that can be fatal. Nitrates are not carcinogenic in themselves, but they may combine with amines in the body to form *nitrosamines*, which are highly potent carcinogens in animals.

Some researchers suggest that nitrates added to smoked fish, a staple of the Japanese diet, are a factor in the high rate of stomach cancer in Japan. Other researchers claim that evidence linking nitrates and nitrites to cancer is inconclusive. They argue that nitrates and nitrites vaporize during cooking, that they occur naturally in saliva anyway, and that the formation of nitrosamines is blocked by vitamin C. Thus, according to these researchers, a glass of orange juice will prevent your breakfast bacon from contributing to the manufacture of carcinogens in your body.

While this controversy continues, the Food and Drug Administration has been acting to limit the addition of nitrates and nitrites to cured meats to just the amount needed to prevent botulism. One California supermarket chain has gone one step further. For several years it has been selling hot dogs containing no nitrates or nitrites at all, with no reported cases of botulism.

Artificial sweeteners such as saccharin and cyclamate have also been indentified as carcinogens. Some years ago the FDA banned the use of cyclamate because high doses induced cancer in animals. Later it ordered saccharin removed from the market for the same reason. These sweeteners are again available, but the basic problems are still unresolved. No one knows whether experimental results with animals suggest a duplicate human response to the same substances. Further, there

Table 18-2   Cancer in the Environment: Ten Suspects

Agents	Where Found	Cancers They May Cause
Arsenic	Mining and smelting industries	Skin, liver, lung
Asbestos	Brake linings, construction sites, insulation, powerhouses	Lung, pleura, peritoneum
Benzene	Solvents, insecticides, oil refineries	Bone marrow
Benzidine (outlawed in Great Britain and U.S.S.R., still used widely in U.S.)	Manufacturing rubber, dyestuffs	Bladder
Coal-combustion products	Steel mills, petrochemical industry, asphalt, coal tar	Lung, bladder, scrotum
Nickel compounds	Metal industry, alloys	Lung, nasal sinuses
Radiation	Ultraviolet rays from the sun, medical treatments	Bone marrow, skin, thyroid
Synthetic estrogens	Drugs	Vagina, cervix, uterus
Tobacco	Cigarettes, cigars, pipes	Lung, bladder, mouth, esophagus, pharynx, larynx
Vinyl chloride	Plastics industry	Liver, brain

Cancer and Personality

Theories about the link between cancer and personality . . . are still . . . controversial. Only recently, for example, has the issue been openly discussed at psychosomatics meetings. In 1957, when a psychologist, Dr. Lawrence LeShan, proposed to study the matter, virtually every hospital and research center in New York he contacted refused to allow him to use its facilities or interview its patients. Finally, the Institute for Applied Biology granted him access to some cancer patients, and he eventually interviewed and tested more than 500. His conclusion: By and large, they psychologically resembled each other in striking ways. Meanwhile, in Philadelphia, Dr. Claus Bahne Bahnson and Marjorie Brooks, studying other cancer patients, had arrived at similar findings.

More often than not, the two sets of research showed, cancer victims reported a disturbed childhood. They had been raised by emotionally distant parents or, early in life, they had either lost a parent or sibling. Although lonely and hurt, they had emerged from their bleak youth as model adults—conscientious, dutiful, solid citizens. (Notes Dr. Bahnson: "Cancer is little known among psychotics and schizophrenics who are at the other extreme, quite emotionally flamboyant.") Often they acquired a particular attachment to a "central relationship," most frequently a spouse or a job that gave new meaning to their lives. They showed an admirable stoicism. "Ask them how they are," says Dr. Bahnson, "and they're always 'just great,' no matter what the truth of the situation is." But clinical studies and psychological tests reveal a very different person behind the composed facade. Their stoicism hides a basic despair, which rises to the surface when the crucial central relationship disappears, when a beloved spouse dies or a job is lost. Within a short time, the studies indicated, the first symptoms of cancer appear.

A typical case concerned a woman who, a decade ago, had been diagnosed as having incurable cancer following her separation from her husband. Their daughter recalls: "My father felt incredibly guilty and finally agreed to move back in. My mother was extremely happy, and her cancer quite unexpectedly went into remission." When the old differences between the couple resurfaced, and the father left once again, the daughter reports, "My mother was quite broken up, and her cancer began to metastasize; she died soon afterward. Some people might call that coincidence. I must say, I don't."

Yet, even those scientists who believe that emotions play a role in cancer emphasize that it is a limited role, modified by genetic predisposition and environmental factors. And there are scientists who have strong reservations about the basic premise. "A lot of these studies have examined people who already have the disease," says Dr. Bernard H. Fox of the National Cancer Institute. "But some cancers are very slow-growing—can take up to 20 years or more before they reveal themselves. Meanwhile, biochemical changes taking place within the person's body may very well have some effect on his personality. So it's rather difficult to tell what he was like before the disease first started." Too many of the psychological studies of cancer are poorly designed, Dr. Fox complains, although he agrees that there is enough "highly interesting material" to warrant further investigation. The uncertainty of many scientists has led to a marked governmental reluctance to fund research into the "psychology" of cancer.

There is another order of concern over the growing public debate over the issue. Some fear that the new emphasis on personality factors will impose an additional burden on those already suffering from cancer, heart disease, or other ailments—a feeling that in some way they are to blame for their own illness. In some instances, as in the case cited above concerning the separated couple, friends or family members of an ill person may blame themselves, or others, for actions they feel contributed to a loved one's death. And scientists have noticed that those untouched by sickness sometimes develop a feeling of moral superiority toward those who are ill—a kind of "healthier-than-thou" smugness. Dr. Bahnson ridicules all such comparisons or notions of guilt. "No one," he says, "is any more to blame for his illness than the features on his face. Disease is so complex that to try to make any moralistic judgments about it is absurd."

Lawrence Cherry
New York Times Magazine

Estrogen
Female sex hormone.

Smog
Fog polluted by smoke and chemical fumes.

Radiation
A type pf energy. Some radiation (e.g., X rays) can damage living cells.

Diagnostic X rays
Photographs produced through radiation for detection and analysis of a disease.

Mammogram
An X ray of the breasts.

Melanoma
A malignant tumor of the skin.

Virus
A microorganism responsible for colds and many other illnesses.

---

may not even be such a thing as a safe dose of a potentially carcinogenic substance. In other words, the whole concept of a safe dose may be erroneous. These and similar problems occupy many cancer researchers fulltime.

Diet Factors   A "fatty diet" (one high in saturated fats such as are found in red meats) appears to contribute to cancer of the intestine and cancer of the breast, two of the most prevalent types of cancer. Scotland has the highest incidence of intestinal cancer in the world, and the Scots eat 20 percent more "fatty" meat than do their English neighbors. In Japan, fish, not fatty meat, is the staple, and intestinal cancer is uncommon. But Japanese who have emigrated to the United States, where fatty meats are an important part of the diet, appear to be as susceptible to intestinal cancer as other Americans.

Some populations, particularly vegetarians, have little or no colon cancer. The vegetarian diet typically is high in fiber, which suggests, according to some scientists, that colon cancer is related to a *lack* of fiber in the diet. Fiber does not supply nutrition; it provides bulk needed to move other foods through the digestive tract. The shorter transit time afforded by a high-fiber diet is believed by some to be an important factor in the low colon cancer rates of vegetarians. A diet high in meats, especially beef and pork, probably causes the digestive tract to work overtime to rid the body of material that is difficult to break down and excrete. Whether a diet high in both meat and fiber can result in a low incidence of colon cancer is still not known.

Breast cancer may also be linked to high fat intake. Scientists suspect that fats overstimulate hormone production or disrupt normal hormone balance.

Alcohol and Drugs   High alcohol intake is correlated to cancer of the mouth, pharynx, esophagus, larynx, and liver. The risk is greatest among drinkers who smoke, which suggests that alcohol and tobacco may interact as carcinogens. Oral cancer deaths are two to six times greater among men who drink more than 1½ ounces of hard liquor a day than among teetotalers, depending on how much tobacco the drinkers smoke. For the heavy drinker and smoker the risk is up to 15 times greater than for the nondrinking nonsmoker.

Certain prescription drugs, especially *estrogens* (female sex hormones) are also suspected of being carcinogenic. Shortly after World War II, DES (diethylstilbestrol) was prescribed for many infertile women. (DES is a synthetic drug that mimics the effects of natural estrogen.) The drug worked—that is, the women conceived—but 15 to 30 years later many of their daughters developed vaginal cancer. DES has also been used in a "morning-after" birth control pill and as a growth-stimulating hormone given to beef cattle. Cancer researchers recommend against the use of DES, but Australia and New Zealand are among only a few countries that have banned its use entirely.

Inhaled Chemicals   Inhaling carcinogenic irritants over a long period of time triggers the cancerous potentials in susceptible lung tissue cells. More Americans die of lung cancer (over 100,000, with the number increasing each year) than are killed in automobile accidents. Cigarette smoking (see Chapter 8) is responsible for at least 80 percent of lung cancer cases, and even people who do not smoke suffer from cigarette smoke in the air. A recently published major study found that women whose husbands smoked more than 20 cigarettes a day had more than twice the incidence of lung cancer as women whose husbands did not smoke.

Smog is another source of carcinogens. Industrial smoke and other pollutants mix with fog to produce smog. The chemicals in this highly irritating mixture contribute to a higher rate of lung cancer among city dwellers than among rural dwellers. Los Angeles and Pittsburgh have the highest death rates from lung and other respiratory diseases—and the thickest smogs.

Many chemicals used in the rubber, plastics, paint and dye, cable, and petrochemical industries have serious consequences for workers and their families (see Table 18–2). Carcinogens such as asbestos, nickel, and arsenic, as well as dusts, gases, and tars, continually irritate the lung tissue and may eventually alter the cell structure. Coal tar and its derivatives account for the largest group of occupation-related cancers.

Workers are not the only ones who suffer from these chemicals. They are also a hazard to people living near factories that use them. New evidence shows that people who live near asbestos plants, copper-smelting facilities,

Interferon Research: New Hope for Cancer Control

Interferon is a natural body substance discovered in 1957 to be effective against viruses and later found to inhibit tumor growth. Compared to other chemicals used to treat cancer, it appears to have few side effects.

Until recently, interferon for humans has been an expensive and scarce commodity produced only from fresh human blood. However, its early promise as an agent to control cancer has sparked interest from government sources, the American Cancer Society, and private industry, resulting in heavy investment in interferon research. Several investigators have reported more efficient and less expensive methods of producing interferon. These include

a chemical synthesis and the use of recombinant DNA techniques to introduce the interferon gene into bacteria that could then serve as "interferon factories" producing unlimited supplies of interferon at low cost.

All cells can produce interferon when they are stimulated by a viral infection. Human cells are known to produce at least three different forms of the substance. One kind is produced by white blood cells and is called *leukocyte interferon.* Another comes from connective tissue cells and is called *fibroblast interferon.* The third human interferon is produced by the T cells of the immune system and is called *T* or *immune interferon;* this type of

interferon may be the most important in cancer control because the immune system is generally thought to play an important role in preventing cancer development.

Although it is too early to tell what the long-term response to interferon will be, a number of patients have had early positive responses, especially to immune interferon, ranging from stabilization of a downhill trend to the complete disappearance of tumors. Interferon has opened the door to a whole new class of compounds called *biologic response modifiers,* which fight cancer by stimulating the body's immune system.

and industries that use vinyl chloride have a significantly increased risk of cancer and other diseases.

Radiation   Radiation can produce chemical changes in cells that can eventually lead to cancer. All sources of *radiation*—including X rays, radioactive substances, and sunlight—are potentially harmful. For example, uranium miners in Colorado have a very high incidence of lung cancer. Victims of the atomic bombs in Hiroshima and Nagasaki continue to suffer radiation effects, in the forms of breast cancer and leukemia, 40 years after the bombing. There is also a high incidence of leukemia among X-ray technicians. And children treated with radiation for tonsillitis and thymus gland diseases during the 1940s and 1950s have higher rates of thyroid cancer than those who were not treated.

Medical researchers cannot agree on the amount of risk involved in the use of *diagnostic X rays.* Some researchers say that a single abdominal X ray with the standard unit of dosage significantly ages the cells it strikes and thus increases the risk of leukemia. And some are convinced that irradiation of men and women during their reproductive years increases the likelihood that the offspring will develop leukemia. The National Cancer Institute now recommends that people below the age of 50 who want to avoid such perils avoid routine screening X rays of all kinds, including the low-dosage breast X rays known as *mammograms.*

Excessive exposure to ultraviolet radiation from the sun is the major cause of skin cancer, especially among fair-skinned people. Skin cancer has a 95 percent cure rate, but it is a common cancer and causes about 5,000 deaths a year. *Melanoma,* one type of skin cancer, is one of the deadliest cancers, and the death rate from melanoma is 75 percent higher in the southeastern states than it is in the less sunny northern states. People with light skin, particularly the freckling type, are about ten times more likely to develop skin cancer after excessive exposure to sunlight than are dark-skinned people. Heavy pigment evidently offers some protection against ultraviolet radiation. Skin cancer usually occurs in people over 50, but people may receive half the ultraviolet rays they will receive in their lifetimes by the time they are 30.

Viruses   *Viruses* cause some types of cancer in animals. Viruses survive by taking over living cells in the body. After the virus cell penetrates the animal cell, it sheds its protein overcoat, freeing its core to take over the functions of the plundered cell. The virus can then do one of several things. The virus can command the cell it has taken over to make more viruses like itself or to slow down its own self-multiplication. It can remain inactive for some time, all the while doubling its numbers with each division of the animal cells. Then, for reasons still unknown, it may suddenly infect the

Herpes simplex
A virus that causes sores or blisters on the skin or mucus membranes.

RNA (Ribonucleic acid)
Acid that is present in all cells along with DNA; plays an important part in protein synthesis.

Breast self-examination (BSE)
A procedure women can use to detect changes in their breasts that might be signs of cancer; done monthly.

Testicle self-examination
A procedure men can use to detect abnormalities in their testicles; done every six to eight weeks.

body. *Herpes simplex,* a disease characterized by "fever blisters," or "cold sores," appears to work this way. However it works, though, the virus robs the animal cell of its ability to make healthy cellular protein and to stick closely to other animal cells.

Table 18-3 Summary of ACS Recommendations for the Early Detection of Cancer in Asymptomatic People

Test or Procedure	Population		
	Sex	Age	Frequency
Sigmoidoscopy	M & F	over 50	every 3-5 years after 2 negative exams 1 year apart
Stool guaiac test	M & F	over 50	every year
Digital rectal examination	M & F	over 40	every year
Pap test	F	20-65; under 20, if sexually active	at least every 3 years after 2 negative exams 1 year apart
Pelvic examination	F	20-40 over 40	every 3 years every year
Endometrial tissue sample	F	at menopause; women at high risk[1]	at menopause
Breast self-examination	F	over 20	every month
Breast physical examination	F	20-40 over 40	every 3 years every year
Mammography	F	between 35-40 under 50 over 50	baseline consult personal physican every year
Chest X ray		not recommended	
Sputum cytology		not recommended	
Health counseling and cancer checkup[2]	M & F M & F	over 20 over 40	every 3 years every year

[1]History of infertility, obesity, failure of ovulation, abnormal uterine bleeding, or estrogen therapy.

[2]To include examination for cancers of the thyroid, testicles, prostate, ovaries, lymph nodes, oral region, and skin.

Acute leukemia, sarcoma, and melanoma are the cancers most likely to be linked to viruses. Breast cancer cells and leukemia cells in human beings contain *RNA* molecules similar to the RNA viruses known to cause similar cancers in animals. Thus far, however, we have no proof that viruses cause cancer in humans.

Detection and Diagnosis

Close self-monitoring is the key to early cancer detection (see Table 18–3). Indeed, one of the difficulties in detecting cancer is that the responsibility lies almost totally with the individual. Signals warning of cancer, unlike those of measles, mumps, or colds, are not apparent to anyone but the victim.

The American Cancer Society has listed seven warning signals that should alert people to the possibility of cancer:

1. Change in bowel or bladder habits.
2. A sore that does not heal.
3. Unusual bleeding or discharge.
4. Thickening or lump in breast or elsewhere.
5. Indigestion or difficulty in swallowing.
6. Obvious change in wart or mole.
7. Nagging cough or hoarseness.

None of these signals is a sure sign of cancer. For example, most breast lumps are not cancerous. But the appearance of any one of the signs should send you to see your doctor. Pain is seldom an early cancer signal, so if you wait until something hurts, it will be too late.

The need for women to practice *breast self-examination (BSE)* is urgent. Breast cancer is the leading cause of cancer deaths among women, and the regular practice of BSE could prevent most of these deaths. The American Cancer Society is making a great effort to educate high school girls to make BSE one of their regular health habits. Women should examine their breasts once a month, after each menstrual period (see page 419).

Self-examinations such as the BSE and *testicle self-examination* (see page 421) and yearly examinations by a physician of the sites especially susceptible to cancer

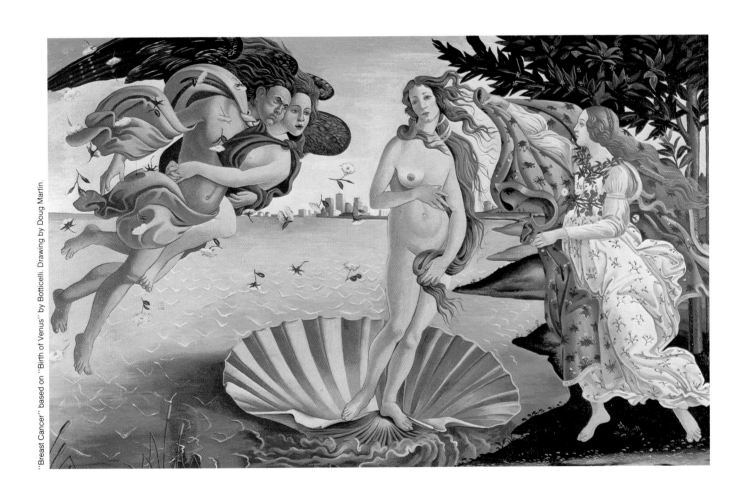

"Breast Cancer" based on "Birth of Venus" by Botticelli. Drawing by Doug Martin.

Thermography
Photographic portrayal of the surface temperature of body parts produced by measuring naturally occurring infrared radiation; used to diagnose cancer and other diseases that cause local changes in temperature.

Buccal smear test
Scraping and examination of cells from inside the cheek for precancerous changes.

> ## If You Won't Read
> ## These 7 Signals of Cancer . . .
> ## You Probably Have the 8th
>
> 1. Change in bowel or bladder habits.
> 2. A sore that does not heal.
> 3. Unusual bleeding or discharge.
> 4. Thickening or lump in breast or elsewhere.
> 5. Indigestion or difficulty in swallowing.
> 6. Obvious change in wart or mole.
> 7. Nagging cough or hoarseness.
> 8. A fear of cancer that can prevent you from detecting cancer at an early stage. A stage when it is highly curable. Everyone's afraid of cancer, but don't let it scare you to death.
>
> American Cancer Society

could save more lives than any other available means. Women and men who are over the age of 40 should have a yearly examination with a proctoscope, a lighted tube for examining the rectum and lower intestine, where cancer often strikes. Women of all ages should have a Pap smear once a year. If all women had this simple test yearly, deaths from cervical cancer would be virtually eliminated.

One of the most promising diagnostic techniques for detecting the early stages of breast cancer is *thermography*. Unlike mammography (breast X rays), thermography does not create risks from radiation. Thermography instead detects heat given off by malignant tumors.

Smokers should have annual examinations for lung and other cancers. Examination of saliva sometimes reveals the presence of precancerous cells. Tissues scraped from the inside of the cheek can also show the existence of cancer cells. This test is called the *buccal smear test*.

Loss of appetite and weight are strong indications of cancer. These effects lead, in turn, to generalized weakness and lack of resistance to disease. Anemia is a common symptom, resulting from malnutrition or

directly from cancer. The body's normal defense mechanisms become less effective, and death can result from bacterial or fungal infection.

Prevention

The belief that cancer strikes people randomly is giving way to a belief that cancer is something we do to ourselves. We may not know—or need to know—*why* we do this to ourselves, but we are learning a great deal about *how*, and we therefore have the means to stop doing it. We can begin to stop by learning all we can about carcinogens in our environment and removing either the carcinogens or ourselves from that environment. You can go a long way toward preventing cancer if you do the following things:

1. Avoid excessive exposure to sunlight to reduce the chances of skin cancer. Protect yourself from direct sun, especially at the beach.
2. Never smoke tobacco. At least 80 percent of lung cancers could be prevented if we gave up all tobacco smoking. Cancer of the mouth, throat, larynx, esophagus, and bladder would also occur less often.
3. Avoid X rays, if possible, to cut the risk of leukemia and cancer of the thyroid, breast, and lungs. Avoid all X rays during pregnancy and otherwise have only as many as are necessary to provide needed medical information.
4. Reduce your intake of foods containing preservatives when possible, particularly foods containing nitrites and nitrates. (*Read the list of ingredients!*)
5. Cut down on fatty meats such as beef, pork, and lamb. Increase your fiber intake.
6. Go easy on sweeteners, both artificial and natural.
7. Refuse to take drugs that may be dangerous, particularly those with high estrogen dosages.
8. Live in a city or—better yet—in a rural area where there is little smog.
9. Choose a job in an industry that does not specialize in producing carcinogens. If you must work in the rubber, plastics, paint and dye, cable, or petrochemical industry, make sure you are adequately protected from inhaling and touching the carcinogens present there.

Breast Self-Examination

Early detection of breast cancer is possible through monthly self-examination. Sit in front of a mirror, raise your arms, and check for unusual dimples in the skin or depression of the nipples (*a*). This check should also be done with the arms lowered. Then lie down and place a flat pillow or a folded towel under the shoulder of the same side as the breast to be examined. Keep the left arm at the side while the left breast is examined. Check the outer side of the breast, moving your hand up into the armpit (*b*). Using the flat part of the fingers, inspect the lower part of the breast (*c*) and then the upper part (*d*). Next, raise the left arm and repeat the procedure, beginning at the breast bone [(*e*) through (*h*)]. Repeat steps (*b*) through (*h*) with the right breast. If you detect a lump or unusual mass, you should contact a doctor immediately. If you find a similar lump or mass in the same place in the other breast, it probably is normal tissue. Breasts should be examined one week after the end of every menstrual period.

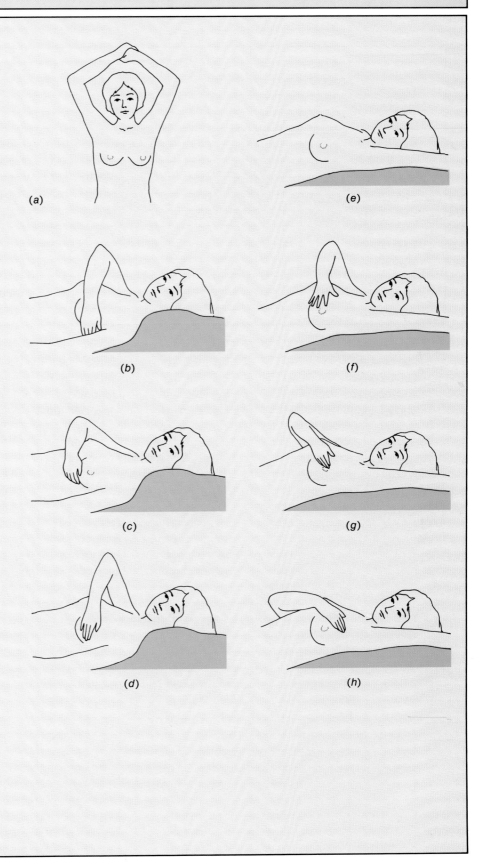

(a)

(b)

(c)

(d)

(e)

(f)

(g)

(h)

Breast Cancer Surgery: From Radical to Conservative

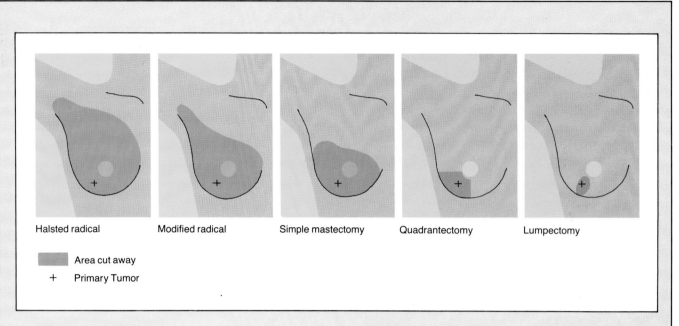

Halsted radical   Modified radical   Simple mastectomy   Quadrantectomy   Lumpectomy

▨ Area cut away
+ Primary Tumor

Mastectomy is the surgical removal of the breast. The oldest form, the *radical mastectomy (Halsted radical)*, introduced 80 years ago, removes the entire breast, the axillary fat and lymph nodes, both pectoral muscles on the affected side, and all overlying fat and skin. In a variation called *extended radical mastectomy,* the internal mammary lymph nodes (under the breastbone) and sometimes a portion of the rib cage may be included. Since 1979, the radical has become much less frequently performed, having been supplanted by the techniques below as well as by breast-preservation procedures, often referred to as "conservative procedures."

Breast-cancer patient Rose Kushner was instrumental in the American Cancer Society's officially condemning the Halsted radical as the routine treatment for breast cancer in favor of the *modified radical,* which involves the surgical removal of the entire breast and some or most axillary lymph nodes. The major pectoral muscle is preserved, but sometimes the pectoralis minor is removed.

Total mastectomy (also called *simple* or *complete*) is the removal of the breast only. Some axillary nodes may also be removed.

Conservative Procedures   The most extensive is the *partial (segmental)* mastectomy, sometimes called *quadrantectomy:* the removal of the tumor plus a wedge of surrounding normal tissue, some overlying skin, and part of the muscle facia (lining). A *wide excision* calls for the removal of the tumor and a margin of adjacent normal tissue only. *Tumorectomy* is a term meaning excision of the tumor only, a procedure that is also known as *lumpectomy.* An *excisional biopsy* is equivalent to a lumpectomy.

These conservative procedures are often accompanied by removal of some or all of the lymph nodes and followed by radiation therapy and, perhaps, chemotherapy as well.

Ruth Spear
New York Magazine

Testicle Self-Examination

Self-examination can permit early detection of testicular cancer. Although this type of cancer accounts for only 1 percent of cancer in men, it is the most common type of cancer in those who are 29 to 35 years old. Males with undescended testicles are at high risk for testicular cancer, and for this reason the condition should be corrected in early childhood.

The American Cancer Society recommends the following:

1. Perform the examination after a warm bath or shower, when the scrotal skin is most relaxed. (*Scrotal* refers to the scrotum, the pouch in which the testicles normally lie.)

2. Cup each testicle in the palm of one hand and examine it by feeling with the fingers of the other hand. The normal testicle is smooth, egg-shaped, and somewhat firm to the touch.

3. At the rear of each testicle is a tube called the epididymis, which carries sperm away from the testicle. This is a normal part of your body; its presence does not indicate cancer.

4. If there is any change in shape or texture of the testicles—or any lumps, especially hard ones—consult a doctor immediately.

Repeat this examination every six or eight weeks. It is important that you know what your own testicles feel like normally so that you will recognize any changes.

Cancer Risk Behavior Scale

Read the following statements carefully. Choose the one in each section that best describes you at this moment and record its score at the right. (For example, "knows the risk factors in cancer" has a score of 5.) When you have identified five statements, total your score and find your position on the scale.

5 knows the risk factors in cancer
4 knows that life-style is implicated in cancer
3 knows that lung cancer is caused by smoking
2 defends cancer risk behaviors such as smoking
1 denies that cancer can be prevented by life-style

Score _____

5 knows the recommendations for early detection of cancer
4 checks breasts or testicles regularly
3 knows cancer's warning signals
2 avoids thinking about cancer detection
1 resists cancer prevention

Score _____

5 avoids excessive sun exposure
4 uses sunscreens when exposed to the sun
3 sunbathes occasionally without protection
2 sunbathes regularly without protection
1 sunbathes frequently without protection

Score _____

5 avoids carcinogens
4 limits X rays
3 limits intake of foods with preservatives
2 prefers cured meats such as ham or bacon
1 eats burnt food

Score _____

5 lives in an area with little smog
4 has a job without exposure to carcinogens
3 has a job with exposure to carcinogens but is protected
2 lives in an area with heavy smog
1 has a job with exposure to carcinogens and is not protected

Score _____

Total score _____

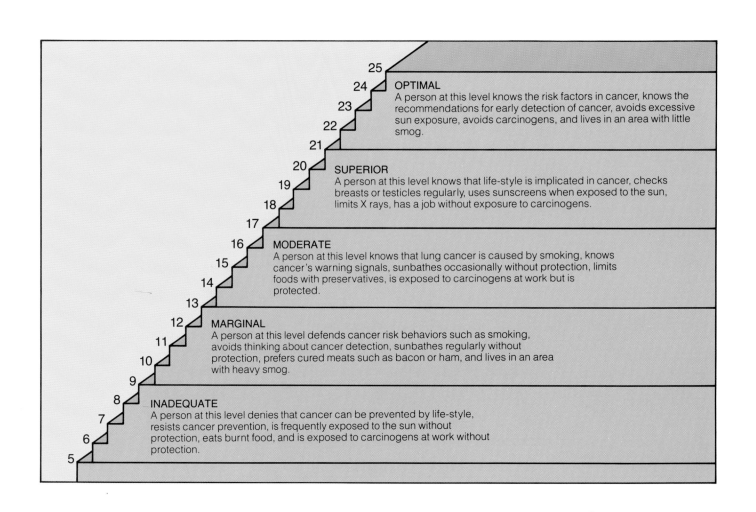

25
24 **OPTIMAL**
23 A person at this level knows the risk factors in cancer, knows the
22 recommendations for early detection of cancer, avoids excessive
21 sun exposure, avoids carcinogens, and lives in an area with little
    smog.

20 **SUPERIOR**
19 A person at this level knows that life-style is implicated in cancer, checks
18 breasts or testicles regularly, uses sunscreens when exposed to the sun,
17 limits X rays, has a job without exposure to carcinogens.

16 **MODERATE**
15 A person at this level knows that lung cancer is caused by smoking, knows
14 cancer's warning signals, sunbathes occasionally without protection, limits
13 foods with preservatives, is exposed to carcinogens at work but is
    protected.

12 **MARGINAL**
11 A person at this level defends cancer risk behaviors such as smoking,
10 avoids thinking about cancer detection, sunbathes regularly without
 9 protection, prefers cured meats such as bacon or ham, and lives in an area
    with heavy smog.

 8 **INADEQUATE**
 7 A person at this level denies that cancer can be prevented by life-style,
 6 resists cancer prevention, is frequently exposed to the sun without
 5 protection, eats burnt food, and is exposed to carcinogens at work without
    protection.

Take Action

Your answers to Probing Your Emotions at the beginning of this chapter and your placement level on the Cancer Risk Behavior Scale will, we hope, encourage you to begin a process of self-exploration and self-discovery that you will continue. Reflect on the entire chapter's content and ask yourself how each point relates to your own life. Then take action:

1. If you recently ate a hot dog or bacon you probably ingested sodium nitrite, which has been shown to be a cancer-causing agent in animals. Contact the American Cancer Society for a list of other such agents. Then make a list of the potential cancer-causing agents you ingested during the past week. Which ones could you have easily avoided?

2. Write a letter to three insurance companies, asking them about the circumstances under which they would insure cancer patients.

3. During the next 30 days keep track of periods of time of over 30 minutes during which you are exposed to the sun. If you feel you have been overexposed, show your records to your doctor and ask his or her opinion.

4. List the positive behaviors that may help you avoid cancer. Consider how you can strengthen these behaviors. Also list the behaviors that tend to increase your risk of cancer. Consider what you can do to change these behaviors.

Before leaving this chapter, review the questions that open the chapter. Have your feelings or values changed? Are you now better equipped to handle the complex and very human problems associated with cancer?

Chapter Nineteen

Infection and Immunity

Probing Your Emotions

1. As you arrive in class one morning, you learn that a friend, who had been in perfect health, has hepatitis. Two days later he is dead. You are brutally reminded of our frail hold on life and of the sea of microorganisms surrounding us. Do you feel your life will be materially altered if you know about the processes of infection and immunity?

2. Suppose the grocer who supplied the food for a party you had given for 30 of your friends about to disperse for summer vacations was reported to be a hepatitis carrier, responsible for infecting many of his customers. Several weeks after the party one friend is severely ill from a virus to which all the others were also exposed. What is your immediate reaction? What should you do? Whose help should you enlist?

3. Has anyone told you that a particular illness you have is "all in your mind," even though the symptoms (nausea, headache, running nose) are clearly real and uncomfortable? Can your mind trigger illness or predispose you to infection by lowering your natural resistance? If so, why has the medical profession expended so little effort in understanding the emotions, motivations, and thoughts of the "patient"?

Chapter Contents

PATHOGENS
Viruses
Bacteria
Fungi
Protozoa
Parasitic worms
DIAGNOSIS OF PATHOGENIC DISEASES
INFECTION: THE BREACHING OF DEFENSES
Body defenses
Scale of infectivity
Breakdown of body defenses
Treatment of infection
IMMUNITY
IMMUNE MECHANISMS
Nonspecific mechanisms
Specific mechanisms
RECOGNITION OF FOREIGN CELLS
IMMUNOLOGY OF CANCER
ALLERGIES
AUTOIMMUNE DISEASE
DO THE EMOTIONS AFFECT
THE IMMUNE RESPONSE?

Boxes

The common cold
Sickle-cell disease
Strange alliance: legions of
   bacteria created to serve man
The mind as healer
A pictorial history of events in infection immunity
Keeping up with the genetic revolution

Parasites
Organisms that feed on other living organisms.

Pathogens
Disease-producing substances or organisms.

Infection
A disease resulting from organisms that enter the body and grow and multiply there.

Enzymes
Proteins in the cells that aid chemical reactions.

Contagious disease
Disease capable of being spread from one person to others.

Herpes
A type of virus or a disease produced by this type of virus. A cold sore is an example of a herpes infection.

Poliomyelitis
An infectious disease that is caused by a virus and can result in temporary or permanent paralysis.

Hepatitis
A disease of the liver that is caused by a virus.

Debilitating
Causing extreme tiredness or weakness.

Infectious mononucleosis
A viral infection that affects white blood cells and gives rise to a feeling of weakness and extreme tiredness.

---

19 We are surrounded and inhabited by a multitude of potential enemies, most of them much too small to be seen. We speak of these organisms, which can take up residence and survive in the living tissue of humans or animals, as *parasites*. When parasites cause a disease they are known as *pathogens*. Disease caused by a pathogen is called *infection*. Who and what are these infective agents? How, being surrounded by them, do we defend ourselves from continuous infection? Under what conditions can pathogens breach your defenses and give rise to an infection? And what means do we have to overcome infections once they have started? This chapter will attempt to answer these questions.

Pathogens

In this section we shall discuss the classes of pathogens and the different ways in which they cause damage to the invaded host. In order of size, from smallest to largest, pathogens are classified as follows:

Viruses: subcellular, semiliving particles

Bacteria: unicellular, plantlike organisms

Fungi: unicellular and multicellular plantlike organisms

Protozoa: unicellular animals

Parasitic worms: multicellular animals

Viruses   Viruses, the smallest of the pathogens, are on the borderline between living and nonliving matter. They are visible only with an electron microscope. The pure virus particle appears to have no metabolism of its own. Viruses lack all the *enzymes* essential to energy production and protein synthesis in normal animal cells, and they cannot grow or reproduce by themselves. They must lead a parasitic existence inside a cell, borrowing what they need for growth and reproduction from the cells they invade. Once a virus is inside the host cell, its genetic material takes control of the cell and tricks it into manufacturing more viruses like itself. The normal functioning of the host cell is thereby disrupted. Different viruses infect different kinds of cells, and the seriousness

of the disease they cause depends greatly on which kind of cell is infected. The viruses that cause colds, for example, attack upper respiratory tract cells, which are constantly cast off and replaced. The disease is therefore mild. Polio virus, in contrast, attacks nerve cells that cannot be replaced, and the consequences, such as paralysis, are severe.

Over 150 viruses are known to cause disease in humans. Illnesses caused by viruses are the most common forms of *contagious disease*. They include most of the minor ailments that cause transitory illness and are rarely precisely diagnosed. Among these are the common cold; a variety of undiagnosed, short-lived respiratory infections; influenza; gastrointestinal upsets that cause diarrhea and can last for only 24 hours; and assorted aches and pains. More serious are the diseases that occur mainly in childhood and frequently cause a severe rash, such as measles, chickenpox, and mumps. Smallpox, which used to be the most severe of these diseases, has now been eliminated thanks to an encompassing vaccination program carried out by the World Health Organization in the 1960s and 70s. Infections from a variety of *herpes simplex* virus (type I) lead to sores that last from a few days to a week or two and appear mainly on the face around the mouth. (Herpes of the eye can be extremely serious and leads to loss of vision.) A second kind of herpes virus (type II) gives rise to a painful genital disease of similar duration.

More severe infections caused by viruses are *poliomyelitis*, a disease of the nervous system, and *hepatitis*. There are two major kinds of hepatitis. One is mainly transmitted by hypodermic injection and is common among drug addicts (hepatitis B), and the other is transmitted through fecal matter and spread through infected food or drink (hepatitis A). The latter is particularly prevalent in areas with poor hygienic conditions, but it can also be spread readily in societies with high hygienic standards via water contaminated with sewage efflux. It can be contracted on contaminated beaches and other swimming areas close to sewage outlets. The disease can be mild, although it is generally *debilitating* and requires a long period of bed rest. If neglected, hepatitis can lead to extensive liver damage and debilitation of the organism that can cause other infections to appear.

Spleen
An organ located in the upper left portion of the abdominal cavity that serves as a blood reservoir and plays an important part in fighting infection.

Warts
A mass on the surface of the skin that is caused by a virus.

Toxins
Poisons.

Impetigo
A serious skin disease that is marked by pus and yellowish crusts.

Acne
An inflammatory disease of the oil glands that is characterized by pimples on the face, chest, or upper back.

Sebum
An oily secretion of the sebaceous glands.

Strep throat
A bacterial infection of the throat.

Bronchitis
An inflammation of the mucus membranes in the lining of the bronchi, which lead to the lungs.

Pneumonia
A serious infection of the lungs.

Tuberculosis
An infectious disease of the lungs that is caused by a bacterium; less of a problem in the United States than in other parts of the world.

In a similar category is the disease of children and young adults—*infectious mononucleosis.* This is a virus infection that affects white blood cells and gives rise to a debilitated condition. With adequate rest, there are no consequences; however, when neglected, the *spleen* may rupture, causing the need for removal of this organ and a life-long increase in susceptibility to infection.

Certain viruses can also cause proliferation of cells. The human disease clearly based on this property is *warts*, which generally is a very mild disease but can become extremely severe if the resistance of the infected individual breaks down. In rodents many viruses can cause cancer, and they are suspected of doing so in humans, but this has not yet been demonstrated.

Bacteria   Bacteria, which can be seen under a light microscope, are generally 100 to 1,000 times larger than viruses. On the other hand, they are considerably smaller than mammalian cells, most of which can hold 50 to 100 bacteria. The three basic shapes of bacteria are shown in Figure 19-1.

Of several thousand species of bacteria, approximately 100 cause disease in humans. Most bacteria are neither parasites nor pathogens, however, and many are quite beneficial. Unlike viruses, many, but not all, disease-causing bacteria do not have to enter cells to cause infection. They generally thrive on, around, and between human cells and can cause harm through the *toxins* and poisonous enzymes that they produce. (Some bacterial toxins are among the most powerful poisons known. One fourth of a teaspoon of a toxin released by the tetanus organism can kill over 10,000 people.)

Some of the toxins and poisonous enzymes bacteria produce work locally, killing and dissolving the cells near the site of the infection. The damaged cells become food for the bacteria. The infection then spreads deeper into the surrounding tissue, giving rise to boils, abscesses, soreness, and the like. Other bacterial products are carried by the bloodstream, causing fever or affecting vital organs and systems (such as the nervous system in a tetanus infection). Some pathogenic bacteria have no specific toxic attributes. They grow to large numbers and cause damage by obstructing vital pathways of the host—the lungs, for example—and by consuming materials needed by host cells for sustenance.

Generally speaking, almost all bacterial infections require attention. Chief among these are skin infections such as small abscesses or boils, which, when unattended, can give rise to major complications. Such superficial skin infections are generally caused by bacteria known as *staphylococci* and *streptococci*. If the infection persists, it may cause a more serious disease known as *impetigo*, which requires a physician's attention. *Acne* is caused by relatively innocuous bacteria growing in hair follicles (pores that give rise to hair). These bacteria plug the pores and produce inflammatory substances that cause pus formation. Good hygiene often can remove *sebum* and other substances that such bacteria require.

Common diseases of the respiratory pathways are *strep throat*, *bronchitis*, and *pneumonia*. These vary in severity. Because they generally respond rapidly to treatment with antibodies, they should be treated early.

Tuberculosis, a disease of the lungs, is caused by a very resistant bacterium and used to be a major problem.

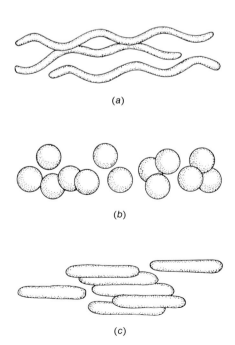

(a)

(b)

(c)

Figure 19-1   The three basic shapes of bacteria: (*a*) spirilla, (*b*) cocci, and (*c*) bacilli.

Periodontal disease
An infection of the gums.

Dental caries
Tooth decay.

Appendicitis
A serious infection of the appendix, which is a small tube that extends from the intestine in the lower right portion of the abdomen.

Diverticulitis
Inflammation of pouches in the intestine.

Salmonellosis
Food poisoning characterized by high fever and caused by salmonella bacteria.

Botulism
Acute food poisoning characterized by weaknesss, dizziness, nausea, and eventually respiratory paralysis and possible death; caused by botulinum bacteria.

Typhus fever
A serious disease that is characterized by a high fever and a dark red rash and is caused by a rickettsia.

Trachoma
A contagious disease of the eye that is caused by a rickettsia.

Candidiasis
A fungal infection that can involve the skin, respiratory tract, or vagina.

Sufferers had to be isolated from the rest of the population during the infectious stage of the disease. The incidence of tuberculosis has significantly declined through the use of certain drugs. Nonetheless, the disease is far from being eradicated in the United States, and it still presents a major problem in many countries of the world.

Periodontal disease, an infection of the gums, attacks over 50 percent of the population. It is caused by a variety of bacteria and can lead to extensive and painful consequences. Probably the most common consequence of bacterial infection is *dental caries,* a scourge known to almost everyone who has ever sat in a dentist's chair. It is caused by products of streptococci, which are related to the organisms that cause strep throat.

Bacterial diseases of the stomach and intestines (gastrointestinal or G.I. tract) are more common in children than in adults. However, localized G.I. infections such as *appendicitis* can occur at any age. In middle-aged and older people another localized form of infection, known as *diverticulitis,* can occur. This results from food caught in little deformations of the intestine known as diverticuli.

Food poisoning is not always a consequence of direct infection. It can be caused by food that has been standing at temperatures that allow bacteria to grow. These bacteria produce toxins that can cause severe illness and high fever, and it is wise not to eat food that has been standing in a warm place for more than six hours. Among foods that can give rise to severe infection are insufficiently cooked poultry, unwashed eggs, and, occasionally, prepared meats, such as sausage. Infec-

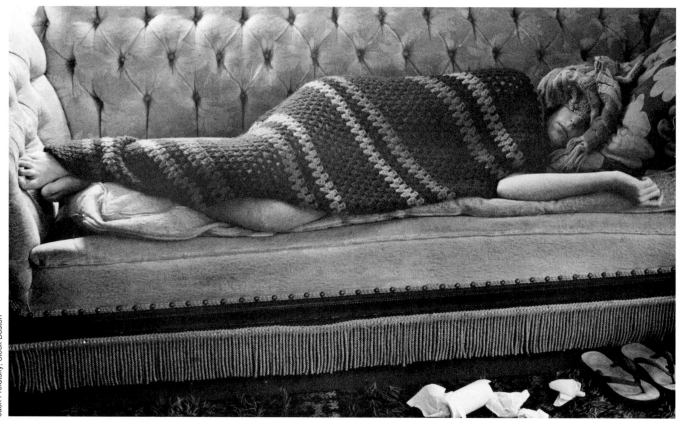

Jack Prelutsky, Stock Boston

Thrush
Common name for candidiasis, particularly in infants.

Athlete's foot
A form of ringworm that affects the feet.

Jock itch
A fungal infection of the skin of the groin area.

Ringworm
Fungal infections of the skin.

Systemic
Throughout the system; affecting the whole body.

Cryptococcosis
A fungal disease that affects the whole body, including the brain.

Coccidioidomycosis
A respiratory infection that results from spore inhalation.

Malaria
A recurrent disease that is marked by high fever and is transmitted by mosquitoes.

African sleeping sickness
A lethal disease transmitted by the tse-tse fly.

Amoebic dysentery
A recurrent disease that is characterized by abdominal pain and diarrhea.

Trichomoniasis
A vaginal infection that causes a discharge and inflammation.

---

tions arising from contaminated food are caused by organisms called salmonella and are therefore known as *salmonellosis*.

The most lethal bacterial poison carried by food is that of the botulinum organism. These organisms grow in the absence of air, and improperly canned food is the main source of them. Home-canned foods are the chief offenders. The early appearing symptoms of botulism—weakness, dizziness, and nausea—soon give way to respiratory paralysis, which can lead to death within 36 or 48 hours after food consumption. Sterilizing foods by cooking prior to canning avoids the growth of the organism. The toxin itself is degraded by boiling the canned food for 10 minutes.

The urinary tract of women is particularly accessible to bacteria, and urine presents a relatively good source of bacterial nutrient. Therefore, bladder infections occur fairly frequently in women. Although these infections are not necessarily severe, they can become so if they are not treated promptly. Such infections can also lead to an ascending infection of the kidneys, which can be extremely serious.

Some bacteria are like viruses in that they can reproduce only within living host cells. A group of these, called rickettsiae, are usually transmitted by insects such as fleas, lice, mites, and ticks. Diseases that are caused by rickettsiae include *typhus fever* and Rocky Mountain spotted fever. Another type of bacterium that needs the host cell causes an eye infection called *trachoma*. The trachoma organism is spread by poor hygienic conditions. It affects over 200 million people in Asia and Africa. In the United States the chief infection due to the trachoma organism (thought to be *chlamydia trachomatis*) is a sexually transmitted disease in women. This disease is difficult to diagnose. It has reached nationwide epidemic proportions, rivaling gonorrhea. (See Chapter 20.)

Fungi   Fungi are primitive plants that may be multicellular (like molds) or unicellular (like yeasts). Mushrooms and the molds that form on bread and cheese are all examples of fungi. Only about 50 fungi of many thousands of species cause disease in humans, and these diseases usually are restricted to the skin, mucous membranes, and lungs. Curing fungal disease is extremely difficult. To defend against treatments, some fungi form spores, which are an especially resistant dormant stage of the organism.

The most common fungal malady is *candidiasis*, a yeast infection of the vagina that can also occur in other areas of the body, especially in the mouth in infants (here it is known as *thrush*). Candidiasis, a relatively mild disease that causes itching, should be examined by a physician. When unattended and persistent, this disease can become severe and involve inflammation of the mucous membranes on which it normally exists. (See Chapter 20.)

Another common group of fungal diseases are diseases of the skin, including *athlete's foot, jock itch,* and *ringworm*, a disease of the scalp. These three are rather mild diseases that, although difficult to treat, rarely give rise to major problems.

Fungi can also cause *systemic* (infecting large portions of the body) disease. Such disease is severe, life-threatening, and extremely difficult to treat. Among the systemic forms of fungal disease are *cryptococcosis* and *coccidioidomycosis*, also known as valley fever because it is most frequently seen in the San Joaquin Valley in California.

Protozoa   The protozoa, microscopic single-celled animals, are associated with such tropical diseases as *malaria, African sleeping sickness,* and *amoebic dysentery*. Many protozoa-based diseases are recurrent. The pathogen remains in the body, alternating between activity and inactivity. Hundreds of millions of Asians, Africans, and South Americans suffer from a protozoal infection. The most common protozoal disease in the United States is *trichomoniasis*, a vaginal infection. (See Chapter 20.)

Parasitic Worms   The parasitic worms are the largest organisms that can enter the body to cause infection. The tapeworm, for example, can grow to a length of several feet. Worms, including such intestinal parasites as the tapeworm, hookworm, and pinworm, cause a

Gonorrhea
A sexually transmitted disease caused by a type of bacteria.

Cilia
Hairlike appendages on certain cells.

Leukocytes
White blood cells.

Adaptive or acquired immunity
Immunity obtained by overcoming a particular disease or by being vaccinated against it.

Vaccination
Producing immunity by injection of attenuated or killed organisms or injection of toxoids.

---

large variety of relatively mild infections. Smaller worms—known as flukes—infect organs such as the liver and lung and can be quite deadly.

Diagnosis of Pathogenic Diseases

Although most fungal and protozoal diseases are relatively easy to diagnose as such, it is frequently difficult to distinguish between viral and bacterial diseases. In general, however, the most common viral diseases are relatively mild and of short duration. The symptoms they produce are usually caused by the reactions of defense systems of the body trying to eliminate the invading virus. Because this defense requires elimination of an invader that inhabits the body's own cells, some tissue destruction results. The severity of the disease is frequently dependent on the extent of the body's own responses. Such tissue destruction is often accompanied by fever. In addition, reflexes such as mucus secretion and coughing, which serve to remove the invading organism, are perceived as noxious by the suffering patient. Fortunately, mild infections are typically of short duration.

The more common bacterial infections, on the other hand, last longer and are usually accompanied by some marked symptoms. There are notable exceptions, however. The most important exception is *gonorrhea*, which, especially in women, may show no symptoms for long periods of time but remain infectious and capable of causing severe problems. (See Chapter 20.) The hallmark of bacterial infections, when they are localized, is the accumulation of pus, which is seldom present with viral infections.

The common fungal and protozoal infections, especially those prevalent in the Western world, are generally marked by their persistence and their mildness. It must be remembered, however, that any mild condition can become severe when it is neglected and allowed to spread or when the defenses that keep it limited break down. It is a sound health principle that any persistent infection condition, even if it is only mildly disturbing to the individual, should be treated.

Infection: The Breaching of Defenses

In discussing infection we must briefly outline the defenses of the body. Later in this chapter these will be more extensively described and discussed.

Body Defenses   The primary lines of defense of the body are the external barriers that prevent ready access to the more vulnerable interior of the body. These consist of the outside skin and the mucous membranes that line the gastrointestinal and respiratory tracts. In addition, special defenses are placed at the most conspicuous points of entrance of microorganisms. The nose and throat secrete mucus and are armed with *cilia,* hairlike appendages that can sweep out substances that attempt to penetrate. The ears secrete wax that prevents a ready access to the interior ear. The eyes have a potent protective mechanism in tears and the continuous sweeping action of the eyelids.

In addition to these physical barriers to penetration, the body has a very sophisticated armament of secondary defenses. Cells that can ingest and digest organisms are present in mucous membrane surfaces and throughout the interior organs and bloodstream. Collectively, they are called "white cells," or *leukocytes.* As explained later, these white cells have additional functions that involve a learning process. They learn to recognize foreign materials and to produce substances and reactions, beyond that of ingestion, that are designed to counter infection at many levels. This ability to retain a memory of previous infections is known as *adaptive* or *acquired immunity.* As we shall see later, such immunity can be acquired either through overcoming the particular disease or through deliberate immunization with the pathogen or its components or products. When this immunization involves injection, it is called (somewhat incorrectly) *vaccination.*

The defenses brought to bear on invading organisms by the mechanisms of acquired immunity are potent and multifaceted. Even in unimmunized individuals, those exposed to the particular disease agent for the first time, these mechanisms come into play progressively as the infection advances, and they constitute the ultimate means of the body of ridding itself of invading organisms.

The Common Cold

Since the discovery of penicillin in 1928 there has been more progress toward the prevention and treatment of infectious diseases than in all the rest of medical history combined. Smallpox has now been eradicated, typhoid fever has become a rarity, and pneumococcal pneumonia is both curable and, now, preventable. And yet no means has been found, to date, to eliminate or cure the common cold, which, it has been estimated, costs $5 billion each year in lost wages and medical expenses.

In fact, the common cold is not a simple matter; rather, it is a complex of symptoms. Caused by any one of a group of viruses (more than 120 different viral strains that produce common cold symptoms in humans have been isolated), the common cold is primarily an infection of the lining membrane of the upper respiratory tract, including the nose, the sinuses, and the throat. This delicate membrane reacts to infection by swelling and by increasing its rate of mucus formation, leading to congestion, stuffiness, and a great deal of nose blowing. Due to loss of the nasal cavity as a resonating chamber, a characteristic change in voice quality also occurs. The increased mucus flow usually causes a postnasal drip, which is irritating and contributes to the familiar ''scratchy'' throat and cough.

The sinuses, which normally empty into the nasal cavity, may become blocked by excessive swelling of the membranes. The resultant increase in sinus pressure may cause a headache. In similar fashion, swelling in the upper part of the throat can block the Eustachian tubes—the two narrow canals that lead to the ears. This blockage can cause accumulation of fluid and pressure in the middle ear, which may be painful. Less commonly, an unpleasant spinning sensation known as vertigo may result.

A cold is usually self-limited, lasting about one to two weeks. At any time during the course of a cold, bacteria (such as staphylococci or pneumococci) can be secondary invaders, bringing on painful infections of the sinuses and ears. However, the old warning that, if you don't take care, a cold will turn into pneumonia, is hardly ever true. Pneumonia and most other infections of the lower respiratory tract begin in the bronchi and the lungs rather than in the upper respiratory tract.

Most people stay home from work or school because of generalized symptoms—muscle aches, weakness, and fatigue. The extent of these symptoms varies from person to person. Although mild elevation of temperature can occur with the common cold, a rectal temperature above 101°F is usually a sign of a more serious viral or bacterial infection. If fever above 101°F, taken rectally, persists beyond two days, medical advice should be sought.

Americans spend more than $900 million a year for cold and cough remedies. Advertisers have claimed preventive and curative virtues for vitamins, alkalizers, lemon drinks, antihistamines, decongestants, timed-release capsules, bioflavonoids, nose drops and sprays, quinine pills, aspirin mixtures, laxatives, inhalers, aromatic salves, liniments, room air sprays, and a variety of other products. There are at least 300 over-the-counter (OTC) products—most of which are a combination of ingredients—marketed for the treatment of symptoms of the common cold. Many of these drugs do neither good nor harm to the cold victim—but there is no doubt that they benefit the drug manufacturers.

Everyone has heard of sure-fire formulas for preventing a cold. Popular home methods include a cold shower, regular exercise, and a hot rum toddy. Some people swear by cod-liver oil, tea with honey, citrus fruit juices (or massive doses of vitamin C), or keeping one's feet dry. At one time, many large firms encouraged their employees to submit to inoculations with cold ''vaccines.'' And splendid results from these programs were regularly reported. But such vaccines, like many other ''scientific'' (or folk) remedies, gradually have been abandoned as experience and controlled testing have proved their uselessness in preventing colds. Now, just as fifty years ago, Americans on the average will suffer two to three colds a year, the acute infectious stages of which will last about a week or two (although a cough or postnasal drip may linger), regardless of any physical measure, diet, or drug used to try to head off the colds. U.S. Public Health Service (PHS) studies show that, during the winter quarter of the year, 50 percent of the population experiences a common cold; during the summer quarter, the figure drops to 20 percent.

It is unfortunate that the name ''cold'' has been given to this common, but minor, malady. The name has led many people to infer that the common cold is somehow caused by walking bareheaded in the rain, not wearing enough winter clothing, or getting caught in a draft. There is as yet no evidence that the common cold ever occurs in the absence of an infecting organism. Moreover, studies have

(continued on next page)

The Common Cold (continued)

shown that chilling does not predispose one to infection with the cold virus (or viruses). The increased incidence of colds in winter reflects the fact that people spend more time indoors, thereby facilitating the transfer of viruses from person to person. In fact, one is less likely to catch a cold after exposure to the elements than after mixing with a convivial group of snifflers and sneezers at a fireside gathering.

The common cold, it is now reasonably certain, is not only spread by sneezing and coughing but also by shaking hands and handling contaminated articles. The home, office, classroom, bus, or any other place where people gather is a good spreading ground. But resistance seems to vary greatly among individuals, so that not everyone exposed to a common source of infection becomes ill. Moreover, the natural factors—whatever they are—that contribute to resistance in an individual may be operative at one time and not at another. Thus it is not uncommon for some unlucky person to have a "bad year," suffering from as many as five or six colds, and then remain in excellent health during the following year or two. These variations in resistance and the irregular pattern in the occurrence of colds make it extremely difficult to evaluate the effect of any medication on the course of the common cold.

Consumers Union
The Medicine Show

Sickle-Cell Disease

Sickle-cell disease is a blood disorder caused by an inherited abnormality in hemoglobin, the part of the red blood cell that carries oxygen to all parts of the body. Hemoglobin has an identifiable biochemical structure determined by the combination of two inherited genes. When the most common or usual hemoglobin gene (Hemoglobin A gene) is inherited from each parent, the hemoglobin structure is called "Hemoglobin AA" to reflect two inherited A genes.

While most people have Hemoglobin AA, abnormal hemoglobins are formed when one or both inherited genes are not of the common A type. Over 320 hemoglobin variations (named by symbols such as C, S, D [Punjab], E, and so on) have been identified. Fortunately, most unusual hemoglobins do not affect the red blood cell or are combined with enough Hemoglobin A to let the blood do the job of carrying oxygen. However, some abnormalities create problems. The most severe effects are those associated with the Hemoglobin S gene or "sickle hemoglobin."

The blood disease sickle-cell anemia results when an S hemoglobin gene is inherited from both parents (Hemoglobin SS). Sickle hemoglobin gets its name from the tendency of this abnormal red blood cell to become elongated or sickle-shaped rather than retaining the flexible disc shape of normal red cells. Sickled cells become too rigid and brittle to pass through small blood vessels in the body. Instead, sickled cells clump together like a logjam in a river and obstruct blood and oxygen flow to the tissues. With oxygen cut off from some parts of the body, the patient with sickle-cell anemia may experience an episode of severe pain called a "crisis" and possible tissue damage. Other medical complications linked to sickled cells include frequent infections, organ damage, and skeletal damage. These may be serious enough to limit activity, interfere with work or schooling, and ultimately shorten expected life span. Because cells with Hemoglobin SS sickle under different conditions and vary in their effects, the clinical course of sickle-cell anemia is unpredictable. Some patients are very ill while others have infrequent difficulty. Increased attention to symptoms and complications allows many children with this condition to live to adulthood and lead productive lives, even though they are restricted in some activities. Yet no cure for sickle-cell anemia is known. It continues to be a serious chronic illness that all too often becomes life threatening.

In addition to the personal suffering that sickle-cell disease inflicts on over 50,000 affected Americans and their families, several commonly held misconceptions about sickle-cell disease are significant in their societal consequences. A first misconception comes from confusion between sickle-cell anemia and sickle-cell trait. What is called "sickle-cell trait" is really a carrier state for healthy persons capable of passing on a sickle-cell gene. It is not a trace or mild form of sickle-cell anemia. A person with sickle-cell trait has inherited a sickle gene from one parent along with a normal A gene from the other (forming Hemoglobin AS). This contrasts

Sickle-Cell Disease (continued)

with the Hemoglobin SS of sickle-cell anemia. With AS hemoglobin, the functions of the red cell continue. People with "trait" have no illness from the hemoglobin structure and may be unaware that their hemoglobin is abnormal. Nevertheless, the common misconception that sickle-cell "trait" is a mild form of sickle-cell anemia has led to discrimination in employment, in obtaining insurance, and in interpersonal relationships.

Being a carrier of the sickle-cell gene is only of concern if two individuals with trait have a child. These parents face a risk of having a child with sickle-cell anemia. A child inherits one gene from each parent. The parent with Hemoglobin AS can contribute *either* a sickle (S) hemoglobin gene *or* a normal (A) gene to each offspring. When both parents have sickle-cell trait (both A and S genes) *and* it happens that they each contribute their abnormal S gene, their child will have sickle-cell anemia (Hemoglobin SS). The chance of this is calculated from the 50 percent chance of passing on the S or A hemoglobin: each child of two AS parents has a 25 percent chance of inheriting Hemoglobin AA, a 50 percent chance of Hemoglobin AS (trait), and a 25 percent chance of receiving the S gene from each parent to form Hemoglobin SS, sickle-cell anemia.

A second misconception about sickle-cell disease is the belief that it only affects blacks. While it is true that sickle-cell disease is most prevalent among people of African descent, hemoglobin abnormalities are found among ethnic groups of African, Mediterranean, and Asian heritage. One explanation for this ethnic pattern comes from the theory that the structure of AS hemoglobin (sickle-cell trait though not sickle-cell anemia) may have

been associated with resistance to malarial-related death in the African and Mediterranean region. In the United States, current estimates of the prevalence are that 1 in 12 American blacks have sickle-cell trait, and 1 in 600 have sickle-cell anemia. These rates vary in different geographical areas, indicating again the genetic nature of the sickle hemoglobin gene.

A third issue in public understanding of sickle cell involves prevention of the condition. Because the genetic transmission is statistically predictable if parental hemoglobin is known, preventing the birth of sickle-cell children has been suggested as the only way to deal with the illness. Mass screening programs targeted at the black population were emphasized when reliable hemoglobin tests became available. The goal was to identify sickle-cell carriers who were unaware of their status because they had no illness but could pass on the gene. (Persons with sickle-cell anemia would already have been detected because they would have experienced illness with the condition.) Supporters of screening programs argued that birth control among those with trait to prevent sickle-cell anemia would reduce needless suffering.

Critics of major screening efforts pointed to the potential use of genetic information to discriminate against individuals or to pressure the reproductive decisions of several racial minority groups. Opponents also suggested that large-scale screening is expensive and tends to be repeated unnecessarily. Unlike blood pressure, hemoglobin type never changes over time. Further, knowledge of sickle-cell trait is only of importance at the time of reproductive choice. It is irrelevant to the very old or very young and

might cause distress if the complex nature of the carrier state is not understood correctly. With increased sensitivity to these concerns, community hemoglobin screening directed at particular racial groups is now less popular. Several states, however, require hemoglobin testing of newborns to identify possible genetic abnormalities without regard to the infant's racial background.

Another approach to preventing sickle-cell anemia involves programs which offer voluntary hemoglobin testing services to any concerned individual. Following testing, persons with sickle-cell trait are counseled about their status as healthy individuals and as sickle-cell carriers. Counseling is intended to allow those of childbearing age to make their own decisions about reproduction based on accurate medical information.

Thus, misconceptions about sickle-cell anemia and confusion about trait make this condition significant for a community larger than those suffering directly from sickle-cell disease. Decisions about appropriate emphasis in screening, the need for availability of testing and counseling, and ethical concerns over reproductive decisions are the societal issues involved in this complex genetic field. Minority concerns about needless discrimination against those with sickle-cell trait and the fear of pressures on any groups at risk for an inherited disease are relevant to all.

Health is increasingly recognized as dependent both on our individual decisions and on the physical structure that we have inherited. Sickle-cell disease brings together these concerns of genetic structure, individual responsibility, and community health.

Katrina W. Johnson

Virulence
The ability of a given pathogen to overcome the immune system and cause disease.

Integrity
Wholeness; here, the ability of the body to defend itself against disease.

Opportunistic organisms
Organisms in the body that are activated by other organisms or conditions to cause disease.

Fecal matter
Bodily wastes that are discharged from the anus.

Bubonic plague
A highly infectious disease that is often carried by rats.

Cholera
A serious infectious disease that is marked by severe diarrhea and vomiting.

Influenza
A highly contagious viral disease that is characterized by aches, pains, and fever.

Most of the time these potent defenses can protect the normal, healthy host from infection. How then do the potential invaders manage to breach these defenses? Their ability to do so depends on their *virulence*, the *integrity* of the defenses of the host, and peculiarities in the host's makeup that are chiefly determined by heredity.

Scale of Infectivity   Organisms can be placed on a scale of infectivity. At the bottom of the scale are the so-called *opportunistic organisms*, those that require a great deal of circumstantial help in order to initiate a disease process. These include a number of the organisms that normally survive in our gut and form part of the *fecal matter*. In this group are a variety of organisms that rarely if ever cause infection by themselves but can superinfect areas that are already infected by other organisms.

Midpoint on the scale of infectivity are organisms that are also normal inhabitants of the body but that become infective when they reach areas in which they do not normally exist. Thus, for example, the organisms that live on the surface of the skin will infect broken skin, particularly in the presence of dead tissue. Here, too, belong many agents that are not infective under normal circumstances but become a threat when they are present in large numbers. It is mainly because of these agents that good hygiene is advisable. Many bacteria and some viruses and fungi fall in this category.

At the top of the scale are the very highly infective organisms. Although virulence, the severity of illness that an organism can produce, does not go hand-in-hand with its infectivity, it frequently parallels it. Thus in this category are the great plagues of mankind, *bubonic plague* and *cholera*. On the other hand, here also we find minor ailments such as *influenza*. The agent causing such disease, and this is particularly true for bacteria, is frequently present in certain geographic areas where it persists in water sources and in animal reservoirs. These bacteria give rise to local epidemics and are called *endemic* in the population or region. Their constant presence can cause immunity in the immediate population, and only their spread to more distant areas will cause such organisms to become epidemic in nature.

The science of *epidemiology*, the study of the spread of disease, is vital to the health authorities who are in charge of the prevention of epidemics. Influenza is one example of an epidemic disease that periodically spreads throughout the world. When authorities determine that an epidemic has begun somewhere on the globe, they direct manufacturers to prepare corresponding vaccines to vaccinate susceptible populations. Since new strains of influenza virus appear continuously, a vaccination is not adequate to protect the population against anything but the current epidemic. Other diseases, particularly the *sexually transmitted diseases*, are of epidemic proportions in the population. Since they are almost exclusively transmitted through sexual contact, the best available means to limit their spread is to avoid infectious contacts or to take anti-infective precautions. Currently, no vaccines are available for such diseases, but there is much work in progress to produce them. (See Chapter 20.)

Breakdown of Body Defenses   As we have seen, infectivity of the organism predicts a probability of infection in conjunction with the integrity of the defenses of the potential host. (See Figure 19–2.) How do these defenses break down? Mechanical factors, such as trauma of the skin, lodging of an object in the intestinal tract with injury to mucous membranes, an anatomical obstruction in the urinary tract, or scarification of the heart valves, can allow organisms that are normally present in small numbers to grow to infective proportions before they can be reached by the defensive white cells or before the mechanisms of acquired immunity come into play. Physical stresses, such as extreme cold, exertion to exhaustion, and shock, can significantly depress these defenses. Psychological stress is thought to effectively decrease resistance to disease, although scientific proof is still rather weak. Statistics show that particular stresses that lead to depression can cause the appearance of infections, especially upper-respiratory infections. Some medical treatments lead to general suppression of the immune mechanism. Outstanding among these are treatments with X rays or anticancer drugs. Cancer patients die more often of infection than they do of the spread of the tumor. Treatment with cortisone, or corticosteroid derivates, which are used in arthritis and inflammation, can also lead to significant

Endemic
Commonly found in a particular geographic area.

Epidemiology
The study of the rates, distribution, and control of diseases.

Sexually transmitted diseases
Diseases transmitted via sexual intercourse or other close physical contact.

Prophylaxis
Preventive treatment against disease.

Immune gamma globulin
A serum used to treat those exposed to a viral disease such as hepatitis or measles.

Serum
The clear part of a liquid separated from its solid part.

---

lowering of immune defenses. Patients under such treatment must be watched carefully for the appearance of infection.

Although it has long been believed that heredity can determine the nature of infections that plague an individual, this belief has only been scientifically verified in very recent times.

Treatment of Infection   The preferred treatment of infection is *prophylaxis*. To this mode of treatment belong efforts of personal and public hygiene, eradication of disease-carrying insects and sources of food for those insects, sewage treatment and controlled release of sewage into public water sources, control of the bacterial contamination of drinking water, and so on. More active and direct intervention is that of vaccination. Vaccination in childhood is common for diphtheria, whooping cough, and tetanus, all of which have virtually disappeared in the United States.

Incidence of the so-called childhood diseases (measles, German measles, and chickenpox) has been significantly reduced, polio has been virtually eradicated, and smallpox has been totally eliminated by means of vaccination. (See Table 19-1, p. 436.) The nature of vacci-

nation and available vaccines will be discussed in the next section.

One particular treatment worthy of mention is that with *immune gamma globulin*. This material is obtained from *serum* (the clear liquid residue that results when blood is allowed to clot) from individuals immune to a given disease. It is most frequently applied today for prevention of hepatitis in individuals who are known to have been exposed to a source of the virus. It has also been used in other limited viral epidemics, in particular in hospitals where there are patients whose immunity is suppressed because of radiation therapy or burn wounds and where a viral epidemic is in progress. Immune gamma globulin has also been used in therapy, but for the moment this is still a relatively restricted area. New developments that allow production of antibodies make it likely that this therapy will become more common in the future.

Active therapy of infectious disease has become progressively more effective over the last 70 years. This is based on the difference in the physiology of parasites and the host, which makes it possible to produce substances that are toxic for one but are not toxic or are only mildly toxic for the other. Because the physiol-

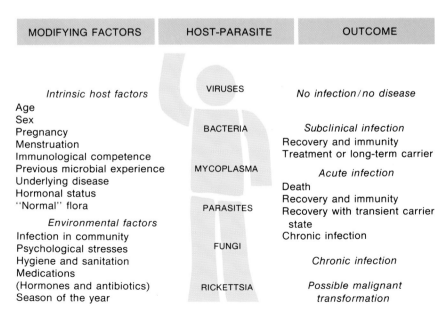

MODIFYING FACTORS	HOST-PARASITE	OUTCOME

Intrinsic host factors
Age
Sex
Pregnancy
Menstruation
Immunological competence
Previous microbial experience
Underlying disease
Hormonal status
"Normal" flora

Environmental factors
Infection in community
Psychological stresses
Hygiene and sanitation
Medications
(Hormones and antibiotics)
Season of the year

VIRUSES

BACTERIA

MYCOPLASMA

PARASITES

FUNGI

RICKETTSIA

No infection/no disease

Subclinical infection
Recovery and immunity
Treatment or long-term carrier

Acute infection
Death
Recovery and immunity
Recovery with transient carrier
   state
Chronic infection

Chronic infection

*Possible malignant
   transformation*

Figure 19-2   The physiological condition of a person (or host) may interact with environmental factors to influence the way in which a person responds to exposure to potential pathogenic microbial organisms.

Antibiotic
A chemical that is capable of inhibiting
the growth of or killing organisms such as
bacteria.

Penicillin
A drug used to treat bacterial diseases.

Table 19-1   Immunizations Available in the United States

Type of Immunization	Who Should Be Immunized	Effectiveness of Immunization and Frequency of Booster Doses
Cholera	Foreign travelers	Only partial immunity; renew every 6 months for duration of exposure
Diphtheria	All adults in good health with no previous immunization; travelers	Highly effective; renew every 10 years
German measles	Mainly for children	Highly effective; need for boosters not established
Influenza	All adults of any age, especially those with chronic disease of the heart, respiratory tract, or endocrine system	Renew every year (because viral strains change easily)
Measles	Mainly for children	Highly effective; usually produces lifelong immunity
Mumps	Most helpful to children and young adults who have not had mumps	Believed to confer lifetime immunity
Plague	Anyone exposed; travelers to Asia, Africa, and Tibet	Incomplete protection; boosters necessary every 3 to 6 months
Polio	All adults, particularly travelers, those exposed to children, and those in health and sanitation industries	Long-lasting immunity; no booster necessary unless exposure anticipated
Rabies	Only those bitten by rabid animal	A vaccination each day for 14 to 21 days beginning soon after the bite
Spotted fever	—	Not very effective
Tetanus	Everyone	Very effective; renew every 10 years or when treated for a contaminated wound if more than 5 years have elapsed since last booster
Tuberculosis	High-risk people; nurses and children in contact with active tubercular cases	Highly effective
Typhoid fever	Anyone exposed; travelers	About 80 percent effective
Typhus	Anyone exposed	Renew every year (if exposed)
Whooping cough	Essential for children by age 3 to 4 months	Highly effective
Yellow fever	Anyone exposed; travelers	Highly effective; provides immunity for at least 17 years

---

ogy is not completely different, however, most drugs
have some residual degree of toxicity for the host as
well as the pathogens and should not be used indiscriminately. Into this category fall the antibiotics.

Antibiotics are substances produced by microorganisms that are toxic to other kinds of microorganisms.
They were discovered by Alexander Fleming, who
found that a fungus growing on a growth medium

that contained bacteria produced a clear zone around
it, in which the bacteria had been killed. From this
fungus he purified a substance that he called *penicillin*,
after the fungus, penicillium. This was the first of a
long series of antibiotics that now include such widely
used drugs as erythromycin, tetracycline, streptomycin,
gentamicin, and the cephalosporins.

Antibiotics are effective only against bacteria and

Strange Alliance: Legions of Bacteria Created to Serve Man

With every new feat of genetic engineering, it becomes increasingly clear that mankind has made one of the strangest and most complex alliances ever achieved with another form of life.

Bacteria, invisible to the eye and feared as the agents of infection, have become workhorses of the revolution in biology. They have been domesticated to do things no microbe ever did in nature.

Among the newest accomplishments reported recently are bacteria redesigned genetically to make substances native only to human brain and blood. These new microbes are chimeras, with traits of different creatures as fantastically mixed as the winged lions imagined by the ancient Greeks, but they are the latest fruits of an alliance that began before history.

Although the ancients were ignorant of microbes, they knew plague and pestilence and spoiled food. But sometimes the food did not spoil. Instead, it changed miraculously into something different and better.

Babylonians and Sumerians unwittingly used yeast to make beer more than 8,000 years ago. About 2,000 years later, the Egyptians knew that yeast could leaven bread. Ancient peoples also used yeasts to make wine, bacteria to make vinegar and yogurt, and various molds and bacteria to make cheese. All of these uses were flourishing thousands of years before Anton van Leeuwenhoek, in the 17th century A.D., first looked through his primitive microscope and actually saw living microorganisms in water and decaying matter.

Humans have improved their stocks of yeasts and other useful microbes, but always, until recent years, in the style of animal husbandry. The best performers were saved and nurtured over and over, producing special strains, just as the cows that produce the most and best milk are bred to get more. But these old microbial techniques seem trivially simple today, compared with the powers of modern biotechnology.

Even the most inspired selective breeding will not make cows produce coffee or tea with their milk. In rough analogy, that is what genetic engineering does. It gives living bacteria and yeasts the ability to produce exotic products they could never make at all in nature.

Calcitonin, a substance that regulates the deposition of calcium in human bones, is being made in bacteria so that it can be tested in patients suffering from Paget's disease and osteoporosis, disorders in which bone formation is affected.

A hormone called thymosin alpha, normally produced only by the human thymus, is to be tried as a cancer treatment because of its possible effects in the patient's immune defense system.

A blood substance called tissue plasminogen activator, a potentially important dissolver of blood clots in conditions such as heart attacks, may replace other substances now used for that purpose.

Human serum albumin, a blood substance that has widespread uses in medicine, is also being produced in bacteria, as is human epidermal growth factor, which shows promise as an aid to wound healing.

Pieces of important human genes can be made in bacteria for use in diagnosis and even, perhaps, for treatment of some human hereditary diseases.

Genetically engineered bacteria and yeasts have also become factories for making substances for vaccines and veterinary and medical products of several kinds. All of these developments are still only in their early stages, their promise for public health still largely to be proved. Meanwhile the research has been accompanied by debates over the safety and desirability of taking such liberties with the heredity of living things. . . .

Harold M. Schmeck, Jr.
New York Times

fungi; with almost no exception, they are totally ineffective against viruses. They may be used prophylactically in viral disease to prevent superinfection of a host by bacteria when immune defenses have been weakened by the virus. There are also a number of excellent synthetic drugs, many of which are based on antibiotics and are a modification of their structure. They can be very effective against bacteria as well as fungi.

Antibiotics and other antimicrobial agents act on a limited range of microorganisms. The physician must choose the drug that best copes with the infecting organism. Equally important, the drug must be well tolerated by the patient. To illustrate, all streptococci succumb to penicillin. This is therefore the drug of choice for strep throat. Some patients, however, have allergic reactions to penicillin, so erythromycin must be used.

Mutation
A permanent transmissible change in genetic material.

Interferon
A substance that is produced by a cell under attack from a virus and that keeps other viruses from infecting the body.

Immune system
Mechanisms that protect the body against invading foreign organisms and substances.

Nonspecific immune mechanism
A mechanism that keeps out invaders regardless of their specific type.

Specific immune mechanism
A mechanism that recognizes specific organisms or substances and defends against them.

Most gastrointestinal and urinary tract infections are caused by organisms that resist penicillin; therefore, a number of other drugs, especially sulfa drugs and tetracycline, must be used instead.

Although bacteria do reproduce true to type, and a bacterial population consists of identical individuals, occasionally (about once in ten million divisions) a *mutation* occurs. Such mutant bacteria can manifest resistance to a drug to which the parents were sensitive. When resistant bacteria appear in a population that is exposed to the drug, they will soon take over because they have no competition for nutrient. The overuse of antibiotics has led to the frequent appearance of resistant strains. This can be particularly disastrous in hospitals, where many drugs are used and susceptible patients abound. Many hospitals now have committees charged with preventing such abuse.

Because of their very close resemblance to the host and their lack of any metabolic activity that might be interfered with by drugs, viruses are considerably more difficult to kill than any bacteria and fungi. Only two effective drugs are currently on the market, but several others are being tested. Since they may interfere with the reproductive apparatus of the cell itself, they are very toxic and present a potential danger. At the moment, a substance produced by the body itself, *interferon* (see page 415), is the best hope for treatment of viral disease.

Immunity

The unicellular (one-celled) organism copes with its environment mainly by trying to ingest everything it encounters. Its "universe" thus consists of two kinds of materials—those that are digestible and those that are not. In contrast, the multicellular (many-celled) organism, being made up of different kinds of cells that have to live together in harmony, must be able to distinguish between what it itself is made of and what is foreign to it. The multicellular organism has to recognize the difference between "self" and "nonself." ("Nonself" refers both to materials that are intrinsically alien to an organism and to materials belonging to other members of its species.) In addition, the multicellular

organism must also be able to recognize those portions of its own original structure that have become useless or detrimental and disturbing to its harmony. To eliminate all harmful materials, multicellular organisms have evolved methods of protection, or immune mechanisms, together called the *immune system.* (See Figure 19–3.) The immune system functions (1) to prevent entry of foreign and undesirable substances, living or dead, into the organism, and to remove any such substances that break through its barriers; and (2) to eliminate certain products of the organism itself—dead cells and cells that have changed and become lethal, such as cancer cells. Certain recognition systems, barriers, and toxic mechanisms have evolved within the organism to accomplish these purposes.

Sometimes, however, the recognition systems and toxic mechanisms themselves can be a problem, possibly a lethal one. They can, for example, make it difficult to perform necessary surgical operations such as blood transfusions and organ or tissue transplants. By attacking basically harmless substances like plant pollens with their full toxic power, they can cause a disease known as an allergy. They may even go totally awry and attack normal and necessary constituents of the body, causing autoimmune disease.

Immune Mechanisms

Immune mechanisms defend the body against infection. The immune mechanisms are generally classified as specific or nonspecific. *Nonspecific mechanisms* keep out all foreign invaders no matter what they are. *Specific mechanisms,* on the other hand, recognize individual organisms and allow the body to focus on any single invader that might be the main threat of the moment. The word *immunity* is frequently used only to refer to specific mechanisms.

Nonspecific Mechanisms   Nonspecific mechanisms include the physiological barriers, secretions and enzymes, and the phagocytic cells. The physiological defenses of the body include the skin, the mucous membranes, secretions such as tears and mucus, certain activities of enzymes, and some organisms, fluids, and biochemical processes of the gastrointestinal tract.

The skin provides a multiple defense. It functions as a physical barrier to the entry of microorganisms, and it also obstructs their entry chemically. The normal weak acidity at the surface of the skin is a poor growth condition for bacteria and fungi. The nonpathogenic bacteria that survive normal skin conditions are still another barrier. These occupy areas needed by attacking pathogens, consume what little food is available, and sometimes even secrete materials toxic to other bacteria.

Mucus membranes are also staunch defenders of the body. Located in the eyes, nose, sinuses, throat, windpipe, bronchial tubes, gastrointestinal tubes, and vagina, all have specific protective functions.

Tears keep the surfaces of the eyeball from drying out; they provide a solution in which protective substances and cells can function; they wash away invaders from the mucous membranes of the eye; and they contain an enzyme that kills certain bacteria.

The mucus that is secreted by the membranes of the nose, throat, and bronchial tubes ensures proper moistening, cleansing, and temperature regulation of the air that is breathed deeply into the lungs. This mucus coating, acting much like sticky flypaper, captures inhaled foreign substances. The membrane of the respiratory tract also has slender microscopic hairlike structures called cilia. As these cilia move, they gradually pass the overlying mucus coating forward and out of the bronchial tubes. When the mucus coating reaches

Figure 19-3   A simplified view of the immune system.

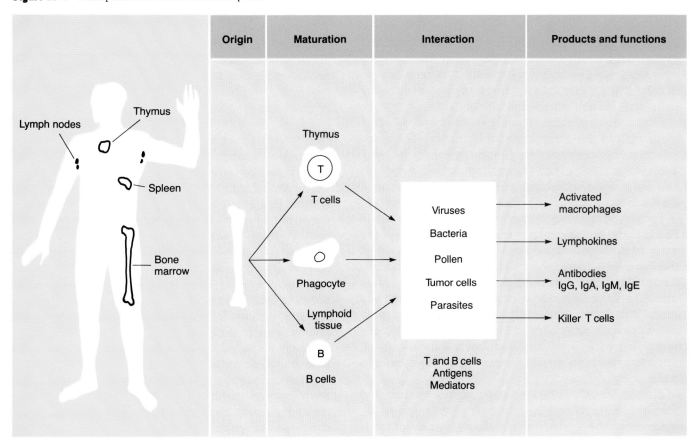

Phagocytes
White blood cells that specialize in ingesting and digesting undesirable matter they come into contact with.

Granulocyte
A kind of phagocyte containing granules.

Macrophage
A kind of phagocyte.

Lymphocytes
Blood elements that produce antibodies and other substances important in immunity.

Platelets
Blood elements that are necessary for the formation of clots.

Plasma
The fluid portion of the blood.

Lymphatic system
The physiological system that includes the lymph nodes, lymphatic vessels, and lymph. Lymphocytes and macrophages are concentrated in this system.

---

the windpipe or voice box, it is coughed out, spat out, or swallowed.

The mucus secretion of the vagina, which has a lubricating function, contributes to the prevention of infection, perhaps by supporting the beneficial bacteria. When this secretion ceases, infections—especially those caused by fungi and protozoa—occur frequently.

Enzymes that exist in the blood act as defense agents by destroying some kinds of bacteria. (This process usually consists of the rupture of the bacterium's outer membrane, causing its contents to spill out.) The clotting of blood around a wound is another form of defense. The scab physically blocks microorganisms from entering the body.

Digestive enzymes, intestinal secretions, stomach fluids, and intestinal bacteria all protect the gastrointestinal tract. If a pathogen is swallowed, strongly acidic stomach fluids usually destroy it. Pathogens surviving the acidic environment of the stomach must pass into the alkaline secretions of the small intestine. There they are attacked by the digestive enzymes, which consume foes as well as foods. Still farther down the intestinal tract resides a large army of intestinal bacteria whose density, living habits, and by-products discourage many pathogens from making territorial claims.

Phagocytes are white blood cells that specialize in ingesting and digesting undesirable matter. (The word *phagocytes* is derived from *phagein*, meaning "to eat," and *kytos*, meaning "cell"; hence, "eater cells.") The two kinds of phagocytes are *granulocytes* (so called because they contain many small granules) and *macrophages.* Both cell types circulate through the tissues and channels of the body, but specialized macrophages also line the walls of the blood vessels and form an integral part of their structure. Macrophages also predominate in cavities of the body, especially in the lungs, where they immediately attack all particulate matter that has managed to pass through the upper respiratory passages. Granulocytes predominate in the bloodstream and thus rapidly reach any area where a breach in the integrity of the body occurs. Granulocytes thus constitute a first line of defense.

Phagocytes, which move along surfaces by changing their shape, travel rapidly through the two major traffic systems of the body: the circulatory system (blood-stream) and the lymphatic system (a network of extremely delicate small vessels). From one-third to one-half of the total volume of blood is made up of blood cells; these are continuously manufactured by bone marrow. Most of these are red cells, which give the blood its color and carry oxygen to the tissues. About 1 out of 500 are white cells, which consist of phagocytes and lymphocytes. (*Lymphocytes* are a kind of white blood cell that is continuously made in lymphoid tissue as well as in bone marrow.) *Platelets,* elements that cause clotting, are also part of the solid constituents of blood. The fluid portion of the blood is called *plasma,* and the liquid remaining after clotting is called serum.

The bloodstream carries white cells to areas of infection. White cells can move through the walls of the blood vessels and through tissues under their own power, sometimes in response to signals that originate at the breakdown site of local tissues. Pus is mostly made up of white cells.

Macrophages and lymphocytes travel through the *lymphatic system.* The liquid content of the lymphatic system resembles plasma. The lymphatic network serves and clears tissue spaces and organs; it ends in the main lymphatic vessel, the thoracic duct, which empties into the bloodstream. At major junctions in the lymphatic network are rice-grain to pea-size structures called lymph nodes. Lymphocytes and macrophages congregate here in great numbers. They enter these nodes directly from the blood stream by passing through vessel walls, by which route they recirculate continuously through the two systems. The lymph nodes are traps for invading pathogens. If the invaders manage to multiply there, a lymph node becomes a major battlefield, aching and swelling. An infected cut on the hand can cause swollen lymph nodes in the armpit.

A microorganism's virulence depends greatly on its ability to breach the body's barriers and to survive these immune systems. Many microorganisms live in one or another area of the body continuously but cause infection only rarely, when barriers are breached by trauma or immune systems are made less effective by environmental stresses that lower the body's resistance. Thus the billions of harmless bacteria that live in the intestine and help us to digest our food will cause a highly dangerous infection if they leak out into the abdominal

The Mind as Healer

Anna had been given three months to live. The malignant tumor, growing rapidly at the back of her neck, had virtually crippled her. Her upper body was hunched over, her head was forced painfully to one side, and her right arm was contracted and paralyzed. The best thing she could do, said her doctor, was to go home and make adequate arrangements for the future of her young son and daughter.

Then, by an extraordinary stroke of good luck, she met psychologist Patricia Norris, clinical director of the Biofeedback and Psychophysiology Center at the Menninger Foundation. They met only three times, but Norris talked to her about a controversial technique called visualization, or imaging. Anna was already doing imaging, but Norris was able to make it more powerful, "more in tune with her emotional values." Armed with this unexpected help, Anna continued to fight her disease.

She visualized the tumor as a dragon on her back; she saw her white blood cells as knights, attacking the tumor with swords. A year later, Norris saw Anna again, and a dramatic change had occurred. "The tumor had shrunk so that her arm was fully mobile again; the next time I saw her, she was in total remission."

Can simple thoughts heal the body? The idea is a radical one, and most scientists are skeptical. The problem is that, so far, nobody has been able to show how imaging works—or even prove that it does. Norris herself points out that her patients follow a program with many other elements besides imaging—among them exercise, diet modification, and counseling—and they continue conventional medical treatment.

Nevertheless, without losing their skepticism, neuroscientists are beginning to discover pathways between brain and body that may show how it is possible for the mind to influence the immune system.

In fact, a whole discipline, with the tongue-twisting name "psychoneuroimmunology," has been created to study these relationships. In the future, this research is likely to change the way we treat diseases such as cancer and, perhaps, AIDS.

The prestigious and conservative National Institutes of Health (NIH) has endorsed the new discipline and its parent field, neuroimmunomodulation. This broad term enfolds a whole range of studies of "the brain as a computer that's involved in all the other reactions of the body," according to Novera Herbert Spector, one of the health scientist administrators of the Fundamental Neurosciences Program at NIH.

In New York City, the Institute for the Advancement of Health has been established by Eileen Rockefeller Growald to focus on the mind-body interaction in health and disease. Norman Cousins, a member of its Scientific Advisory Board, has twice startled both the public and the medical world by his own invocation of the mind's influence on the body. He claims first to have cured himself of a crippling disintegration of the connective tissue in his spine, and second, to have brought himself back from a massive heart attack. "What is significant," he says, "is that there is recognition that the endocrine system, the nervous system and the immune system are part of a totality." No less an authority than Nobel laureate Joshua Lederberg has called the institute "a most important step in joining the motives and methodology of 'humanistic

medicine' and rigorous laboratory science."

The new science actually began years ago, when scientists first started to understand the stress response as a mind-body connection. In the fight-or-flight response, defined by physiologist Walter Cannon in the 1920s, the brain perceives stress and signals the sympathetic branch of the autonomic nervous system, which regulates much of the "automatic" machinery of the body. The result? Rapid heartbeat and breathing and a rush of blood away from skin, hands, feet and digestive organs toward the deep muscle tissue, carrying needed oxygen for the muscles' use in either fight or flight in the stressful situation that has arisen.

Along with these familiar changes come some that are far subtler: Nerve endings in target organs, such as the stomach and intestines, release norepinephrine, a neurotransmitter. The usual job of neurotransmitters is to carry messages from one neuron to another; in the brain, these chemicals make thinking and feeling possible. But in the body, when the same chemicals are released by an organ into the bloodstream, they may be called hormones. Epinephrine (also known as adrenaline), for instance, is a neurotransmitter—but in the fight-or-flight response it is released in massive amounts as a hormone by the adrenal glands.

A region of the brain also sends a message (via neurotransmitters) that ultimately travels to the adrenal glands and signals them to send out cortisol, a major stress hormone, in massive amounts.

These hormones are important because it has been established that they can affect the immune

(continued on next page)

The Mind as Healer (continued)

system. "The net effect of stress," says biochemist Nicholas Hall, of George Washington University in Washington, D.C., "is a depression of immunity."

Another important discovery that helped lay the foundations for the new science came in the 1940s, when Swiss Nobel-prize-winning physiologist Walter B. Hess found that the hypothalamus, the area of the brain that signals the stress response to start, can also signal the opposite reaction. Cardiologist Herbert Benson, of the Harvard Medical School, calls this the "relaxation response": Heart rate, respiration, and bodily metabolism slow down, and the whole sympathetic nervous system is quieted.

The next step was taken when experimental psychologist Neal Miller, now professor emeritus at Rockefeller University in New York

City, and other scientists demonstrated that the sympathetic nervous system can be controlled through biofeedback.

In treating disease, imaging takes the evidence for control of the sympathetic nervous system and makes what until now has been a leap of faith to the idea of directly helping the immune system. "We do have an immune system," says Norris, "and it's effective against disease. So we try to enhance the immune system; to reengage it, to get it back to doing its own work.

"You do this," she says, "by helping people overcome depression or a feeling of helplessness. You give them a feeling of empowerment, help them to get healthy again—and simultaneously give them some definite psychophysiological skills: to be able to reduce sympathetic activity, to reduce

tension and anxiety, to feel calm."

According to psychiatrist Steven Locke, of Harvard Medical School and Boston's Beth Israel Hospital, "Teaching people relaxation technique, self-hypnosis and biofeedback is now becoming widespread in medicine." But the idea of enhancing the immune system through relaxation, through a feeling of empowerment or by overcoming depression is one that many "hard" researchers still consider very soft indeed. And softest of all is the idea that the immune system will respond to pictures in the mind of someone who's ill. Nevertheless, research scientists are beginning to provide hard evidence that could eventually bear these theories out.

Signe Hammer
Science Digest

---

cavity as, for example, through a hole caused by a bullet. The most virulent bacteria, such as those that cause cholera or bubonic plague, infect a large proportion of people who come in contact with them. Many pathogens, however, are intermediate in virulence.

The body's natural defenses can cope continuously with a small number of pathogens, but minor breakdowns in immune defenses lead to infection. Defense barriers are also relatively ineffective in preventing viral infection, and viral diseases spread quite easily among humans. The nonspecific defense mechanisms we have described so far are not adequate for coping with many infections. Highly specific mechanisms have evolved to fill the gap. These mechanisms can "learn" quickly to respond with vigor to a particular invader. The specific mechanisms are capable of reproducing themselves rapidly; they have "memory"; and they can draw on other systems to increase their ability to defend. This specialized process is the adaptive immune system.

Specific Mechanisms   Adaptive immunity and vaccination are essential to the immune system.

Adaptive Immunity   Adaptive immunity is a function of the lymphocytes. There are two types of lymphocytes:

B cells and T cells. The B cells carry on their surface a kind of molecule known as *antibody*. There are perhaps a million different kinds of antibody molecules, but those that occupy a single B cell (about 100,000 to 500,000) are all identical and are the only kind which that particular B cell can manufacture. The antibody molecules are about one-twentieth the size of the smallest virus. The million or so kinds of antibodies differ from each other chiefly in a certain tiny portion of the molecule known as the antibody-combining site. The antibody-combining site is able to locate and react with a specific molecular pattern that may exist as part of a larger carbohydrate or protein molecule. It may recognize, for example, such particular molecular patterns as a segment of the protein that constitutes the outside, or "coat," of a virus particle, or components of the cell walls of bacteria. The molecular patterns that antibody-combining sites can recognize are called *antigenic determinants*. The molecule, particle, or organism carrying the antigenic determinants is called the *antigen*. Antibody tends to be highly specific. It will only recognize and react to (that is, combine with) the matching structure (or antigenic determinant) of the antigen. When the antigen contacts an antibody-combining site that is specific for it, antigen and antibody stick together at this

Antibody
A molecule that will react specifically with molecules of a single kind. Gamma globulin, a material prepared from blood serum, contains all the antibodies.

Antigenic determinants
Molecular patterns on the antigen that the antibody reacts to.

Antigen
The molecule, particle, or organism carrying the antigenic determinants that the antibody reacts to.

Primary response
The first response of the immune system to an antigen.

Secondary response
The subsequent stronger response of the immune system to an antigen.

Neutralization
Binding of an antibody to an antigen in such a way that the antigen is no longer harmful.

Agglutination
The action of antibodies to make bacteria or other particles clump together.

Complement fixation
A process that helps to make antigen-antibody complexes easier for phagocytes to digest.

---

site. The combination of antibody with antigen leads to the inactivation and removal of parasites, especially bacteria and viruses. The million or so kinds of antibody molecules (and corresponding B cells) have the ability to recognize as many antigenic determinants. Any foreign invader presents many antigenic determinants, and one (or more) of these is certain to come into contact with B cells carrying the antibody that will combine with it.

Interaction of antigen with the B cell stimulates the B cell to release antibody into the surrounding tissue. At the same time, and sometimes aided by the T cells, a B cell will begin to grow and divide, yielding first two new B cells, then four, then eight, and so on. The new B cells release antibody of the same type as the original. Soon there is a larger number of B cells of the same kind, with many identical antibody molecules. These antibodies aid in the removal of accumulated toxic antigen. Antibody is circulated through the blood and seeks out any antigen that may have moved from the point of entry. When the antigen is removed, the B cells stop dividing and producing antibody, and in 3 to 12 months all antibody has left the bloodstream. However, a much larger number of B cells is now present, and if the antigen reappears, antibody production begins almost immediately, achieving high levels quickly. The body is thereby protected against a recurrence of the same infection. The response to the first encounter with antigen is called the *primary response*. Subsequent, intensified responses are called *secondary responses.*

T cells also react to antigens, and like B cells, they divide and proliferate in contact with them. One kind of T cell releases a number of substances that act on phagocytes and accelerate the removal of antigen. Another T cell releases other substances that stimulate the B cell to divide and produce antibody. Yet another kind of T cell is particularly good at eliminating foreign cells from the body. T cells may have evolved as a mechanism for removing those changed cells, such as cancer cells, that could menace the body's integrity.

Two additional kinds of T cells require mention, although their dynamic of action in the body is not fully understood. The first such type of T cell is the so-called "natural killer" (NK) cell. Natural killer cells in some way recognize foreign cells, in particular tumor or virus-infected cells, and kill them. The importance of this mechanism may lie in defending the body from an occasional cancer cell that arises through mutation. A second, better understood type of T cell is the so-called suppressor T cell. This cell appears during a developing immune response and serves to terminate the response by killing the cell, either T or B, that is reacting to a foreign antigen. It is now thought that on occasion the healthy body reacts against one or the other of its own normal components. Suppressor T cells then suppress this particular reaction. As we shall see, this reaction against normal cell components can turn into disease. This disease is now thought to be due to the inability to form suppressor T cells against the particular autotoxic (autoimmune) response. Fortunately, suppressor T cells seem to be much shorter lived than the memory B or T cells, so that when the body sees an antigen for a second time, a secondary response can arise and, at least at the onset, not be suppressed by suppressor T cells.

When T cells interact with antigens, they directly secrete a number of important defensive substances. One such substance attracts macrophages and retains them in the needed area. In addition, T cells, because of their ability to identify changes in cell surfaces, can actually bind to areas of change caused by virus infection and destroy the altered cell before it finishes manufacture of complete viruses.

Antibody and T cells employ several mechanisms in protecting the body against infection. For example, the enzymes and toxins released by bacteria cause damage by acting on specific tissue. Such molecules when attached to antibody frequently become incapable of attacking their target. Similarly, antibodies, though smaller than viruses, can stop viral infection by binding to small, specific areas in the virus that the virus needs to attach itself to the cell. This simple action of antibody is called *neutralization.*

Occasionally, antibody can prevent bacteria from multiplying by binding directly to their surfaces. More frequently, antibodies bind bacteria together in relatively large bunches by an action called *agglutination.* The phagocytes can ingest the bunches of bacteria more easily than they can ingest individual organisms.

Much of the effectiveness of antibody defense depends on a process it activates called *complement*

A Pictorial History of Events in Infection Immunity (Highly Schematic and Simplified)

Note that items are not drawn to scale and may vary from drawing to drawing. The relative size of antigenic determinants and that of antibodies is particularly exaggerated. Real sizes relate approximately as follows: Length or diameter: Cell ≈ 10 × microorganism ≈1,000 × antibody.

1. A lymph node prior to first exposure to the microorganism, which is entering the scene at bottom right. T cells are yellow, B cells dark blue. Note that they are clustered separately. There are very few cells with receptors (not shown) on their surface that fit X, Y, or α, three of many kinds of determinants on the surface of the microorganism as shown in 1a.

1a. Antigenic determinants are arranged in clusters and repeated many times. To these determinants correspond receptors on . . .

1b. The "specific" T (yellow) and B (dark blue) cells. Receptors on B cells are antibodies that fit either the X or the Y determinant. Each B cell carries only one kind of receptor, and there are 100,000 to 500,000 per cell. T cell receptors fit the α determinants. Their nature is not known, but there seem to be fewer than there are antibodies on B cells. Note that the antibodies are firmly attached to the B cell surface until profound changes occur in the cell due to the interaction with antigenic determinants (2).

2. Instead of interacting with antigen directly, B and, particularly, T cells frequently must react with antigen sitting on the surface of a macrophage in order to be activated. For the sake of simplification, this is not depicted here. X1 and Y1 are the respective parent cells, which have been stimulated by antigens. The cells begin to divide and to release their respective antibody into the surroundings. α-specific T cells are also stimulated to divide by contact with antigen. They give off a material (fine black-dotted lines) that causes B cells to divide. This process starts in earnest about 24 hours after the first encounter of cells and antigen, and the first phase is complete in about 72 hours. From then on, divisions of cells and production of antibody speed up enormously and an effective defense is mounted by day 7.

3. On day 7 the small area of the lymph node we have focused on is now chock full of lymphocytes, and almost all of them are X- or Y-specific B cells or α-specific T cells. The microorganisms (seen only in 4) are coated by free antibody molecules or attached to specific cells. The black dots are materials produced by T cells; the brown dots, materials produced during complement activation. These materials act as shown in 4.

4. The antibodies, through their two attachment sites, link microorgan-

isms into bundles. The process is called agglutination. The organisms are prevented from multiplying, and agglutinates are preferred food for the phagocytes ("eating cells"). These cells are attracted by the materials given off by complement, which is activated by the antibody when it attaches to the microorganism, and by materials that come from T cells. Phagocytes attach preferentially to complement-coated organisms.

5. Sometime after the infection has been defeated—3 months to 20 years, depending on the individual, the microorganism, and the severity of the infection—most of the free antibody has vanished, as have many of the specific cells. However, there are many more present now than there were prior to infection (1). In addition, they don't require the 24- to 72-hour "activation" period. If the body is invaded by the same microorganism, the immune defenses go into accelerated action immediately and infection does not take place. The animal has acquired immunity. In addition, the animal can now cope more readily with all organisms that have either the X, the Y, or the α determinant. This is the principle on which most vaccines work.

fixation, a process in which other protein molecules are attached to the antigen-antibody complex. Complement fixation helps to make antigen-antibody complexes easier for phagocytes to digest, and it also attracts large numbers of these cells to the invaded site. The power of antibody as protective agent is thus largely due to its ability to increase phagocytic removal of pathogens.

An overview of immune system activity can be seen in the events following infection of the throat with streptococcus bacteria. The organisms, finding no resistance, settle in the mucus membrane and, while multiplying, release enzymes that attack the surrounding tissue. The decaying tissue causes an influx of phagocytes, which are defeated by the toxins produced by the

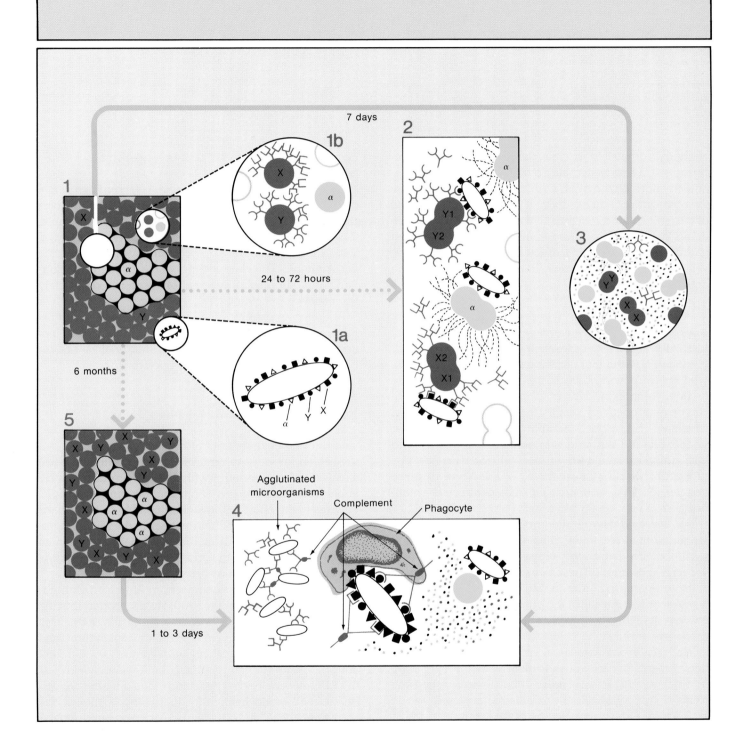

growing bacterial population. Some of these toxins reach T and B cells, which contain antibody receptors directed against them, and antibody manufacture begins. Meanwhile, dead bacteria and bacterial breakdown products, both with some intact antigenic determinants, are carried by macrophages. These also reach specific B and T cells, stimulating them to proliferate and to secrete. Some live

bacteria may also have reached the lymphatic vessels, been transported into the nearest lymph node, and settled there. The lymph node then becomes a battlefield, as evidenced by painful swelling. Increasing amounts of antibody and numbers of T cells now come to the sites of infection. Antibodies neutralize the toxic enzymes, thereby sustaining cell survival. Antigen-

Attenuated organisms
Organisms that are similar to virulent pathogenic organisms in terms of their antigenic determinants, but are not virulent themselves. Such organisms can often be bred in the laboratory, starting with a disease-producing organism and selecting offspring that are less and less virulent until after many generations an organism that is suitable for vaccination is obtained.

Toxoid
A toxin (natural poison) that has been modified so that it loses its toxicity but still has its antigenic determinants.

---

antibody complexes activate the complement fixation process. This activity, along with T cell secretions, attracts more phagocytes, whose job is made easier by the complement that has formed. Soon the site is cleared of bacteria and tissue debris. If the same kind of bacteria enters the body in the future, it returns to an environment harboring large numbers of specific B and T cells that will recognize and destroy it before it can become entrenched.

Vaccination   The protective power of the secondary response can be taken advantage of through vaccination. Late in the eighteenth century, Edward Jenner, an English physician, noticed that occasionally the hands of people who milked cows showed a pox infection similar to the dreaded smallpox. Jenner observed that victims of cowpox, a relatively mild disease, never contracted smallpox. He rubbed scrapings from infected cow udders into the skin and skin abrasions of people who had not had smallpox to see whether or not this procedure would protect them. It did. None of these people—the first to be vaccinated—contracted smallpox.

No one understood the process of vaccination in Jenner's time. We know now that both cowpox and smallpox are caused by viruses, called, respectively, vaccinia and variola. These viruses have certain antigenic determinants in common. When the body successfully overcomes infection by one, the immune system prevents infection by the other by setting up a secondary response.

We can breed viruses that carry many antigenic determinants but are not as virulent as their progenitors. In other words, we can breed mild disease organisms from severe ones. Such organisms are said to be *attenuated*. Oral polio vaccine is an attenuated virus. Attenuated organisms are generally the best possible means of immunization. One of their major advantages is that the process of immunization occurs via the same routes that the virulent organism would have had to traverse.

Sometimes it is not possible to breed attenuated organisms that retain enough of their original structure to confer immunity against their more dangerous progen-itors. When this situation arises, organisms are killed and used for vaccination.

When the toxicity of an organism is limited to a single product, immunization against the single product gives complete protection against the organism. For example, if the tetanus toxin is treated with formaldehyde, it will lose its toxicity without significant change in its antigenic determinants. This detoxified *toxoid* is used for vaccination, and successful vaccination protects completely from tetanus infections.

Adaptive immunity also defends the body against fungi, protozoa, worms, and the like, but we do not understand these processes nearly as well as we do those involved with viruses and bacteria.

Recognition of Foreign Cells

One of the oldest pursuits of medical science has been the search for ways to replace organs and limbs. Blood was the first "tissue" with which transfers were attempted—because the surgical procedure is simple. Failures in the effort to transfer animal blood to humans may be documented all the way back to the Middle Ages. Many attempts to transfer blood from one human to another were made at the end of the nineteenth century, but the results were unpredictable.

Karl Landsteiner, an Austrian-born American pathologist, solved the problem in 1900. He discovered that the surfaces of red blood cells contain antigen systems that vary from person to person. The major such system (and there are at least 12 others with about 100 different antigens), and the first one described by Landsteiner, is the ABO system. Each letter stands for a different antigen on the cell surface. Each individual's blood contains one or two of these three antigens. A person with type A blood cannot be given a transfusion of type B blood—because his or her immune system will reject it. Military personnel and others who have a high risk of injury are routinely blood-typed and carry this information on their persons. Anyone would be well advised to do the same. Rejection of blood of the same ABO type is rare, and safe transfusion is usually ensured by cross matching the donor's and recipient's blood in a test tube.

Rejection
An immune response that causes transplants of foreign tissues to be attacked by the immune system and destroyed.

Immunosuppression
Temporarily weakening the immune response with drugs or radiation in order to keep transplants from being rejected.

One other blood-group system of medical significance is the Rh blood-group system. This system was first described by Karl Landsteiner and Alexander Wiener and independently by Paul Levine in 1940. The mother's immunization is believed to occur at the birth of her first child, when red blood cells from the fetus enter her bloodstream. If the fetus and the mother have different types within this group, the mother may become immunized to the fetus's blood. If in a later pregnancy, the fetus has the same Rh as the earlier fetus, a secondary response will cause Rh antibodies to cross the placenta and destroy the fetal blood cells. The resulting Rh disease is sometimes fatal to the fetus. It is therefore common practice to administer antibody to the mother at the time of first birth where the mother and child have opposing Rh factors.

If the fetus has Rh positive blood, the mother is given the antibody to Rh positive blood, which immediately destroys any fetal blood cells that might cross into the mother's bloodstream, thus preventing the mother from forming her own immune response to them. This practice has reduced the incidence of Rh disease by 90 percent.

Although the immunology of blood cells has been understood for many years, similar insight into other kinds of cells is a recent occurrence. The surgical techniques required for skin transplants have existed for some time, but the phenomenon of rejection has prevented the transplanting of skin from one individual to another. The causes of rejection became clear through the work of Sir Peter Medawar and his associates in the 1940s and 1950s. *Rejection* is an immune response resulting from differences in the tissue cell antigens, which are much like antigens on red blood cells. Inbred mice do not have such differences, and skin transplants among them are possible.

The surgical techniques for performing organ transplants were known long ago, but it was not known how to control the immune factor. Once researchers began to understand immune rejection, several kidney transplants between identical twins were successful. The next step, now widely practiced, was to suppress the immune response with a variety of drugs and corticosteroids (hormones that are produced by the adrenal cortex). This procedure is called *immunosuppression*. Immunosuppression is itself risky, however, and should be used only for a limited time. It weakens or abolishes the natural defenses of the organism. The current techniques maximize interference with tissue rejection and minimize suppression of the body's defenses.

If we knew as much about matching tissue antigens as we do about matching blood cell antigens, successful organ transplants would be much easier. The organ tissue can be typed directly from blood samples because most of the relevant tissue antigens are present on white blood cells. But the match between donor and recipient is never complete; surgeons can only seek the closest available match. The greater the antigenic similarity, the more successful the transplant. In tissue cells as in blood cells, some antigens stimulate the immune system more strongly than others, and the best match of these antigens is usually the primary goal.

Greater success in organ transplants will come from increasing our ability to deceive the immune system into recognizing the transplanted organ as "self." The present method of achieving this deception involves using immunosuppression drugs to suppress the immune response and gradually reducing the dosage as the transplant "takes hold." This approach has resulted in many successful transplants of kidneys. Some patients having this operation have survived for more than 15 years. Heart transplants have been less successful, but survivals of 10 years or longer are on record. A new drug, cyclosporin A, is the most effective immunosuppressant known and is beginning to increase the success of organ transplants.

Immunology of Cancer

Cancer is generally defined as cells proliferating out of control. Normally, cells contain mechanisms that limit growth. For example, when the body sustains an injury, a scar forms over the area. Eventually the scar is replaced by normal tissue and covered by skin. This repair process stops as soon as normalcy is restored. We do not know why the skin stops growing when the repair is made. It is possible that cells of similar composition

Allergy
A disease such as hives or hay fever that results when immune mechanisms over-respond to innocuous substances in the environment.

Mast cell
A cell that contains a toxic substance called histamine, which, when released into the blood, causes an allergic reaction.

Histamine
A chemical that is released into the blood and is involved in allergic reactions.

can recognize one another's surfaces and that when they get close enough to one another the recognition mechanism within them stops further growth.

Cells that are cancerous, however, may have their normal surface recognition mechanisms altered; that is, they may have changed antigenically. Ordinarily, the immune system would be quite able to recognize such a change. Why does it accept cancer cells rather than reject them?

One possible explanation is that cancer cells differ so little antigenically from the native cells that the immune system does not react enough to cause rejection. Another possibility is that the immune system may be suppressed by environmental stresses to the point where it is too weak to combat the cancerous condition.

Two current theories have given rise to much research and some treatments to combat cancer immunologically. One theory holds that cancerous cells are continually appearing in the organism and continually being combated by the immune system. The immune system is successful in eliminating most such intruders. When the cancerous cells do establish themselves, however, perhaps due to temporary suppression of immunity, they may grow so rapidly that the immune mechanism can no longer cope with them. T cell responses have been shown to be extremely weak in people with advanced cancer. One cancer therapy consists of administering substances known to cause proliferation of T cells, since these cells seem to be most relevant in the response to cancer.

A second theory holds that many cancers are caused by viruses. Attempts are under way to isolate such viruses from human cells and produce vaccines against them. (Figure 19–4 shows the probability of an American's developing cancer.)

Allergies

The adaptive immune defenses cannot distinguish between potentially noxious materials and those that are harmless. The adaptive system also cannot distinguish between living and nonliving material. The unpleasant aspects of disease, such as fever, discomfort, abscess formation, and inflammation, are as much caused by the

actions of immune defenses as they are by invading toxins, but these unpleasantries aid in fighting the invading organisms. Many bacteria, for example, do not withstand the temperature reached by the body during fever bouts. Inflammation and abscesses localize the invaders, making it difficult for them to spread through the body. Even discomfort may be useful in that it forces the body to avoid stress and hoard its energies, which are needed for defense.

But when the material the immune mechanism responds to is an innocuous and common substance such as house dust or pollen, the defense becomes a disease known as an *allergy.*

Allergies are poorly understood. Their manifestations cover a wide range, from hives to respiratory difficulties to cardiac arrest (stopping of the heart). Allergies are grossly divided into two types: those due to B cell action (that is, antibodies) and those based on toxic materials released by T cells. Which system predominates in the allergy depends to some extent on the antigen that causes it. The allergies related to T cells are chiefly due to certain compounds—for example, metals, oils present in plants like poison oak, dyes, and the like. The chief causes of allergies related to B cells are plant pollens (ragweed and many kinds of grasses, for example), house dust (in which the active ingredient is probably some insect by-product), insect toxins such as those left by bee stings, and many foodstuffs. These are all materials that almost everyone can come into frequent contact with. Why, then, do only 10 to 15 percent of us suffer from allergies?

The total answer is not known, but parts of it have become clear. The tendency to acquire allergies is hereditary. It may also have something to do with an individual's ability to produce a particular kind of allergic antibody in large quantities. The main property of this allergic antibody is its ability to attach itself to a type of cell called a mast cell.

Mast cells contain substances that are toxic when released. These substances can cause spastic contraction of certain muscle tissues of the lungs, heart, and intestines and can increase the permeability of small blood vessels. The toxic substances (*histamine*, in particular) are released when the allergic antibody attached to the outside of the mast cell is contacted by antigen of an allergenic material. The respiratory system is the principal portal of entry of a number of allergenic materials, and many allergies manifest themselves as respiratory disturbances: coughing, mucus secretion, sinus congestion, and so forth. Toxic substances can travel from one part of the body to another, so even when the antigen enters through other portals, such as the skin, the eyes, or the gastrointestinal tract (following ingestion), respiratory symptoms frequently occur. Food allergies frequently manifest themselves by the appearance of hives, which can either be restricted to small areas or can cover the whole body.

A variety of treatments have been used for allergies related to B cell action. Drugs that interfere with the action of histamine (called antihistamines) are well known. More modern treatments have used compounds that prevent the release of the toxic materials from mast cells. The most common treatment consists of frequent injections of the material to which the patient is allergic, but in amounts too small to cause allergic reactions.

The allergies based on T cells have different symptoms from those based on B cell action. Certain of these allergies are referred to as contact sensitivity, or contact allergy. The most common is poison oak. Oils present in the poison oak plant attach to the skin components, modifying them and causing an immune response to the oil. No symptoms appear at first since the immune response takes time to develop. On the second exposure, however, greatly increased numbers of T cells bring about a toxic reaction that causes local inflammation. Allergies of the T cell type are usually treated with corticosteroids. These reduce inflammation in various ways (one of which involves the destruction of white blood cells).

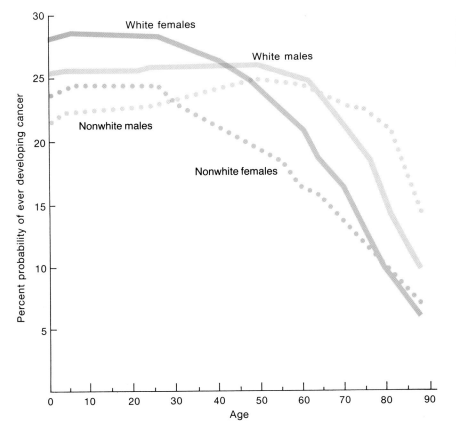

Figure 19-4   The lifetime probability that a person in the United States will develop cancer of any site, except skin, according to age, sex, and race.

Keeping Up with the Genetic Revolution

Of the estimated 100,000 genes found tucked up inside a human cell, some 800 have now been tracked to their chromosomal locations, with new genes being mapped at a rate of 200 per year. According to Dr. Frank Ruddle, professor of biology and human genetics at Yale University, this rate will accelerate exponentially over the next few years so that "by the turn of the century, the major outline of the human gene map should be known."

. . . Already the molecular cartography of animal and human genes heralds startling advances in health care:

■ Vaccines. [In October 1983], scientists of the New York State Health Department announced they had used the manipulation of genetic material—genetic engineering, as it is commonly called—to develop vaccines that protect rabbits against hepatitis and mice against a type of herpes. They held out hope that tests could begin in three years or so on similar vaccines that might protect humans from the same afflictions. In the same week, a New York City team announced it had isolated the gene for a substance that may cause toxic shock syndrome. A vaccine to guard against that condition, too, might possibly result.

■ Early warning for adult diseases. In the brief interim since the genetic origins of many cancers first came to light, scientists have succeeded in isolating specific snippets of genetic material that may predispose individuals to heart disease and emphysema. Medical sleuths are now hot on the trail of genes that have emerged as likely culprits in diabetes, allergies, peptic ulcers, and other common diseases of midlife, a trend that may shift the central thrust of medicine from treatment to prevention.

■ Understanding the basis of inherited diseases. The blood disorders sickle-cell anemia and beta thalassemia, and over a dozen other hereditary diseases, have now been traced to specific "spelling errors" in the genetic code, shedding new light on the underlying causes of hereditary afflictions.

■ Prenatal screening. Old limitations of prenatal diagnosis are being overcome by new techniques that enable clinicians to analyze directly the genetic makeup of developing fetuses. By the late 1980s, experts predict, these methods will permit fetuses to be screened early in pregnancy for such lethal hereditary diseases as cystic fibrosis, muscular dystrophy, and Huntington's chorea.

■ Therapy. Within the last year, doctors at the National Institutes of Health in Washington reported using a revolutionary gene therapy to ease the effects of two hereditary blood disorders, a historical first that suggests that the power to alter our biological destinies may be fast approaching.

■ Natural drugs. Genetic formulas are being used increasingly by the pharmaceutical industry to prepare potent natural medicines never before available for routine clinical use.

Along with the anticipated benefits, however, has come a barrage of worries and uncertainties, including the familiar questions about just where all the ground-breaking research is leading.

Of all the ethical dilemmas raised by genetic science, none is more pervasive than the public's fear that we may soon be tempted to "play God." Last June, a group of 64 religious leaders and several prominent scientists asked Congress to ban experiments that could alter man's inheritable traits. The question of when, or if, it is morally acceptable to modify human genes is certain to remain the focus of debate well into the next century.

Within medical circles, meanwhile, there is concern that people may come to expect too much too soon. Specialists point out that the age of genetic discovery is still in its infancy; major obstacles will have to be overcome before our newfound knowledge is translated into treatments and other useful applications. Others observe that advances in genetic science may tend to confirm belief in man's fate and lack of free will.

Kathleen and Sharon McAuliffe
New York Times Magazine

Autoimmune
Immune reactions directed against the body's own tissue.

Rheumatoid arthritis
A disease that results in inflammation and stiffening of the joints.

Multiple sclerosis
A chronic progressive disease in which patches of tissue harden in the brain or spinal cord and cause partial or complete paralysis.

Schizophrenia
A mental disorder characterized by a disturbance in thinking and perceiving reality.

Asthma
A disease characterized by wheezing and labored breathing.

In vitro
In an artificial environment.

Steroid hormone
A chemical that suppresses the immune system.

Many allergies are of a mixed type, showing both kinds of symptoms. Corticosteroids are often used to treat allergies in general, but they can have serious side effects that make prolonged use inadvisable.

Autoimmune Disease

Fairly often, the body's self-recognition mechanisms break down. When such failures happen, the immune system may attack one of the organs of the body. One of the diseases that results from this phenomenon is Hashimoto's disease. In Hashimoto's disease the organism produces both T cells and antibodies that are directed against the thyroid gland. The thyroid gland itself may eventually be destroyed. Administration of corticosteroids is successful for a time, but the treatment is limited by serious side effects. *Autoimmune* responses are suspected in many diseases, including *rheumatoid arthritis, multiple sclerosis,* and even *schizophrenia.* Proof of the autoimmune origin of disease is, however, extremely difficult to come by.

Control of the immune response is clearly the key to controlling many of the diseases that still plague humankind. Our present notions about the cellular interactions involved in the immune response have been shown by recent studies to be greatly oversimplified. The actual interactions are complex, specific, and full of feedback controls that have evolved over many millions of years.

Do the Emotions Affect the Immune Response?

We have already mentioned findings that show that during states of stress, particularly during depression, infectious diseases are more likely to occur in humans.

Emotions are even more clearly associated with the manifestations of allergy, especially *asthma.* Today it is widely recognized that treatment of a disease should in many cases include or even be based on psychiatric treatment of the patient. This can be easily understood by the observation that the response to the toxic agents released by cells in an allergic condition, in particular histamine, varies widely from individual to individual. Thus, given the same underlying immune conditions, one person can become severely ill during an immunological reaction, while another will "shrug it off" as a minor irritation. It has been shown that some reactions can be totally abolished by hypnotism, proof positive that they are under the control of the mind. It has also been shown conclusively in animals that both autoimmune diseases and cancer can be accelerated or even brought on in susceptible strains by stress. *In vitro* experiments accompanying these observations indicate that T cell deficiency may be brought on by stress. It must be remembered that NK cells, which are presumed to be the prime defense against spontaneously arising cancer, and suppressor cells, which prevent the appearance of autoimmune disease, are both T cells. It has been shown by direct experiments that NK cells can be suppressed by stress in mice. One of the pathways through which the mind may affect T cells is the *steroid hormones,* which are elevated in stress conditions. We know that these hormones can destroy or interfere with the action of T cells and that NK cells are especially susceptible to this action. Meanwhile, further research on the effects of emotions on the immune response is being conducted.

Immunity Behavior Scale

Read the following statements carefully. Choose the one in each section that best describes you at this moment and record its score at the right. (For example, "knows that colds are caused by viruses" has a score of 3.) When you have identified five statements, total your score and find your position on the scale.

5 is well educated about causes of infection
4 is informed about causes of infection
3 knows that colds are caused by viruses
2 is confused about causes of infection
1 is totally ignorant about causes of infection

Score _____

5 washes hands vigorously before handling food
4 washes hands before meals
3 usually washes hands before meals
2 occasionally washes hands before meals
1 rarely washes hands before meals

Score _____

5 brushes teeth after eating
4 brushes teeth at least once a day
3 usually brushes teeth every day
2 brushes teeth irregularly
1 rarely brushes teeth

Score _____

5 recognizes spoiled food
4 refrigerates perishable foods
3 throws out moldy food
2 eats food that has not been washed
1 will eat moldy food

Score _____

5 keeps personal immunization history
4 has been immunized against major diseases
3 has been immunized against some diseases
2 doesn't know immunization history
1 has never or rarely been immunized against disease

Score _____

Total score _____

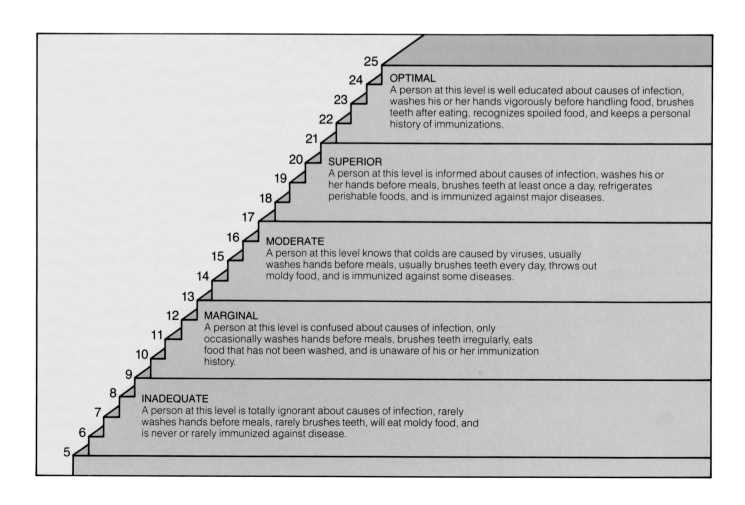

25
24
23   OPTIMAL
22   A person at this level is well educated about causes of infection, washes his or her hands vigorously before handling food, brushes teeth after eating, recognizes spoiled food, and keeps a personal history of immunizations.
21

20   SUPERIOR
19   A person at this level is informed about causes of infection, washes his or her hands before meals, brushes teeth at least once a day, refrigerates perishable foods, and is immunized against major diseases.
18
17

16   MODERATE
15   A person at this level knows that colds are caused by viruses, usually washes hands before meals, usually brushes teeth every day, throws out moldy food, and is immunized against some diseases.
14
13

12   MARGINAL
11   A person at this level is confused about causes of infection, only occasionally washes hands before meals, brushes teeth irregularly, eats food that has not been washed, and is unaware of his or her immunization history.
10
9

8   INADEQUATE
7   A person at this level is totally ignorant about causes of infection, rarely washes hands before meals, rarely brushes teeth, will eat moldy food, and is never or rarely immunized against disease.
6
5

Take Action

Your answers to Probing Your Emotions at the beginning of this chapter and your placement level on the Immunity Behavior Scale will, we hope, encourage you to begin a process of self-exploration and self-discovery that you will continue. Reflect on the entire chapter's content and ask yourself how each point relates to your own life. Then take action:

1. Find out what diseases you have been immunized against and list them in your Take Action notebook.

Include the dates and note whether any further boosters are required.

2. Pretend you are Alexander Fleming about to discover penicillin. Put some food, such as a crust of bread, in a small dish and observe daily changes until it becomes moldy. Note how long it takes before observable changes occur. Suppose you fail to notice mold on some food you eat. What are the consequences?

3. Carefully observe the times you get a cold or cold symptoms. Note the date, time of day, actual symptoms, and your emotional state,

e.g., depressed, bored, and so forth. Also note how long it takes for the cold to run its course. Do you find any associations between your emotional state and the length of your colds?

4. List the positive behaviors that help you avoid or resist infection. Consider how you can strengthen these behaviors. List the behaviors that tend to block your positive behaviors. Consider which of these you can change.

Before leaving this chapter, review the questions that open the chapter. Have your feelings or values changed? Are you now better equipped to handle the complex and very human problems associated with infection and immunology?

Chapter Twenty

Sexually Transmitted Diseases

Probing Your Emotions

1. In applying for your marriage license, you and your fiancé must take a screening test for sexually transmitted diseases. The results of your test are fine, but your partner's test is positive. How does this make you feel? Why do you feel this way? Will your feelings toward your fiancé be different?

2. You have noticed symptoms that may indicate you have contracted gonorrhea, and your physician has just confirmed it. How do you feel about this? Do you feel differently than you would if you had contracted influenza? If so, why?

3. A couple is about to engage in sexual intercourse. One of the partners asks the other, "Do you have a sexually transmitted disease?" How would you feel if someone asked you that in similar circumstances? Is it realistic to expect that such a question would be asked? Would you ask it?

4. You are a woman and realize that women frequently do not experience observable signs of a sexually transmitted disease. During a regular physical examination you realize your doctor will not routinely test you for exposure. What do you say to the doctor? Will you be able to ask for appropriate tests? Why do you suppose your doctor does not make the inquiry?

Chapter Contents

CAUSES OF THE PREVALENCE OF SEXUALLY TRANSMITTED DISEASES

WHAT THE INDIVIDUAL CAN DO
Education
Prevention
Diagnosis and treatment

MAJOR SEXUALLY TRANSMITTED DISEASES
Gonorrhea
Nongonococcal urethritis (NGU)
Syphilis
Pelvic inflammatory disease (PID)
Herpes
Trichomoniasis
Candida albicans
Pubic lice
Scabies

OTHER SEXUALLY TRANSMITTED DISEASES

Boxes

Doctoring VD stereotypes
The VD National Hotline
Dealing with sexually transmitted diseases
Twenty prominent victims of syphilis
Acquired Immune Deficiency Syndrome (AIDS)

Gonorrhea
A sexually transmitted disease caused by a type of bacteria.

Syphilis
A sexually transmitted disease caused by a certain type of spiral-shaped bacteria.

Nongonococcal urethritis (NGU)
An infection in the urethra that cannot be related to a specific organism.

Herpes
A type of virus or the disease produced by this virus. A cold sore is an example of this type of virus infection. May or may not be a sexually transmitted disease.

Trichomoniasis
A vaginal or penile infection caused by a certain one-celled microorganism.

---

20 Despite the efforts of medical science, a number of communicable diseases still exist, some at epidemic levels. Among these are the 20 or so known as sexually transmitted diseases (STDs) or, more commonly but less accurately, as venereal diseases (VD).

Each year over two million new cases of *gonorrhea* and 100,000 new cases of *syphilis* are reported in the United States—and the incidence is undoubtedly much higher because many cases are never reported. Conservative estimates indicate that over ten million people are afflicted annually with STDs, and health officials predict that this number will double in the years ahead. The combined case rate of these diseases is already more than four times that of arthritis or lung diseases and ten times that of diabetes or heart diseases.

Unlike some of the other communicable diseases, such as childhood diseases, flu, or the common cold, STDs if left untreated can exact a heavy toll. Consequences of untreated sexually transmitted diseases to the affected individual may include disfigurement, infertility, damage to the urinary tract and central nervous system, blindness, sterility, and even death. More poignant perhaps is the risk to unborn and newborn children, who may suffer mental retardation, congenital deformities, and many other kinds of damage. In their first few days of life, over 8,000 infants born of infected mothers die annually.

Needless pain, anguish, and suffering can be avoided if we will only recognize the seriousness of the STDs and help to reduce the barriers to seeking and obtaining information, early diagnosis, and proper treatment.

tions. *Trichomoniasis*, the most common protozoal disease in the United States, was not granted STD status until less than ten years ago.

Another cause may be the greater societal acceptance of premarital sex, accessibility of contraceptive information and methods, influence of the women's movement on greater sexual freedom and later marriage (married people have a lower incidence of STDs), and pressures by advertising and the mass media to be "popular, sexy, and part of the 'in' crowd."

A third factor that has contributed to the epidemic proportions of some STDs is the biophysical changes that have occurred in some disease organisms. The best known of these changes is the emergence of antibiotic-resistant bacterial strains. Some of these strains cause minimal or no apparent symptoms (thus turning their hosts into unknown carriers), while other strains cause damage much more quickly than earlier versions did. The relatively recent strain known as "Viet Nam Rose" developed as a result of self-administered, often black-market penicillin that killed only the initial weakened bacteria and permitted a stronger, more resistant strain to take its place.

Because the STDs are almost always contracted through intimate contact with an infected person, sexual behavior is called into question. For a teenager, admission of such a disease may mean parental disapproval. For a single person, it may mean religious disapproval or an undesired admission of sexual activity. For a married person, it may signal infidelity. For these and other reasons, some people resist seeking proper diagnosis and treatment.

Causes of the Prevalence of Sexually Transmitted Diseases

Many causes have been suggested for the current high incidence of STDs. One of the most significant causes is the relatively recent identification of diseases other than gonorrhea and syphilis that are sexually transmissible. Although gonorrhea and syphilis remain problems, incidence of *nongonococcal urethritis (NGU)* is five times that of gonorrhea, and there may be ten times that number of sexually transmitted cases of *herpes* infec-

What the Individual Can Do

There are at least three major areas in which the individual can take responsibility for his or her own health and a general reduction in the number of cases of sexually transmitted diseases: education, prevention, and diagnosis and treatment.

Education A basic tenet of health behavior is that the individual be knowledgeable about his or her susceptibility to various diseases. Many people mistakenly be-

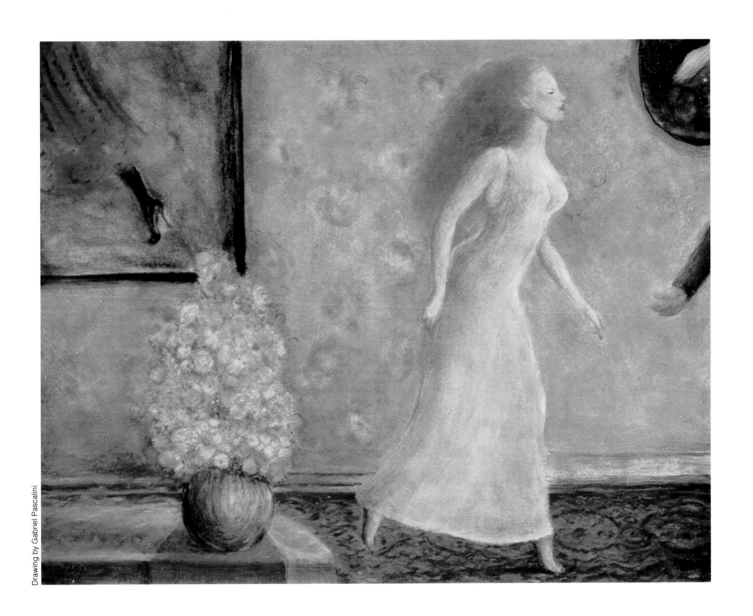

457

Doctoring VD Stereotypes

Squares Are Not Immune

College students who have had a sexually transmissible disease, such as syphilis or gonorrhea, are often stereotyped as irresponsible social deviants. That stereotype may be grossly unfair, says an assistant professor of health education at Purdue University.

His research suggests that college women who have had such infections are more serious, forthright, and trusting than those who have not. His study also indicates that male students who have had a sexually transmissible disease may be more sensitive and practical than those who have not.

William L. Yarber, H.S.D. (doctor of health science), a health and sex educator at Purdue, bases his findings on a recent study of students from seven colleges and universities in the east, west, and central parts of the U.S. "Measured against students who had never had an infection, the personality differences of those who had been infected fell within the average personality range for college students," he reports.

The undergraduate students in his study, which was conducted with Robert Kaplan, professor of health education at Ohio State University, were given a personality scale that measures the major factors differentiating people.

Of the students studied, 49 males and 47 females reported having been treated for infections at some time in their pasts. In addition to syphilis and gonorrhea, among the sexually transmissible infections reported were nongonococcal urethritis, herpes simplex genitalis, cytomegalovirus, and trichomoniasis. These subjects were compared to an equal number of college students who had not had previous infections. Differences were apparent in only a few areas. The males who had infections were more relaxed and assertive than those who had not. The females who reported having had an infection were more self-assured, serious, and forthright than the women who had never been infected.

Yarber says that the students in

both groups did not show differences in intelligence or in being in control of themselves. Also, they were equally outgoing and venturesome. The females in both groups were on the same par moralistically, and the males who had had a previous infection were just as conservative, self-assured, emotionally stable, and happy as those who had not. "The traditional stereotypes for those who had had infections—that they are irresponsible, immature, and have extremely radical life-styles—just didn't hold up," Yarber reports. "Contrary to previous studies in this area, we found that those who had had infections at some time in their lives did not have any more or fewer psychological difficulties than those who never had an infection. However, such differences might be found in studies of the general population that lacks the homogeneity of the college population."

Human Behavior

---

lieve that sexually transmitted diseases simply could not happen to them. Yet the STDs are among the most democratic of illnesses. Men, women, and children of any age, race, or economic status can contract a sexually transmitted disease. Sexual intercourse is not necessarily a prerequisite, but direct physical contact is.

If each of us recognizes that anyone who is physically intimate with another human being is at risk each time he or she makes contact, we will be more willing to do something about it. (See Figure 20–1.) We can, for instance, ask questions of our sex partners, take certain precautions before and after intercourse, practice monogamy, and so forth.

It is also important that we become knowledgeable about the nature and severity of the STDs. Some of the consequences of sexually transmitted diseases left unchecked and untreated have already been noted. In

the discussions of specific STDs that appear later in this chapter, others are outlined. It is the responsibility of each of us to learn not only the causes and nature of these diseases but also their potential effects on us personally, on our children, and on others with whom we share relationships.

Prevention   The second area in which the individual can make a difference is prevention. Methods of preventing sexually transmitted diseases can be mechanical, emotional, or a combination of the two, depending on the individual's preference.

Mechanical methods, not always completely effective, include male use of the condom during sexual intercourse and urination immediately after and the practice of washing thoroughly after any kind of intimate contact. Although condoms are often effective in preventing

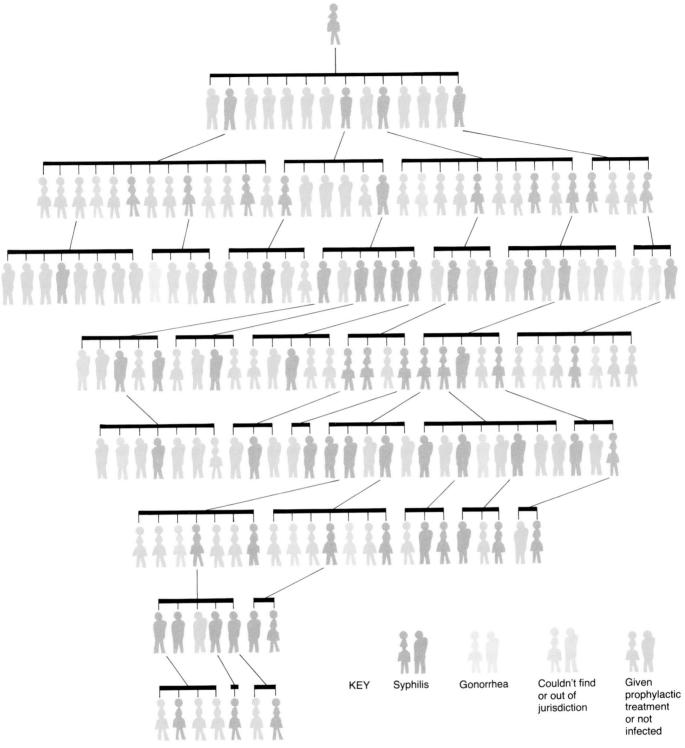

KEY   Syphilis   Gonorrhea   Couldn't find   Given
                                or out of   prophylactic
                                jurisdiction   treatment
                                                 or not
                                                 infected

Courtesy of American Social Health Association.

Figure 20-1   This diagram shows how a sexually transmitted
disease spread from a 17-year-old girl who had secondary syphilis. Investigators found and examined all but 15 of 141 people.
Of the 126 examined, 34 were found to have syphilis or gonorrhea. The average age of those infected was 18.4 years; the
youngest was only 6 years old.

The VD National Hotline

There appear to be four main reasons why young people remain at highest risk from venereal disease:

1. They don't realize how serious VD can be.
2. They don't know where to go for medical help.
3. They are afraid their parents will find out if they *do* go for help.
4. They don't know enough about the signs and symptoms that indicate they *should* seek help. (To make matters worse, most girls and women do not have symptoms, and an increasing number of males are also asymptomatic.)

For these reasons the VD National Hotline, sponsored by the Center for Disease Control and a core program service of the American Social Health Association, was established in October 1979.

Trained volunteers are available from 8 A.M. to 8 P.M. (Pacific time) Monday through Friday to provide free, confidential information and referral service to callers from the 48 continental states.

Anyone wishing to ask a question pertaining to VD or wanting to know where to go for diagnosis and treatment can call 800-227-9822; in California 800-982-5883.

gonorrhea, they will not help to prevent diseases that are contracted from direct contact with sores on the mouth, anal area, and so on. For men, urinating immediately after having had sex can flush bacteria from the urethral opening, but this by no means eliminates all risk. Washing with soap and water can remove bacteria from the surface of the skin but obviously is not effective against bacteria that have entered the body.

It should be pointed out that women are at a disadvantage in terms of anatomical structure. This highlights the importance of telling a woman if she has been exposed to an STD. Women also often have no symptoms with some of these diseases, but they can have relatively rapid and severe complications. Furthermore, women who have an unsuspected and therefore undiagnosed disease run the risk of passing it on to their unborn children.

Emotional methods are another means of preventing STDs. People form relationships for a variety of reasons: to have pleasant times, to avoid loneliness, to develop intimacies, to have sex, to have families. The decision to have any physical relationship with another person carries with it an array of uncertainties and risks, including intimacy itself, pregnancy, and disease. Such a decision may be dealt with subconsciously, superficially, or with deliberate thought. Crucial to the last of these are mutual respect and open communication. To begin with, we ought to care enough about ourselves and the other person to know our own and that person's physical condition. In terms of STDs we must care enough to ask questions and to be aware of signs and symptoms. Certainly it may be momentarily awkward to do these things, but if we think about the danger, to others as well as ourselves, of possibly transmitting as well as contracting a disease, temporary embarrassment seems well worth the cost. If a person thinks less of us for being concerned about and openly discussing such matters, perhaps that person is not really one we want a relationship with.

Diagnosis and Treatment A third area in which the individual can take responsibility in regard to sexually transmitted diseases is diagnosis and treatment if the possibility of having contracted such a disease exists. Warning signals can come from the alert of a partner or any indication of unusual pains, sores, rashes, or discharges. Before a person can know for sure if he or she has an STD, proper tests must be made. In almost all instances, the person to do this should be a qualified health professional (physician, nurse, public health official, or other allied health practitioner) working in the proper setting (physician's office, health center or clinic, or other licensed health facility).

If diagnosis confirms the presence of an STD, the affected individual should inform any sex partners, refrain from any physical contacts, and seek immediate treatment. Specific kinds of medication are available for treating, and in most cases curing, all of the STDs. Medication may come in the form of injections, pills or capsules, salves or lotions. Regardless of the kind of medication prescribed, all accompanying instructions should be followed exactly.

In nearly all cases, the individual should also be sure to have follow-up tests after treatment is complete to ensure that the disease is gone and that it can no longer be transmitted to another person.

Major Sexually Transmitted Diseases

Gonorrhea Of the 50 or more infectious diseases on which the U.S. government's Centers for Disease Control keep statistics, gonorrhea (sometimes called the clap or

Asymptomatic
Without symptoms.

Pharyngeal
Relating to the pharynx, which lies
between the mouth and the esophagus.

---

drip) is ranked number two, exceeded only by the common cold. It is caused by the bacterium *Neisseria gonorrhoeae,* one of the most sensitive of disease-causing organisms. Because these bacteria cannot live very long outside the warm, moist environment of the human body, it is highly unlikely that anyone can contract gonorrhea from toilet seats or towels. It is primarily transmitted by sexual contact.

A male exposed to gonorrhea during vaginal intercourse has a 20 percent chance of developing the disease. However, a female who is exposed in the same manner has an 80 percent chance of developing gonorrhea even though no symptoms may be present. Risks of contracting the disease through oral-genital or anal intercourse are similar.

The organism grows well in mucous membranes, including the moist linings of mouth and throat, vagina, cervix, urethra, and anal canal, and the particularly sensitive eyelids of newborn babies.

The incubation period for gonorrhea is usually short (three to five days), although it can be as long as 30 days. One attack of the disease does not grant immunity.

In a male, burning on urination is usually the first symptom if the penis is the primary site of infection. Most men with gonorrhea will also notice a discharge from the penis. Within a day or two this discharge becomes thick, heavy, and creamy. The color varies from white to yellow or yellow-green. The lips of the urethral opening become swollen and protrude. The lymph glands in the groin may also become enlarged and tender. In some uncircumcised men, the bacteria may multiply under the foreskin and cause irritation and redness of the glans penis. In many cases symptoms disappear without treatment, and these males may then become asymptomatic carriers.

In a female, pus may be discharged through the cervical opening. Unlike a male, in whom a discharge is obvious, a female may not observe this early sign of infection. Some women may notice a green or yellow-green vaginal discharge that can be irritating to the vulva. This discharge is rarely heavy, and it, too, may go unnoticed unless some other infection is also present.

It has been estimated that 80 percent of the infected female population are *asymptomatic* carriers of gonorrhea, whereas only about 20 percent of the infected male population have no signs or symptoms.

It is not known how long an infected individual may remain asymptomatic, how long he or she may be infectious, or what triggers the onset of symptoms.

Diagnosis A smear of the discharge from the penis of the male is generally sufficient to diagnose gonorrhea. However, if the organisms are not discovered, further cultures from the urethral, anal, and *pharyngeal* exudates should be made, and the bacteria identified microscopically.

Gonorrhea in women is more difficult to diagnose because approximately 80 percent of infected women have no symptoms. The only defense women have is to go for an examination and a culture within a week to 10 days after sexual contact they consider suspicious. Cultures are taken from urinary sediments, the cervix, and the anus.

Should arthritis or dermatitis develop, treatment is indicated. If left untreated, severe complications may develop in as few as three weeks. If pain and swelling of joints, fever, or rashes occur, hospitalization may be warranted. Fluid from swollen joints is removed to reduce pain and obtain samples for laboratory testing. Blood samples and joint fluid are then cultured for gonorrhea. Samples of pus from skin rashes should also be examined.

All patients with proven gonorrhea should also be tested for syphilis before treatment is begun. This is especially necessary since syphilis mimics a dozen other diseases.

Treatment Anyone who even suspects gonorrhea should remember two facts. First, gonorrhea is easy to cure when it is treated early. It is a dreadful, chronic, sterility-producing disease when it is treated late. Second, anyone seeking treatment for gonorrhea (or any sexually transmitted disease) will be treated with utmost confidentiality at any medical facility from free clinic to private office.

Penicillin is the preferred drug for the treatment of acute, noncomplicated gonorrhea. The drug probenecid is also given to keep penicillin in the system long enough to effect a cure. For those people who are allergic to penicillin or probenecid, tetracycline is used for a longer period of time, although tetracycline should not be administered to pregnant women.

Dealing with Sexually Transmitted Diseases

How do you tell your partner that you not only were unfaithful but you also exposed him or her to a sexually transmitted disease? You know that you should tell your partner immediately, that the consequences of an untreated or advanced STD can be very serious. Yet this is often easier to say than to do.

Since gonorrhea and nongonococcal urethritis (NGU) are usually asymptomatic in women, meaning that women will not be aware of the presence of an infection until it is too late, and since most males are symptomatic, the male usually has the responsibility of informing his partner or partners of exposure.

There are a number of ways in which people avoid their responsibility to their partners. Some never tell them. They devise ingenious methods for attempting to deal with a very delicate situation. On a two-week sales trip, for example, a man met a woman at a bar, went to her place, and had sex. A few days later he returned home. The salesman noticed a slight discharge, but since he had been away for a while he nevertheless had sex with his wife. His symptoms increased and he went to a doctor, who diagnosed him as having gonorrhea and gave him penicillin. The salesman realized that he had exposed his wife to the disease but did not want to tell her he was unfaithful. In our counseling session he asked, "Since I have penicillin in my medicine chest, can I give it to my wife in her food?" The obvious answer was no. The penicillin (which, when stored for a period of time, loses potency) could have been inadequate and served only to hide or mask the symptoms, in which case the disease would re-incubate later and cause much more serious problems. The question

I asked him was, "When you and your wife face any type of problem, how do you handle it?" His response was that they don't talk about their problems.

In this couple's relationship, problem-solving mechanisms, namely, interpersonal communication, trust, and values, were not considered viable or adequate to solving the predicament. When a relationship is built without problem-solving techniques, it is considerably more difficult to solve a problem that cannot be dismissed easily because of its serious health consequences. In short, when couples do not normally practice open communication, it becomes much more difficult to do so in a crisis situation. When a crisis does occur, family counseling or marriage counseling may be a starting point for resolving the crisis. In this instance it was evident that the parties involved had been practicing a noncommunicative relationship for many years, and to change their life-style would be extremely difficult.

In another case a 17-year-old male confronted the problem of telling his girlfriend that he had exposed her to gonorrhea. As we talked about his problem, he asked, "How do I tell my girlfriend that I gave her VD?" He was planning to tell her that he had the flu and in order for her not to catch it she would have to go to the clinic and get two shots of penicillin. I told him that a clinic would not substantiate his story and that he would have to inform her that she had gonorrhea. At that point he realized that he would have to tell her the truth himself and that he would have to work through the relationship and hope for the best.

In yet another case a man contracted gonorrhea on his travels. He

went to a doctor and was diagnosed and treated, but *before* he did this he had sex with his wife and exposed her to the infection. His solution to the problem was to try to reverse the situation. After he had been to the doctor and was treated, he thought he would wait a few days and then have sex with his wife, who would then *reinfect* him; his position would be that she was not faithful to him and had exposed him to the infection!

Each of these three people had some understanding or perception of the severity of STDs. However, in each case the person's first choice was the easy way out: hiding penicillin in food, getting a friend to be immunized for the flu, and reversing the situation and blaming the partner.

The two married couples had a long-established pattern of lack of communication. They were unable to deal with sensitive issues and had developed no problem-solving skills. In addition, other considerations compounded the problem: questions of fidelity, trust, security, fear, and a need to step outside the relationship, perhaps to achieve feelings of self-worth, to reaffirm their sexuality, and so on. These considerations must also be examined and dealt with.

In the case of the 17-year-old man, behavioral patterns revolving around relationships were just being developed. Granted, these dynamics probably began long before they were applied to the relationship, but they were at this point being tested, and the young man realized that an honest, open relationship was perhaps painful but nonetheless the only way out of the predicament.

Dealing with STDs, either from the standpoint of telling someone that you exposed him or her or getting the news that you were exposed, raises a number of emotions, including anger, guilt, shame, low self-esteem. These emotions are natural and can motivate a person to act in his or her own best immediate interest. But they can also be turned inward against the self and against the partner, in which case dire consequences can occur.

For example, a female client I had occasion to talk with said that she had been exposed to herpes simplex virus and that she had an extremely severe case. Her reaction to her partner was that she never wanted to see him again and for good measure never wanted to see any man again. For three years she had no social or sexual contacts. During our conversation I found that she had a lot of misinformation about the disease and that once she understood the etiology of it, her anger, fear, and feelings of guilt and low self-worth would subside. I had occasion to talk with her a year later, and she informed me that she was getting married. After getting help with her problem, she was better equipped to deal with the situation and her life.

Remy Lazarowicz

It is vitally important that people who have been treated for gonorrhea return to their health care professional for follow-up examination and tests. Cultures should be taken 3 to 10 days after completion of treatment. Intercourse and other close sexual contacts should be avoided until the results are confirmed as negative. Many infections that continue after adequate treatment are in reality due to reinfection.

Sexually active men and women should consider having a gonorrhea screening every six months. Men and women should also take responsibility for their behavior by communicating with their partners if they do develop gonorrhea, or any sexually transmitted disease, so that everyone involved can be effectively treated.

Nongonococcal Urethritis (NGU)   Nongonococcal urethritis (NGU) is rapidly becoming one of the most common sexually transmitted diseases. It is estimated that 2.5 million Americans are infected annually.

NGU is an inflammation or infection of the urethra that is caused by something other than the organism that causes gonorrhea. It is suspected that NGU is caused by several different organisms.

Chlamydia trachomatis is suspected of causing 49 to 51 percent of all nongonococcal urethritis cases. This organism is only slightly larger than a virus, difficult to isolate, and expensive to diagnose. If left untreated, chlamydial infections in women can cause pelvic inflammatory disease (see next section), and are often responsible for pneumonia and eye infection in newborn infants whose mothers are infected.

T-strain mycoplasmas, which are also thought to cause some nongonococcal urethritis, are similar to bacteria but closer in size to viruses. Also difficult and expensive to diagnose, these, too, may exist normally in the vagina, as well as in the urethra of the male, and only trigger the disease in particularly susceptible individuals. Undiagnosed T-strain mycoplasmas are being considered as a possible cause of infertility when other causes have been ruled out.

It has been suggested that some men become allergic to the vaginal secretions of their sexual partners and that in such cases NGU is an allergic response. It is also possible that the urethra can become irritated by the use of certain soaps, deodorant sprays, clothing dyes, and vaginal contraceptives.

In males, symptoms of NGU include a discharge from the penis, which may be thin and watery or thick and white, and a burning and itching around the opening of the penis. Sometimes symptoms appear only in the morning. Approximately 10 percent of afflicted males have no symptoms at all.

Because the disease is internal, women sometimes do not get obvious symptoms. However, pain, itch, or burning around the vagina or any discharge may be a sign of NGU.

If left untreated, because of a lack of symptoms or reluctance on the part of an individual with mild discomfort to seek medical attention, NGU can have serious consequences. Among these may be sterility in both men and women, pelvic inflammatory disease in women, and serious difficulties for a newborn child whose mother remains untreated.

Diagnosis   Diagnosis may be undertaken initially by excluding the presence of gonorrhea. Absence of the gonococcus, however, does not mean that the person is *not* infected. If there is reason to believe that NGU may be present, further testing should be carried out or a course of antibiotic therapy should be initiated.

Microscopic examination of any discharge and an

Chancre
The sore produced by syphilis in its earliest stage.

Twenty Prominent Victims of Syphilis

1. Charles Baudelaire, French poet
2. Ludwig van Beethoven, German composer
3. Al Capone, U.S. gangster
4. Lord Randolph Churchill, English statesman
5. Christopher Columbus, Italian discoverer of America
6. Capt. James Cook, English mariner and explorer
7. George Armstrong Custer, U.S. army officer
8. Paul Gauguin, French artist
9. Johann Wolfgang von Goethe, German poet and scientist
10. Henry VIII, king of England
11. "Wild Bill" Hickok, U.S. frontier marshal
12. John Keats, English poet
13. Louis XIV, king of France
14. Ferdinand Magellan, Portuguese navigator
15. Mary ("Bloody Mary"), queen of England
16. Napoleon, French emperor
17. Friedrich Nietzsche, German philosopher
18. Peter the Great, czar of Russia
19. Marquis de Sade, French writer of erotica
20. Robert Schumann, German composer

David Wallechinsky et al.
The Book of Lists

---

analysis of the first urine sample in the morning should be made in order to identify the disease-causing organism.

Treatment   NGU is usually treated with tetracycline or erythromycin. Penicillin and some of the other antibiotics are of no value in the treatment of NGU.

Follow-up tests should be taken after treatment, and the affected individual should abstain from sexual contact until these tests are negative. Sexual partners should also be treated to avoid reinfection and to prevent complications.

Syphilis   Syphilis (also known as *evil pox, great pox,* or *the great imposter*) is considered to have the most severe complications of the sexually transmitted diseases if left untreated. Complications may result in blindness, paralysis, insanity, or death.

Syphilis is caused by the *Treponema pallidum,* a very thin, corkscrew-like organism that has the capacity to move steadily by rotating on its long axis. Warmth and moisture are essential to its survival, and it dies very quickly outside the human body.

The organism can be transmitted through an opening or break in the skin or mucous membranes by means of kissing or vaginal, oral-genital, or anal intercourse.

The incubation period for syphilis can range from 10 to 90 days, although the average is 21 days. However, an individual with untreated syphilis can remain contagious for as long as 18 months.

Primary Syphilis   As early as 10 days or as late as 90 days after contact with an infected person, the first sign of syphilis, an open sore commonly known as a *chancre,* appears at the location where the organism entered the body (usually on the genitals but sometimes on the cervix, anus, lips, mouth, throat, or breast). The chancre may be painless, and if left untreated, it heals within one to five weeks.

Secondary Syphilis   Generally two weeks to six months after the chancre appears, symptoms of secondary syphilis develop. During this time some people have no apparent symptoms. In about 25 percent of the cases, however, there is a general feeling of poor health, which may include a combination of headaches; loss of appetite; nausea; constipation; pain in the long bones, muscles, or joints; and a low-grade, persistent fever. Hair may fall out in patches, and the lymph glands may be swollen and tender.

Among the classic symptoms of secondary syphilis is a rash that may appear anywhere on the body, particularly on the palms of the hands and the soles of the feet. The rash may also affect the mucous membranes of the lips, cheeks, tongue, tonsils, throat, and vocal cords. In these areas, grayish-white mucus patches surrounded by a dull-red border appear. These sores break down and ooze a clear fluid that contains large numbers of the organism, making this a highly contagious stage.

Pelvic inflammatory disease (PID)
An infection that progresses from the vagina and cervix and eventually moves into the pelvic cavity.

With or without treatment, the rash of secondary syphilis disappears within two to six weeks. This does *not* mean that the disease is gone or the individual is cured.

Early Latent Syphilis   After 12 to 18 months, an individual with syphilis is no longer considered infectious, except in the case of pregnancy, during which a mother can infect her unborn child. Approximately two-thirds of those who do not receive treatment can live the remainder of their lives without any other problems. However, the remaining one-third will develop complications.

Late Latent Syphilis   Signs of late latent syphilis, which is not infectious, may appear two or more years after initial infection. Major manifestations include damage to the central nervous system, the digestive organs, the liver, lungs, eyes, brain, heart, blood vessels, muscles, and bones. In some cases such damage can lead to death.

Diagnosis   Although syphilis can produce symptoms similar or identical to many other diseases, it is crucial for anyone who thinks that he or she may have syphilis to go to a doctor, health clinic, or whatever medical facility is available. In the case of primary syphilis a technician or doctor lifts the crust off the chancre and extracts the clear fluid from the center. The fluid is then examined under a special microscope. In the case of secondary syphilis, diagnosis is made by blood tests. Two or three tests are used, the most usual being the Veneral Disease Research Laboratory (VDRL) and the fluorescent treponema antibody (FTA) reaction. A test of the spinal fluid should, at this stage, show a negative result. A negative finding means that the central nervous system has not yet been invaded.

Syphilis in Pregnancy   The *Treponema pallidum* organism can invade the placenta of an infected mother after the tenth week of gestation, although this generally takes place after the eighteenth week. If the mother is not treated before this time, the probability of stillbirth or congenital infection and deformities exists. Possible damage includes crippling, blindness, deafness, and facial abnormalities. Children who are born with syphilis are contagious only while lesions are present. These

children do not pass their syphilis on to the next generation because they are usually not infectious by the time they reach puberty.

Treatment   Primary, secondary, and latent syphilis of less than one year's duration are treated with penicillin. For patients allergic to penicillin, tetracycline is effective. Latent syphilis of more than one year's duration is treated with a combination of antibiotics, including penicillin, tetracycline, and erythromycin.

Follow-up tests should be performed four weeks after the completion of treatment and every three months thereafter for a year. A person who has had syphilis should not have sexual contact with others until at least one month after treatment is completed and he or she is participating in follow-up testing.

Pelvic Inflammatory Disease (PID)   The Center for Disease Control estimates that of at least 2.7 million cases of gonorrhea that occurred in the United States in 1976, 10 to 17 percent of those occurring in women resulted in *pelvic inflammatory disease (PID)*. PID occurs when infection progresses from the vagina and cervix into the uterus and Fallopian tubes, subsequently spilling out of the open ends of the tubes into the pelvic cavity. (See Figure 20–2.) Symptoms may include one or more of the following: pelvic pain, chills and fever,

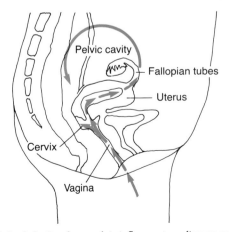

Figure 20-2   Infection from pelvic inflammatory disease can move from the vagina and cervix to the uterus, Fallopian tubes, and, finally, the pelvic cavity.

Polymicrobial
Marked by the presence of several species of microorganisms.

Ectopic pregnancy
Fertilization of the ovum in a place such as a Fallopian tube where the fetus cannot develop normally.

---

irregular menstrual periods, and lower back pain. Although usually dramatic, the symptoms may be intermittent at first. Reported cases of asymptomatic PID with resultant tubal damage have led to use of the term *silent PID.*

Studies of the causes of PID are still inconclusive, but agreement exists as to the implication of organisms other than the gonococcus. The nature of the disease has been described as *polymicrobial.* Reinforcing this description are studies that show that when gonorrhea is cultured from the cervix, other microbes are also present in the genital tract. It is thought that the gonococcus may initiate an infectious process and pave the way for other infection or that the infection may have been caused by nongonococcal organisms from the beginning.

Certain risk factors may make some women more vulnerable to PID than others. Prolonged or repeated bouts of PID predispose women to chronic infection; damaged Fallopian tubes are more susceptible to further infection; the use of an IUD results in a three-to-nine-times greater risk of infection. It is both the patient's and the physician's responsibility to be aware of medical history when PID is suspected.

Complications of PID can be serious and irreversible. Scarring in the tubes, often a product of abscesses due to infection, can cause reproductive organs to adhere to other proximal or adjacent organs. Chronic pelvic pain and/or painful intercourse often occurs as a result of these adhesions, and surgical correction is often necessary. Scarring in the tubes can also prevent the passage of the ovum into the uterus. This can result in *ectopic* (tubal) *pregnancy,* which usually ends in spontaneous abortion but may require surgery. Furthermore, PID and its complications can be responsible for premature sterility in a significant number of young women.

Diagnosis and Treatment Consideration of the most effective treatment of PID depends on identification of the specific organism(s) responsible. The implications for diagnostic surgical procedures are highly controversial and presently under study.

Herpes Estimates are that at least 20 million people in this country are suffering from genital herpes and that about 500,000 new cases occur each year. This makes herpes a major sexually transmitted disease. Media coverage of the disease has sensitized the public to the proportions and severity of its problems and has also generated a sense of anxiety in some areas. (*Time* magazine labeled herpes the "new sexual leprosy.")

Herpes is caused by a virus, either the herpes simplex virus type I or type II. *Facial herpes,* generally caused by type I, affects the lips, mouth, face, and sometimes the eyes, while *genital herpes,* type II, usually affects the genitals, buttocks, and thighs. The virus enters the body when an individual comes into direct contact with someone who is infected and is shedding the virus. Therefore sexual contact, including kissing, should be avoided at this time.

Either type I or type II herpes can and does occur genitally or facially. It is important to point out that someone with facial herpes does not necessarily have an STD. If and only if the disease has been transmitted by sexual contact is it considered to be an STD. Facial herpes, or "cold sores," are *very* common. Also very common is the infection of a partner by engaging in oral-genital sex when a cold sore is in full bloom.

Typically, a herpes infection appears 2 to 20 days after exposure. Symptoms can include one or more sores on or around the face or sex organs. The sores are often painful, blisterlike lesions filled with fluid. They may be accompanied by swollen glands, general muscle aches and pains, fever, a mild burning sensation, and, in women, a vaginal discharge.

Some women have internal herpes lesions, with the cervix or vagina being the only site of infection. Because there are no nerve endings on the cervix, these women may be unaware of the lesions and exhibit no noticeable symptoms.

The virus is still present in the body and enters a dormant phase. In the case of facial herpes the virus may enter nerve endings and lodge in nerve cells lying in the cheek. In the case of genital herpes the virus retreats to the nerve cells outside the spinal canal, far removed from the original site of active infection. While dormant, the virus appears to remain in the cells without causing any damage to these nerve fibers.

Once infected, a person may be prone to recurrences of the disease if the virus reactivates, and the symptoms will appear much the same as in the initial stage. Some

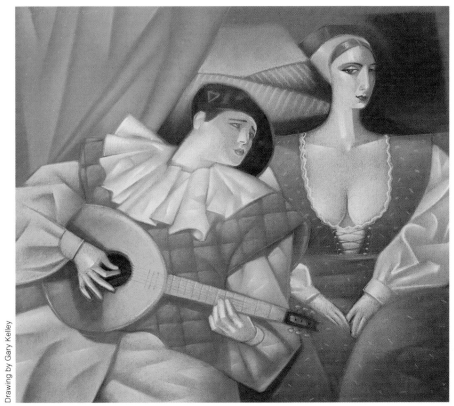

467

individuals never experience a recurrence; some, only infrequently; others, regularly. What triggers a reactivation of the virus is not clearly understood. However, it is believed that generally poor health, low resistance, physical trauma, and even emotional stress may be contributing factors.

Although a direct relationship between the herpes virus and cancer is yet to be established, women with genital herpes are five to eight times more likely to develop cervical cancer. It is recommended that women who have had genital herpes inform their doctor and be sure to obtain a Pap smear every six months.

Even more serious are the complications and the risks to newborn babies whose mothers have active genital herpes. Pregnant women should inform their physician if they have had herpes so that proper precautions can be taken prior to the delivery of the child. If genital lesions are present during the time of delivery, it is recommended that the child be delivered by Caesarian section. Should an infant come in contact with herpes lesions while passing through the birth canal, there is a 50 percent chance that the baby will then become infected. Of such infected babies, 50 percent suffer serious brain damage or die. Care should also be taken to ensure that no family members or friends who may have active facial herpes expose the infant to the disease by kissing and fondling.

Diagnosis Ninety percent of the herpes cases seen by medical practitioners are diagnosed on the basis of sores or lesions and other characteristic symptoms accompanying the lesions. Fever, swollen lymph nodes, and pain or itching of the sores are common. If there is any doubt that the disease is herpes, such visual diagnosis is not enough, however. A tissue culture, although still relatively expensive, can yield a more definitive diagnosis. Because the virus must be grown on live tissue, this test is difficult to obtain. Many facilities simply do not have the capability to conduct live-tissue cultures, although select hospitals and clinics across the country are beginning to provide this test. A specific antibody filter test can also be conducted to demonstrate the presence of the herpes antibody in the blood. But, again, this test is expensive and not yet readily available.

Presently there is no herpes screening test for people who have no lesions.

Treatment Herpes, both facial and genital, can be treated. At the present time researchers are just beginning to experiment with drugs that may attack this virus. Because no specific drug or treatment has yet been discovered to cure the disease, the prescribed therapy is to deal with the symptoms, while the body itself marshalls its reserves to fight the virus.

Treatment and care are directed at relieving pain, itching, and burning and at preventing the sores from becoming infected or being spread to other parts of the body. Bathing with soap and water or other drying agents such as epsom salts or Burrow's solution is helpful in preventing secondary infection and the spread of lesions and speeds drying of the lesions.

Trichomoniasis Trichomoniasis is caused by a one-cell organism, *Trichomonas vaginalis*, a pear-shaped protozoan with a moving membrane and four flagella that whip back and forth to give the organism a capacity for rapid, jerky movement. It can remain alive on external objects for 60 to 90 minutes, in urine for three hours, and in seminal fluid for six hours. The organism is usually transmitted sexually and may be present along with other STDs, especially gonorrhea. Twenty-five percent of women harbor this organism, but not all of them have a reaction.

Although many females show no symptoms, in as few as four days or as many as 28 days, some women with trichomoniasis experience a greenish vaginal discharge and severe itching. In some cases the discharge is white or yellow and frothy, with an unpleasant odor, and frequently irritates the vagina and vulva, which may become red and painful. In many women with trichomoniasis, bright red, slightly raised spots can be seen on the vaginal walls and cervix.

Although most males show no symptoms (the organism can survive under the foreskin of the penis without causing any symptoms), some males may experience slight penile itching, a clear penile discharge, and painful urination.

Acquired Immune Deficiency Syndrome (AIDS)

Acquired Immune Deficiency Syndrome (AIDS) is the nation's number one public health concern. It is a fatal condition that affects the immune system (the body's natural defense against disease), making an otherwise healthy person susceptible to a variety of infections and certain forms of cancer. As of September 24, 1984, there were 6,122 cases nationwide and 2,734 deaths, and the number of new cases was doubling every seven to nine months. AIDS patients have been identified in 45 states, plus Puerto Rico and Washington, D.C., and in at least 20 other countries.

The largest group of AIDS patients (approximately 73 percent) is made up of homosexual and bisexual males. The second largest group of patients (17 percent) is intravenous drug abusers. Smaller percentages are found among persons who have received blood or blood products donated by people infected with the disease, the sexual partners (and their offspring) of persons from the high-risk groups, and a few individuals with no apparent risk factor. There have also been a number of cases among Haitians newly arrived in the United States. It appears that they are at risk because of their lifestyle, not because they are Haitian.

The probable cause of AIDS is a variant of the human cancer virus called HTLV III, or human T-cell leukemia virus. HTLV III is a retrovirus, so named because of its ability to convert ribonucleic acid (RNA) into deoxyribonucleic acid (DNA), which is the chemical constituting the genes of human and animal cells. This virus uses the genetic machinery of the cells it infects to make the protein it needs for survival.

Common to all AIDS patients is a significant impairment of the body's immune system. Within this system, there are helper T cells, which marshal the defenses against infection; there are also suppressor T cells, which prevent the formation of antibodies. Generally, individuals with normal immune function have about twice as many helper as suppressor T cells. In AIDS patients, however, there is often a reversal of this ratio.

It is believed that blood and blood-contaminated fluids of the body can carry the causal agent. In homosexual and bisexual males, transmission can occur through sexual activity that involves the exchange of body fluids and their entry into the blood system. The route of transmission among intravenous drug users is the sharing of contaminated needles or syringes. Hemophiliacs who develop AIDS are probably infected by contaminated blood from a donor carrying AIDS—even though they are treated for their condition with a product prepared from the blood of as many as a thousand donors.

Once a person is infected, the incubation period for AIDS ranges from about four months to as long as five years. Less than 10 percent of patients with AIDS has survived for more than three years following the diagnosis, and none has recovered cellular immune function. It is therefore assumed that AIDS is universally fatal.

Signs and symptoms suggestive of AIDS include unexplained swollen glands, night sweats, fever chills, weight loss (unrelated to illness, dieting, or increased physical activity), of more than ten pounds in less than two months, and fatigue. Obviously, some of these signs and symptoms can occur with minor colds or stomach flu ailments.

The infection most commonly seen in patients with AIDS is Pneumocystis carinii, a pneumonia producing shortness of breath, a persistent dry cough, sharp chest pains, and, in severe cases, difficulty in breathing. Kaposi's sarcoma is the second most common problem seen in AIDS patients. It is a form of cancer that produces purple or brownish lesions that resemble bruises but are painless and do not heal. They may occur anywhere on the skin or inside the nose, mouth, or rectum.

The risk of AIDS transmission to individuals not in the high-risk groups is very small. Basically, the disease has confined itself to the high-risk groups. Even doctors and nurses who have been working with AIDS patients for the past four to five years have not contracted this tragic disease. Therefore, no one should fear having casual contact with a person who has AIDS.

Because the probable cause has been identified, it is hoped that a cure and a vaccine to prevent future infections will be forthcoming. However, this breakthrough may take as long as five years. Therefore, the most important action that people in the high-risk groups can take is to prevent the exchange of body fluids between individuals. The two fluids considered most highly contagious are blood and semen.

Many forms of treatment have been tried, but none (including Interferon and Interleukin II) has successfully brought about a reversal of the suppressed immune condition. Although physicians have been successful in treating the infections and cancer that attack AIDS

(continued on next page)

Acquired Immune Deficiency Syndrome (AIDS) (continued)

patients, the body is eventually overpowered and succumbs. Other care includes counseling, in-home services, and hospice services.

What does the future hold? In the immediate future, the number of new cases will continue to rise at an alarming rate. The long incubation period makes it unlikely that preventive actions already undertaken will produce a decline in that rate within the next two years. However, research to find a vaccine and a cure will bring us closer to understanding the mysteries of the immune system, and, possibly, success with AIDS will lead to some answers relating to cancer.

Regardless of the potential accomplishments at some future time, education must be the cornerstone in the prevention of the spread of this disease. Because the highest-risk group spreads AIDS through sexual contact, educational programs must be implemented in a sensitive and relevant manner. The social and psychological implications of this disease make it necessary to tailor education programs very carefully so that misinformation and unnecessary anxiety within the *general* community are minimized and awareness of the seriousness of the disease in the *affected* communities is maximized.

There must be a modification of behavior, and this change must continue into the foreseeable future. It is well known that fear has a short-lived impact on behavior. Therefore, positive approaches to behavior change must be implemented to motivate the continued involvement of individuals in safe and healthy practices. With intensified research into the cause, cure, and vaccine for AIDS, and a comprehensive educational program, we may by the end of this decade be able to look back at AIDS as a *historical*, albeit tragic, phenomenon.

Mervyn Silverman, M.D.
Director of Health
City and County of San Francisco

Diagnosis and Treatment   The simplest diagnostic test is a slide prepared from the vaginal or penile discharge. If *T. vaginalis* is found, the drug metronidazole (Flagyl) should be taken orally by the person affected, as well as by all sex partners. A condom should be used until the infection is gone. Alcoholic beverages should be avoided during treatment because, when metronidazole is in the body, alcohol is not metabolized normally and produces unpleasant side effects.

Candida Albicans   *Candida albicans*, a microscopic, yeastlike fungus, is present in the vaginal tract of most women. Several factors can make a woman more susceptible to a vaginal infection caused by increased fungus production. These include pregnancy, diabetes, use of birth control pills, antibiotic therapy, and lowered resistance.

Symptoms include intense vaginal and vulval itching and a thick, white, and curdy vaginal discharge that resembles cottage cheese. The vagina becomes red and dry, and sexual intercourse may be painful.

Diagnosis and Treatment   Diagnosis is made by microscopic examination of the discharge. The antibiotic nystatin, in the form of vaginal tablets, is generally prescribed. Treatment usually lasts for four weeks, and further testing should be done if the condition continues.

Pubic Lice   *Pubic lice*, also known as crabs, are a type of louse that has three pairs of claws in front and four pairs of small legs in back; they are a pest, not a disease.

Pubic lice are often the color and size of small freckles and are difficult to see on light skin. After the lice have eaten, they are swollen with blood and can be seen more easily.

Although pubic lice usually infest the pubic hair, they can also infest other hairy areas of the body, including the head and underarms and even eye lashes, moustaches, and beards. Separated from humans, lice are able to live about 24 hours.

Most people who have pubic lice experience intense itching, a response to the bites of the lice. Usually transmitted by person-to-person contact, pubic lice may also be transmitted via infected clothing, towels, bedding, and toilet seats.

Diagnosis and Treatment   Diagnosis is confirmed by finding lice or lice eggs attached to body hairs. Pubic lice are easily treated. Several over-the-counter medications for lice infestation are available at the local pharmacy. These come in shampoo or lotion form, and some include a very fine-toothed "nit" comb. If directions are followed carefully, the lice and nits will be killed on contact. Washing of infested linen and clothing is essential in preventing reinfestation. For stubborn cases,

Candida albicans
A vaginal infection caused by a fungus.

Pubic lice
Insects that infest the hair of the pubic region.

Scabies
A contagious skin disease caused by a type of mite.

Larvae
The immature, wingless forms that hatch from the eggs of many insects.

Contact dermatitis
Inflammation of the skin that results from contact with material to which a person is allergic.

Chancroid
A sexually transmitted disease caused by a bacterium and characterized by a soft chancre.

Lymphogranuloma venereum (LGV)
A sexually transmitted infection that causes swelling of the lymph nodes.

Acquired immune deficiency syndrome (AIDS)
An often fatal new disease that primarily affects male homosexuals, intravenous drug users, and hemophiliacs. Victims lose the ability to fight infections and usually die from cancer or any of a host of rare diseases that almost never afflict people with normal immune function. Believed to be caused by a virus carried in blood or semen.

---

the drug gamma benzine hexachloride, or Kwell, can be used. Also available as lotion or shampoo, Kwell can only be obtained by prescription. Gamma benzine hexachloride is a known central nervous system toxin and should be used with caution, particularly where children are concerned.

Scabies   *Scabies,* also known as "the itch," is caused by the mite *Sarcoptes scabiei* or *S acarus.* The pregnant female mite burrows under the skin and deposits her eggs. The resulting *larvae* hatch within a few days and congregate around hair follicles.

Itching, especially at night, is present wherever the burrowing parasite is found. Usual sites of infestation are between the fingers and on the wrists, armpits, breasts, buttocks, thighs, penis, scrotum, and, occasionally, female genitals.

Scabies is easily transmitted, often through an entire household, by contact with an infected individual. In some instances it is transmitted by sexual contact.

Diagnosis and Treatment   Diagnosis of scabies is made by finding the actual mite, eggs, or larvae in scrapings taken from the burrows in the skin. Standard treatment is a prolonged hot bath with vigorous cleansing of affected areas and application of benzyl benzoate emulsion or Kwell lotion. If inflammation and itching

persist after treatment, they are probably the result of a scratch or *contact dermatitis,* a secondary infection. Calamine lotion or a lotion containing one percent menthol and one percent camphor is usually effective in reducing inflammation and itching. Starch baths may also help.

Other Sexually Transmitted Diseases

Several other sexually transmitted diseases are considered minor in terms of their prevalence in the United States but certainly not in terms of their severity. Among these are *chancroid, lymphogranuloma venereum,* and *granuloma inguinale.* As with any communicable disease, these should be carefully diagnosed and treated (usually with proper antibiotics) because they can be confused with each other or with syphilis.

The *acquired immune deficiency syndrome* commonly known as *AIDS* is a relatively new STD. Its cause is not known, but many researchers believe that it is brought on by a virus that attacks the immune system. Although AIDS is not very prevalent among the general population, the fatality rate among AIDS victims is high. See "Acquired Immune Deficiency Syndrome (AIDS)," page 469, for a detailed discussion.

STD Behavior Scale

Read the following statements carefully. Choose the one in each section that best describes you at this moment and record its score at the right. (For example, "uses contraceptives to prevent STDs" has a score of 3.) When you have identified five statements, total your score and find your position on the scale.

5 refrains (or would refrain) from physical contact if infected
4 refrains from sexual contact if infected
3 uses contraceptives to prevent STDs
2 takes few precautions to avoid STDs
1 takes no precautions to avoid STDs

Score _____

5 seeks (or would seek) immediate treatment if infected
4 seeks treatment if infected
3 seeks treatment for an STD only after extensive symptoms
2 doesn't voluntarily seek treatment for STDs
1 deliberately avoids treatment for STDs

Score _____

5 discusses STDs openly with others
4 discusses STDs openly with sexual partner(s)
3 prefers not to discuss STDs openly
2 rarely discusses STDs openly
1 refuses to discuss STDs

Score _____

5 educates others about STDs
4 is familiar with STD hotline
3 is willing to be educated about STDs
2 relies on friends for STD information
1 has no sources of STD information

Score _____

5 knows sexual partner(s) very well
4 knows sexual partners fairly well
3 avoids one-night stands
2 has occasional one-night stands
1 prefers one-night stands

Score _____

Total score _____

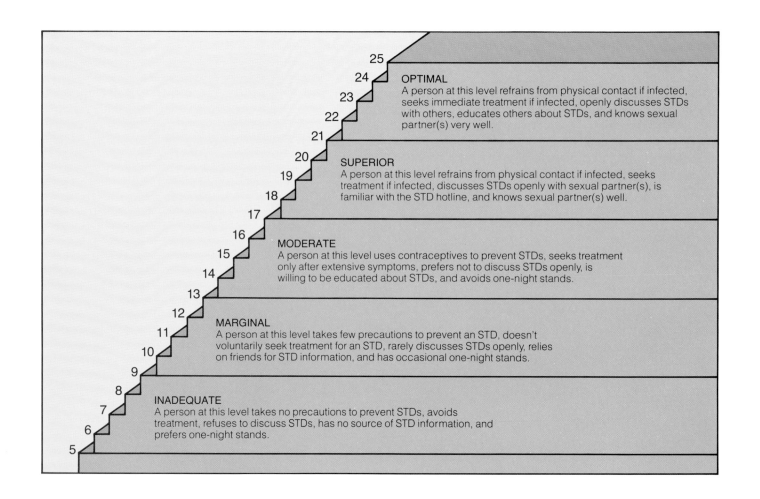

25
24 **OPTIMAL**
A person at this level refrains from physical contact if infected, seeks immediate treatment if infected, openly discusses STDs with others, educates others about STDs, and knows sexual partner(s) very well.
23
22
21

20 **SUPERIOR**
A person at this level refrains from physical contact if infected, seeks treatment if infected, discusses STDs openly with sexual partner(s), is familiar with the STD hotline, and knows sexual partner(s) well.
19
18
17

16 **MODERATE**
A person at this level uses contraceptives to prevent STDs, seeks treatment only after extensive symptoms, prefers not to discuss STDs openly, is willing to be educated about STDs, and avoids one-night stands.
15
14
13

12 **MARGINAL**
A person at this level takes few precautions to prevent an STD, doesn't voluntarily seek treatment for an STD, rarely discusses STDs openly, relies on friends for STD information, and has occasional one-night stands.
11
10
9

8 **INADEQUATE**
A person at this level takes no precautions to prevent STDs, avoids treatment, refuses to discuss STDs, has no source of STD information, and prefers one-night stands.
7
6
5

Take Action

Your answers to Probing Your Emotions at the beginning of this chapter and your placement level on the STD Behavior Scale will, we hope, encourage you to begin a process of self-exploration and self-discovery that you will continue. Reflect on the entire chapter's content and ask yourself how each point relates to your own life. Then take action:

1. In your Take Action notebook list the positive behaviors that help you avoid exposure to sexually transmitted diseases. Consider what additions you can make to this list or how you can strengthen your existing behavior. Don't forget to congratulate yourself for these positive aspects of your life. Also list the behaviors that block your maintaining wellness. Consider each of these behaviors. Which ones can you most easily change? Start with these.

2. Go to the drugstore and peruse the contraceptive section. Read the labels on various packages. What if anything do they tell you about STDs? Ask the pharmacist what he or she would recommend to prevent STDs.

3. Call the VD National Hotline (see page 460). Ask the trained volunteer a question about something you personally would like to know or confirm about STDs.

Before leaving this chapter, review the questions that open the chapter. Have your feelings or values changed? Are you now better equipped to handle the complex and very human problems associated with sexually transmitted diseases?

Chapter Twenty-One

Aging

Probing Your Emotions

1. Consider spending a Saturday afternoon visiting a nursing home or convalescent hospital. What do you imagine such a visit would be like? What emotions would you have to confront in such a situation? Do you fear old age?

2. A friend of yours is in his mid-twenties. You learn during a conversation with him that he is very much involved with a woman and hopes to marry her. In the course of the conversation you learn that she is 43 years old. What would your reaction be? Why? What would you say to your friend?

3. How do you feel about the indisputable fact that you are growing older every day? Why do young people generally find it difficult to conceptualize their own old age?

4. Can you imagine what retirement will be like for you? At what age would retirement be a good idea? Is chronological age a reasonable gauge to answer such a question, or would your degree of work satisfaction be a better one? Suppose you truly enjoyed your work; how would you feel if you *had* to retire?

Chapter Contents

THE GOAL OF GERONTOLOGY
America's aged minority
Increased life expectancy:
  the myth and the reality
The search for lasting youth

THEORIES OF AGING
Food restrictions
Brain chemistry
Errors in DNA and RNA duplication
Hormone imbalance

THE ETHICS OF TAMPERING
WITH THE AGING PROCESS

LIFE-EXTENDING MEASURES
Don't smoke cigarettes
Control drinking
Eat wisely
Control your weight
Keep physically fit
Detect and control hypertension
  and diabetes
Recognize and reduce stress
Use it or lose it
Be involved

AGING: A POSITIVE EXPERIENCE

Boxes

Aging and health:
  an anthropological point of view
Parent abuse
Senility
Gray power

21 Many older people are happy, healthy, and self-sufficient. Changes that come with age, including negative changes, normally occur so gradually that the majority of people adapt easily and gracefully. Only 5 percent of people over age 65 in the United States are being cared for in institutions, and generally the rest continue to live meaningful and independent lives. Even so, most people in America do not look favorably on the prospect of growing old. They may dread it, feel that being old is somehow shameful or something to be regretted, or treat it with self-conscious humor. We laugh at old age jokes to make ourselves somehow feel more comfortable about aging. Culture in America is oriented toward youth, and it discriminates against the aged as mercilessly as it discriminates against other oppressed minorities. Yet all people age—no matter what their color, their religion, or their sex—and each of us is likely to become a victim of "ageist" discrimination.

What we overlook is that the process of aging is not limited to the elderly. It begins at conception and continues until death. Looked at in one way, aging is no more than the changing of structure and function over time. In *Stress of Life,* Canadian biologist Hans Selye points out, "there is little doubt that under constant use with the passage of time, every construct, living or inanimate, wears out or, if you will, 'ages.' This is true of human beings, insects, autos, civilizations, volcanoes, and tornados alike."

Most of us do not understand what aging is all about. We also are not aware that we can have some control over the length and the quality of our lives. We shall try here to explore some of the ways in which we can make the most of our individual potentials for long and meaningful lives. After all, as a wit once said, "Growing old is not so bad when you consider the alternative."

The Goal of Gerontology

Gerontology is the study of aging. Human gerontology is the study of *aging* in people. Such study is aimed toward adding years to people's lives and "life" to those years. The goal is not to keep old, decrepit bodies alive at all costs but to bring as many people as possible to later life as vibrantly alive, experienced, growing, and involved as possible. People should be able to live long and well and then die with dignity. This outcome does not happen by accident. It depends on circumstances in the environment, and these circumstances can be controlled, at least in part. Aging is not just important to people middle-aged or older; it is important to all of us. What we are and do in later life is greatly affected by what we are and do in earlier life.

America's Aged Minority There is no precise age at which a person becomes "old." Some people are "old" at 25; others are still "young" at 75. Although Congress has upped the mandatory retirement age for nongovernment employees from 65 to 70, age 65 has usually been taken as the dividing line. People over 65 have been considered "aged." People 65 and older are a large minority in the American population—25 million people, or 11 percent of the total population, in 1980. As birth rates drop, the percentage also increases dramatically. Longer life expectancies do not contribute much to overpopulation, however, in spite of what many people think. Overpopulation is the result of young people having too many babies who grow up to have too many babies, not the result of longer life expectancies. The greater numbers of older people who are often ill and dependent do, however, create major social and economic problems. (See Figure 21–1 for age distribution trend.)

Whatever the American dream may have been, for some older citizens it has faded. Forced or persuaded into retirement, they find their incomes reduced to the point where they can barely exist. They are also likely to feel as if they have become worthless. Americans are conditioned in a thousand ways to value only what is shiny and new. Objects lose their value once they acquire a few scratches or scuffs or become a little worn around the edges. So, apparently, do people. Similarly, in this youth-oriented culture, the changes in a person's appearance brought about by age are usually seen as negative. The ways of urban life and the *nuclear family* worsen the effects of these attitudes on older people. In cultures that have *extended families,* older people stay active in society generally and in caring for children. Here, they often face lonely isolation, or institutions, or

Gerontology
The study of changes in structure and function with aging.

Aging
Changes that occur with the passage of time.

Nuclear family
The family unit consisting only of parents and children.

Extended family
The nuclear family along with its relatives by blood or marriage; generally refers to a family in which in-laws and/or grandparents live in the same house with the nuclear family.

Life expectancy
Expected average years of life for a species within a given environment; usually calculated from birth.

geriatric ghettos, bleak downtown hotels or posh retirement cities.

Illness sometimes makes the later years little more than a miserable prolonged wait for death. Medicare does not change this basic fact, although for some people the wait is made "easier." The same is true with the aged as with other oppressed minorities. Older people are like other people and need what all people need. They need to have their basic requirements satisfied, and they need a chance for a meaningful existence. More and more these needs are being considered basic human rights.

Increased Life Expectancy: The Myth and the Reality
Life expectancy at birth in the United States, an average figure, has increased dramatically from 49 years in 1900 to about 74 years in 1980. This increase does not mean that each and every individual American adult is now living much longer. It does not mean, either, that in 1900 everyone simply dropped dead the minute they blew out the candles on their forty-ninth birthday cake. What it does mean is that far fewer people are dying young, because childhood and infectious diseases are much better controlled than they were in 1900. (For

an even broader view of life expectancy through the ages, see Figure 21-2 on page 480.)

The young have benefited from modern medical and public health measures far more than the elderly. As late as 1980, a person of 65 could expect to live only about six years longer than a person of 65 in 1900. In 1977, however, the U.S. Census Bureau reported a dramatic 3 percent decrease in death rates for the three preceding years: The life expectancy of women was raised to 78 years and that of men to 70 years. These are all-time highs for Americans and reflect both new successes in medical care and health payoffs from early identification and treatment of high blood pressure, more prudent diets, and less cigarette smoking among middle-aged adults.

Another significant fact of life expectancy is that as one gets older and survives the hazards to life of younger years, he or she gains statistical life expectancy. For example, life expectancy for males born in 1980 is 70 years, but for men who were 20 in 1980, the expected remaining number of years of life is 52.5, or a total of 72.5 years (20 + 52.5). For a female born in 1980, life expectancy is 78 years, but for women who were 30 *(text continues on p. 480)*

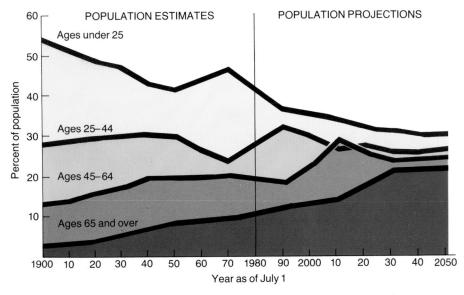

Figure 21-1 Trend in age distribution of United States population,* 1900-2050.

Source: Adapted from various reports and unpublished data of the Bureau of the Census.

*Including Armed Forces overseas.

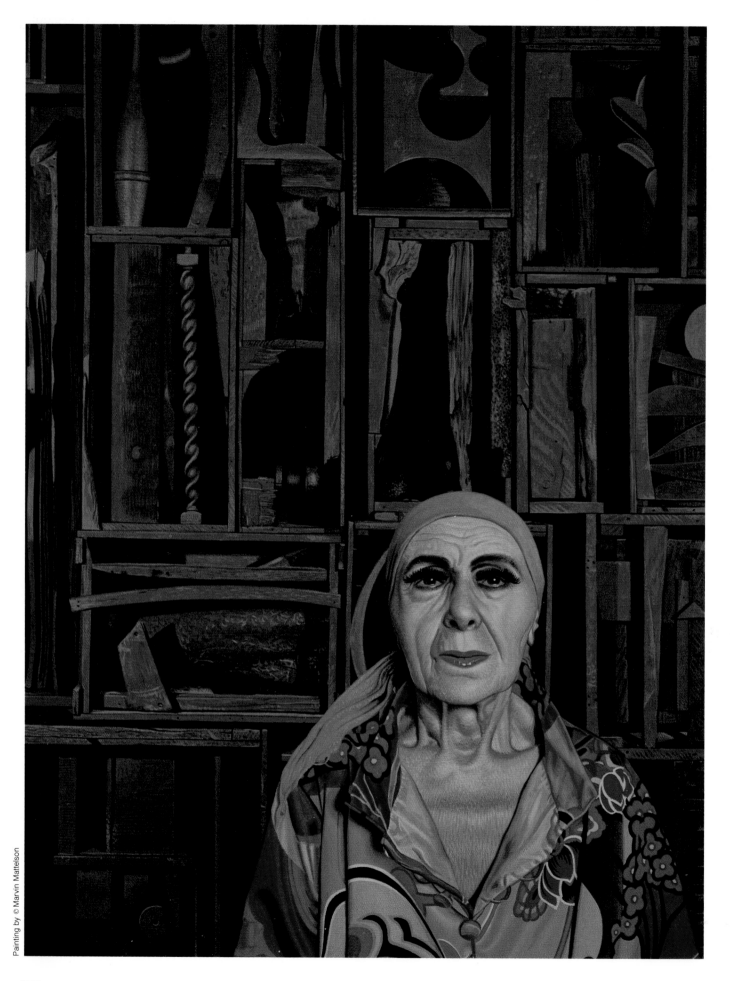

Aging and Health: An Anthropological Point of View

Aging should be just another word for growing, for we are designed to grow (increase in amplitude) and develop (increase in complexity) all the days of our lives. When I say "designed" I mean precisely that, for the scientific evidence clearly shows that just as we have evolved physically, retaining our neotenous (or childlike) traits—for example, the large brain, the high forehead, the flatness of the face, and small teeth—so we are designed behaviorally by retaining the behavioral potentialities of the child. Those childlike traits are:

the need for love

friendship

sensitivity

the need to think soundly

the need to know

to learn

to work

to organize

curiosity

wonder

play

exercise

imagination

creativity

enthusiasm

spontaneity

touch

speech

fantasy

self-esteem

trust and honesty

openmindedness

flexibility

experimentalmindedness

explorativeness

resiliency

sense of humor

joyfulness

laughter and tears

optimism

compassionate intelligence

dance

song

These are our inbuilt system of values which tell us what we ought to do: to grow young, to grow in health, to die young (as late in life as possible), and to live as if to live and love were one. To grow young means to grow and develop in the spirit of the child, in the childlike

basic behavioral traits. To grow in health means to develop the ability to love, work, play, and use one's mind as a fine instrument of precision. If one will do these things one will certainly grow older with time, but one will never grow old.

The quality of life is a matter of the spirit, and all the evidence indicates that where the spirit is happily realized the body will be too, for spirit, mind, and body are simply various faces of the same organism that is the human being. Certainly physical and physiological changes will occur during our life, but many of these are avoidable. Unfortunately the mythology that surrounds aging has resulted in a self-fulfilling prophecy which has deceived many, nay, almost everyone, into believing that growing older is a descent into senility and decrepitude. The old are expected "to act their age," to retire into nonentityism and anecdotage. Older people are made to feel old, to believe that they *are* old, and to fulfill only those requirements that are expected of them, to walk, talk, sit, think, rise and move as old people should. Dr. Gay Luce in her inspiring book, *Your Second Life* (New York, Delacorte, 1979), has listed the stereotypes of our culture relating to "old age":

- Old people should be dignified and circumspect.
- Old dogs cannot learn new tricks.
- Old people are close-minded, set in their ways, slow, senile.
- Old people are ugly.
- There is no future for old people. Why teach them?
- Old people don't want to use or touch their bodies.
- Old people like to sit still and be quiet.

These myths about old people are all false and very damaging.

Nevertheless, our culture has forced millions of wonderful human beings into the tragedy of acting out the stereotypic roles expected of them, much of the time not altogether unwillingly, for the old have come to accept the mythology of aging quite as much as the young. In this way too many people have been shipwrecked by "old age" simply because they have never learned to navigate the waters in which they suddenly find themselves. They find themselves in unfamiliar territory, traumatically displaced persons consigned to the very outskirts of the society in which they were once full members; forced into a life-style for which they have not been prepared, a life-style of unstructured time and reduced input from the world with which they were once familiar.

The results are abandonment, rejection, and a kind of exile or excommunication.

Those who retain their youthfulness into the later years are the biologically elite, not simply because they have survived, but because they have attained that weathered wisdom that only they can possess. The truth is that age is in no way connected with feeling old, but in every way with feeling young. There is an untouched freshness that comes to us when we are old, which need not for a moment ever waver, but keep us buoyant all the days of our lives, bringing to others that wisdom and that other gift which is the true vocation of the "old," love.

The whole of life is a journey toward youthful old age, toward self-contemplation, love, gaiety, and in a most fundamental sense, the most gratifying time of our lives. Growing older should mean reach-

(continued on next page)

Aging and Health: An Anthropological Point of View (continued)

ing one's full behavioral potential, a completeness.

Our preoccupation with youth has made us forget that people considered "too old" often have the youngest ideas of all. "Old age" should be a harvest time when the riches of life are reaped and enjoyed, and shared, while it continues to be a special period of self-development and expansion, instead of a half-life waiting to die. And in that connection, one needs a special strength to die, rather than a special weakness, and that strength can only come to us by dying young, at whatever age that may be, neither surprised by time nor attenuated by it.

And finally: always remember that the fountain of youth resides in yourself.

Ashley Montagu
Healthline

---

in 1980, the expected remaining number of years of life is 50, or a total of 80 years. Statistically, one never runs out of life expectancy. Even at age 85, men and women still have an expectation of 5.3 and 6.8 more years, respectively.

So how long could humans expect to live under the best of circumstances? It now seems likely that genetically our maximum potential *life spans* are from 100 to 120 years and that failure to achieve such life spans in good health results largely from the destructive environmental and behavioral factors—factors over which we could exert considerable control. It is a mistake to think that prolonging life automatically prolongs old-age disability. People often live longer because they have been well longer. In other words, a healthy, productive old age is often an extension of a healthy, productive middle age.

The Search for Lasting Youth A huge variety of "magic" preparations, devices, and practices for preserving youth have been invented—and believed in—by people throughout history. Lotions, potions, and baths have all been tried, as have spells, chants, and rituals. None of these has worked. More recently, science has not been idle in this area. Some scientific research is being directed toward learning more about the aging process, and researchers believe they are close to breakthroughs that may permit people to have longer lives and maintain much of their youthful vigor.

Some scientists believe aging is genetically programmed; a necessary process by which the older members of a species make way for the younger members. According to this thinking, a person might be likened to a spaceship that has been designed to fly past Mars but has no built-in instructions beyond that point. The

Figure 21-2 Life expectancy.

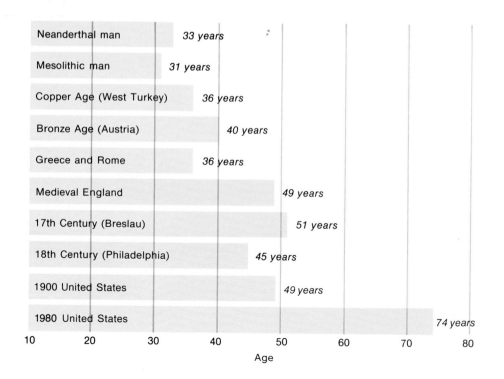

	Age
Neanderthal man	33 years
Mesolithic man	31 years
Copper Age (West Turkey)	36 years
Bronze Age (Austria)	40 years
Greece and Rome	36 years
Medieval England	49 years
17th Century (Breslau)	51 years
18th Century (Philadelphia)	45 years
1900 United States	49 years
1980 United States	74 years

Life span
The average length of life for a given species.

Environmental medicine
The study of environmental causes of disease. Studies of the effects of cigarette smoke on the lungs and the effects of stress on the heart are examples of kinds of problems dealt with in environmental medicine.

DNA (Deoxyribonucleic acid)
Acid that is the part of the genetic material which determines heredity and, therefore, controls the development of the whole organism. It is found in large amounts in the chromosomes of all cells.

ship will keep on going, but its various systems will begin to break down and continue until the breakdown is total.

Theories of Aging

The effects of aging have been characterized as "a decline with time in the production of the necessary free energy for the individual to function," and as "the increasing inability of the body to maintain itself and to perform the operations it once did." (See Figure 21-3.) As people lose their ability to withstand the stresses of the environment, they become more and more susceptible to certain diseases, particularly to what we can call the mass killers, heart attack and cancer. Researchers in the field of *environmental medicine* are turning up evidence that environmental factors trigger many of these diseases.

It is clear that the way we live has much to do with how long we live. The human organism has marvelous powers, but if we treat ourselves badly, we certainly will not perform as well as we would otherwise and we will break down sooner. Subjecting ourselves to environmental stress is one example of bad treatment that may be unavoidable. But sometimes we choose to mistreat our bodies, as we almost certainly do when we smoke cigarettes, eat too much, take too many drugs or the wrong kind, and do not exercise enough.

Aging does occur, however, even with the best behavior in the best environment. It is the result of biochemical processes that we do not yet understand. None of the existing theories of aging fits all the facts, so it is likely that aging is caused by a variety of different processes. No one yet knows enough to construct a completely workable theory. The genetic makeup of the cell largely controls aging. This factor explains why fruit flies can only live at the most about 100 days, dogs 30 years, humans 120 years, and giant tortoises 180 years. Some scientists believe that every organism has so-called aging genes, which control its rate of aging. Experiments give some support to this concept. For example, certain cells from the lung tissue of a four-month-old human embryo have been observed to multiply only about 50 times before they die. According to established opinion, they should have multiplied indefinitely. In addition, about the thirty-fifth time they multiplied, these cells began to show "signs of age."

Another popular theory is that in aging, the *DNA*, or genetic material, somehow becomes defective. Defective DNA, in turn, results in the synthesis of defective protein,

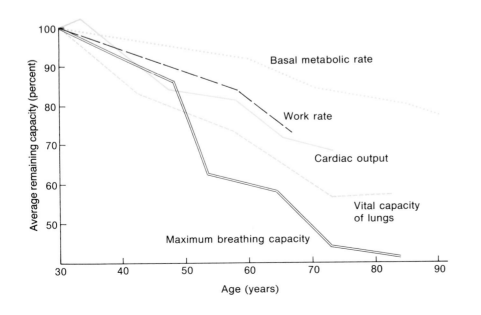

Figure 21-3   Decline of basic physiological capacities with age.

Protein synthesis
The chemical process of making complex protein molecules out of simpler molecules (amino acids). Proteins are crucial to the development and functioning of all bodily processes.

Longevity
Length of life.

which means that the organism cannot function normally, and it deteriorates.

A third theory suggests that for some (unknown) reason the body begins to make errors in *protein synthesis* and produces different, changed proteins. The body's immune mechanism reacts against its own changed protein just as it would against a foreign substance. The result—destruction of cells and impaired body functions—may be a primary factor in aging. Increasing incidence of diseases as people get older may be due to yet another dysfunction of the immune system, in which the production of antibodies is significantly reduced, thereby making people increasingly vulnerable to disease. Drugs that promise to reinforce faltering

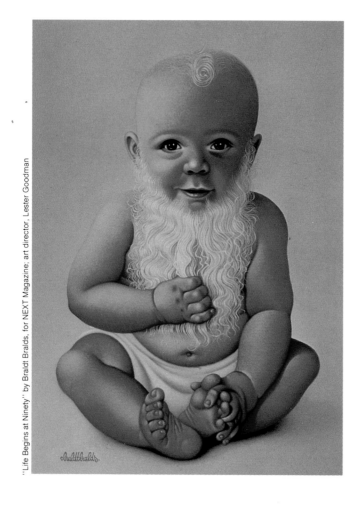

"Life Begins at Ninety" by Braldt Bralds, for NEXT Magazine; art director, Lester Goodman

immune systems are now being tested in research studies and soon will be used routinely in medical treatment of disease.

If people in countries like the United States would avoid rich diets, cigarette smoking, and tension, and if they would exercise more, they would, on the average, live 90 years or more. This fact would not make any difference in the maximum *longevity*, however. Few people would live to be 100. If science could unravel the biological mystery of aging and control the aging process, the picture would be quite different. A greater number of people would live much longer lives. People may achieve dramatically longer lives even in this century. There are reasons for this optimism.

Food Restrictions In 1927 Clive McCay of Cornell University started the most significant of the experiments suggesting that the 100- to 120-year barrier can be broken. He fed white rats enough vitamins, minerals, and proteins to keep them alive, but he did not give them enough calories to grow normally. He fed another group of rats the same diet, but these rats were allowed to eat as much sugar and lard as they wanted. The animals on the diet with fewer calories did not grow as fast as the others, and they kept their youthful appearance even after the normally fed rats were dead (after about 1,000 days). Then he gave animals that had been "fasting" full rations. These animals developed to almost normal size, and some lived for as long as 1,400 days, or about 50 percent longer than the rats who ate the standard diet throughout their lives. This experiment is important because it was the first time the environment was manipulated to change the "fixed" life span of a mammal.

No one has seriously suggested withholding food from human infants and children to delay their growth and ultimately increase their life span, but certainly feeding them too much during their developmental years is not healthy for them, and parents would be wise to avoid it.

Brain Chemistry Aging may be caused by a lack of coordination among the various tissues of the body. According to this theory, a many-celled organism can die if its control systems fail. That its vital cells are still alive makes no difference. In this theory, aging is directly

Parent Abuse

When her son walked out and left Sarah Clark to the mercies of his angry family, the 75-year-old widow kept her fears to herself. She didn't complain when her daughter-in-law, Nancy, began to shout drunkenly: "Since we can't take it out on your good-for-nothing bastard of a son, we'll just have to take it out on you." Nor did the frail old woman seek help even when Nancy made good on the threats: blackening her eyes, bruising her arms, and forcing her to grovel for food. The concern of a sharp-eyed Massachusetts neighbor and a persistent visiting nurse eventually ended Mrs. Clark's ordeal—but only after three years of repeated abuse. Her terrified rationale for silence, according to Boston elderly-rights advocate James Bergman: "No matter what, the daughter-in-law was her sole provider."

Now that Americans have finally faced the appalling realities of battered children and wives, a shocking new family secret is coming to light: the abused parent. Elderly and dependent, these long-silent victims are being physically assaulted and psychologically degraded by their own resentful children or even grandchildren, a problem geriatrics specialist Diana Koin calls "the King Lear Syndrome" (after Shakespeare's aging monarch who fell afoul of his two scheming daughters). Like Mrs. Clark, many abused parents are reluctant to complain, fearing they will lose their source of support—or be shuttled off to an institution that could be still worse. Due to that reticence, their real numbers are not yet known. But at least one expert estimates that between 500,000 and one million aged parents are abused in any given year—and that number may well worsen as inflation drives more old people to move in with their families.

Some researchers say the abusers were once abused by these same parents, and now want their measure of vengeance. But many are not as monstrous as they seem. They may find tending to a senile, bedridden, bedwetting parent an unbearable financial and emotional burden just as their own children are growing up. Meanwhile, they are torn with guilt over the temptation to commit the invalid to a nursing home. "It may be a question of reaching a breaking point," says Marilyn Block, of the Center on Aging at the University of Maryland. "The children want to do right, but they find they can't cope."

Transferring the responsibility, however, is often impossible. "You can't divorce your parents," says sociologist Richard J. Gelles, co-author of *Behind Closed Doors,* a study of family violence. . . . "As stressful as it may get, this is not a relationship that society allows you to break." In her own study of the King Lear Syndrome, Diana Koin discovered that the stresses usually grew out of long-term family conflicts. The tensions cut across socioeconomic lines, she discovered—and so did the resultant abuse. "Professional families did it, working-class families did it, black families did it, and white families did it," says Koin, who is chief of geriatric medicine at St. Luke's Hospital in Denver.

Pressured Few public-counseling, financial-aid, or day-care programs are available to ease the pressure on children, and few laws adequately protect their parents. Only eleven states now have laws requiring physicians and other professionals to report elderly abuse cases to legal authorities; another eleven are considering them. Where there are other legal remedies, moreover, they are often difficult to enforce. On the federal level, no abuse law, specifically protects the elderly, although a domestic-violence bill now pending before the Senate could provide assistance.

The State of Connecticut is a leading exception to the general rule of government neglect. Since 1978, anyone who regularly deals with the elderly must report suspicious occurrences or risk a $500 fine. Five ombudsmen from the Department on Aging check out complaints and arrange social services as needed; about one-third of the 1,000 cases reported in the first year involved physical abuse. In one chilling instance, a boy called police and said his grandmother was being beaten. When investigators arrived, they found the woman bruised and chained to a chair, but still refusing to give up her Social Security check. Her son was arrested.

Gray Power Even without much help from the government, the elderly are starting to fight back. Groups like the American Association of Retired Persons are lobbying for such services as senior-citizen daycare, and they expect to pick up power as the aged population continues to grow. But to rescue the victims, the law must first find them, and almost by definition, most are elderly shut-ins, hidden away from prying eyes. "Even a battered child is more protected," declares John Von Glahn, executive director for the Family Service Association of Orange County, California, which specializes in family-abuse problems. "During the course of their activities they come in contact with all kinds of people—schoolteachers, nurses, and doctors. About the only place many of the elderly can call for help is the police department, and few will sign an arrest warrant for their own son or daughter." The ironic truth may be that, for all their fears, a nursing home could well provide a safer refuge for aged parents than the bosom of their own family.

Newsweek

Neurotransmitter
A substance that transmits nerve impulses.

Dopamine
A neurotransmitter located in the brain.

Thyroid
A gland at the base of the neck that affects growth and metabolism.

Thymus
A gland in the upper chest that affects the immune system.

Lymphocytes
Blood elements that produce antibodies and other substances important in immunity.

RNA (Ribonucleic acid)
Acid that is present in all cells along with DNA; plays an important part in protein synthesis.

Testosterone
A male sex hormone.

Menopause
The time when menstruation stops permanently.

Dehydroepiandrosterone (DHEA)
A hormone formed in the adrenal glands of the fetus and believed to have some influence on the aging process.

---

related to chemical neurotransmitters in the brain. *Neurotransmitters* are substances that transmit nerve impulses. They are responsible for keeping the tissues of the body as finely tuned as the instruments of a symphony orchestra must be. In old age the neurotransmitter in the brain, *dopamine,* is commonly greatly reduced. Insufficient dopamine prevents the hypothalamus from signaling the pituitary to produce the hormones necessary for the *thyroid* and *thymus* glands to function. Reduced thyroid impairs cell maintenance in the brain and elsewhere. Reduced thymus function lowers production of T cells, one type of *lymphocyte,* which are linked to immunity to cancer and other disorders. Takashi Makinodan at the National Institute on Aging has dramatically increased life spans of rats in two ways. One is by transplanting young thymuses into older animals. The other is by storing lymphocytes from young rats and transfusing those lymphocytes back into the same animals when they are older. As part of an effort to slow down pathological aging, drug experiments aimed at maintaining certain levels of brain dopamine are currently underway.

Errors in DNA and RNA Duplication   A change in DNA molecules may contribute to the aging process. DNA molecules contain the basic genetic instructions for the orderly behavior of the cell. According to one Soviet gerontologist, aging is caused by errors in the various stages of the genetic replication process. Aged insects and experimental animals have been shown to have decreased amounts of *RNA* in their brain cells. If a similar condition occurs in aged human beings, preservation of the RNA of the brain would be an effective way to slow down aging. Recent drugs developed to improve memory by increasing RNA could perhaps be applied to slow down the aging process.

Hormone Imbalance   The theory that aging is caused by hormonal imbalance was first advanced by a French professor named Brown-Séquard. Perhaps he was motivated by the fact that he was 72 years old and married to a young woman. In any case, he tried to overcome the obstacles of age by injecting himself with extracts from the testicles of dogs and guinea pigs. He was not successful, but he was on a promising trail.

Testosterone, the male sex hormone, first became available for therapy in 1935. Patients were able to supplement their own production of testosterone with injections. Testosterone increases the production of protein, and men taking it experienced new vigor and better muscle tone. It is possible though that testosterone may promote cancer and other diseases. For that reason testosterone treatment is not common. Hormone therapy is, however, often used with women to treat disturbances associated with *menopause,* including osteoporosis, a softening of the bones.

Recently, the hormone *dehydroepiandrosterone* (*DHEA*) has been receiving increased attention among gerontologists. It appears that DHEA falls sharply with age and is drastically reduced in women prone to breast cancer and in men who have heart attacks. In experimental animals, artificially administered DHEA has prevented immune system declines, lowered serum cholesterol, and blocked growth of induced cancer. There is also evidence that DHEA levels increase significantly with calorie-restricted diets. Work now under way with humans may verify that DHEA is of pivotal importance in the aging process or in the prevention of some age-related diseases.

The Ethics of Tampering with the Aging Process

Should we try to lengthen our lives? Significantly extended life spans will undoubtedly bring great social changes, but we will have to deal with them. The wheels are already turning, and such extension appears to be inevitable. We could delay the process by cutting back on research funds, and we could accelerate it by making more funds available, but it is coming. The effects of slowing down the aging process will vary depending on which diseases are eliminated. If, for example, diseases of the blood vessels now associated with aging were wiped out, people on the average might expect to live 11 years longer. With the most usual causes of death eliminated, however, many more people would then die of remaining causes, and many more would survive only to face long exposure to environmental hazards and

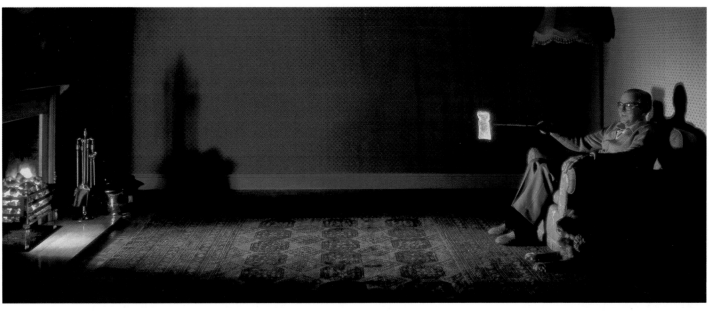

accumulated stress. These people would suffer even greater disability and dependence during the added years.

Scientific advances in making longer lives possible must be matched with better control and understanding of environments and life-styles. Researchers are aware of the problems, and they do not aim to prolong lives that are nothing more than living death. We can hope that this situation will not happen and that the added years will, instead, be productive and fulfilling. (See "Gray Power," page 488, for positive steps in this direction.)

Life-Extending Measures

All kinds of life-extending miracles are doubtless on the way. But some people will not live long enough to see them. They will die or suffer disabling diseases when they could have stayed alive and healthy if only they had paid attention to what we already know. Throughout this text facts and cues suggest actions that people can take in order to avoid diseases, disabilities, and premature death. Some of these actions, however, are directly and profoundly related to health in later life and are, therefore, highlighted here.

Don't Smoke Cigarettes   Former Surgeon General William Stewart called cigarette smoking the nation's leading preventable cause of disability and death. It has also been singled out as the only factor that can account for the unusually large death rate among older men in 17 Western countries. The average pack-a-day smoker can expect to live, on the average, 5.5 years less than the person who does not smoke cigarettes. Smokers also suffer more illnesses that last longer, and they are subject to respiratory disabilities that limit their total vigor many years before their death. Even young cigarette smokers suffer respiratory impairment, some within a year from the time they first start smoking. Premature skin wrinkling has been linked to cigarette smoking. Smokers at age 50 have the wrinkles of a person of 60. More details (for these, see Chapter 8) do not change the picture: Smoking is not part of the long or good life.

Control Drinking   Alcohol impairs both liver and kidney function. Evidence is accumulating that heavy drinkers suffer brain damage, too. Alcohol taken in excess is directly destructive to life, but besides this aspect, it is a major factor in accidents. More than 25,000 traffic deaths per year involve a drinking driver or pedestrian.

Eat Wisely   Nutrition is a key to successful aging and longevity. Health at any age is facilitated by a varied diet that includes

1. Generous amounts of fruits and vegetables
2. Whole-grain cereals and cereal products
3. Nonfat milk products
4. Fish, poultry (no skin), vegetable protein (beans, nuts) in place of red meats and eggs most of the time
5. Low intake of table sugar and sugar products
6. Low intake of salt, including canned and prepared foods high in salt
7. Caloric intake not in excess of need for maintenance of ideal weight

The need for taking extra vitamins and minerals to supplement the diet is highly controversial. Such supplements in the form of low-dosage, multiple-vitamin-mineral pills, however, are inexpensive and probably harmless, and they may be of some value to people who are careless in their eating habits.

Control Your Weight   People who are fat are greatly handicapped, both socially and psychologically. Obesity is also not healthy physically. The fatter people of all ages are, the more likely they are to die, but as people get older, the risks are much greater. Adults who have been obese since infancy are not usually very successful in achieving normal weight, but their health risks seem to be less than those faced by people who become obese in adulthood. People can control their weight, although it takes time and it is not easy. A sensible program of either cutting down on calories or using more (through exercise) or a combination of both will work for most people who want to lose weight, but there is no magic formula for anyone.

Senility

The dictionaries coolly define senility as ''the sum of the physical and mental changes occurring in advanced life'' or as ''the physical and mental infirmity of old age.'' But for the more than two million Americans who suffer the ravages of intellectual decline—and for the families who care for them—the word often connotes deep despair. In recent years, medical and social scientists have become more informed about the mental problems of aging—and increasingly more aggressive in the search for ways to reverse or even cure some problems of aging formerly dismissed as ''simple senility.'' The purposes of this essay are to describe these developments and to highlight some of the common ''reversible'' causes of senility.

Definition   The more specific word for the condition most people label as senility is dementia—the usually gradual development of widespread intellectual impairment including failing attention, memory loss, decreased ability to handle numerical calculations, and loss of orientation for time and place. Personality changes (irritability, diminished humor, etc.) usually accompany these intellectual deficits. In addition, some elderly persons may enter a mental state of delirium—the usually abrupt development of dramatic changes including confusion, hallucinations, and rather sudden fluctuations in alertness. Delirium is more likely to have reversible causes—infection, a new medication, alcohol withdrawal—though it may also be another part of the process of gradual intellectual deterioration. Whatever the definition used, however, the practical questions

remain the same: What is causing the problem? Can anything be done to reverse the situation?

Causes   While exact statistics are hard to come by, it is generally estimated that about 80 percent of all dementia in persons over age 65 is due to two irreversible conditions. *Alzheimer's disease*—by far the most common—is a disorder of unknown cause associated with progressive dementia leading to death within five to ten years. At autopsy, the brain shows characteristic microscopic abnormalities in the cerebrum—the largest, ''intellectual'' part of the human brain. Though many tantalizing research leads are under exploration, *no treatment for this condition has yet proved to be effective*. The other major cause of irreversible dementia among the elderly is a phenomenon usually known as *multi-infarct dementia*—meaning many small strokes, each of which destroys a small area of brain tissue. The treatment of existing high blood pressure is often helpful in preventing further ''ministrokes.'' Treating hypertension in the elderly can be very tricky since over-treatment can also lead to brain damage due to insufficient blood flow.

That's the bad news. The relatively good news is that approximately 10–20 percent of persons over age 65 with mental deterioration have underlying causes that may be partially or completely reversed—including the following:

1. *Inappropriate drug ingestion:* This cause is put at the top of the list to emphasize the increasing recognition of excessive and inappropriate drug use by the elderly. Some of this stems from the prob-

lems of dementia itself (forgetfulness as to when the last dose was taken, confusion about how long medication should be taken) or a tendency to try something suggested by a friend. However, much of the blame must be laid at the doorstep of physicians who too readily prescribe drugs without carefully checking what the person is already taking or who spend too little time to consider (and explain) the special problems that many common drugs might cause older people. Indeed, one of the first steps in evaluating the development of dementia in anyone is to review all medications carefully, including nonprescription drugs. In some cases it may be necessary to check the medicine cabinet at home rather than rely on a verbal report. The discontinuation of drugs should be done under the supervision of a physician since serious withdrawal problems can occur.

2. *Unrecognized depression:* At any age, serious underlying depression may be missed in the midst of intellectual deterioration. There is a special danger of this happening to an elderly person—given the easy explanation of ''senility'' for such deterioration and the erroneous assumption that elderly persons are not likely to become depressed. Indeed, during depression they are likely to deny mood changes and focus instead on bodily complaints. Depression is being increasingly identified as the basis for impaired mental function in elderly people. Proper treatment can lead to striking improvement.

3. *Underlying physical disease:* This category is all-inclusive and runs the gamut from alcoholism or malnutrition to infection, low thyroid func-

(*continued on next page*)

Senility (continued)

tion, or an unrecognized blood clot next to the brain. A recent task force sponsored by the National Institute of Aging listed fifty "reversible causes of mental impairment." The important issue, of course, is that these causes must be considered if they are to be discovered. And it is still too easy to dismiss changes in mental function as a matter of "growing older."

4. _Loss of social support:_ Older people are particularly vulnerable to changes in their social environment. Loss of loved ones, moving to an unfamiliar place, or increased social isolation (as often occurs in hospitals) can lead to mental deterioration that is potentially preventable or treatable.

Which brings us to the all-important question of when and where to seek evaluation for someone with changing mental function.

Diagnosis and Treatment   There is obviously a fine line between doing too much and too little for those we love—between frantically seeking further opinions and possible cures for a situation that is beyond medical help, versus too quickly assuming that nothing can be done. Ultimately, the best answer to this dilemma is to find a qualified person or institution that takes a special interest in evaluating problems relating to the elderly. In the past, such resources were often lacking in many communities, and in many major medical centers. Today there is a great interest in teaching physicians about the special medical and social problems of the elderly, and expertise will be increasingly available in the near future. Wherever help is ultimately sought, the medical evaluation can be expected to include the following:

1. _A careful history_ of past and current problems with special emphasis on tendencies to depression and a survey (including a home check, if necessary) of all drugs used.

2. _A thorough physical exam_ with particular attention to abnormalities of the nervous system and tests of mental function.

3. _A thoughtfully chosen set of laboratory examinations_ which typically will include not only familiar studies (blood and urine) but almost always a so-called CAT (computerized axial tomography) scan for structural abnormalities of the head and brain. Indeed, because of its safety and effectiveness, the CAT scan is one of the most important advances of the past decade in evaluating intellectual impairment in the elderly.

Avoiding unnecessary tests is important for the patient and family. But given the legitimate hope that reversible causes of dementia might be found, the emphasis today should be on thorough initial evaluation rather than casual dismissal of the problem as "old age."

Harvard Medical School Health Letter

Gray Power

Founded by Maggie [Kuhn] in 1970, the Gray Panthers are a coalition of both young and old dedicated to the fight against "ageism," or discrimination based on age, in the U.S. And although their initial focus was mainly on the needs of the elderly, Gray Panthers have evolved more comprehensive goals. They now define their purpose as "advocacy for social change to benefit the larger public good."

Maggie reiterates this broader perspective when asked about the impact of the Gray Panther movement on society. Could the effect be as great as that of the women's movement or the civil rights movement? "Only if we don't narrow our objectives to include only the interests of the old," she answers. "We must, instead, consider the needs of society as a whole. . . .

"This is a new age, an age of sweeping change and liberation, of self-determination; a new kind of freedom for all of us who dare to take risks. And I see us as a new breed of old people."

Maggie Kuhn is the embodiment of the "new breed." When forced into mandatory retirement after 25 years of service with the Presbyterian Church, she rebelled. She thought mandatory retirement unfair and set out to organize other old people against their enforced lifestyle. Thus, by retiring, she took on a much larger task. . . .

Gray Power (continued)

And what is the root of ageism? In Maggie's view, it is "society's refusal to take responsibility for the old. And on a personal level, it is the fear of middle-aged people about becoming old and the self-hate of old people in being old."

Gray Panthers are working hard to dispel the negative attitudes about old age. One method is through the media; they publish their own newspaper and have radio programs in some cities. But even though they work through media, Panthers recognize it as one of the prime promoters of ageist attitudes. As a result, a group of Panthers formed Media Watch. Volunteers monitor television programs and file complaints about those that are objectional from an age point of view. Specific complaints have included youth-oriented commercials, negative stereotypes of old folks in certain comedy routines, and the almost total absence of any older emcees and news anchor people. . . .

While Panthers are striving to rid American society of negative ageist stereotypes, they are also trying to replace them with positive images. "We must give old people new images of themselves as functioning individuals of value to society," says Kuhn.

Such new images involve the creation of new roles and functions. Kuhn perceives old people in monitoring roles: watchdogs of utility commissions, city councils, hospital boards, the courts, corporations. She also envisions them as advocates for consumer rights: patient advocates in nursing homes and hospitals, advocates for those with impaired hearing, advocates for constructive activity in various civic Senior Centers. . . .

Much nursing home reform, especially in regard to patients' rights, has been accomplished through a cooperative effort with Ralph Nader and his Retired Professional Action Group.

The lifting of the mandatory retirement age from 65 to 70 was a substantial credit to Panther effort. Since their founding, Panthers have made mandatory retirement their special legislative issue. They are not satisfied yet, however. Says Kuhn, "We want to knock it out entirely. We do not regard age as a criterion for measuring competence, productivity, or creativity. It's just not relevant. Society has made it so, but such a standard has little to do with the facts."

As for the argument that young people will be robbed of jobs or promotions because of an older work force, Kuhn has this to say: "People must realize that the population pyramid is shifting; the number of people over 65 is increasing rapidly. If we continue to waste the experience and talent of the older population, we will become a dying society."

Maggie envisions an important political coalition between young and old. Apparently young people share her view; about 25 percent of the Gray Panthers are under 30. "Both the young and the old can afford to take risks for social change, because both have little to lose," she explains. . . .

Maggie thinks that old people ought to go back to college or at least participate in the many continuing education programs now going on.

"Education has traditionally been deemed for the young. Work is for the middle years, and leisure for the later years. Life, which is a continuum, has been chopped up into age-segmented pieces. Instead, education, meaningful work, and leisure should all be lifelong experiences."

"Radicals"—sometimes the Panthers are so called. But Maggie Kuhn is not bothered by the term. "We are radical," she says, "in the classical sense. A radical, by definition, is the person who looks to the roots of the problem."

The individuals in contact with Maggie also have to deal with her unsettling probes. "What have you done with your life so far?" is one of her favorite openers when she faces a Gray Panther "consciousness-raising" group. In conjunction with its answer, members are instructed to do a "life line," writing the year of their birth at one end, a purely assumed year of their projected death at the other, and a "present-day status" point in-between. Above the line, they list the high points and traumas of their personal lives: marriage, first job, biggest failure, major illness, etc. Below the line they list the societal events that were happening concurrently: wars, natural disasters, recessions, moral changes, etc. Seeing this analysis reduced to a single page startles most individuals into recognition of the many changes they have witnessed, the many traumas they have survived, both in society and in their personal lives. As Maggie puts it, "It's exciting and invigorating to get a historical perspective on one's own life."

At this point Maggie Kuhn usually asks her favorite final question—unnerving to us all—which sums up her own measure of individual and social worth: "What will you do with the rest of your life?"

Rebecca Blalock
Saturday Evening Post

Hypertension
Abnormally high blood pressure.

Vascular system
The heart and blood vessels.

Diabetes
A chronic disease characterized by too much sugar in the urine.

Keep Physically Fit   Exercise can benefit every system of the body in some way. The best kind of exercise for combating bodily deterioration associated with aging, however, is the kind that builds endurance in the cardiovascular and respiratory systems. We know that normal men and women can achieve and maintain endurance fitness even into their 70s and 80s. Continuous, rhythmic, controlled, mild exercise such as walking, jogging, bicycling, and swimming produces endurance fitness. Besides benefiting the cardiovascular system, it slows down the degeneration of muscular, skeletal, digestive, and other systems. Remarkable recent studies with aging animals have demonstrated that youthful brain cell morphology is maintained in physically trained subjects as opposed to degeneration of brain cells in sedentary subjects.

Detect and Control Hypertension and Diabetes   The victim of *hypertension,* or high blood pressure, does not notice it in the early stages. It can take a terrible toll in premature disability and death, but it can be successfully controlled if the person will take medication and change his or her living habits. Without control, wear and tear and finally breakdown of *vascular systems* is much accelerated. A simple check of blood pressure, which takes only a few minutes, will show if a person has hypertension. Blood pressure higher than 140/90 is abnormal for anyone, and even small increases in blood pressure reduce life expectancy considerably.

Diabetes can escape detection for years. It accelerates the breakdown of body organs and systems, especially the circulatory system, and increases the risk of hypertension, heart attack, and strokes. When diabetes is diagnosed and treated early, however, the diabetic has an improved chance of living a full life span.

Recognize and Reduce Stress   The business executive facing a production deadline, the taxicab driver caught in a traffic jam, the factory worker exposed to continuous high noise levels—all are victims of stress. Blood pressure probably goes up, heart rates quicken, and body chemistries change. Primitive people needed these changes to provide more strength and energy for "fight

or flight." Neither fight nor flight is the answer in most situations today, so most of the time these physical changes do not serve any purpose. One popular theory holds that changes in body chemistry caused by stress increase wear and tear on the system. (See Chapter 2.)

Future living and working environments may be designed so they are less stressful. Until they are, we can personally try to cut down on the stresses in our life. Living within bicycling distance of work and shopping areas will reduce the stress of driving, for example. We might also choose less stressful occupations and recreations and generally develop less stressful lifestyles.

Use It or Lose It   All of the body's systems thrive when they are used and degenerate when they are not. Muscular strength and bone hardness, for example, reduce very gradually in individuals who continue to work and play hard physically, but deteriorate early and rapidly in people who are not very active and spend most of their time sitting. Likewise, frequent sexual activity helps maintain both the quality of genital organs and the capacity for sexual response.

Intelligence test scores were once thought to reach their highest point in people in their mid-20s. Now we know that test scores continue to improve in mentally active individuals until they are at least 50. And except for the effects of some diseases there is little or no decline in intellectual functioning before the age of 70. In fact, people who are intellectually active usually show continuing intellectual development until advanced old age. Many older people do, however, experience mental impairment beginning in some cases as early as the fifth decade of life. Such impairment is often reversible when it occurs as a result of conditions such as pneumonia, high fever, dehydration, thyroid problems, anemia, heart disease, depression, kidney disease, or adverse drug reactions. When the condition is resolved and rehabilitative therapy is applied, improvement in mental functioning occurs, sometimes dramatically.

The myth that age means sexual impotence has only recently begun to fade. Most people feel sexual desire and have the capacity for sexual activity well into old age, although the sex drive does gradually become less

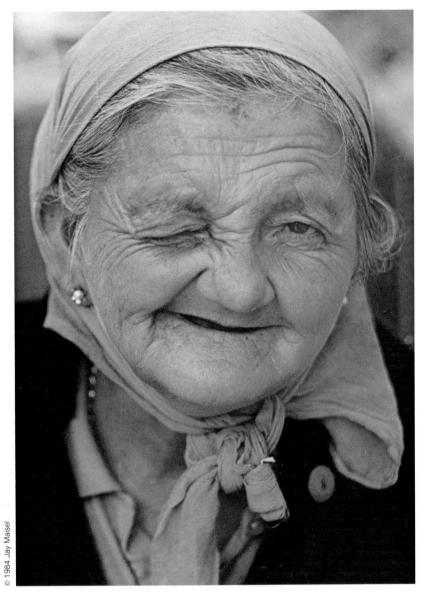

intense. Totally unrealistic stereotypes of the very old (and of the very young) have given many Americans the idea that people between adolescence and early middle age are the only ones interested in sex. Older people who believe these stereotypes without examining the evidence of their own senses may be declaring themselves candidates for an early grave—one of the spirit, if not of the body.

Be Involved   People who continue to be involved in useful activity are more likely to enjoy long, meaningful lives than are those who "drop out." The person who withdraws from life invites passivity, meaninglessness, and premature disability and death. We can benefit from the experience older people have accumulated in a lifetime of living. Traditional retirement from work might well be replaced by retirement to social, political, and other activity that makes use of a valuable and underrated human resource.

Aging: A Positive Experience

In a culture that discriminates against age, it is not easy to perceive much that is positive about getting older. If we can disentangle ourselves from the artificial values and stereotypes surrounding aging, however, we can become free to experience each stage of life as a challenge and an adventure through which we continue to grow and to become more and more complete individuals. Perhaps the most valuable human resource is our *time* in life. Long life at least represents an abundance of this resource available for our continuing development. The quality of life, of course, remains another matter.

Probably before the year 2000, science will have discovered how to slow down primary aging, the "normal" changes that take place with the passage of time. Other institutions, educational, political, and technological, should make headway in dealing with changes resulting from disease, stress, and self-destructive behavior. Birthrates in the developed countries should continue to decline, and life expectancy should increase dramatically. The population will, on the whole, be older, and we shall see revolutionary social and economic changes.

The other side of the coin is the individual struggle for life, health, and meaning. We all must face the fact that we are aging. A very involved older woman, a member of the Gray Panthers, illustrated this fact well. During a militant demonstration for the rights of older people, she poked her finger into the chest of a young Capitol guard and said, "Zap! You're getting old."

Aging Attitude Scale

Read the following statements careful-ly. Choose the one in each section that best describes you at this moment and record its score at the right. (For example, "seldom thinks about old age" has a score of 3.) When you have identified five state-ments, total your score and find your position on the scale.

5 considers aging a natural life process
4 regards old age as another stage in life
3 seldom thinks about old age
2 worries about getting older
1 finds the idea of becoming old painful

Score _____

5 views older people as valuable human resources
4 feels older people can make sig-nificant contributions
3 feels older people without resources should be subsidized
2 feels older people burden the community
1 views older people as hopeless burdens on society

Score _____

5 believes physical and mental decline can be avoided in old age
4 believes mental decline can be avoided in old age
3 believes severe physical and mental decline can be delayed
2 believes severe physical decline is inevitable
1 believes severe mental and physi-cal decline is inevitable

Score _____

5 feels retirement age requirements should be eliminated
4 feels retirement age requirements should be raised
3 feels retirement age requirements are just about right
2 feels retirement age requirements should be lowered
1 feels older people should retire to make way for younger people

Score _____

5 enjoys older people
4 likes spending time with older people
3 doesn't mind spending time with older people
2 reluctantly spends time with older people
1 resents spending time with older people

Score _____

Total score _____

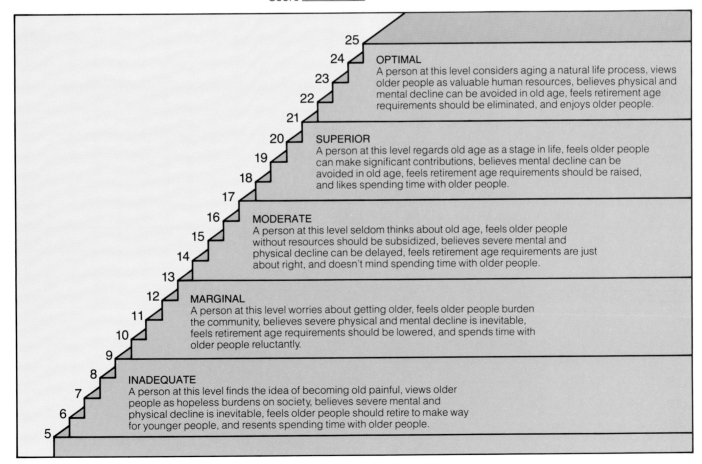

25
24 OPTIMAL
23 A person at this level considers aging a natural life process, views
22 older people as valuable human resources, believes physical and
        mental decline can be avoided in old age, feels retirement age
21 requirements should be eliminated, and enjoys older people.

20 SUPERIOR
19 A person at this level regards old age as a stage in life, feels older people
18 can make significant contributions, believes mental decline can be
        avoided in old age, feels retirement age requirements should be raised,
17 and likes spending time with older people.

16 MODERATE
15 A person at this level seldom thinks about old age, feels older people
        without resources should be subsidized, believes severe mental and
14 physical decline can be delayed, feels retirement age requirements are just
13 about right, and doesn't mind spending time with older people.

12 MARGINAL
11 A person at this level worries about getting older, feels older people burden
10 the community, believes severe physical and mental decline is inevitable,
        feels retirement age requirements should be lowered, and spends time with
9   older people reluctantly.

8   INADEQUATE
7   A person at this level finds the idea of becoming old painful, views older
6   people as hopeless burdens on society, believes severe mental and
        physical decline is inevitable, feels older people should retire to make way
5   for younger people, and resents spending time with older people.

Take Action

Your answers to Probing Your Emotions at the beginning of this chapter and your placement level on the Aging Attitude Scale will, we hope, encourage you to begin a process of self-exploration and self-discovery that you will continue. Reflect on the entire chapter's content and ask yourself how each point relates to your own life. Then take action:

1. Imagine yourself as elderly. You have just made the decision to live in a retirement or nursing home. Visit such a home. Interview the manager and one or more residents. Write down your reactions in your Take Action notebook. Would you eventually want to live in such a home? Would you recommend it to an elderly relative or friend?

2. At what age should people retire? Survey five college students in their late teens or early twenties and five older people. Did the answers of the two groups vary?

3. What are the most pronounced differences between a 20-year-old and a 70-year-old? List the differences in your Take Action notebook, and ask your grandmother or some other older person if he or she agrees. What are the similarities between a 20-year-old and a 70-year-old?

Before leaving this chapter, review the questions that open the chapter. Have your feelings or values changed? Are you now better equipped to handle the complex and very human problems associated with aging?

Chapter Twenty-Two

Death and Dying

Probing Your Emotions

1. Think back to your childhood. Can you remember the first time someone close to you died? Was it a person? A pet? How old were you? How did you feel about it at the time? How does recalling that death make you feel right now?

2. Consider your own death for a few minutes. Is this difficult for you to do? What emotions are you experiencing?

3. What would be your feelings if someone you loved were terminally ill and in pain and asked to be allowed to die, not to be kept alive by artificial means such as a respirator? What would you say to this person? What would you do?

4. Suppose a friend of yours who is a medical student asked you to sign a card stating that upon your death you wished to donate your body to medical research. What would be your immediate reaction to this request?

Chapter Contents

WHAT IS DEATH?

WHY IS THERE DEATH?

DENYING DEATH IN AMERICA

THE PROCESS OF DYING
When and how to die
Being with a dying person
Letting people die

THE HOSPICE

DEAD BODIES AS RESOURCES

GRIEF

COMING TO TERMS WITH DEATH
Five stages
Beyond death
The walking dead
Facing death as a way to renew life

Boxes

Definitions of death
Elements of a hospice program
About memorial societies
Life after death: the growing evidence

Electroencephalogram
Records of the fluctuating electrical potentials of the brain (brain waves) as recorded from electrodes on the scalp.

Species
A distinct kind of plant or animal whose population evolves independently of other such populations.

Nuclear family
The family unit consisting only of parents and children.

22 There is a very old story about a man who was hiking on a high mountain trail when he suddenly lost his footing and found himself hurtling toward certain death. As he plummeted past a small bush growing out of the sheer rock wall, he caught a berry in his hand and ate it. It was the most delicious berry he had ever eaten. This man's condition is the same as yours or mine or anyone else's. Each of us is hurtling toward certain death and how we deal with it has a lot to do with how freely and rewardingly we live our lives.

What Is Death?

Death, like life, is change. Matter and energy are never destroyed. They merely change from one form to another. When the body is no longer able to resist unhealthy changes in itself, or when it is mechanically broken beyond repair, or when it is poisoned by the environment, it ceases to function and dies.

Traditionally, death has been defined as occurring when the heart stops beating. Scientists now agree, however, that the brain continues to function for a short time (less than 10 minutes) after the heart stops beating. Scientists also now agree that the brain, not the heart, is the key to human life. Once the brain stops functioning, the person is medically and in some states legally dead. Brain death is most reliably shown by a flat tracing on an *electroencephalogram*. Most states either have already adopted or are considering legislation that redefines death in this way. (See "Definitions of Death," page 498.) There are a few exceptions, however. Overdoses of certain depressant drugs can produce a flat electroencephalogram trace. Some people have shown no brain life after such overdoses, yet they have recovered. A stilled heart is not always final, either. Some patients recover when their hearts are directly massaged or otherwise manipulated.

Why Is There Death?

Death permits the renewal and evolution of the *species*. The normal life span is long enough to ensure that we reproduce ourselves and that our species continues. It

is short enough to allow new genetic combinations to be tested. This fact means that we, as a species, can adapt better to changing conditions in the environment. Looked at from the viewpoint of species survival and improvement, the arrangement makes sense. Unnecessary and wasteful death, however, is another matter.

Denying Death in America

In the United States we try to deny that death exists. This denial is not new. It has been going on for several generations. During the Victorian era (about the last half of the nineteenth century) people referred to death—like sex—only in euphemisms, if at all. Euphemisms are "nice" words used to describe unpleasant reality. For example, people "pass away" instead of dying. In numerous ways we continue to avoid the reality of death. The *nuclear family* system common in the United States keeps older people at a distance from the young. When a grandparent dies, for example, children are not likely to be around. They usually do not see what happens when a person dies. They may be told, but the subject is considered awkward and requires much hedging. Many Americans, both adults and children, have never seen someone die, which makes it difficult for them to understand that they, too, will die.

We hide death in many ways. Besides "protecting" children from the actual, physical fact of it, the dead body, we present false ideas of it. Death, the real thing, its finality, its aftermath of grief, is largely taboo, but fake death is a game that is played all over our TV and movie screens. The movie only lasts two or three hours at the most, and when it is over, we continue our daily lives. Children playing war or cops and robbers or cowboys and Indians play the game, mimicking the actors, suddenly gasping and sprawling on the ground, "dead." In just a minute, they get up and play the same scene over again. Our death taboo is in some ways like our sex taboo. The version of sex that is offered for public consumption is also distorted. Many times, in both cases, natural events are either presented out of context or are hidden, especially from children.

Our modern urban life prevents many people from tangible experience of the workings of nature. Most of us are as insulated from death as we are from birth.

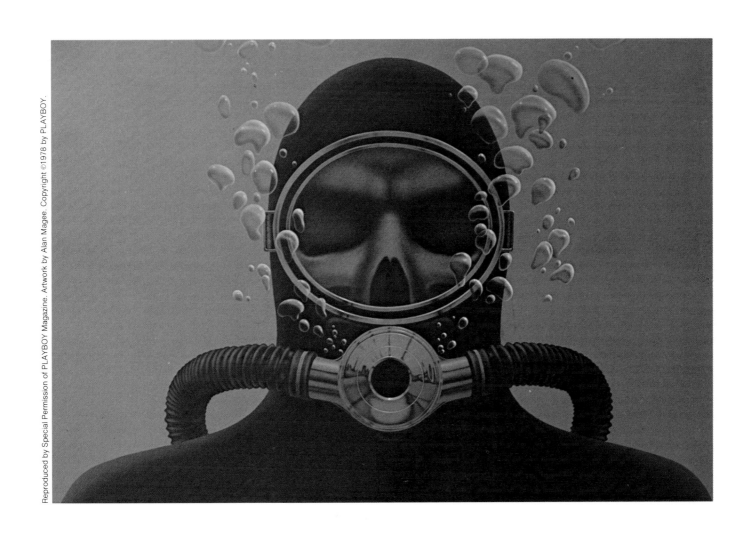

Definitions of Death

Somatic Death "Somatic death is the cessation of all vital functions such as the heartbeat and respiration. Molecular or cellular death follows. Many cells in the body will continue to live for some time after somatic death. . . . Groups of cells may be removed from a body after death and kept alive, sometimes indefinitely, in tissue culture. The rate at which cellular death occurs varies in different organs. The more specialized the organ, the more rapidly its cellular death follows somatic death. The advent of organ transplantation surgery has greatly increased the importance of death."

A. Keith Mant
The Medical Definition of Death

Cardiac Death   Cardiac death occurs "when a patient's heart [has] stopped beating and he [has] ceased to breathe. Death might be verified by electrocardiogram."

Robert Glaser
Innovations and Heroic Acts in Prolonging Life

Brain Death   Four elements comprise brain death: "unreceptivity and unresponsivity; no movements or breathing; no reflexes; and flat electroencephalogram."

Harvard Medical School's Ad Hoc Committee to Examine the Definition of Brain Death

"Although the beating heart remains for some a symbol of life and love, its role has been put into perspective scientifically. The brain is our master control; the heart is just a pump."

Robert Glaser
Innovations and Heroic Acts in Prolonging Life

Biological and Clinical Death
"Physicians are likely to define two levels of physical death: biological death, which occurs when the organs cease to function, and clinical death, which occurs when the organism ceases to function as an organism."

Richard Kalish
Life and Death: Dividing the Indivisible

When someone in the family dies, if there is time, the event is usually removed to a hospital. If there are children, they are with the babysitter or farmed out somewhere. Most of us grow up feeling we are immortal, and it is not surprising. We feel that death happens to someone else. It does not happen to you or me. Or if it looks like it might happen, there will be a magical rescue at the eleventh hour. We cannot even imagine our own deaths because we are alive doing the imagining. It seems we cannot make death real.

Perhaps these are some of the reasons why people refuse to use seat belts in their cars even though they know that seat belts save lives. Perhaps these reasons also explain the person who continues to smoke cigarettes, even after he or she has developed *emphysema* or some other quite possibly fatal disease.

The Process of Dying

Most people, when they think of death at all, have very definite ideas on when and how they want to die. Regardless of whether or not they have those choices, it is becoming increasingly apparent that those who are dying benefit from having others around them—to listen, to share, to care. What is not so clear is the morality of mercy killing and the suspension of artificial life-support treatment.

When and How to Die   People think it is more fitting to die when they are old than when they are young. Living to a ripe, old age seems both just and fair, something that is our due. To the question "When and how would you prefer to die?" most people say something like, "I would prefer to die quickly after a long and meaningful life." Unfortunately, we may not have a choice. To have been conceived, to have been born, and to be alive now are three miracles all living persons share. Beyond these three conditions, certain events are likely, but none is guaranteed. Scientists and researchers—genetic, environmental, medical, and behavioral—are constantly improving our chances, it is true. To be alive, however, is to be always vulnerable to the possibility of one's own death. When one dies—no matter why, how, what might have been or should have been—it is done.

At first thought, most people say they prefer a sudden death to a lingering one. For many, however, especially

Emphysema
A lung disease that often results from cigarette smoking.

Terminal
Term used to describe a disease that will shortly end in death.

Life-support technology
The use of artificial body parts without which the patient would die. Artificial kidneys are an example of life-support technology.

Euthanasia
Hastening the death of an ill person in a painless way by doing or failing to do something.

---

those who have help from family, friends, and professionals who care, dying can be an adventure filled with meaning. Many even gracefully accept the challenge of enduring the pain and suffering while keeping themselves intact and aware. Often the dying person feels freed from trivial concerns and is able to express the best that is in her or him.

Being with a Dying Person   Modern medicine is able to predict earlier and earlier and more and more accurately when an illness will be *terminal*. Increasing numbers of people can know in advance that they or others will die in weeks or months. Now, more than ever before, people have a chance to help others to experience dying gracefully and with dignity. Important parts of the process are establishing or maintaining physical and emotional closeness with the dying person and honest and open communication. There is no rule about who tells a person that he or she is dying. Sometimes the doctor does it, or a family member, or a friend. Other times the dying person figures it out and asks if his or her suspicions are true. From this point on, the dying person is given support and help in taking care of his or her unfinished business and in dealing with the complex emotions involved.

Terminally ill people often testify that they have had the most significant experiences of their lives after they found out they were soon to die. Aware of their limited time, they often become better able to take delight in the experiences of life that are open to them and to find greater meaning in everything. They become more aware of what they are to lose and are able to appreciate small events that might have seemed insignificant before. Some people find a deep meaning in putting their business affairs in order and finally saying to loved ones all the important things they want to say.

The dying person's needs are no different from anyone else's, but they are more urgent. Dying people need to know that they are valued, that they are not alone, that they are not being judged, and that those around them care and are trying to understand and to learn about this thing just as they are. Dying people often need someone to listen to them while they talk their way through the experience. Friends are as important to dying people as they are to others. As with any friendship, there are opportunities for growth on both sides.

Letting People Die   Thousands of people are alive and well today under conditions that would normally be fatal. Anyone who is using a heart pacemaker or an artificial kidney is receiving the benefit of advanced *life-support technology*. Even severely disabled people, such as those who do not have the use of any of their limbs, are being helped to maintain meaningful lives.

In spite of these success stories, many critics are raising serious questions about the medical tradition of keeping people alive by any means and at any expense. Should a patient who cannot possibly recover, one who is not capable of leading a meaningful life, be kept alive? Some families are emotionally and financially ruined while a loved one (or anyone they are responsible for) is maintained in a seemingly endless coma or in a "vegetable" state.

Two different issues are involved. One is the rightness or wrongness of *euthanasia,* which is often called mercy killing. Few cases of euthanasia have ever been reported. Dying patients are often so heavily dosed with potentially dangerous drugs that it is not always possible to tell exactly what caused death. Helping someone to die, however, even at that person's request, is against the law and very risky. Criminal prosecution may be the result.

The second issue deals with a more widely accepted practice. When the dying person no longer has any chance to recover or live a meaningful life, the artificial life-support treatment may be withdrawn. This procedure—often called *passive euthanasia*—may or may not be legal. The question has not been finally decided. When it is possible, though, more and more doctors are letting families of patients make this decision and even the patients themselves when they are able to. A growing number of people are making their personal wishes known by drawing up a "living will" such as the one shown in Figure 22–1.

People who are terminally ill now have a perfectly legal way to let themselves die: They can choose to leave

Hospice
A community-oriented treatment facility for the dying; provides social and psychological support in addition to medical care.

Cornea
The transparent part of the coat of the eyeball that admits light to the interior of the eye.

the hospital and spend their last days at home with their families and friends. In the United States there is no law that says a terminally ill person must stay in a hospital.

The Hospice

It has long been recognized that the special needs of dying people are not well served by most regular hospitals. Neither the primary objectives of such hospitals, the orientation of the professional staffs, the social mix of patients, nor economic realities provide the best context. To better serve the needs of dying patients, their families, and their friends, the idea of a special institution called a *hospice* was successfully developed some years ago in England. Now hospices are beginning to be established in the United States. Here, a team usually

consisting of medical, social work, mental health, legal, and spiritual practitioners provides support, comfort, and resources for resolving the many unique problems of dying. Patients, families, and friends typically experience death and the prospect of death as a tolerable reality at worst and as a challenging growth experience at best. Since the hospice provides few expensive life-extending medical services and since volunteers are used widely, costs are greatly reduced.

Dead Bodies as Resources

A dead human body is a valuable resource. Many of its parts can be used to help the living. Eye *corneas* can be transplanted to give sight to the blind. Kidneys can be used to give years of vigorous life to people who have

Figure 22-1   Euthanasia Educational Council's "Living Will" can clarify your wishes in case of terminal illness or trauma. (Copies can be obtained by writing the Council at 250 W. 57th St., New York, NY 10019.)

TO MY FAMILY, MY PHYSICIAN, MY LAWYER, MY CLERGYMAN
TO ANY MEDICAL FACILITY IN WHOSE CARE I HAPPEN TO BE
TO ANY INDIVIDUAL WHO MAY BECOME RESPONSIBLE FOR MY HEALTH, WELFARE OR AFFAIRS

Death is as much a reality as birth, growth, maturity and old age—it is the one certainty of life. If the time comes when I, _____ can no longer take part in decisions for my own future, let this statement stand as an expression of my wishes, while I am still of sound mind.

If the situation should arise in which there is no reasonable expectation of my recovery from physical or mental disability, I request that I be allowed to die and not be kept alive by artificial means or "heroic measures". I do not fear death itself as much as the indignities of deterioration, dependence and hopeless pain. I, therefore, ask that medication be mercifully administered to me to alleviate suffering even though this may hasten the moment of death.

This request is made after careful consideration. I hope you who care for me will feel morally bound to follow its mandate. I recognize that this appears to place a heavy responsibility upon you, but it is with the intention of relieving you of such responsibility and of placing it upon myself in accordance with my strong convictions, that this statement is made.

Signed _____

Date _____

Witness _____

Witness _____

Copies of this request have been given to _____

_____

_____

_____

Autopsy
Examination of the body after death.

Bereaved
Deprived of a loved one by death.

Eulogy
Praise of a person who has died.

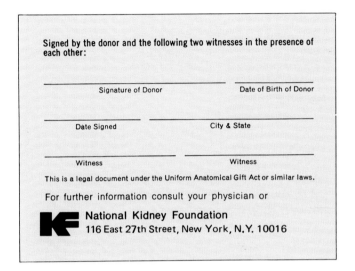

Figure 22-2

kidney disease. Human skin is the best dressing for wounds of burn victims. Bones can be used for grafting. Pituitary glands are desperately needed to make it possible for some children to grow normally. In some parts of the world undiseased blood from dead bodies is used for transfusions. Even jaws are sometimes used to train dentists. People who are horrified at the thought of this "mutilation" often change their minds when they learn how routine *autopsies* are done and how bodies are usually prepared for burial.

Several organizations are trying to make the use of human body parts easier. The simplest and most widely used plan at the moment is the Uniform Donor Card. This card is available from the National Kidney Foundation. (See Figure 22–2.) In some states, permission to "harvest" usable tissues after death is communicated by a signed card attached to the driver's license.

Grief

It is a deep loss when someone close dies, and it is emotionally very painful. If people can allow themselves to feel and express that pain, they will be more able to accept the loss and free themselves to continue with their lives.

When a loved one dies after a long illness, people usually have mixed feelings. They feel relief that "it's over" but pain as they try to adjust. The dead person is just that, dead. When people die suddenly, the thought that they did not suffer may be comforting. But it is still necessary to deal with the shock of sudden and unexpected loss.

Again, people should be encouraged to feel and express their grief—by talking about it, crying about it, reminiscing, or whatever they need to do. They should not try to hold back their feelings and be strong and brave; and no one should expect them to. Many *bereaved* people would rather be private about their grief or share it only with certain people. This choice is their right, but they still need to be reassured that others care and will help if their help is needed or wanted.

Ceremony appears to be useful in helping the bereaved accept and deal with their loss. Evidence from nearly all human cultures suggests this fact. Many people consider the traditional funeral with casket, burial, flowers, family, friends, and *eulogy* to be the only proper way to observe a person's death. Others no longer feel this way. More and more people are using the funeral as a time to celebrate the dead person's life rather than just to mourn his or her loss. There is also a trend toward simpler, less expensive funerals. The living sometimes

---

Elements of a Hospice Program

The most common indication for admission to hospices—in some 40 percent of cases—is the need to give respite to relatives. On the other hand, 20 percent of admissions are social isolates with no one able or willing to care for them. At the same time, 60 percent of admissions need help with better control of their pain. Thus, hospice patients represent a mix of social and clinical need.

A hospice program, then, is not just a program that purports to care for the terminally ill. It is a program for meeting a wide range of physical, psychological, social, and spiritual needs, a program of health care delivery consisting of ten clearly identifiable elements:

1. Service availability to home care patients and inpatients on a 24-hour-a-day, seven-day-a-week, on-call basis with emphasis on availability of medical and nursing skills

2. Home care service in collaboration with inpatient facilities

3. Knowledge and expertise in the control of symptoms (physical, psychological, social, and spiritual)

4. The provision of care by an interdisciplinary team

5. Physician-directed services

6. Central administration and coordination of services

7. Use of volunteers as an integral part of the health care team

8. Acceptance to the program based on health needs, not ability to pay

9. Treatment of the patient and family together as the unit of care

10. A bereavement follow-up service

Not all existing hospice programs incorporate all ten of these elements. For example, some are entirely home care oriented, while others are exclusively institution based with no home care services; some have very limited bereavement follow-up service, while others have extensive bereavement service; many have services available on a 24-hour-a-day, seven-day-a-week basis; while some have more limited hours. Nevertheless, the ten elements represent the ideal to be achieved by any hospice program.

Kenneth P. Cohen

---

seem to see funerals as a chance to impress others, but this behavior does not appear to be happening as often as it once did. Many times, too, the funeral industry presents the funeral as the bereaved's last chance to "do something" for the person who has died. This practice is questionable and is beginning to meet some resistance.

Coming to Terms with Death

If one learns one is to die, one must face it and deal with it. Doing so may be the most difficult experience a person ever has. Most people can adapt and learn and grow if they have enough time and help, but it is a gradual process.

Five Stages   In her book *On Death and Dying* (1969), Elisabeth Kübler-Ross identified five stages of this learning process. She used the observations of hundreds of dying people to define these stages.

Stage One: Denial and Isolation   Stage one is a temporary state of shock in which the person denies the fact and isolates himself from further confrontation with it. He says, "Not me" and "You're wrong" and insists that "It cannot be." This is a useful stage because the denial acts as a buffer against shocks and gives the person time to collect himself and mobilize other defenses.

Stage Two: Anger   When the person can no longer deny the truth, anger often follows. He asks, "Why me?" and tends to lash out at family, physicians, the hospital, blaming them for the situation. Anger at this stage is also a normal response to disability and losing control of one's situation.

Stage Three: Bargaining   As one method for marshalling remaining hope, a person may set himself to work to discover a way out; making promises to God in return for a prolonged life is common. Grasping at any straw of hope for recovery is also typical and makes one especially vulnerable to quackery and to charlatans.

Stage Four: Depression   At this stage the dying person accepts his fate, often reacts by being depressed about problems he is leaving behind and unfinished work. Depression is also a kind of grief that he experiences to prepare himself for the final separation from this

About Memorial Societies

Q What is a memorial society?
A A memorial society is a voluntary group of people who have joined together to obtain dignity, simplicity, and economy in funeral arrangements through advance planning.

Q What happens when you join?
A The society lets you know what kinds of funeral service are available and at what cost. You talk it over in your family and decide on your preference, then fill out forms provided by the society.

Q Can these plans be cancelled or changed?
A Certainly. Any time.

Q How does preplanning help at time of death?
A In several ways:
  1. You know what you want, how to get it, and what it will cost. You don't have to choose a casket or negotiate for a funeral.
  2. Your family understands what is being done. Simplicity will reflect dignity rather than lack of respect.
  3. By accepting in advance the reality of death, and by discussing it frankly, you and your family will be able to meet it when it comes.

Q Does planning really save money?
A The amounts vary greatly, but memorial society members usually save several hundred dollars on a funeral. One large society estimates that its members save a total of $850,000 a year by belonging to the organization.

Q What is the basis of these savings?
A Simplicity. A dignified and satisfying funeral need not be costly if you are not trying to demonstrate social status or compete with the neighbors. There is also the element of collective bargaining in your favor and the advantage of knowing where to go to get the desired services at moderate cost.

Q How do I join a memorial society?
A Phone or write the nearest society and ask for their literature. They will send you information about the help they can give you and the membership fee.

Q What does a memorial society have to do with funeral directors?
A Some societies serve only in an advisory capacity, informing their members where specific services may be had at specific costs. Most societies, however, have contracts or agreements on behalf of their members with one or more funeral directors.

Q Does the society handle the business details of a funeral?
A Not ordinarily. The society commonly brings the family and the funeral director together on a prearranged understanding of services and terms. The family itself deals directly with the funeral director.

Q Are funerals necessary?
A Survivors have important social and emotional needs which should not be ignored. A funeral is one way of meeting some of these needs.

Q Are there other ways?
A Yes. Disposition of the body can be made immediately after death and a memorial service held later.

Q What is the difference?
A In a funeral the center of attention is the dead body; the emphasis is on death. In a memorial service the center of concern is the personality of the individual who has died, and the emphasis is on life. In addition a memorial service generally involves less expense and can be held in a greater variety of locations.

Q Is embalming mandatory?
A If the body is to be kept several days for a funeral service, or is to be transported by common carrier, yes. Otherwise embalming

serves no useful purpose and except in one or two states is not legally required.

Q Why then is embalming usually practiced in this country?
A Funeral directors presume that unless otherwise advised, there will be viewing of the body, and a service in its presence, and that embalming and ''restoration'' are desired. If this is not the case, the funeral director can be instructed to omit embalming.

Q What appropriate disposition can be made of a body?
A There are three alternatives:
  1. Earth burial was once the simplest and most economical arrangement. With increasing population, rising land values, cost of caskets, vaults, and other items usually required, it is becoming more and more costly.
  2. Cremation, a clean, orderly method of returning the body to the elements, is economical and is rapidly increasing in use.
  3. Bequeathal to a medical school performs a valuable service and saves expense. In many areas there is a shortage of bodies for the proper training of doctors. Many public-spirited people leave their bodies for this purpose. A number of body parts can now be transplanted or otherwise used to promote medical research, restore sight, or save a life. To facilitate the gift of body parts at time of death, a ''Uniform Anatomical Gift Act'' has recently been passed by most states and provinces. Everyone is encouraged to cooperate.

There are now memorial societies in 120 cities in Canada and the U.S., representing some half a million members.

Ernest Morgan

Transcend
To go beyond the ordinary or normal limits of something.

Reincarnation
Rebirth in some other form after death.

Cosmic
Relating to the entire universe.

Mystics
People who claim to commune directly with God or to experience truths beyond human understanding.

---

world. While this is often a painful stage emotionally, it is an appropriate step in the process and is eased considerably when the person is allowed to express his sorrow in an atmosphere of nonjudging support and care.

Stage Five: Acceptance   If the earlier stages are worked through successfully, the person reaches a point at which he is no longer angry, nor hoping for a miracle, nor depressed; he is resigned and acknowledges he is powerless and may as well make the best of it. He may or may not want to talk with visitors or attendants. For some this is a predeath withdrawal from life, making the ultimate withdrawal easier.

While the stages are fairly typical of the process of a person's coming to terms with death, there are wide variations in individuals. Many people experience the stages in different sequence, or they skip some stages, or they experience some stages simultaneously.

Beyond Death   Most religions take note of the fact that people die. In one way or another they also set forth the hope that people can *transcend* death. The Judeo-Christian tradition is the most usual tradition in the United States. It is based on both Judaism and Christianity, and its fundamental belief about death is that the body is only a temporary house for the soul. The body dies, but the soul is immortal. It lives forever.

Then there is the idea of *reincarnation*. This idea appeals to some as a way to cheat death. The actual goal in religions that include a belief in reincarnation, however, is a state in which there will be no more rebirths. Still another belief has to do with the individual ego. That each of us is a separate self with a private consciousness is thought to be an illusion. According to this belief, consciousness is in fact a *cosmic* consciousness that we all share. Even though a person dies, the consciousness lives on. This idea has long been popular

with *mystics*. Do humans have a common consciousness? We do not know, but life does go on. It has for millions of years—in a seemingly endless cycle from birth to death to birth to death. The more we live apart from nature, the more difficult it is for us to be aware of this continuity and accept our part in it. Life and death do involve sadness, but this condition is natural, not wrong or unhealthy.

The Walking Dead   All who live, die. No one can control the process, so the best that anyone can do is to live fully. This course does not mean clutching at life in a frantic effort to squeeze out the last ounce of pleasure or meaning or accomplishment. It does mean being aware, open, sensitive, and able to experience the pain and joy of existence. Unfortunately, many people turn themselves off from life when they are quite young. They are alive only in a technical sense. One needs only to compare the faces and bodies of a crowd of adults on their way to work with the faces and bodies of two- and three-year-olds to see the difference. The real tragedy in life is not to live and die. It is to die without ever having lived.

Facing Death as a Way to Renew Life   A confrontation with death makes us aware of the preciousness of life. European writers in the period following World War II expressed this theme over and over again. Many of them had had the experience of being condemned to death and forced to await execution. Without exception these people found the confrontation with death to be a liberating experience. Why? Most of us live much less than full lives because we are afraid or inhibited. Once death is upon us, we somehow begin to see how trivial our other fears are. Facing the fear of death often gives people the courage to live more fully. They can dare to feel and dare to take the risks that are part of any real involvement with life.

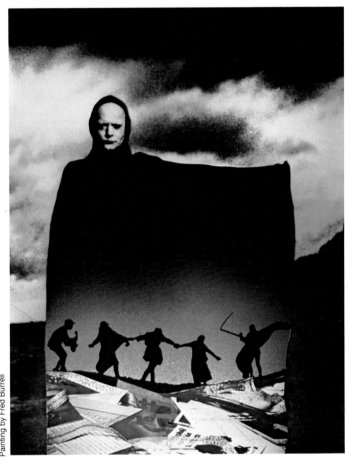

Painting by Fred Burrell

Life After Death: The Growing Evidence

. . . In the course of his research, [University of Connecticut psychologist and professor Kenneth] Ring found that his subjects—men and women of a wide range of age, education, background, and temperament—all spoke of what he came to call a "core experience," which occurred when they were close to death or "clinically dead." They told of floating up and away from their bodies, of communicating with loved ones who were already dead, of gliding down a dark tunnel toward a lustrous light, of reaching a place they sensed was a threshold but from which they were drawn back, sometimes by a sense of responsibility toward others. Although there were variations in the accounts—not everyone told of the happenings in the same sequence, or experienced all of them—the feeling was always the same: There was a sense of great comfort and even bliss in which the person longed to remain and whose positive intensity was carried back to affect the rest of that person's life in the "earthly" world. Regardless of what their attitudes had been before—and their religious beliefs varied widely—these people were convinced that they had been in the presence of some supreme and loving power and had been given a glimpse of a life yet to come.

Throughout his research, Ring checked certain factors to make the accounts more complete. Could these stories have been induced by drugs or anesthesia? Possibly, but in many instances the subjects had had no drugs at all; in other cases, the anesthesia and medications used seemed unlikely to have caused reactions like the ones described. (If anything, Ring believes, it is possible drugs and anesthetics may block these experiences and cause a person to forget a near-death experience he might otherwise remember.)

Were these experiences hallucinations brought about by toxic shock? Again, this could be a factor, but hallucinations are rambling and unconnected and differ widely, depending on the individual; these stories were clear and consistent and grounded in a sense of reality. As a psychiatrist who had one of these experiences told Ring, she was well aware of what constituted a dream or hallucination—and this was neither.

Do people facing the end of their lives see what they *want* to see? Not necessarily. Some of Ring's subjects had no advance warning that their lives were in danger, and many of them had done no wishful thinking about a pleasant afterlife (this was true in particular of 36 attempted suicides Ring studied—most of whom had hoped to end their consciousness altogether).

Finally, was this "glimpse of death" just a brief, bizarre episode—something like a flash of extrasensory perception before the phone rings? Apparently not. These experiences seemed to cause a transformation in the lives of those who went through them. Friends and associates verified the subjects' claims that the near-death experiences had had a deep and positive effect on their attitudes and values, their inclination to love and help others. . . .

What specifically interests Dr. Michael Sabom [assistant professor of cardiology at Emory University] are out-of-body experiences—in which people report leaving their unconscious bodies to observe from another vantage point, usually from above, what is happening. In some cases, a disembodied person even moves to another place and gives a detailed account of what is happening there. "When I started to check these stories out," Sabom says, "I thought I'd find fuzzy, inaccurate stories about things patients saw or heard while unconscious that would be like something they saw in a doctor show on television. To my surprise, I found that some of the patients could tell me in detail, in the correct sequence, exactly what had really happened on the operating table. In about fifteen cases, after hearing the patient's version of what he or she observed, I literally retraced the events and pieced together what had actually gone on. And they all checked out. In the case of one man, he described in visual detail how he floated above his body and watched the operating team at work. He described the instruments, how the heart looked and the operative procedure itself. I was amazed—this man was from rural Florida; there was nothing in his background to indicate that he could have picked up this medical knowledge otherwise. I visited him many times after that, and at no time did I ever detect that he'd surreptitiously read anything in a medical text to explain his knowledge. In another case, a man's heart stopped beating for four to five minutes, and he described—exactly—what went on during that time. To me, this is the strongest evidence that these weren't just hallucinations or fantasies.

"A lot of these people are my patients. I've kept in touch with them over the years so I know their backgrounds. And the thing that impressed me is that here are ten, fifteen, twenty people saying things that I can go back and substantiate. After a while, it all becomes more and more difficult to shrug off.

There's something going on here, and it can't be explained in traditional ways."

But disbelievers do try to explain it. Among the theories are these: that the brain, deprived of oxygen, conjures up hallucinatory visions; that electrical seizures quiver through the dying nervous system and set off patterns of light and music; that a sense of isolation and anxiety in the strange surroundings of a hospital send the mind into protective shock to make the trauma bearable; that the ego, faced with destruction, reacts to the unbearable stress with a last mighty act of denial. It's a mirage, skeptics say, a programmed flood of personal memories and primal responses that come from the storehouse of the unconscious. An even more specific variation on this theory is that the powerful trauma of death triggers the powerful memory of birth; and the movement down a tunnel of darkness to an awaiting light is only a flashback to another time of transition.

However, serious near-death researchers say such answers are superficial and simplistic—and easier for critics to deal with than examining new and "unacceptable" information. Sociologist John Audette is executive director of the International Association for Near-Death Studies, an organization of physicians, scholars, and near-death experiencers whose purpose is to encourage the study and sharing of information on this topic. Audette has directed his own near-death studies at two major medical centers in Illinois, and has approached his research with a cold eye.

"I'm so scientifically minded that I've been the first to point out all the possible clinical explanations for what's happening," he says. "It's true that some of the cases can possibly be explained by biochemical or physiological conditions. For instance, the body is capable of producing substances called endorphins that have a morphinelike effect and can block pain in times of trauma. But such facts don't begin to explain the full scope of these experiences—and if skeptical researchers would study our cases in depth, they too would see that. It's simply impossible to account for the large number and wide range of these stories by using traditional areas of knowledge.". . .

Researchers see these cases as lessons for the living. It is why they hope the public will evaluate these stories thoughtfully, and not rush to romanticize death. Or even to seek it out. "You can't skim over the surface of these stories and say, 'Hey, if that's what death is like, I want to get on with it,'" Kenneth Ring says. "One result of these experiences is that people 'come back' convinced that human life is precious, that it's wrong to violate the natural order of things by ending your own life deliberately.". . .

Another hope is that interest will not be focused on an aspect that is unanswerable except in religious terms: the issue of life after death. "The people we're talking about have been very close to actual physical death," Michael Sabom says, "and their reports are the closest we have to what happens to many people at this time. But whether these experiences continue after a certain point is pure speculation. It does bring up the possibility that something will persist after death. As far as these people who have had the experiences are concerned, there's no doubt about it— they're convinced that what happened was a look at what is to come. They're utterly freed from the fear of dying, and it's allowed them to focus on the here and now.". . .

Over the past ten years, Dr. Ian Stevenson, Carlson professor of psychiatry at the University of Virginia Medical Center, has studied many cases of near-death experiences; his reports have been published by the *Journal of Nervous and Mental Disease* and the *American Journal of Psychiatry,* as well as by university presses.

"People sometimes ask me if I believe in rebirth and survival after death," he says. "But that's the wrong kind of question. People shouldn't ask what I believe, they should ask what *they* believe. Our job is not to convince or convert anybody, but simply to chart the evidence and present it in a form that people can judge and grapple with for themselves. It's possible that researchers will one day decide that life after death isn't the best explanation for the evidence we have—but it's just as possible that they will decide it *is*. It's a leap of faith, of course. But I think all scientific advances involve a leap of faith."

Personally, Dr. Stevenson speaks for many of those who have closely observed this phenomenon when he says that "there is increasing evidence that we do live after death. I think it prudent to prepare for the eventuality."

Mary Ann O'Roark
McCall's

Death and Dying Attitude Scale

Read the following statements carefully. Choose the one in each section that best describes you at this moment and record its score at the right. (For example, "accepts death as a part of life" has a score of 5.) When you have identified five statements, total your score and find your position on the scale.

5 accepts death as a part of life
4 recognizes that everyone must die
3 seldom thinks about death
2 feels that death is something that happens to others
1 denies that everyone must eventually die

Score _____

5 feels and expresses grief unashamedly
4 cries openly at funerals
3 is somewhat inhibited about expressing grief
2 holds back feelings of pain and loss
1 is embarrassed to show feelings of loss and mourning

Score _____

5 feels the dead human body is a valuable resource
4 encourages people to donate organs after death
3 agrees to permit own organs to be used after death
2 is uncomfortable about donating organs after death
1 feels people should be buried intact

Score _____

5 feels that funerals should celebrate a life
4 feels that funerals help the living
3 feels that funerals provide a chance to honor the dead
2 feels that funerals are useless
1 uses funerals to impress others

Score _____

5 knows the costs of and how to plan funeral arrangements
4 knows the options for appropriate disposition of the body
3 is willing to learn about planning for death
2 is not interested in learning about planning for death
1 is unwilling to consider planning for death

Score _____

Total score _____

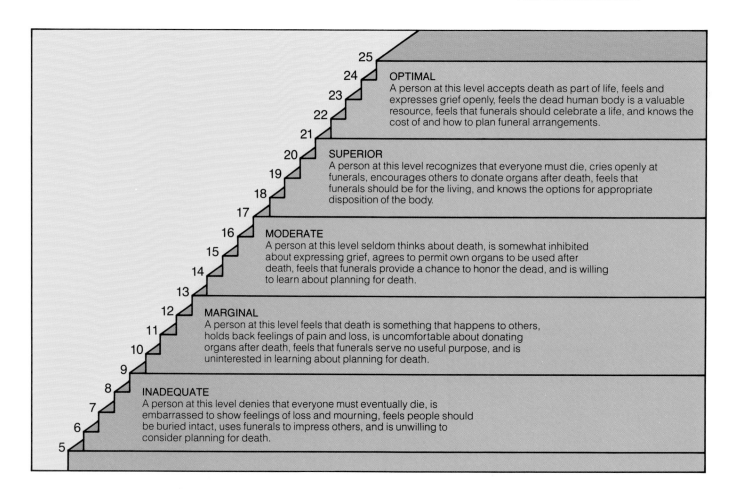

25
24   **OPTIMAL**
23   A person at this level accepts death as part of life, feels and
22   expresses grief openly, feels the dead human body is a valuable
21   resource, feels that funerals should celebrate a life, and knows the
     cost of and how to plan funeral arrangements.

20   **SUPERIOR**
19   A person at this level recognizes that everyone must die, cries openly at
18   funerals, encourages others to donate organs after death, feels that
17   funerals should be for the living, and knows the options for appropriate
     disposition of the body.

16   **MODERATE**
15   A person at this level seldom thinks about death, is somewhat inhibited
14   about expressing grief, agrees to permit own organs to be used after
13   death, feels that funerals provide a chance to honor the dead, and is willing
     to learn about planning for death.

12   **MARGINAL**
11   A person at this level feels that death is something that happens to others,
10   holds back feelings of pain and loss, is uncomfortable about donating
9   organs after death, feels that funerals serve no useful purpose, and is
     uninterested in learning about planning for death.

8   **INADEQUATE**
7   A person at this level denies that everyone must eventually die, is
6   embarrassed to show feelings of loss and mourning, feels people should
5   be buried intact, uses funerals to impress others, and is unwilling to
     consider planning for death.

Take Action

Your answers to Probing Your Emotions at the beginning of this chapter and your placement level on the Death and Dying Attitude Scale will, we hope, encourage you to begin a process of self-exploration and self-discovery that you will continue. Reflect on the entire chapter's content and ask yourself how each point relates to your own life. Then take action:

1. Write to the National Kidney Foundation at 116 East 27th Street, New York, N.Y. 10016, requesting a uniform donor card. When you receive it, consider the advantages and disadvantages of an after-death donor plan.

2. Find out what resources are available in your community to counsel the dying. Write an evaluation of the service.

3. Find out what resources if any are available in your community for counseling the bereaved. If none is locally available, find out where this service is offered and inform the appropriate local community agency.

Before leaving this chapter, review the questions that open the chapter. Have your feelings or values changed? Are you now better equipped to handle the complex and very human problems associated with death and dying?

Index

Boldface numbers indicate pages on which glossary definitions appear.

ABO blood system, 446
Abortions, 144, **146**-149
    spontaneous, **128**
Absenteeism, job, 36, 196
Absorption, 212, **213, 231**
Abstinence, **134**
Acceptance stage, in dying, 504
Acid, **357**
Acne, **83, 427**
Acquired Immune Deficiency Syndrome (AIDS), 469-470, **471**
ACTH (adrenocorticotropic hormone), **31**
Active variance, sexual, 117-118
Acupuncture, **329**
Acute disease, **196**
Adams, Anthony, 266, 267
Adaptive energy, 30, **31**, 39
Adaptive immunity, **430**, 442-446, 448. *See also* Immunization
Adaptive reactions, **24**, 27, 29, 33-35, 39. *See also* Defense mechanisms
Addiction, **187, 231**, 242
    to cocaine, 239
    to depressants, 234
    to opioids, 231-232
    to tobacco, 186, 187, 188-190, 200, 202, 204
Additive effect, of smoking, 196
Additives, food, 259-260, 336, **337, 412**
Adipose tissue, **333**, 397
Adjustment, mental health and, 54
Alder, Alfred, 62
Adolescence, 65, 81, 82, 83
Adrenal glands, 31
Adulterated products, **337**
Advertising
    cigarette, 199
    of health care and products, 337, 345, 347, 348, 350
Aerobics, **303**-304, 309-311, 319, 398, 490
Affectionateness, sex differences in, 85-86
Affection needs, during pregnancy, 160
Africa, 429
African sleeping sickness, **429**
Age
    and high blood pressure, 394
    of mentally ill persons, 56, 67
    of obese persons, 285
    retirement, 476, 489
Ageism, 476, 488-489

Agglutination, **443, 444**
Aggression, sexual, 117
Aging, 33, 475-494
    defined, **477**
AIDS (Acquired Immune Deficiency Syndrome), 469-470, **471**
Alarm reaction, in stress response, 30
Alcohol, 17, 209-225, 232, 234, 357
    abuse of, **216**-220, 486
    cancers from, 195, 215, 414
    defined, **210**
    dependency on (alcoholics/alcoholism), 56, **215, 216**-220, 221, 234
    drugs with, 354, 470
    smoking with, 188
    time-action function with, 213, 228-230
    vitamins depleted by, 352
Alcoholics Anonymous, 200, 204, 220
Aldosterone, 396
Alienation, **36**, 66-**68**
Alkali, **357**
Allemanni tribe, 212
Allergies, 195, 438, **448**-451, 463
Allopathy, **327**, 328
Alpern, David M., 148
Altered states of consciousness, **237**
Alternative Birth Centers (ABCs), **173**-176
Altruistic love, 98
Alzheimer's disease, 487
Amenorrhea, **160**
American Association of Retired Persons, 483
American Cancer Society, 294, 338, 366, 410, 415-421 passim
American College of Sports Medicine, 309, 310
American Druggist Counterdose Chart, 357
American Heart Association, 338
American Hospital Association, 381
American Indians, 32-33, 184, 216, 238
American Medical Association (AMA), 241, 327, 329, 338
American Osteopathic Association, 327
American Psychiatric Association, 216
American Red Cross, 357
American Social Health Association, 459, 460
Amino acids, 252, **253**
Ammonia, 198
Amniotic fluid, 148, **149**
Amniotic sac, 148, **149, 156**, 157, 167
Amoebic dysentery, **429**
Amphetamines, 234, 235-236
Amphigenital sex, 117

Amygdalin, 332, **333**
Amytal, 232
Andes Mountains, 236
Androgens, 312
Anemia, **253**, 350, 352
Anesthetics
    cocaine and, 237
    during labor, 167
    near-death and, 506
Aneurysm, 194, 400, **401**
Anger
    dying stage of, 502
    in intimate relationships, 95, 104-105
Angina pectoris, **194**, 215-216, 391, **398**
Angiotensins, 396
Anonymity, social, **33**
Anorexia nervosa, 284
Antabuse, 220
Antibiotics, 18, **327, 371, 436**
    infection treated with, 371, 436-437, 438, 465, 470
    rheumatic fever prevented by, 402
Antibodies, **170**, 372-374, 442-**443**, 444-451 passim
    aging and, 482
    and atherosclerosis, 389
    with blood transfusions, 165, 372-374, 447
    in mother's milk, 170
Anticipatory stress, 46
Anticoagulants, **350**
Antidepressants, 244
Antigenic determinants, 442-**443**, 444, 445, 446
Antigens, **372**, 442-**443**, 444, 445-446, 447, 448-449
Antihistamines, **350**, 351, 449
Antihypertensive drugs, **397**, 404-405
Antipsychotic drugs, 242
Anus, sexual sensors in, 105
Anxiety, **68**
    anxiolytic drugs and, 244
    caffeine and, 235
    sexual, 113-114
    socially inhibiting, 74-75
    test, 38
Anxiolytic drugs, **244**
Aorta, **194**
Aortic aneurysm, 194
Apisate, 235
Apnea, 174
Appendicitis, **428**
Appetite suppression, through drugs, 235, 290

Approach-approach situations, 68
Approach-avoidance situations, 68
Archetype, **62**
Ardell, Donald, 5, 6, 45
Aristotle, 122
Armoring of the ego, **62-64**
Aronow, W. S., 199
Aronson, Elliot, 200
Arteriogram, **370**
Arthritis, 333, **451**
Arthritis Foundation, 333
Asia, 216, 429. *See also* China; Japan
Aspirin, 350, 352, 354-356
Association of American Medical Colleges, 327
Association of Physical Fitness Centers, 308
Asthma, **451**
Asymptomatic diseases, **461**
Atherosclerosis, **194, 388**-393, 396, 398, 400
Athlete's foot, **429**
Attenuated organisms, **446**
Audette, John, 507
Auscultation, **368-369**
Australia, 126, 414
Authenticity, personal, **57**
Authority, between compatible intimates, 91
Autoimmune disease, 438, **451**
Autonomic nervous system, 30, **31**, 43. *See also* Sympathetic nervous system
Autophilic intimacy needs, 116
Autopsy, **501**
Autosexuals, **116**
Aversion therapy, 220
Aversive smoking, 207
Avoidance-avoidance situations, 68
Awake and Aware, 169

Babylon, 212, 437
Bach, George, 66
Back trouble, 305
Bacteria, 371-372, 426-448 passim, 461
Bahnson, Claus Bahne, 413
Bakersfield, California, 147
Balsam of Life, 344
Baltimore, 56
Balzer, Harry, 264
Barbiturates, **232**, 234
Bargaining stage, of dying, 502
Barnett, L. Walker, 17
B cells, 442-449 passim
Beer, 210, 212

Behavioral change strategies, 5-19, 383
for exercise, 318-320
against heart disease, 48-51, 404-405
with loneliness, 74-75
for medication, 361-362
for nutrition, 273-274
with sexual dysfunction, 101-102
against smoking, 206-207
for weight control, 285, 293, 296-297
Behavioral effects
of alcohol, 211-212, 214
of amphetamines, 235, 236
of barbiturates, 234
of mental illness, 66, 67, 284
Behavioral patterns. *See* Coping; Habit patterns; Life-style
Behaviorist model, of human nature, 61-62, 68, 71
Behavior modification/therapy, 49, **61**, 71, 72, 284, **293**, 296
Bell, Daniel, 26
Belladonna, 344, 350
Bem, D. J., 87
Bem, S. L., 87
Benefit-risk ratio, 336, **337**
Benign tumors, **408**
Benson, Herbert, 442
Benzedrine, 235
Benzodiazepines, 244
Bequeathal, after death, 500-501, 503
Bereavement, 40, 56, **501**-502
Bergman, James, 483
Bibliotherapy, sex, 102
Bierman, Edwin, 390
Billings method, 136, **137**
Biochemical effects, **230**
of drugs, 230
of stress. *See under* Defense mechanisms
Biofeedback, 404-405, 442
Biological death, 498
Biological evolution, 24-27
Biological model, of human nature, 59-61, 71
Biological sex differences, 80-85, 89, 158
Biological therapy, 71, 72. *See also* Drug treatment
Biologic response modifiers, 415
Biopsy, **375**
Birth, 167-169, 171. *See also* Childbirth process
Birth control, 121-151
Bisexuals, **116, 469**
Bizarre behavior, 66

Black, Helen, 255
Blackmun, Harry, 147
Blacks
alcohol use among, 216
cancer among, 409
mental illness among, 56
and sickle-cell disease, 433
Bladder cancer, 195
Bladder infections, 429
Blalock, Rebecca, 489
Blanchard, Edward, 405
Blastocyst, 156
Bleeding, in pregnancy, 160
Block, Marilyn, 483
Blocks, mental, 64
Blood alcohol concentration (BAC), **211**
Bloodletting treatment, 326
Blood plasma, **374, 389**, 390, **440**
Blood pressure, 368, 393, 394, 490. *See also* Hypertension
Blood tests, 372-374, 375
Blood transfusions, 165, 372-374, 446-447, 469, 501
Blood vessels, 236, 388. *See also* Cardiovascular system
Blue babies, 85, **402**
Body fat, of overweight people, 276, 278, 286, 290
Bohmbach, Dwight, 266
Bone, 83, 162, 437, 490, 501
Boredom, 28
Boston Women's Health Collective, 124
Botulism, **428, 429**
Brain cell damage, 241, 398, 400
Brain chemistry, with aging, 482-484
Brain death, 496, 498
Branch, Laurence G., 17
Breast cancer, 125, 409, 414, 415, 416, 420
Breast feeding, 138, 154, 170
Breast self-examination (BSE), 366, **416**, 419
Breathing
smoking and, 193, 194, 198
sudden infant death syndrome and, 174
Breslow, Lester, 336
Brewing beer, 212
British Medical Journal, 203
Brody, Jane E., 256, 260, 269, 392
Bronchitis, **186**, 190, **193**, 196, **427**
Brooks, Marjorie, 413
Brown-Séquard, Charles Edouard, 484
Bubonic plague, **434**
Buccal smear test, **418**

Buddy system, 15
Buerger's disease, 188-190
Bulimia, 284
Burial, after death, 503
Burtoff, Barbara, 92-94
Business Week, 367

Cadmium, 397
Caesarean section, 148, **149, 167,** 171
Caffeine, 44, 234-235, 236
Calamine lotion, 357
Calcitonin, 437
Calcium, 44, 350
Calcium carbonate, 357
Calendar rhythm method, 134-136
California, 147, 172, 203, 380, 429, 483
California Council Against Health Fraud, 334
California Department of Consumer Affairs, 349
Calories, **250, 278**-280, 286, 296, 304
Cameron, Ewan, 268
Campbell Soup Co., 267
Canadian memorial societies, 503
Cancers, 366, 375, 407-423, 434, 449
    of AIDS patients, 469
    alcohol and, 195, 215, 414
    defined, **186, 408**
    diet and, 294, 414, 418
    imaging with, 441
    immune system and, 415, 434, 437, 441, 447-448, 484
    oral contraceptives and, 125, 126
    quackery and, 332-333, 334
    smoking and, 184-202 passim, 409, 414, 418
    viruses and, 414, 415-416, 427, 448, 468
    vitamin C and, 268-269
Candida albicans, 470, **471**
Candidiasis, **428,** 429
Cannabis sativa, 240-242
Cannon, Walter, 441
Carbohydrates, **252,** 294, 312
Carbon monoxide, 186-**187,** 191, 194, 196
Carcinogens, **186,** 411, 412-414, 418
Carcinoma, **409**
Cardiac death, 498
Cardiorespiratory endurance exercise, **303**-305, 309-311, 319, 398, 490
Cardiovascular diseases, **187, 388.** *See also* Heart disease
Cardiovascular system, **215, 388**
Carotene, 257
Carrot preparation, 257

Catecholamines, **303**
Catasexual, **116**
CAT scan, 488
Cellulite, 333
Census Bureau, U.S., 477
Centers for Disease Control, U.S., 460, 465
Central nervous system (CNS), **26,** 27, **211, 228**
    angiotensins and, 396
    depressants of, 211, 214, 232-234, 354
    stimulants of, 228, 234-237
    syphilis and, 465
Cerebral cortex, **187**
Cerebral embolism, **398**
Cerebral hemorrhage, **398**-400
Cerebral thrombosis, 388, **398**
Cerebrovascular occlusion, 398
Cervical cancer, 125, 418, 468
Cervical cap, 132
Cervix, **127, 162**
Chabon, Irwin, 169
Chancre, **464**
Chancroid, **471**
Character Analysis, 62
Checkups, **364**-366, 416-418
Chemicals, carcinogenic, 411-415
Chemical tests, 374-375, 378
Chemistry, brain, 482-484
Cherry, Lawrence, 413
Chewing tobacco, 198
Childbirth process, 154, 158, 164, 165-169, 171-176. *See also* Pregnancy
Childbirth Without Fear, 169
Childhood
    of cancer victims, 413
    hypertension acquired in, 396-397
    obesity in, 281
    vaccination in, 435
Children
    authenticity of, 57, 59
    bacterial diseases of, 428
    cancer in, 409
    and drugs, 235, 354, 356
    heart disease of, 402
    hyperactive, 235
    institutionalized, 40
    parenting of, 85-87, 135-136, 175-176, 178
    and sexuality, 80-87 passim, 118
    STD affecting (through parents), 456, 463, 465, 468
    sudden infant death syndrome in, 174, 195
    See also Childbirth process

China, 36, 144, 146, 329
"Chipping," with drugs, 231
Chiropractics, 327, **329**-331
Chlamydia trachomatis, 429, 463
Chlordiazepoxide, 220
Cholera, **434**
Cholesterol, 18, 35, **304, 389,** 390-393
Chorion, 156
Christian Medical Research League, 333
Christian Scientists, 331, 379
Christian traditions, and death, 504
Chromosomes, 80-81, 155, **238,** 241, **408**
Chronic alcohol users, 212
Chronic bronchitis, **193**
Chronic cough, 190, 193, 194
Chronic diseases, 33, 40, **196, 213**
Cigarettes, 190, 191, 193-198, 202, 390, 392. *See also* Smoking
Cigar smoking, 191, 193, 194, 198
Cilia, 193-194, **430**
Cincinnati, 36
Circulation, 162, 190, 204, 398
Circulatory system, in pregnancy, 162
Circumcision, **129,** 154, 169
Cirrhosis, **216,** 218
City living, 33-35, 56
Clark, Sarah, 483
Client-centered therapy, 72
Clinical death, 498
Clinical programs, **17**
Clitoris, **105**
Coagulant, **215**
Coca-Cola, 237
Cocaine, 234, 236-237, 239-240
"Cocaine helpline," 239
Cocarcinogen, **186**
Coccidiodomycosis, **429**
Cocoa, 234, 236
Coffee, 44, 188, 234, 236
Cohen, Kenneth P., 502
Coitus, **114**
Coitus interruptus, 136-138
    defined, **137**
Colas, 234, 236, 237
Colds, common, 268, 269, 426, 431-432
Cold sores, 466
Collateral circulation, **398**
Colleges
    dating at, 74-75
    dormitory crowding at, 35-36
    health centers at, 329
Colon cancer, 414
Color Additives Amendment, 259

Colorado, 415
Colostrum, **162**
Coming of Post Industrial Society, 26
Commitment
    to behavior change, 13–15, 200
    to growth, 91
Communication, intimate, 95, 462
Companionate love, 98
Companionship marriage, **96**
Compatibility, intimate, 91–95
Complement fixation, **443**–444, 446
Compulsive acts, 66, **67**
Computers, 253, 379
Conception, **122, 156**
Conditioning, **61**
Condoms, 122, **129**–131, 458–460
Conflict, mental, 68
Conflict management, interpersonal, 95–96
Congenital defects, **85, 158,** 402. *See also*
    under Fetal development
Congestion, body, **193**
Congestive heart failure, 400–**401**
Congress, U.S., 336, 337, 338, 340, 347, 476
Connecticut, 56, 483
Consciousness, 43, **62,** 237, 504
Constantinople, 184
Consumer Product Safety Commission, U.S.,
    338
Consumer protection, in health care and
    products, 336–338, 344
Consumer Reports, 203, 262, 338
Consumers, medical care, 170–176,
    321–383
Consumers Union, 338, 356, 432
Contact dermatitis, **471**
Contagious disease, **426**
Continuation rate, of contraceptives, **126,** 129
Contraceptives, 122–144
Contractions, uterine, **164,** 165, 166–167
Contracts, 8, 10–11, 308. *See also* Self-con-
    tracts
Cooking, 252, 256, 266
Cooper, Kenneth, 303, 319
Coping, 41–47, 66, 237
Copper 7, 127
Copper T, 127
Copulation, **111**
Cornea, **500**
Coronary artery disease, 199, 398
Coronary bypass surgery, 391
Coronary heart disease (CHD), **194,** 400
Coronary occlusion, **398**
Coronary thrombosis, **388,** 398
Corpus luteum, **122, 162**

Corticosteroids, 449, 451
Cosmic consciousness, **504**
Cost
    of cardiovascular health, 391, 392, 402
    of cocaine, 237, 240
    of cold remedies, 431
    health care (general), 324, 330, 333,
        338–340, 345
    memorial societies and, 503
Cough, chronic, 190, 193, 194
Cough suppressants, 351
Cousins, Norman, 44–46, 441
Cowpox, 446
Creams, spermicidal, 129, 131, 133–134
Creativeness, 59
Cremation, 503
Crib death, 174, 195
Crisis of transformation, 26
Cross-tolerance, **237**
Crowding, social, 35
Cryptococcosis, **429**
CT scans, **370,** 379
Cultural lag, **26**
Culture (bacterial), **372**
Culture (social)
    on aging, 33, 476, 479
    evolution in, 24–27
    primitive, **39,** 326, **344**
    sex roles in, 80, 85–89, 96
    See also Social environment
Cyclamate, 412
Cyclosporin A, 447
Cytology, **375**

Daffy's Elixir, 344
Dalkon Shield, 127
Danaher, B. G., 7, 11, 207
Data, **347**
Dating, college-student, 74–75
Death, 379, 495–509
    definitions of, 496, 498
Death rates, 18, 477
    alcohol drinking and, 486
    from barbiturate overdose, 234
    from cancer, 409, 415
    and smoking, 18, 184, 191, 193, 194, 486
    social supports and, 41
    STD-related, 456, 469
    from sterilizations, 141, 142
Debilitating diseases, **426**
Decongestants, 351
Defense mechanisms
    of body, 24, 28–32, 430–451 passim. *See*
        also Immune systems

of mind, **62**–64
Deficiency disease, 267–271, 352
Degenerative diseases, **303**
Degree mills, in nutritional counseling, 334
Dehydration, **286,** 290
Dehydroeplandrosterone (DHEA), **484**
Delaney clause, 259
Delirium, 242
Delirium tremens (DTs), **218,** 234
Dementia, 487–488
Demonic theory, **326**
Denial and isolation stage, of dying, 502
Dental caries, **428**
Department of Agriculture, U.S., 263
Department of Health and Human Services,
    U.S., 336, 338
Department of Health, Education, and
    Welfare, U.S., 128
Department of Labor, U.S., 36
Dependency, **187**
    alcohol, 215, **216**–220, 221, 234
    drug, 231, 236
    See also Addiction
Depersonalization, **237,** 240
Depressants, **211,** 214, **230,** 232–234, 236
Depression, 56, **68, 244,** 487
    dying stage of, 502–504
    and infection, 434, 451
    postpartum, **170**
Dermatitis, contact, **471**
Desensitization, **61, 75**
Deutsch, Ronald, 66
Dexedrine, 235
Dextroamphetamine, 235
Diabetes, **490**
Diagnosis, medical, 363–383
    and cancer, 366, 375, 409, 415, 418
    of dementia, 488
    of STD, 374, 460–471 passim
Diagnosis-related groups (DRGs), 340
*Diagnostic and Statistical Manual of Mental
    Disorders,* 216
Diaphragms, 122, **131**
Diaries, health, **5**–6, 12
    of body weight, 296
    of drinking, 223
    of exercise, 313, 318–319
    of smoking, 7, 206, 207
    of social activity, 75
Diastole, **393**
Diastolic blood pressure, **368,** 394
Diazepam, 220
Dick-Read, Grantly, 169
Diehl, H. S., 198–199

Diet, 249–274, 294, 304, 312–313, 418, 486
  and aging, 482, 486
  anorexia nervosa and, 284
  atherosclerosis risk with, 390–393
  and cancer, 294, 414, 418
  fad, 289, 333–334
  and hypertension, 41, 397
  and overweight causes, 278–280, 304
  in pregnancy, 160, 164
  and stress, 41, 44
  weight loss, 281–289 passim, 333–334
  See also Minerals; Vitamins
Diet Center, 288-289
Diethylpropion, 235
Diethylstilbestrol (DES), **126, 412,** 414
Digestion, 252, **253,** 414
Dilatation and curettage (D and C), 148, **149**
Diseases, 324–332 passim, 364
  aging and, 481, 482, 487
  amphetamines and, 236
  autoimmune, 438, **451**
  degenerative, **303**
  diagnosis of. *See* Diagnosis, medical
  exercises reducing risk of, 303
  nutritional deficiency, 267–271, 352
  overweight and, 294
  sex differences in vulnerability to, 85
  sexual dysfunctions from, 101
  smoking related to, 184, 188–196, 198–199
  stress-linked, 30, 33, 36, 38–41
  terminal, **499**
  vasectomy and, 141
  See also Cancers; Heart disease; Infections; Mental illness; Sexually transmitted diseases
Disorientation, **33**
Distillation, **210**
Distress, **28,** 29, 41, 313
Disulfiram, 220
Ditran, 238
Diuretics, **164, 290,** 397
Diversions, from stress, 43
Diverticulitis, **428**
Divorce, 96–98
DMT (dimethyl-tryptamine), 237, 238
DNA (deoxyribonucleic acid), **481**
Doctors. *See* Physicians
Dopamine, **484**
"Dope fiend" stereotype, 237
Dose-response relationship, **211–212, 228**
Douching, **138**
Driving
  alcohol and, 219
  marijuana and, 241

Drug abuse, 56, **288,** 232–234, 235, 239–240, 244, 469. *See also* Dependency
Drug companies, 347
Drugs, 343–362
  contraceptive, 122–126, 144
  genetic formulas for, 450
  near-death affected by, 506
  over-the-counter, 235, **348–357,** 431
  See also Psychoactive drugs
Drug treatment, 343–362
  cancer-causing, 414, 418
  cholesterol-lowering, 392, 393
  for hypertension, 397, 404–405
  dementia from, 487
  immune systems affected by, 434–435, 482
  for infection, 435–438, 461, 464, 465, 470, 471
  of obesity, 290
  with psychoactive drugs, 72, 228, 232, 235, 238, 240, 241, 244
  See also Antibiotics; Over-the-counter drugs
DTs (delirium tremens), **218,** 234
Dubos, René, 28
Dundas, Michael, 266
Dying, 379, 498–500, 502–504. *See also* Death
Dynamic Theory of Personality, 68
Dysentery, amoebic, **429**
Dysfunction, sexual, 101–102

Eagleton, Thomas, 54
Ectopic pregnancy, **466**
Eddy, Mary Baker, 331
Education
  for old people, 489
  about STD, 456–458
Educational level
  and intimate compatibility, 91
  and mental illness, 56
Egg (ovum), **80,** 154–155
Egypt, 212, 437
Ejaculation, **82,** 101, 102, **129,** 154
Electrocardiogram (EKG or ECG), **370,** 371, 378
Electroencephalogram (EEG), **370,** 371, **496**
Electromyogram (EMG), 370–371
Embalming, 503
Embolus, 398
Embryo, **155–157**
Emotional intimacy, **59**
Emotions, 19, 30, 46, 59, 68

and cancer, 413
  in dying stages, 502–504
  exercise affecting, 300–303
  and immune response, 451
  in intimate relationships, 95, 104–105
  and overweight, 283–285, 293, 297
  See also Mental illness
Emphysema, **193,** 199, 498, **499**
Empirical approaches, **326,** 344
Encounter groups, 71, 72
Endemic organisms, 434, **435**
Endocardium, 388
Endometrium, **156**
Endorphins, **31, 231,** 507
Endurance exercise, 303–305, 309–311, 319, 398, 490
Energy
  adaptive, 30, **31,** 39
  nutritional, 250, 252. *See also* Calories
Energy balance concept, in weight control, 296
Energy level, of compatible intimates, 91
England, 40, 203, 223, 344, 414, 500
Enkephalin, **303**
Environment, 481
  cancer caused by, 411, 414–415, 418, 481
  heart disease caused by, 396–397, 481
  pollution in, 193, 198, 199
  for quitting smoking, 12
  See also Social environment
Environmental medicine, **481**
Environmental Protection Agency, 199
Enzymes, 252–**253, 374,** 396, **426,** 427, 440
Epicardium, 388
Epidemics, 434
Epidemiology, 434, **435**
Episiotomy, **167,** 171
Equipment, exercise, 306
Erection, 101, 102, **105–107**
Erikson, Erik, 65
Erythromycin, 464, 465
Escapism, 36
Essential hypertension, 396, **397**
Essential nutrients, **250–263.** *See also* individual nutrients
Estrogen, 85, **122,** 126, **414**
Ethics
  of genetic science, 450
  of life-lengthening processes, 484–486
  of placebos, 345
Ethnic groups, alcohol use among, 216. *See also* Blacks; Whites
Ethyl alcohol, 210

Eulogy, **501**
Euphoria, **231**, 237
Europe, 118, 184, 212, 409. *See also*
    France; Great Britain
Eustress, **28**, 29
Euthanasia, **499**
Euthanasia Educational Council, 500
Evolution, biological vs. cultural, 24-27
Excitement stage, sexual, **109**
Excretion, bodily, **350**
Exercise
    aerobic, 303-304, 309-311, 319, 398,
        490
    after childbirth, 170
    and death rate, 18
    and heart disease, 303, 304, 392, 397,
        398
    intensity of, 309-311
    during pregnancy, 165
    and stress, 13, 32, 303, 313
    weight loss with, 278-296 passim
Exhaustion stage of, stress response, 30
Exhibitionism, **116**
Existential therapies, 71, 72
"Experience of Living in Cities," 35
Exponential curves, 26
Extended family, 476, **477**
External cues, 284-**285**
Extradition, **337**
Eye infection, 429. *See also* Vision

Facial herpes, 466
Fad, **326**
Fad diets, 289, 333-334
Fair Oaks Hospital, Summit, N.J., 239
Faith healing, **331**
Fallopian tubes (oviducts), **154**
False labor, **164**
Family life, 40, 476, 477, 483, 496
Family Planning Services and Population
    Research Act, U.S., 128
Family Service Association of Orange
    County, California, 483
Fast foods, 261-262, 263, 294
Fat, body
    in overweight people, 276, 278, 286, 290
    sex differences in, 83, 276
Fathers, at childbirth, 154, 169, 172
Fatigue, in pregnancy, 160
Fats, food, 18, **252**, 294, 414, 418
FDA, *See* Food and Drug Administration
Fear
    vs. anxiety, 68
    of death, 504

Fecal matter, **434**
Federal Trade Commission (FTC), U.S.,
    336, 337, 348, 350
Federal Trade Commission Improvements
    Act, 337
Fee-for-service system, 338-340, 345
Feiffer, Jules, 33
Females
    alcoholism in, 216
    biological sex characteristics of, 80-85,
        158
    birth control responsibilities of, 143
    body fat percentage of, 83, 276
    cancer in, 409
    high blood pressure in, 394
    infections of, 429, 458, 460, 461, 462,
        463, 465, 470
    life expectancy of, 83, 477
    marijuana effects on, 241
    mental illness among, 56
    pelvic examination of, 369
    sex roles of, 80, 85-89, 96
    sexual dysfunction of, 101, 102
    smoking by, 199, 409
    See also Pregnancy; Sexual relations
Fermented substances, **210**, 211
Fertility, **125**
Fertilization, **81**, **154**-155
Fertilized egg, **154**-155
Fetal alcohol syndrome, **215**
Fetal development, 85, 155-159, 163, 450
    alcohol affecting, 215
    and congenital heart disease, 402
    marijuana affecting, 241
    Rh blood and, 165, 447
    STD affecting, 456, 463, 465, 468
Fetus, **155**-156, 158-159, 163. *See also*
    Fetal development
Fiber, dietary, 414, 418
Fibroblast interferon, 415
Fight-or-flight reaction, **28**, 303, 441, 490
Flashbacks, after psychedelics, 238
Fleming, Alexander, 436
Fleming, Alice, 212
Flexibility, exercise for, 305, 311-312
Foam, spermicidal, 130, 133-134
Focused smoking, 207
Follicles, **154**
Food, 44, 256-271 passim, 294, 412, 418.
    See also Diet
Food additives, 259-260, 336, **337**, **412**
Food Additives Amendment, 259
Food and Drug Act, 259
Food and Drug Administration (FDA), U.S.,

        336-337, 347, 348, 349
    and additives, 259, 336, 412
    and DES, 126
    and Nicorette, 202
Food composition tables, 256-257
Food, Drug, and Cosmetic Act, 347
Food poisoning, 428-429
Fortified wines, **210**, 211
Fox, Bernard H., 413
Fox, S. M., 304
Fracastoro, 327
France, 136, 216, 344
Free people, 57
French, R. de S., 74-75
Freud, Sigmund, 38, 62, 72, 188, 236
Freudian model, of human nature, 62-64
Freudian slip, 62
Fried, Sandra, 266
Friedman, Meyer, 49, 401
Friendship development, 74-75
Froeb, H. F., 199
Fuchs, Victor R., 345
Funerals, 501-502, 503
Fungi, 125, 426, 429, 430, 437, 438, 470

Gall bladder disease, 125
Gamma benzine hexachloride, 471
Gangrene, 190
Garfinkle, Lawrence, 191
G.A.S. (general adaptation syndrome), 30, **31**
Gastric aspiration, **375**
Gastrointestinal tract, **26**, 27, **290**
Gelles, Richard J., 483
General anesthetic, **167**
General Mills, 266
Genes, **80**-81, 450, 481, 484. *See also*
    Chromosomes
Genesis, Book of, 136
Genetic code, **155**, 156
Genetic determinants, of sex differences, 80-83
Genetic engineering, 437, 450
Genetic predisposition, **39**, 435, 450
    to alcoholism, 218
    to allergies, 448
    to cancer, 409
    to hypertension, 396-397
    to mental illness, 60-61
    to obesity, 280-281
    to sickle-cell disease, 432-433
Genital herpes, 466
Genitals, **80**, 81, 158
German measles, 158, 402
Gerontology, 476-481
    defined, **477**

Gestalt therapy, 72
Ginott, Haim, 178
Glass, David, 48
Glucose level, tests of, 374
Glycogen, 312, **313**
Goal setting, 8
Gold, Mark S., 239
Goldmann, Carole, 176
Gonads, **80**, 81
Gonorrhea, **169**, **430**, **456**, 460–463, 465, 466
Gossypol, 144
Gräfenberg, E., 126
Granulocyte, **440**
Granuloma inguinale, 471
GRAS list, 259
Gray Panthers, 488–489
Gray power, 483, 488–489
Grazing, 266–267
Great Britain, 118, 136, 414. *See also* England
Grief, 40, 56, 501–502
Gross, Leonard, 316
Group marriages, 99
Group therapy, 71, 72
Group treatment, of obesity, 290–293
Growald, Eileen Rockefeller, 441
Growth commitment, of compatible intimates, 91
Growth media, **372**
Gum, nicotine-containing, 200–204
Gum disorders, 195, 428

Habit patterns, 5–7, 188–190, 324. *See also* Dependency; Self-management/Self-monitoring
Hahnemann, Samuel, 331
Haitians, 469
Hall, Nicholas, 442
Hall, Trish, 267
Hallucinations, **218**, **350**, 506
Halo effect, 304
Hammer, Signe, 442
Hammond, E. Cuyler, 186, 193
Happiness, mental health vs., 54
Harrison, Beppie, 91
Harvard Medical School Health Letter, 312, 372, 488
Harvard University, 396
Hashimoto's disease, 451
Hashish, 240
Haskell, W. L., 304
Hatcher, Robert, 133
Health clubs, 308

Health Letter, 199
Health maintenance organization (HMO), 330, 338–340
Health Maintenance Organization Act, 338
Health Systems Agencies (HSAs), 340
Heart attacks, 388–400 passim
Heart disease, 387–405
    alcohol and, 215–216
    amphetamines and, 236
    diet and, 294, 390–393, 397
    exercise and, 303, 304, 392, 397, 398
    marijuana smoking and, 241
    and smoking tobacco, 184, 186, 187, 191, 194, 195, 199, 204, 390, 392
    from stress, 33, 36, 39–40, 41, 49, 392
    See also Hypertension; Strokes
Heart transplants, 427
Hegsted, Mark, 278
Help, 16, 71. *See also* Therapy
Hemoglobin, 432
Hepatitis, **426**
Herba panacea, 184
Herbert, W., 191
Heredity. *See* Genetic predisposition
Hernia tests, 369
Heroin, 17, 188, 202, 231, 232, 236
Herpes, **426**, **456**, 466–468
Herpes simplex, **416**, 426, 463, 466
Hess, Walter B., 442
Heterophilic intimacy needs, 116
Heterosexuals, **87**, **116**
"High," **230**
High blood pressure. *See* Hypertension
High-density lipoproteins (HDLs), 215, 304, **390**
Hipp, Frederick R., 267
Hippocampal gyrus, **104**
Hippocrates, 122, 126, 250, 326
Hiroshima, 415
Histamine, **448–449**
History, medical, **366–368**, 488
Holistic medicine, **332**
Holmes, Thomas H., 29, 30
Home births, 172
Homeopathy, **331**–332
Homeostasis, **24**, 46
Homophiles, **99**, 116
Homosexuals, 99, **116**, 118, 469
Hormones, **81**, **160**
    aging and, 484
    during breast feeding, 170
    fatty diets and, 414
    kidneys and, 162, 396
    in pregnancy, 160, 162

sex, 80–85 passim, 122, 125, 126, 143, 144, 312, 414, 484
steroid, 312, **451**
stress, 31, 41, 85, 303, 441–442
tests of levels of, 374
thyroid, 290, 484
Horowitz, L. M., 74–75
Hospices, **500**, 502
Hospitals, 367, 438
Houlihan's, 267
Howard, Jane, 40
Howard, Theodore, 148
Hoxsey, Harry, 333
HTLV III (human T-cell leukemia virus), 469
Human Behavior, 458
Human epidermal growth factor, 437
Humanist-existential therapies, 71, 72
Humanist model, of human nature, 60, 62, 64–65, 71
Humanitarianism, 35
Human nature, models of, 59–66
Human serum albumin, 437
Human Sexual Response, 101, 109
Humor, and stress, 44–46
Humoral theory, **326**, 331–332
Hunger
    global, 267, 269–271
    smoking affecting, 187
Hunt, William A., 17
Hydrogen cyanide, 187
Hyperactive children, 235
Hypercholesterolemia, **390**
Hypertension (high blood pressure), 393–397, 404–405, 487, **490**
    pill and, 125
    stress and, 41
    stroke with, 393, 394, 398, 400
Hyperthyroidism, **352**
Hypochondriacs, **378**
Hypothalamus, 31, **104**, **280**, 442
Hypotheses, **324–326**
Hysterectomy, **143**
Hysterotomy, 147, 148, **149**

Ianni, Elizabeth, 106
Ianni, Francis, 106
Identity
    in psychosocial development, 65
    sex, 80, 85
Imaging, healing with, 441, 442
Immigrants, stress of, 33
Immune gamma globulin, **435**
Immune interferon, 415
Immune systems, 430–451 passim

Immune systems (*cont.*)
aging and, 482, 484
AIDS and, 469
and cancer, 415, 434, 437, 447–448, 484
defined, **194, 438**
diagnostic tests of, 372–374
and fetal development, 159, 165, 447
marijuana and, 241
tobacco and, 195
Immunization
contraceptive, 144
against infections, 430, 436, 446
See also Vaccination
Immunosuppression, **447**
Impetigo, **427**
Implants, contraceptive, 143
Incest, **116,** 117
Incidence, **39**
Indians, American, 32–33, 184, 216, 238
Infections, **158, 426**–451 passim
with oral contraceptives, 125
stress and, 33, 434, 451
tests for, 371–374, 465
See also under Pathogens; Sexually
transmitted diseases
Influenza, **434**
Informed consent, **379**
Infusion, **344**
Inhaling, **186,** 239, 242
Inheritance. *See* Genetic predisposition
Inhibition, 74, **211**
Injections
contraceptive, 143
psychoactive drug, 231, 235–236, 237
See also Vaccination
Injuries
from exercise, 316
plaques caused by, 389
Inner-directed people, **57**
Input overload, **26,** 27–28, 33–35
Inspection, in physical examination, **368**
Institute for Applied Biology, 413
Institute for the Advancement of Health, 441
Institutionalized children, 40
Institutional marriage, **96**
Integrity, **434**
Intelligence, 490
Interactions, drug, **348**–350
Interferon, 415, **438**
Internal cues, bodily, 283–**285**
International Association for Near-Death
Studies, 507
International Planned Parenthood Federa-
tion (IPPF), 128

Interpersonal relations
mental health and, 59, 66, 68–70, 74–75
parenting, 85–87, 135–136, 175–176, 178
and stress, 28, 40–41, 46, 68, 74–75,
96–98
See also Intimacy; Support, social
Intestinal cancer, 409, 414
Intimacy, 59, 89–102, **114**–116. *See also*
Sexual relations
Intoxicant, **210**
Intoxication, 41, **210,** 212, 230
Intrapsychic model, of human nature, 71
Intrauterine devices (IUDs), **126**–129, 466
"Invitation to Die," 57
In vitro, **451**
Irish alcoholism, 216
Iron, in nutrition, 252–253
Isolation, social, 40
Israeli Medical Research Foundation, 333
Izard, C. E., 104

Jackson, Edgar N., 147
Jacobson, Michael, 260
James, William, 33
Janda, Louis, 113
Japan, 36, 256, 412, 414, 415
Jefferson, Mildred F., 147
Jehovah's Witnesses, 379
Jelly, spermicidal, 129, 131, 133–134
Jenkins, David, 48
Jenner, Edward, 446
Jobs
carcinogens in, 414–415, 418
during pregnancy, 165
smoking affecting, 196
stress in, 36–38
Jock itch, **429**
Jogging, 278–280
Johns Hopkins University, 56
Johnson, G. Timothy, 367
Johnson, Katrina W., 433
Johnson, Virginia, 101, 102, 109
Joint Commission on Accreditation of Hos-
pitals, 367
Joint stiffness, 305
Jourard, Sidney, 57
Journal of Human Stress, 29n
Journal of Psychosomatic Research, 30
Judeo-Christian tradition, and death, 504
Jung, Carl, 62
Junk food, 44, 261, 263, 264

Kaiser-Permanente medical centers,
376–378

Kalish, Richard, 498
Kaplan, Robert, 458
Kaposi's sarcoma, 469
Kefauver-Harris Amendment, 347
Kesten, Deborah, 260, 269
Ketamine, 242
Keys, Ancel, 276
Kidneys
alcohol and, 215, 486
donation of, 500–501
and hypertension, 396, 397
infections in, 429
during pregnancy, 162
transplants of, 447
King Lear Syndrome, 483
Kinnick, Nile, 315–316
Kisses, 105, 106
Koch, Robert, 327
Koch, William F., 333
Koin, Diana, 483
Knee-jerk reflex, 369
Knowledge, 344
Krebiozen, 333
Krebs, Ernest, Jr., 332, 333
Kübler-Ross, Elisabeth, 502
Kuhlman, Katheryn, 331
Kuhn, Maggie, 488–489
!Kung people, 35
Kuntzleman, Charles T., 308
Kushner, Rose, 420
Kwell, 471

Labels, drug, 349
Labor, in childbirth, 154, 158, **164,**
165–169, 171–172
Laboratories, sports medicine, 313
Laboratory examinations, diagnostic,
369–375, 488
Ladies' Home Journal, 289
Laetrile, **332**–333, 334
Laing, R. D., 64
Lamaze method, **169**
Landsteiner, Karl, 446, 447
Laparoscopy, **142**–143
Larvae, **471**
Larynx, **193**
Lasagna, Louis C., 191
Laughter, 44–46
Lavoisier, Antoine L., 250
Laxatives, 352
Lazarowicz, Remy, 463
Learning, sex-role, 85–86, 87
Lederberg, Joshua, 441
Leg circulation, 190

Leo (A. B.) company, 202
LeShan, Lawrence, 413
Leukemia, **409**, 415, 416
Leukocyte interferon, 415
Leukocytes, **430**
Levine, Paul, 447
Lewin, Kurt, 68
Librium, 220, 244
Lice, pubic, 470-**471**
Lichtenstein, E., 7, 11, 207
Life after death, 506-507
Life events, and illness, 30
Life expectancy, **83**, 193, 196, 336, **447**-480, 486
Life spans, 480, **481**, 482, 484, 496
Life-style, 5, 278, 303, 401, 411. *See also* Habit patterns
Life-support technology, **499**
"Light" cigarettes, 191
Lightening, in pregnancy, **164**
Lillard, Harvey, 329
Lind, James, 250
Lindsey, J. Stephen, 330
Linea nigra, 162
Lip cancer, 193, 195
Lipids, **304**
Lipoproteins, 215, **304, 390**
Lippes loop, 127
Liqueurs, 210
Liquors, 210, 347
Lithium, 72
Lithium salts, 244
Little, William, 148
Liver condition
alcohol and, 214-215, 218, 486
pill and, 125
Living together, 99
"Living wills," 499, 500
Lochia, **170**
Loci, **329**
Locke, Steven, 442
London, England, 40, 203
Loneliness, 74-75
Longevity, **482**
Los Angeles, 414
Love, 90-91, 98
Low-density lipoproteins (LDLs), 304, **390**
LSD (lysergic acid diethylamide), 237, 238
Luce, Gay, 479
Lumbar puncture, **375**
Lungs
cancer of, 191-193, 199, 202, 409, 414
heart disease and, 194, 400
marijuana and, 240-242

in pregnancy, 162
tests of, 375
tobacco smoking and, 184, 191-193, 199, 202, 409, 414
Lutenizing hormone-releasing hormone (LHRH), 144
Lymphatic system, **440**
Lymph nodes, 440, 444, 445
Lymphocytes, **440**, 442-451 passim, 469, **484**
Lymphogranuloma venereum (LGV), **471**
Lymphoma, **409**
Lyons, Richard D., 240

Macbeth, 214
Macrophages, **194, 440**, 445
Magic, 344, 480
Magnesium, 44
Maharishi Mahesh Yogi, 43
Mahoney, K., 297
Mahoney, M. J., 7, 16, 297
Mail fraud, medical, 337-338
Makinodan, Takashi, 484
Malaria, **429**
Males
alcoholism of, 216
biological sex characteristics of, 80-85, 158
birth control responsibilities of, 143
body fat percentage of, 83, 276
cancer in, 409
in childbirth process, 154, 169, 172
hernia tests on, 369
high blood pressure of, 394
life expectancy of, 83, 477
marijuana effects on, 241
mental illness among, 56
sex roles of, 80, 85-89, 96
sexual dysfunctions of, 101, 102
smoking disorders among, 199
and STD, 458-460, 461, 462, 463, 469
See also Sexual relations
Malignant tumors, **408-409**, 441. *See also* Cancers
Malnutrition, 236, **257**, 267-271, 352
Mammograms, **414**, 415
Mandrake root, 344
Mania, **244**
Manic-depressives, 60-**61**, 244
Manipulation, interpersonal, 68-70
Manipulative therapy, **327**
Man the Manipulator, 70
Marcus Aurelius, 24
Margen, Sheldon, 268

Marginality, social, 40
Marijuana, 230, 240-242, 354
Marital status, and death rates, 41
Marriage, 96, 98, 99, 135
Martial arts, 44
Maslow, Abraham, 54, 59, 60, 64, 74
Massachusetts, 380
Mast cells, **448-449**
Mastectomy, 420
Masters, William, 101, 102, 109
Masturbation, 102, **111**
Maudsley Hospital, 203
Maximum oxygen consumption (MOC), **310**
Maximum pulse rate, **310**
Mayer, Jean, 401
Mayo Clinic, 268
McAuliffe, Kathleen, 450
McAuliffe, Sharon, 450
McCay, Clive, 482
McQueen, Steve, 324, 332
Measles, German, 158, 402
Meats, 294, 414, 418
Mechanistic model, of human nature, 64
Medawar, Peter, 447
Media Watch, 489
Medicaid, 338, 380
Medical diagnosis. *See* Diagnosis, medical
Medical establishment, 324-326
alternatives to, 329-332
orthodox, 327-329
prospective parents and, 170-176
See also Physicians; Treatment, medical
Medical history, **366**-368, 488
Medical research, 324-327
Medicare, 338, 340, 477
Medicine Show, The, 356, 432
Meditation, 43-44
Melanoma, **414**, 415, 416
Memorial services, 503
Memorial societies, 503
Memory, burdening of, 46
Men. *See* Males
Menopause, **484**
Mensinga, Wilhelm, 131
Menstruation, **81**-82, 143, 160, 170
Mental health, 53-75, 487-488, 490. *See also* Emotions; Psychological factors
Mental illness, 56, 66, 67
in eating behavior, 284, 293
genetic factors in, 60-61
physical illness following, 30, 434
therapy for, 71-72, 238, 242-244, 284, 293
See also Depression; Psychosis

Meperidine, 231
Merrell Dow Pharmaceuticals, Inc., 202, 203
Mescaline, 238
Metabolic pathways, **348**
Metabolic rate, **83**
   resting, **281**-283
Metabolism, **24, 162, 252**-253
   of alcohol, 212-213, 214, 230
   in drug tests, 347, 348
   and overweight, 281-283
   in pregnancy, 162
   sex differences in, 83
Metabolization, **213, 230, 347**
Metagenital sex, 117
Metastasizing, **408**
Methadone, 231, 232
Methamphetamine, 235
Methaqualone, 232, 234
Methedrine, 235
Methylphenidate, 235
Metronidazole, 470
Microscope tests, 374-375
Midwives, 172-173
Migrants, stress of, 33
Milgram, Stanley, 35
Milk of magnesia, 357
Miller, Neal, 442
Minerals, 44, **252,** 264-267, 350, 353, 486
Minipill, 122
Mischel, Harriet N., 60
Mischel, Walter, 60
Mnemonic formula, 7, **16**
Mobility, stress from, 33, 41
Mononucleosis, infectious, **426,** 427
Monotony, job, 36
Montagu, Ashley, 481
Morehouse, Lawrence, 316
Morgan, Ernest, 503
Morgan, Karen, 267
Mormons, 41, 411
"Morning-after" pill, 126
Morphine, 231
Morris, Betsy, 264
Motivation, **62**
Motor skills, psychoactive drugs and, 219, 241
Mouth disorders, 193, 195, 428
Mucocutaneous system, 105
Mucus defenses, 193, 439-440
Mucus membranes, STDs in, 461, 464
Mucus method, cervical, 136, **137,** 138
Mucus plug, 167
Multi-infarct dementia, 487
Multiple sclerosis, 376, **451**

Murad IV, 184
Murphy, Dianne, 311
Murphy, Tom, 311
Muscles, 83, 109, 162, 305, 311-312, 490
Musk perfumes, 107
Mussel remedy, 333
Mutation, **438**
Myocardial infarction, 194, **398**
Myocardium, **194,** 388
Mystics, **504**
Myths, about sex, 107

Nader, Ralph, 489
Nagasaki, 415
Nathanson, Bernard, 147
National Academy of Sciences, 191, 256
National Better Business Bureau, 338
National Cancer Institute, 415
National Health Planning and Resources
   Development Act, 340
National Health Survey, 196
National Heart, Lung, and Blood Institute
   (NHLBI), 391, 392, 396-397
National Institute of Aging, U.S., 488
National Institute of Mental Health (NIMH),
   U.S., 56
National Institute on Drug Abuse (NIDA),
   U.S., 234, 241
National Institutes of Health (NIH), U.S., 396,
   441, 450
National Kidney Foundation, 501
National Survey on Drug Abuse, 234
Native North American Church, 238
Natural childbirth, 154, 167, **169**
Natural killer (NK) cells, 443, 451
Naturopathy, **332**
Naughton, J. P., 304
Nausea, in pregnancy, 160
Navajo Indians, 32-33
NBC News poll, 147
Negation, drug, **348,** 349
Neisseria gonorrhoeae, 461
Nembutal, 232
Neoplasms, 408
Nervous system, in sex, 104-109. *See also*
   Autonomic nervous system; Central
   nervous system
Neuroendocrine systems, **26,** 27
Neurosis, 66, **67,** 244
Neurotic needs, **57**
Neurotransmitters, 441, **484**
Neutralization, **443**
New cortex, **104**
New England Journal of Medicine, 199

New Haven, Connecticut, 56
New Jersey, 239, 340
New Yorker, 27
New York State Health Department, 450
New York Times, 195
New Zealand, 35, 126, 414
Niacin, 253
Nicorette, 202-203
Nicotiana tabacum, 184
Nicotine, 184, **186,** 187, 188-190, 191,
   196-204 passim, 234
Nipple-areola system, 107
Nisbett, Richard, 284
Nitrates, 412, 418
Nitrites, 412, 418
Nitrosamines, **412**
No-Doz, 234, 236
Nongonococcal urethritis (NGU), **456,** 462,
   463-464
Nonspecific immune mechanisms, **438**-442
Norepinephrine, 441
Normality, **54**
Norris, Patricia, 441
NPD Group, 264
Nuclear family, 476, **477, 496**
Nursing homes, 483
Nurturance, 98, **99**
Nutrition, 44, 249-274, 333-334, 351-352,
   486
   defined, **250**
   See also Diet
Nutritional consultants, 334
Nyerges, Christopher, 302
Nymphomania, 118
Nystatin, 470

Obesity, 276-293, 486
Obsessive acts, 66, **67**
Office of Population Affairs, U.S., 128
O'Grady, Kevin, 113
Old cortex, **104**
Olfactory nerve, 104
On Death and Dying, 502
Opioids, 231-232, 235
Opium, 231
Opportunistic organisms, **434**
Oral contraceptives, **122**-126
Oral Roberts University, 331
Orgasm, 101, 102, **104,** 109, **111,** 114
O'Roark, Mary Ann, 507
Orthodox medicine, 327-329
Orthogenital sex, 117
Oski, Frank A., 195
Osler, William, 332

Osteopathy, **327**–328
Outer-directed people, **57**
Out-of-body experiences, 506–507
Ovarian hormones, **125**
Ovaries, **80**, 154, 409
Overdose, drug, 357
Over-effort, at exercise, 315–316
Overfat, **276**
Overload, input, **26**, 27–28, 33–35
Over-the-counter (OTC) drugs, 235, **348**–357, 431
Overweight, 41, 275–297, 304, 397, 486
    defined, **276**
    See also Weight loss
Oviducts (Fallopian tubes), **154**
Ovulation, 81–82, **122**, 170
Ovum (egg), **80**, 154–155

Pairing, 66
Palinopia, **238**
Palmer, Daniel D., 329
Palpation, **368**
Pancreas, 195, 215, 409
Pap smear, **366**, **409**, 418
Paragenital sex, 117
Paranoia, 219, 235, 236, **237**
Parasites, **426**, 429–430
Parasympathetic nervous system, 30, **31**
Parent abuse, 483
Parenting, 85–87, 135–136, 175–176, 178
Parents, single, 99
Passamani, Eugene, 391
Passive euthanasia, 499
"Passive smoking," 196–198, 199
Passive variance, sexual, 117
Pasteur, Louis, 327
Patent medicine, 237, **344**–347
Pathogenic model, **326**–327
Pathogens, **426**–430, 439, 440–442, 444, 468. *See also* Bacteria; Fungi; Viruses
Paul, Saint, 106
Pauling, Linus, 268, 269
Pavlov, Ivan, 61
Peak experiences, 74
Pedophilia, 118
Peer group, sex-role learning in, 87
Pellagra, **253**, 269
Pelvic examination, for women, 369
Pelvic inflammatory disease (PID), 128, **129**, 463, **465**–466
Penicillin, **436**, 437–438, 461, 465
Penis, **105**
Peptic ulcers, **196**
Perceptional changes, **237**

Perceptiveness, **59**
Periodontal disease, **428**
Persona, **62**
Personal contracts, **8**, 10–11. *See also* Self-contracts
Personality
    and disease susceptibility, 39–40, 48–51, 401, 413, 458
    in senility, 487
Peter Principle, 36
Phagocytes, **440**, 444, 446
Pharmacological factors, 228–**230**. *See also* Drugs
Pharyngeal exudates, **461**
Phencyclidine (PCP), 242
Phenmetrazine, 235
Phenylpropandamine (PPA), 290
Phenylpropanolamine, **350**
Pheromones, 107
Phlegm production, smokers', 190, 193, 194
Phobias, 56, **72**
Phosphorus, 350
Physical activity, for weight control, 285, 292. *See also* Exercise
Physical advantages, of exercise, 303–305
Physical appearance, and friendship development, 74
Physical dependence, **187**. *See also* Addiction
Physical examination, 368–369, 488
Physical fitness, **300**, 313, 316
Physical stresses, and body defenses, 434
Physicians, 324, 327–329, 330, 345, 363–380 passim
    cancer detection by, 366, 416–418
    childbirth-related, 164, 172
Pill, birth control, 122–126
Pipe smoking, 191, 193, 194, 195, 198
Pittsburgh, 414
Pituitary gland, 31, 501
Placebo effect, **326**, 345
Placenta, **156**, 157, 158, 169
Planned Parenthood Federation of America, 128
Plaques, **194**, **304**, **388**, 389–390, 396
Plasma, **374**, **389**, 390, **440**
Plateau stage, sexual, **109**
Platelets, **389**, **440**
Plato, 122
Platt, John, 26
Play plans, for weight loss, 292
Pleasure, 46
Pneumonia, **427**, 431, 469
Poisoning

drug, 357
food, 428–429
See also Toxicity
Poison oak, 449
Police jobs, 36
Poliomyelitis, **426**
Pollin, William, 239
Pollution, air, 193, 198, 199
Polyaromatic hydrocarbons, 241
Polymicrobial disease, **466**
Postal Service, U.S., 336, 337–338
Postpartum depression, **170**
Postural muscles, **109**
Potassium, 44
Potentiation, drug, **348**–349
Poultice, **344**
Powell, Anne, 266
Pregnancy, 159–165
    during breast feeding, 170
    German measles during, 158, 402
    with IUD, 129
    Rh blood during, 165, 447
    psychoactive substances during, 195–196, 215, 238, 241, 244
    STD and, 465, 466, 468
    See also Fetal development
Preludin, 235
Premature ejaculation, 101, 102
Premenstrual tension, **85**
Prescription drugs, 347–348, 414. *See also* under Drug treatment
Preservatives, **412**, 418
Pressure-sensitive receptors, sexual, 105–107
Prevalence, **39**, 285
Preventive medicine, **304**
Primary response, **443**
Primary tumors, **408**
Primitive cultures, **39**, 326, **344**
Probenecid, 461
Problem solving, 15–16, 462
Professionals
    childbirth-related, 164, 172–173
    mental health, 72
    See also Physicians
Professional Standards Review Organizations (PSROs), 338
Progestasert, 127
Progesterone, 85, **122**, **143**
Prolactin, 170
Proof value, of alcohol, **210**, 211
Prophylaxis, **435**
Prostaglandins, **144**, 148
Prostate cancer, 409

Proteins, 252, **253**, 294
Protein synthesis, **482**
Protozoa, 426, 429, 430, 468
Psora, 331
Psychedelics, 237-238, 240
Psychic changes, with psychedelics, **237**
Psychoactive drugs, 188, 227-246
  defined, **184, 210, 228**
  See also Alcohol; Tobacco
Psychoanalysis, **62**, 68, 71, 72
Psychological Care of Infant and Child, 61
Psychological factors
  after abortion, 149
  and body defenses, 434
  in cancer victims, 413
  with cocaine abuse, 239
  in development, 65
  in drug use, 230
  in sexual dysfunction, 101
  in stress, 32-38
  See also Emotions; Mental illness; Personality
Psychometric measurement, **188**
Psychoneuroimmunology, 441-442
Psychoneurotic disorders, 66, 67, **244**
Psychoprophylaxis method, **169**
Psychosis, 66, **67, 235**, 242. *See also* Schizophrenia
Psychosomatic symptoms, **35**
Psychotherapy, 71-**72**, 238, 293
Puberty, **81**, 82, 83
Pubic lice, 470-**471**
Public Health Service (PHS), U.S., 184, 190, 196, 431
Puerperium, **169**-170
Pulmonary heart disease, 194, 400
Pulse rate, **310**
Punishments, behavior modification with, 61-62
Pure Food and Drug Act, 347
Pus, 440

Quaalude, 232
Quackery, **326**, 332-338
Quicksall, Brad, 267
Quinine, 331, 344

Race, and alcohol drinking, 216. *See also* Blacks; Whites
Radiation, **414, 415**
Radioactive isotopes, **369**
Radiopacity, **369**
Rahe, Richard H., 29, 30

Raleigh Hills alcoholism treatment, 220
Rank, Otto, 62
Rape, 117
Reality, mental health and, 54, 57, 65-66
Recall, of consumer products, 337
Receptors, **105**-109
Recommended daily allowances (RDA), 256, **257**, 267, 268, **352**
Records. *See* Computers; Diaries, health
Reflexes, 158, 369
Refractory period, **112**
Regier, Darrel A., 56
Regression, **332**
Reich, Wilhelm, 62-64, 72
Reincarnation, **504**
Reinforcers, **61**, 188
Rejection
  interpersonal, 66-68
  tissue, **447**
Relapse, **17**
Relationships. *See* Interpersonal relations
Relaxation, 43, 45, 442
  and heart disease, 40, 397, 404-405
  and smoking, 206, 207
  and weight control, 297
Religion
  and cancer incidence, 411
  and death observances, 504, 507
  and death rate, 41
  humanist model and, 64
  of obese people, 285
Remarque, Erich Maria, 46
Remission, **332**
Renin, 396
Repressed ideas/feelings, **68**
Reproductive process, 80-82, 154-155, 162. *See also* Childbirth process
Research, medical, 324-327
Resistance stage, of stress response, 30
Resolution stage, sexual, **111**-114
Respiratory system, **186**, 191, 193-194, 204, 449. *See also* Cardiorespiratory endurance exercise
Responsibility
  healthy people taking, 57
  in intimate relationships, 89
  parents teaching, 178
  patient, 379-380, 383
Resting metabolic rate (RMR), **281**-283
Retired Professional Action Group, 489
Retirement, 476, 488, 489, 492
Rewards, behavior modification with, 8-12, 61-62, 297, 319-320
Rh blood, 165, 447

Rheumatic fever, **402**
Rheumatic heart disease, 402
Rheumatoid arthritis, **451**
Rhythm method, of contraception, **134**-136, 137
Richmond, Julius B., 354
Rickettsiae, 429
Rifkind, Basil M., 392
Rights
  of aged people, 477
  in intimate relationships, 89
  patient, 379-381
Ring, Kenneth, 506, 507
Ringworm, **429**
Risk behavior, **5**
Risk ratio, of high blood pressure, 394-396
Ritalin, 235
RNA (ribonucleic acid), **416, 484**
Robbins, Howard J., 367
Roberts, Oral, 331
Rogerian therapy, 72
Rogers, Carl, 59, 72
Role models, 15, 87
Role playing, **64**, 65, 66
Roles, 24, 80, **85**-89, 96
Romantic love, 98
Romney, Ronna, 91
Rooming-in, after childbirth, 170
Rosenman, Ray, 49, 401
Roskies, Ethel, 49
Rubin, David, 333
Ruddle, Frank, 450
Rusk, Howard A., 32
Ryan, Kenneth J., 147

Sabom, Michael, 506-507
Saccharin, 412
Saf-t-coil, 127
St. Louis, 56
Salicylamide, **350**
Saline method, of abortion, 148, 149
Salmonellosis, **428**, 429
Salt intake, 397
Sample, **372**
Sanger, Margaret, 128
San Joaquin Valley, California, 429
Sarcoma, **409**, 416, 469
Satyriasis, 118
Saxton, Lloyd, 98
Scabies, **471**
Scale of infectivity, 434
Scheider, William L., 289
Schizophrenia, 60, **61, 451**
Schmeck, Harold M., Jr., 437

School, sex differences in, 87. *See also* Education
Science News, 56
Scotland, 414
Screening examination, **376**
Sebum, 83, **427**
Seconal, 232
Secondary hypertension, 396, **397**
Secondary reinforcers, **188**
Secondary response, **443**, 446
Secondary sex characteristics, **81**
Secondary tumors, 408, **409**
Second opinions, 380
Sedation, **211**, 216, 240
Sedative-hypnotics, **232**, 234
Self-actualized people, **54**, 59, 60, 64, 74
Self-contracts, 8
    exercise, 319–320
    for quitting smoking, 10–11
    weight-control, 297
Self-esteem, of compatible intimates, 91
Self-examination, of breasts and testicles, 366, **416**, 419, 421
Self-image, **57**
Self-management/self-monitoring, 5–6, 12–13, 71, 383
    of anxiety, 74–75
    of cancer signals, 416–417
    of exercise, 313, 318–319
    of weight control, 296–297
    See also Behavior change strategies; Diaries, health
Self-medication, 348–359, 361–362
    defined, **352**
Self-statements
    in exercise program, 319
    in weight-control program, 297
Sellery, Stephen, 266
Selye, Hans, 29–30, 32, 41, 46, 476
Semen, **82**
Senility, 487–488
Sensors, 27, **105**–109
Septum, **104**
Sergovich, Fred, 81
Sernylan, 242
Serum, **374**, **435**, 440
Serum cholesterol level, **35**
Set, of drug user, **230**
Set point, of body weight, 280–281
Setting, for drug use, **230**
Seventh-Day Adventists, 41, 411
Sex differences
    biological, 80–85, 89, 158
    cultural, 80, 85–89, 96

vs. individual differences, 87–89
    See also Females; Males
Sex identity, 80, 85
Sex roles, 80, **85**–89, 96
Sexual feelings, armoring against, 64
Sexual love, 98
Sexually transmitted diseases (STDs), **129**, 429, 434, **435**, 455–473
    gonorrhea as, 169, 430, 456, 460–463, 465, 466
    herpes as, 426, 456, 463, 466–468
    tests for, 374, 465
Sexual needs, 114–**116**, 490–492
Sexual relations, 96, 103–120, 490
    aging and, 490–492
    alcohol affecting, 214
    dysfunction in, 101–102
    parenting affecting, 135
    during pregnancy, 160–162
    See also Birth control
Sexual taboos, **116**, 117, 118
Shadow, in Jungian theory, **62**
Shakespeare, William, 13, 214
Shanor, Karen, 92, 93
Shapiro, Leo, 266
Shellock, Frank G., 309
Shock treatments, 72
Shoes, exercise, 306
Short, John, 148
Shostrom, Everett, 70
Shyness, 74–75
Sickle-cell disease, 432–433
Sickle-cell trait, 432–433
Side effects, **125**, 347
    of antihypertensive drugs, 404
    of appetite suppressants, 290
    of birth control pills, 125
    of corticosteroids, 451
    of marijuana, 242
"Sidestream" smoke, 196–198, 199
Silberner, J., 392
Silence, 57–59
Silver, Bernard, 405
Silverman, Mervyn, 470
Singleness, 99
Single-parent households, 99
Sinusitis, **196**
Sitting position, for childbirth, 171
Skill development exercise, 312
Skills-deficit perspective, 74
Skin
    cancer of, 199, 415, 418
    defense provided by, 439
    donation of, 501

infections of, 427, 429
    during pregnancy, 162
    sex differences in, 83
    tests on, 372
    transplants of, 446
Skinfold calipers, **278**
Skinner, B. F., 61–62
Sleepiness, in pregnancy, 160
Sleep patterns, of alcohol drinkers, 214
Smallpox, 426, 446
Smell sense, 104, 107
Smith, Adam, 43
Smog, **414**, 418
Smoking (tobacco), 17, 184–207, 215, 241, 486
    and cancer, 184–202 passim, 409, 414, 418
    contracts about, 10–11
    death rate and, 18, 184, 191, 193, 194, 486
    diary of, 7, 206, 207
    and heart disease, 184, 186, 187, 191, 194, 195, 199, 204, 390, 392
Smoking and Health, 190
Snacking, 267
Snuff, 198
Social environment, 23–51, 54, 65
    alcohol and, 218, 219
    drug use and, 230
    overweight and, 283–285
    and sexual dysfunction, 101
    stressors of, 32–38, 40–41
    See also Interpersonal relations; Support, social
Social Readjustment Rating Scale (SRRS), 30
Social Support Scale, 40, 42
Socioeconomic status
    of compatible intimates, 91
    inconsistencies in, 40–41
    of obese persons, 285
Sodium, 85
Solitude, 57–59
Solvents, **357**
Somatic changes, **237**
Somatic death, 498
Somatic features, sex-differentiated, 80, **81**, 83
Sounds, sexually arousing, 107
South America, 236, 429
Spartans, ancient, 147
Spear, Ruth, 420
Specialization, medical, 327, 328, 367
Specialized cells, **156**
Species, **496**

Specific immune mechanisms, **438**, 442-446
Specimen, **372**
Spector, Novera Herbert, 441
"Speed freak" syndrome, 235
Sperm cell, 80, 82, **154**
Spermicides, 129, **130**, 131, **132-134**
Sphygmomanometer, **393**
Spleen, **427**
Sponge, contraceptive, **132**
Spontaneous abortion, **128**
Sports medicine laboratories, 313
Spotting, 124, **125**
Stanford University obesity study, 278
Staphylococci, 427
Starch blockers, 290
Starvation, for weight loss, 286, 290
Statistical concept, **54**
Statistical correlation, **198**
STDs. *See* Sexually transmitted diseases
Sterility, STD causing, 463, 466
Sterilization, surgical, 125, **140-143**, 144
Steroid hormones, 312, **451**
Steroids, 312
Stevenson, Ian, 507
Stewart, William, 486
Still, Andrew T., 327
Stimulants, **211**, **230**, 232, 234-237, 240
Stimuli, **26**, 27-28, **61**
Stimulus-response bit, **61**
Stomach cancer, 409, 412
Stone, Irwin, 268
STP (dimethoxy-methyl-amphetamine), 237, 238
Stramonium alkaloids, **350**
Strength, exercise for, 305, 311
Strep throat, **427**, 428, 444-446
Streptococci, 427, 428, 444
Streptomycin, 347
Stress, 13, 23-52, 67, 68, 74-75
    and aging, 33, 490
    alcohol abuse during, 216
    anxiolytic drugs for, 244
    breast feeding and, 170
    defined, **24**, 29
    divorce, 96-98
    exercise and, 13, 32, 303, 313
    and heart disease, 33, 36, 39-40, 41, 49, 392
    immune response and, 434, 441-442, 451
    premenstrual, 85
Stress of Life, 29, 46, 476
Stressors, **28**, 32-38, 40-41, 44

Stress point, 32, 41-43
Strokes, 194, 388, **398-400**, 401
    amphetamines and, 236
    dementia from, 487
    with hypertension, 393, 394, 398, 400
Strychnine, **357**
Stuart, Richard, 293
Stunkard, Albert, 296
Stupor, **211**
Sucking reflex, **158**
Suction curettage, 146-148, 149
Sudden infant death syndrome (SIDS), 174, 195
Sugar, 44, 260
Suicide, 66, 234
Suicide prevention centers, 66
Sulfanilamide Elixir, 347
Sumerians, 437
Sun exposure, 415, 418
Superstition, 344
Supplements, nutritional, 334, 486. *See also* Minerals; Vitamins
Support, social, 15, 30, 40-41, 42, 160, 488
Supportive care, by physicians, 324
Suppressor T cells, 443
Supreme Court, U.S., 147
Surgery
    for abortion, 147, 148
    for breast cancer, 420
    heart, 391, 402
    for obesity, 290
    second opinions on, 380
    for sterilization, 125, 140-143, 144
Sweeteners, artificial, 412, 418
Symbolism, 62
Sympathetic nervous system, 30, **31**, 396, 442
Sympathomimetics, 351
Symptoms, 54, 72, **364-366**, 368
Syndrome, 212, **213**
Synergy, 196, 256, **257**
Synesthesia, **237**
Synthesis, **252**, 482
Synthetic compounds, **122**, **235**, 237
Synthetic diets, 256, **257**
Syphilis, 374, **456**, 461, 464-465
Systematic desensitization, 75
Systemic disease, **429**
Systole, **393**
Systolic blood pressure, **368**, 394

Table wines, **210**, 211
Take It Off and Keep It Off, 296
Tampons, prostaglandin, 144

Tar, tobacco, **186**, 191, 196, 198, 199, 202
Target behaviors, 5-6, 71
Target pulse rate, **310**
Tastes, of compatible intimates, 91
Taste sense, 107, 187
Tax Equity and Fiscal Responsibility Act (TEFRA), 340
T cells, 442-451 passim, 469, 484
Tea, 234, 236
Tears, body defense by, 439
Technology, 24-26, 324, 327, 499
Temperature, body
    alcohol and, 215
    rhythm method by, 134-136
Tenuate, 235
Terkel, Studs, 36
Terminal disease, **499**
Terry, Luther, 202
Test anxiety, 38
Testicles, **80**
Testicle self-examination, 366, **416**, 421
Testing
    diagnostic, 369-378, 465, 488
    of prescription drugs, 347-348
Testosterone, 83, **144**, **484**
Tetanus, 446
Tetracycline, 352, 461, 464, 465
Thalamus, **109**
Thalidomide, **347**
Tharp, R. G., 71
THC, 240
Theoretical effectiveness, of contraceptives, **126**, 130, 131
Theories, 344
Therapist, **72**
Therapy
    aversion, 220
    gene, 450
    for mental illness, 71-72, 238, 242-243, 284, 293
    sex, 102
    for type A individuals, 40, 49
    See also Drug treatment
Thermography, **418**
Thoresen, Carl, 40
Throat
    cancer of, 195
    strep, **427**, 428, 444-446
Thromboembolism, 125
Thrombosis, 125, 388, 398
Thrush, **429**
Thymosin alpha, 437
Thymus, **484**
Thyroid, **290**, 451, **484**

Tieffer, Leonore, 106
Time-action function, of drugs, **213**, **228**-230, 237
Time magazine, 466
T interferon, 415
Tissue plasminogen activator, 437
Tobacco, 183-207. *See also* Smoking
Tobacco amblyopia, 195
Tobacco and Your Health, 198-199
Tolerance, **187, 213, 231**
    to depressants, 212, 218, 232-234
    to marijuana, 242
    to nicotine, 187
    to opioids, 231
    to psychedelics, 237
    to stimulants, 235, 236
    to vitamins, 352
Tolerant attitudes, in intimate relationships, 91
Tomkins, S. S., 104
Tonic, **344**
Tonometry, **375**
TOPS (Take Off Pounds Sensibly), 290
Touching, 85-86, 107, 109
Toward a Psychology of Being, 54, 59, 64
Toxemia of pregnancy, **164**
Toxicity, **252**, 264, **347**, 436
Toxic shock syndrome, **132**
Toxins, **427**
Toxoids, **446**
Toynbee, Arnold, 401
TPI (*Treponema pallidum* immobilization), 374
Trachoma, **428**, 429
Training effect, **310**
Tranquilizers, 72, 242
Transactional analysis (TA), 71, 72
Transcendental meditation (TM), 43
Transcending, **504**
Transplants, 447
Trauma, **39**
Treatment, medical, 18, 326-338, 434
    alcohol for, 215-216
    of hypertension, 397, 404, 487
    for infection, 371, 435-438, 460-470 passim
    for obesity, 290-293
    for STD, 434, 460-471 passim
    See also Drug treatment; Therapy
Treponema pallidum, 374, 464, 465
Triceps, **278**
Trichomonas vaginalis, 468, 470
Trichomoniasis, **429, 456**, 468-470
Triglyceride, **304**

Trimesters, **155**-160
Trippett, Frank, 46
T-strain mycoplasmas, 463
Tubal sterilization, **142**-143
Tuberculosis, 372, **427**-428
Tuinal, 232
Tumors, **408**-409, 441. *See also* Cancers
Turlington, Robert, 344
Turner's syndrome, 81
Twain, Mark, 46, 202
Type A behavior, **39**-40, 48-51, 401
Type A Behavior and Your Health, 401
Type B behavior, **39**-40, 48-51, 401
Typhus fever, **428**, 429

UCLA, 203, 336
Ulcers, 36, 196
Umbilical cord, **156**
Unconscious, **62, 68**
Uniform Anatomical Gift Act, 503
Uniform Donor Card, 501
United States
    abortion in, 146, 147
    age distribution in, 476, 477
    alcohol abuse in, 216, 219
    birth control in, 126-127, 128, 131, 132, 133, 140, 141, 414
    cancer in, 409, 414, 449
    childbirth in, 169, 171
    cocaine use in, 239
    colds in, 431
    consumer protection agencies of, 336-338, 348, 350. *See also* Food and Drug Administration
    costs of health in, 324, 333, 338-340, 402, 431
    death attitudes in, 496, 504
    and DES, 126, 412, 414
    dietary guidelines in, 256, 263
    drug ingredients in, 348
    food consumption surveys in, 264-267
    food supply in, 264, 267
    heart diseases in, 392, 393, 402
    homosexuality in, 118
    hospices in, 500
    housework time in, 136
    hunger and deficiency disease in, 267, 269
    hypertension deaths in, 393
    infections in, 428, 429, 456, 465, 466, 469
    life expectancy in, 477
    marijuana use in, 241
    memorial societies in, 503

    misemployment in, 36
    overweight in, 276, 278
    patent medicines in, 344
    retirement age in, 476
    senility in, 487
    sickle-cell trait and anemia in, 433
    sudden infant death syndrome in, 174
    tobacco subsidies by, 200
    tobacco use in, 184, 190, 196
United Way, 16
University of California, 199, 203, 336
University of Chicago, 284
University of Pennsylvania, 112, 398
University of Pittsburgh, Western Psychiatric Institute and Clinic, 90
Urge diary, smoking, 7, 207
Urinary infections, 429
Urination
    in pregnancy, 160
    to prevent STD, 460
Urine tests, 374, 375
Use effectiveness, of contraceptives, **126**, 129, 130, 131-132, 134, 139, 140
Uterus, **126, 154**, 156, 159, 165, 170, 409

Vaccination, **430, 442**, 450
    against infections, 430, 434, 435, 444, 446, 450
    Rh blood and, 165
Vacuum aspiration, **146**-148, 149
Vagina, **105**, 429, 440
Vaginal ring, 143-144
Valium, 220, 244
Valley fever, 429
Values, of compatible intimates, 91
van Leeuwenhoek, Anton, 437
Variance, sexual, **116**-118
Vasa deferentia, **140**, 141
Vascular systems, **490**
Vasectomy, **140**, 141-142
VD National Hotline, 460
Vegetarian diets, 263, 414
Venereal disease (VD). *See* Sexually transmitted diseases
Veterans Administration Medical Center, Brentwood, California, 203
Vickery, Donald M., 18
"Viet Nam Rose," 456
Vikings, 212
Villi, chorionic, 156
Vinyl chloride, 415
Virulence, **434**, 440-442
Viruses, **414**, 426-427, 430, 431, 442, 443, 446

Viruses (*cont.*)
  and cancer, 414, 415–416, 427, 448, 468
  drug treatment for, 415, 437, 438
  in fetal development, 158
  herpes, 416, 426, 456, 463, 466–468
Visceral receptors, 109
Vision
  alcohol affecting, 219
  sexually relevant, 107
  smoking affecting, 187, 195
  tests of, 375
Vitamin A, 257, 350
Vitamin B, 44, 253, 256, 350, 352
Vitamin B$_{12}$, 350
Vitamin B$_{17}$, 332, 333
Vitamin C, 44, 46, 256, 268–269, 350, 352
Vitamin C and the Common Cold, 268
Vitamin D, 312, 350, 352
Vitamin E, 352
Vitamin K, 352
Vitamins, **252**, 256, 264–267, 350–352, 353, 486. *See also individual vitamins*
Von Glahn, John, 483
Voyeurism, **116**, 117
Vulva, **105**

Wallace, Jane, 266–267
Wallechinsky, David, 464
Warm-up, before exercising, 306–309
Warts, **427**

Washington University, 56
Washton, Dr., 239
Water drinking, with exercise, 312–313
Watson, D. L., 71
Watson, John, 61
Weepiness, in pregnancy, 160
Weight
  and drug effects, 230
  ideal, 276, 277
  See also Overweight; Weight loss
Weight loss, 281–293, 296–297, 486
  with amphetamines, 235, 236
  diets for, 281–289 passim, 333–334
Weight Watchers, 290–293
Wellness behavior, **5**, 54–57
Wells, Theodora, 86
Wendy's International, Inc., 267
Wet dream, **82**
"What We Must Do," 26
White, J. R., 199
Whites
  cancer among, 409
  mental illness among, 56
Wiener, Alexander, 447
Wills, euthanasia, 499, 500
Wines, 210–211
Withdrawal, **232**
Withdrawal symptoms, **188**, **218**
  from amphetamines, 236
  from caffeine, 235

from depressants, 218, 232–234
from smoking, 188, 202, 207
Wolfe, Sidney M., 367
Women. *See* Females
Women's movement, 33
Wood, Peter, 278, 292
Working, 36. *See also* Jobs
World Health Organization, 426
World War II, 40
Worms, parasitic, 426, 429–430

X chromosomes, 80–81
X rays
  diagnostic, **369–370**, 372, 378, **414**, 415, 418
  therapeutic, 434

Yale University, 56
Yankelovich, Skelly, and White, 300
Yarber, William L., 458
Y chromosomes, 80–81
Yeast fungus, 125, 429, 437, 470
Yellow Pages, 16
Your Second Life, 479
Youth-oriented culture, 33, 476, 479

Zen, 43–44, 46
Zinc, 44
Zygote, **80**

Credits and Sources (continued)

Page 212   Excerpted from the book *Alcohol: The Delightful Poison* by Alice Fleming. Copyright © 1975 by Alice Fleming. Reprinted by permission of Delacorte Press.

Page 221   Reprinted from *Mental Hygiene*, 23 (1939): 80-86.

Pages 239-40   From "Cocaine Survey Points to Widespread Anguish" by Dr. Richard D. Lyons, *New York Times*, January 4, 1984. Copyright © 1984 by The New York Times Company. Reprinted by permission.

Page 241   From "The Marijuana Problem" in *The Health Letter* (June 11, 1982). Reprinted by permission of Communications, Inc.

Page 255   Copyright © 1980 by Bull Publishing Company, Palo Alto, Calif. Reprinted by permission of the publisher from *The Berkeley Co-op Food Book* (p. 67), edited by Helen Black.

Page 256   From *Jane Brody's Nutrition Book* by Jane E. Brody. Copyright © 1981 by Jane E. Brody. Reprinted by permission of W. W. Norton & Company, Inc.

Page 259   From "Additives: Friend or Foe?" by Deborah Keston, *Healthline* (June 1983), pp. 19-20. Reprinted with permission of the Robert A. McNeil Foundation for Health Education, San Mateo, Calif.

Page 260   From *Jane Brody's Nutrition Book* by Jane E. Brody. Copyright © 1981 by Jane E. Brody. Reprinted by permission of W. W. Norton & Company, Inc.

Pages 261-62   Copyright © 1984 by Consumers Union of United States, Inc., Mount Vernon, NY 10550. Reprinted by permission from *Consumer Reports* (July 1984), pp. 369-70, 372.

Page 264   From *The Wall Street Journal*, February 3, 1984. Reprinted by permission of The Wall Street Journal. Copyright © Dow Jones & Company, Inc., 1984. All rights reserved.

Pages 266-67   From *The Wall Street Journal*, April 6, 1984. Reprinted by permission of The Wall Street Journal. Copyright © Dow Jones & Company, Inc, 1984. All rights reserved.

Pages 268-69.   "The Vitamin C Controversy" by Deborah Kesten, *Healthline* (April 1983), pp. 12-13. Reprinted with the permission of the Robert A. McNeil Foundation for Health Education, San Mateo, Calif.

Page 288-89   From *Ladies' Home Journal* (February 1984), pp. 93, 122. Copyright © 1984 by Family Media, Inc. Reprinted with permission of Ladies' Home Journal and the Diet Center.

Page 289   From William L. Scheider, "Evaluating a Fad Diet," *Nutrition: Basic Concepts and Applications* (New York: McGraw-Hill, 1983). Reprinted by permission of McGraw-Hill Book Company. Copyright © 1983 by McGraw-Hill Book Company.

Page 292   From *The California Diet and Exercise Program* by Peter Wood. Reprinted by permission of Anderson World Books, Inc.

Page 302   From *Los Angeles Times*, February 8, 1981. Reprinted with permission of the author. Nyerges is also the author of *A Guide to Wild Food* (Survival Services, 1980) and *Urban Wilderness* (Peace Press, 1980).

Page 308   From *Rating the Exercises* (pp. 300–301) By Charles T. Kuntzleman and the Editors of *Consumer Guide*. Copyright © 1978 by Publications International Limited. By permission of William Morrow & Co.

Page 309   From Frank G. Shellock, "Physiological Benefits of Warm-Up," *The Physician and Sportsmedicine*, 2 (October 1983), a McGraw-Hill publication.

Page 311   From Tom Murphy and Dianne Murphy, "The Five Principles of a Safe and Effective Exercise Program," *The Personal Fitness Workbook* (San Diego: Avant Books, 1983), p. 14. Copyright © 1983 by Fitness Publications.

Page 312   Excerpted from the October 1983 issue of *The Harvard Medical School Health Letter*. Copyright © 1983 by the President and Fellows of Harvard College.

Pages 315-16   Reprinted from *Maximum Performance* (pp. 22-25) by Laurence E. Morehouse, Ph.D., and Leonard Gross, by permission of Simon & Schuster, Inc. Copyright © 1977 by Laurence E. Morehouse, Ph.D.

Page 330   Reprinted by permission from the June 1978 issue of *Life & Health*. Copyright © by the Review and Herald Publishing Assocation.

Page 345   Reprinted from Victor R. Fuchs, *Who Shall Live?* Copyright © 1974 by Basic Books, Inc.

Page 356   Reprinted from *The Medicine Show* (pp. 29-33). Copyright © 1980 by Consumers Union of United States, Inc., Mount Vernon, NY 10550.

Page 367   Reprinted from the July 7, 1975, issue of *Business Week* (pp. 59-60). Copyright © 1975 by McGraw-Hill, Inc., New York, NY 10020.

Page 372   Excerpted from the November 1978 issue of *The Harvard Medical School Health Letter*. Copyright © 1978 by the President and Fellows of Harvard College.

Page 381   Reprinted with the permission of the American Hospital Association. Copyright © 1972.

Pages 391-92   From "Is Bypass Surgery Needed?" by Jane E. Brody, *Science Times*, November 1, 1983. Copyright © 1983 by The New York Times Company. Reprinted by permission.

Page 392   Reprinted with permission from *Science News* (January 21, 1984), the weekly newsmagazine of science; copyright © 1984 by Science Service, Inc.

Page 393   Copyright © 1983 by the American Heart Association. Reproduced with permission.

Page 413   From "How the Mind Affects Our Health," by Lawrence Cherry, *New York Times Magazine*, November 23, 1980. Copyright © 1980 by The New York Times Company. Reprinted by permission.

Page 420   Copyright © 1984 by Ruth Spear. Originally appeared in *New York Magazine*, January 16, 1984, p. 27.

Pages 431-32   Reprinted from *The Medicine Show* (pp. 34-37). Copyright © 1980 by Consumers Union of United States, Inc., Mount Vernon, NY 10550.

Page 437   From "Strange Alliance: Legions of Bacteria Created to Serve Man" by Harold M. Schmeck, Jr., *New York Times*, January 4, 1984. Copyright © 1984 by The New York Times Company. Reprinted by permission.

Pages 441-42   Exerpted from "The Mind as Healer" by Signe Hammer. First appeared in *Science Digest* (April 1984). Copyright © 1984 by The Hearst Corporation.

Page 450   From "Keeping Up with the Genetic Revolution" by Kathleen and Sharon McAuliffe, *New York Times Magazine*, November 6, 1983. Copyright © 1983 by The New York Times Company. Reprinted by permission.

Page 458   Reprinted by permission of *Human Behavior* magazine (January 1979). Copyright © 1978.

Page 465   "Twenty Prominent Victims of Syphilis" from *The Book of Lists* by David Wallechinsky, Irving Wallace, and Amy Wallace. Copyright © 1977 by David Wallechinsky, Irving Wallace, and Amy Wallace. By permission of William Morrow & Company.

Pages 479-80   From "Aging and Health: An Anthropological Point of View" by Ashley Montagu, *Healthline* (November 1983). Reprinted